J. E. Richardson, —
— 1972 —

NEUROTRANSMITTER–RECEPTOR
INTERACTIONS

NEUROTRANSMITTER-RECEPTOR INTERACTIONS

D. J. TRIGGLE

*Department of Biochemical Pharmacology
School of Pharmacy and The Center for
Theoretical Biology, State University of New
York at Buffalo, New York, U.S.A.*

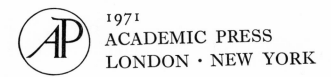

1971
ACADEMIC PRESS
LONDON · NEW YORK

ACADEMIC PRESS INC. (LONDON) LTD
Berkeley Square House
Berkeley Square,
London, W1X 6BA

U.S. Edition published by
ACADEMIC PRESS INC.
111 Fifth Avenue,
New York, New York 10003

Library of Congress Catalog Card Number: 76-141729
ISBN: 0-12-700350-9

PRINTED IN GREAT BRITAIN BY
WILLIAM CLOWES & SONS LIMITED,
LONDON, COLCHESTER AND BECCLES

PREFACE

The problem of the mechanism of action of neurotransmitters is one that has occupied the attention of workers in several disciplines for many years: chemists, biochemists, pharmacologists and physiologists have all made their contributions. In my opinion, however, there exists a definite and quite general lack of communication between these various disciplines that are focussing on a common problem: this is a great pity for an effective understanding of the actions of neurotransmitters will require collaboration and effective communication between many workers in many areas.

In writing this book I have, therefore, attempted to discuss the chemical, biochemical, physiological, pharmacological and biophysical implications of neurotransmitter-receptor interactions and to show, wherever possible, how the various fragments of knowledge obtained from individual approaches may complement one another. I have, furthermore, taken the view that there are two broad areas into which our knowledge of neurotransmitter-receptor interactions must be incorporated and from which we shall continue to derive new insight into the molecular basis of macromolecular interactions of biological significance. These areas are the regulatory control of macromolecules and membrane structure and function. Hence in organizing this book, I have devoted the first two chapters to a rather general treatment of these two topics. Subsequent chapters employ the general concepts so developed and deal with the biochemical, chemical, ionic and potential implications of neurotransmitter-receptor interactions, with excitation-contraction coupling and finally with the problems of receptor isolation and characterization. Of necessity, in a book of this size it has not been possible to cover comprehensively all of these topics and in any event discussion is essentially limited to acetylcholine and norepinephrine as transmitters in the peripheral nervous system. I have, however, endeavoured to provide sufficient documentation so that the interested reader may pursue topics in greater detail. I also wish to take this opportunity of thanking a number of people who have contributed directly and indirectly to this book: Professor N. K. Adam and Professor N. B. Chapman who contributed greatly to my undergraduate and graduate education, Professor B. Belleau whose influence continues past the enjoyable years I spent in his laboratory, to Professor J. F. Danielli who has continually encouraged and supported my work, and Dr. J. F. Moran with whom I have had many stimulating discussions relating to various aspects of this book. My thanks are also due to Mrs. Enez King who typed most of the manuscript and Mrs. Evelyn Wood who made the drawings. My thanks are due to Academic Press for their continual helpfulness in the production of this book. Needless to say, however, all errors and omissions are the sole responsibility of the author.

March 1971

D. J. TRIGGLE

CONTENTS

ACKNOWLEDGMENTS

We express our sincere appreciation to the various authors, publishers and organizations who generously gave permission to reproduce figures from their publications. The authors and the sources of each figure are noted individually in the text. Our acknowledgments are due also to the following organizations as copyright owners: The American Association for the Advancement of Science for Figs V-17, V-23 and VII-1, 2, 4 and 9; The American Chemical Society for Figs I-15-19, I-28, I-36, I-56, I-58, II-20, II-22, IV-17, IV-19, IV-21, VI-16 and VI-17; The American Institute of Physics for Figs I-4 and I-10-14; The American Heart Association for Figs VI-13 and VII-13; The American Physiological Association for Fig. V-7; The American Association of Biological Chemists (*Journal of Biological Chemistry*) for Figs I-29, I-30, I-35, I-60, II-36, II-47, VI-9 and VI-10; Cambridge University Press (*Journal of Physiology and Quarterly Reviews of Biophysics*) for Figs II-6, II-7, II-18, II-21, II-23, II-29-31, VII-6-9, VII-11 and VII-18-20; The Federation of American Societies for Experimental Biology for Figs II-39, II-49, V-4, V-5 and VII-26; Little Brown and Co. and The New York Heart Association for Figs II-17 and II-18; McGraw-Hill Book Company for Figs II-23-26; Macmillan Journals (*Nature, London* and *British Journal of Pharmacology*) for Figs I-7, I-26, II-43-45, IV-2, IV-12, IV-31, IV-32, IV-69, V-31-33 and VI-12, The National Academy of Sciences for Figs I-57, II-10, II-13, II-49, II-50 and V-12; The National Research Council of Canada for Fig. IV-25; The New York Academy of Sciences for Figs II-11, IV-24, IV-29, IV-57, V-19, V-20 and VI-6; the North-Holland Publishing Company (*European Journal of Pharmacology*) for Figs II-37, II-38 and IV-52-55; Pergamon Press, Ltd. for Figs IV-50, IV-51, IV-74, IV-75, V-11, VI-1 and VII-30; Rockefeller University Press (*Journal of General Physiology*) for Figs II-32, VII-12, VII-14 and VII-23; The Royal Society for Figs I-48 and V-26-29; The Williams and Wilkins Company for Figs VI-14, VI-15, VII-15, VII-16, VII-27-29 and VII-34; J. Wiley and Co. for Fig. I-22.

This book is dedicated to
Andrew, Jocelyn and Maureen

Read not to contradict and confute, nor to believe and take for granted, nor to find talk and discourse, but to weigh and consider.

Francis Bacon

Chapter I

THE MOLECULAR BASIS OF BIOLOGICAL INTERACTIONS

INTRODUCTION

Biological systems are composed of highly organized macromolecular assemblies, of which an essential feature is a susceptibility to change both in the long term response to the pressures of natural selection and in the more immediate context of biological regulation, that is, the ability of the macromolecular assembly to respond rapidly to modulating influences (1). Since biological function is an intrinsic property of the integrated macromolecular organization it is susceptible to modification by any agent or influence that perturbs the regulation of the organization. The mechanisms for regulation are themselves properties of the organized system and can only be understood in terms of the organization of their respective macromolecular assemblies. In general terms, however, continuing biological function must relate to the existence and persistence of a given organizational pattern, the free energy of which must be at a minimum relative to other potentially stable patterns. Furthermore, if biological organization, and hence function, is to be readily responsive (to exist in a dynamic state) to various controlling influences it will be dependent upon the coordinated involvement of many weak intermolecular forces rather than a few powerful interactions. Such coordination will ensure that the macromolecular organization is a sensitive function of environmental interactions, that perturbations of the organization are likely to be small and thus that upon removal of the perturbing influence a spontaneous reversal to the original organization will occur.

The actions of the neurotransmitters with which this book is largely concerned are examples, in common with many other agents, of molecules that serve a regulatory function. To understand such regulatory functions it is necessary to consider not only the specific cellular components with which such agents directly interact, but also the organization and integration of such components in relation to the total cellular response initiated by this primary interaction.

It is clear that the organization of any state of matter is determined by the interactions between its constituent parts and that the uniqueness of biological organization rests in large part on the complex inter-relationships existing between the various possible interactions. In particular, it must be emphasized that no discussion of the molecular organization of biological systems can be complete unless related to the structure and function of water, both macroscopic and microscopic, since water constitutes the bulk of the biological environment.

INTERMOLECULAR INTERACTIONS

A summary of the various intermolecular interactions is presented below in the order of decreasing strength and decreasing range of action. A fairly full discussion of the nature, origin and magnitude of these various interactions has been presented by Webb (2) and at this stage is offered merely a discussion of some aspects of the interrelationships between these forces and their interactions in relation to the biological environment.

$$\text{Ion–ion} \propto 1/dD \qquad \text{(I)}$$
$$\text{Ion–dipole} \propto 1/d^2 D \qquad \text{(II)}$$
$$\text{Dipole–dipole} \propto 1/d^3 D \qquad \text{(III)}$$
$$\text{Ion–induced dipole} \propto 1/d^4 D \qquad \text{(IV)}$$
$$\text{Dipole–induced dipole} \propto 1/d^6 D \qquad \text{(V)}$$
$$\text{Fluctuation dipole–induced dipole} \propto 1/d^6 \qquad \text{(VI)}$$

All of the above expressions, save that for the dispersion interactions, involve the dielectric constant of the medium, signifying not the macroscopic, but a microscopic dielectric constant describing the medium in the immediate vicinity of the interacting species. There have been several approaches to the determination of this microscopic constant (2–6): Conway (7) and Webb (2) have described the variation of dielectric constant with distance (d) from a univalent ion according to the expression

$$D = 6d - 7$$

so that D will have a value of 3–5 at a distance some 2–3 Å from the ion. The dielectric modification plays an importance role in determining the magnitude of polar interactions: Fig. I-1 shows the enormous effect of dielectric variation on the association constant for an ion pair interaction at an interionic distance of 5 Å.

Values for the various interaction energies can be calculated for various sets of conditions (Webb (2) gives a detailed discussion), according to the assumptions that it is desired to make. Thus the interaction of oppositely charged univalent ions *in vacuo* will yield an interaction energy of substantially over 100 kcal mole^{-1}: in the aqueous environment, however, such interaction may range from 2–20 kcal mole^{-1} depending upon local environment effects. Other ion–dipole or dipole–dipole interaction energies will be correspondingly less except for hydrogen bonds which, while formally an example of a dipole–dipole interaction, are much more important probably because the small size of the hydrogen atom allows a closer approach of the interacting electronegative atoms. Calculations of the maximum dispersion inter-action energy for two —$(CH_2)_n$— chains oriented for closest fit yield a maximum energy of 0·76 kcal mole^{-1} CH_2 group (8) but it is unlikely,

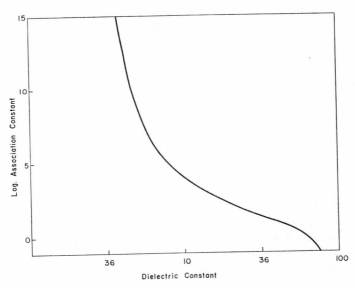

FIG. I-1. Association constants for a pair of oppositely charged ions at 5 Å separation as a function of the dielectric constant.

save in the most favorable circumstances, that this value is reached. In any event, it is somewhat misleading, at least for systems of biological interest, to consider separately each type of interaction energy: it will become apparent that the specificity of biological interactions is deter-mined by the total contribution of all such interactions. Thus the contributions of ionic interactions alone to ligand binding in aqueous systems are, despite their potentially great strength, likely to be small because of the competition for binding by the water molecules. Similarly, it will be anticipated that dipolar interactions will also occur in com-petition with solvent interactions and will be of little significance alone. The dispersion interactions between nonpolar groups are, in contrast, not reduced through competition with water and are also the most specific in the sense that dispersion interactions fall off more rapidly with distance than the ionic or dipolar interactions. Because of this latter factor dispersion interactions are unlikely to be of importance in the long range biological recognition process (9): the key to the general problem of the operation of specific molecular recognition processes lies in the operation of the so-called hydrophobic interaction, an entropy driven association of nonpolar surfaces occurring with expulsion of partially structured water (see section on p. 16). As will be seen from subsequent discussion of water structure, the hydrophobic interaction provides a general basis of molecular interaction in the environment of which other, and more specific, recognition forces become fully operative. It will become increasingly apparent that the role of water in determining the thermodynamics of ligand–macromolecule and macromolecule–macromolecule association and dissociation reactions through its ability to associate with and dissociate from solute molecules represents a major contribution to biologically important molecular interactions. Indeed, according to Szent-Gyorgi (10), "Biological functions may actually consist of the building and destruction of water structures, water being part and parcel of the living machinery and not merely its medium."

THE STRUCTURE OF WATER AND WATER–SOLUTE INTERACTIONS

Since water constitutes the bulk environment of biological systems any discussion of the forces determining biological organization will require some considerations of the structure of water and the nature of its involvement with various solutes.

THE STRUCTURE OF WATER

The vast amount of literature dealing with the structure of liquid water (reviewed in refs 11–19) precludes all but a brief survey of this area. Of the several theories available concerning the structure of water, all retain to a greater or lesser extent, the concept of a hydrogen bonded network of water molecules. This concept derives, in part, from consideration of the existence of the tetrahedrally-directed hydrogen bonded network in ordinary ice (ice I, Fig. I-2), although this does not necessarily imply that any structure found in liquid water be that of ice I, but rather that order conferred by extensive hydrogen bonding is found in both ice and liquid water.

Most treatments of water structure assume the existence of at least two types of water molecule. The treatments associated with Samoilov (20), Forslind (21), Pauling (22), Marchi and Eyring (23) and Frank and Quist (24) assume that water may be regarded as "loosened ice" or "clathrate ice" in which monomeric water molecules are occupying the interstices of the hydrogen bonded lattice.

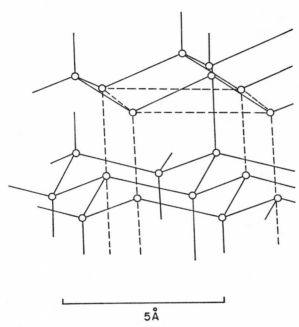

5 Å

FIG. I-2. The structure of ice I showing tetrahedral arrangement: dotted lines indicate part of unit cell which contains four molecules.

In contrast, the model of Frank and Wen (25) stresses the discontinuity of the hydrogen bonded structures in liquid water. At the present time this model and its variations appear to be the most widely accepted and the most developed particularly with regard to solute–water interactions. Frank and Wen argued that the formation of a hydrogen bond between two water molecules involves partial charge separation and that consequently the making (and breaking) of hydrogen bonds

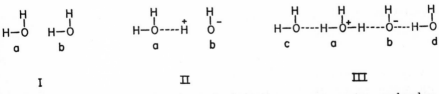

FIG. I-3. Cooperative hydrogen-bond formation among water molecules: formation of II from the unbonded water molecules I facilitates the formation of III and higher aggregates.

will be a cooperative process (Fig. I-3). Consequently several hydrogen bonds will be made or broken at the same time giving rise to areas of short-lived (average lifetime 10^{-10}–10^{-11} sec) hydrogen bonded regions, referred to as "flickering clusters" (Fig. I-4; a schematic comparison

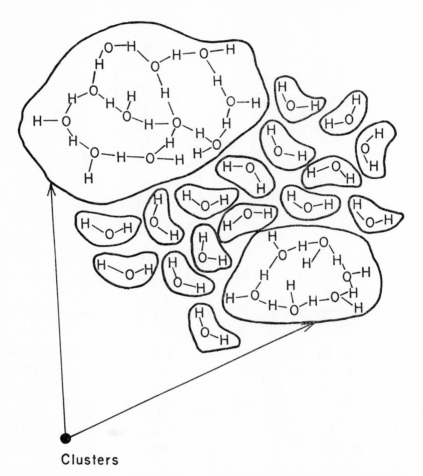

Clusters

FIG. I-4. Representation of the structure of liquid water according to the treatment of Némethy and Scheraga (61). Reproduced with permission.

of various proposed water structures is presented in Fig. I-5). Qualitatively, the Frank-Wen model is in accord with most experimental data for water and aqueous solutions including heat capacity, dielectric relaxation, thermal conductivity, ionic mobility and NMR studies (14–16, 24).

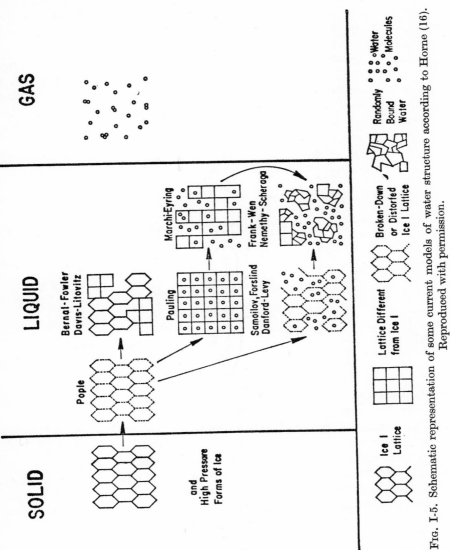

Fig. I-5. Schematic representation of some current models of water structure according to Horne (16). Reproduced with permission.

The Frank–Wen concept has been developed by Némethy and Scheraga (11, 13) whose statistical thermodynamic treatment affords generally good agreement with the experimentally determined thermodynamic parameters of water. In the Némethy–Scheraga treatment, the non-clustered water is assumed to be "monomeric unbonded water" but which is nevertheless involved in dipolar and van der Waals interactions with its neighbors. The total water is assumed to be present in five energy levels depending upon the number of hydrogen bonds in which a molecule participates (Fig. I-6); the spacing of these levels representing the differences causing the breaking of a hydrogen bond (energy $= E_H$). The average cluster size is calculated to range from 91 to 25 over the

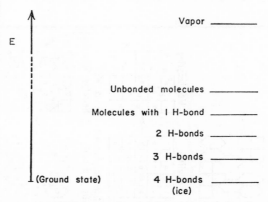

FIG. I-6. Representation of energy levels for water molecules in liquid water according to the treatment of Némethy and Scheraga (61). Reproduced with permission.

temperature range 0–70° with the mole fraction of non-hydrogen bonded molecules ranging from 0·25 to 0·39.

In this model, no definite structure is assigned to the clusters beyond the assumption that the cluster is as compact as possible, that is, involves the formation of the maximum number of hydrogen bonds. The term "ice like" has been applied to the structure of these clusters and the term "melting" to describe the disordering effects of temperature, added solutes, etc. (11, 13, 25): it must be re-emphasized that these terms are merely intended to refer to the ordered nature of the structure produced by hydrogen bonding and to its subsequent disordering by temperature and other variables, and not to signify that the clusters have the structure of ice I. In point of fact it seems unlikely that the clusters can have significant ice I structure since it would then be extremely difficult to observe supercooling of water. It should be emphasized that there is certainly no complete agreement on the structure of liquid water and the widely quoted "flickering cluster" model does not accord quantitatively with all experimental data (16–19).

Finally, no discussion of liquid water is complete without reference to the subject of "anomalous" liquid water. Water condensed in quartz

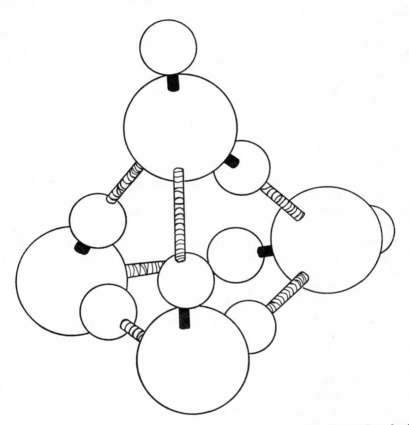

FIG. I-7. Proposed tetrameric model for anomalous water (28). Reproduced with permission.

capillaries under specified conditions is found to have, compared with ordinary water, a lower vapor pressure, higher density, viscosity and thermal expansion coefficient (26, 27). There have been several theoretical discussions of the possible structure of this material (27–29); Bolander et al. (28) have suggested the existence of tetrahedrally hydrogen bonded clusters (Fig. I-7) the formation of which is catalysed by the geometry of oxygen atoms on the surface of silica tetrahedra.

However, some evidence exists to suggest that many of the "anomalous" properties of this water may arise from the presence of very significant quantities of inorganic material (30).

WATER–SOLUTE (IONIC AND POLAR) INTERACTIONS

The effect of the medium in determining the energy of ionic interaction finds a general expression in the dielectric constant as discussed previously (see section on p. 2). Quite simply, interactions between charged or polar species become energetically more favorable with decreasing polarity of the medium. It may readily be envisaged that two organic polar species, for example, an organic base and a negatively charged protein component, may undergo an ionic interaction in a virtually nonpolar environment created by the association of nonpolar groups (see section on p. 52), this energy of interaction being substantially greater than the corresponding event in an aqueous medium. This point will be reconsidered later since it unquestionably represents a major consideration in any discussion of ligand binding processes.

However, as previously noted the bulk dielectric constant is not appropriate for any quantitative discussion of interaction energies since the interacting species will, through their influence on local water structure, substantially modify this bulk constant. It is necessary therefore, to relate both polar and nonpolar interactions of biological significance to the structure of water and its modification by the solute.

According to the model developed by Frank and Wen (25) and which is supported quite substantially by several lines of experimental evidence (14, 15, 17, 25, 31–34), hydration of ions is best characterized by the surrounding presence of two distinct water structures: a tightly bound, highly ordered, electrostricted layer(s) immediately surrounding the ion and a second layer which is less structured than bulk water and in which greater mobility of the water species is found relative to the bulk state. The relative importance of these two zones (Fig. I-8) of water structure is, of course, a function of the ionic species in question. From studies on viscosity, entropy, heat capacity and NMR relaxation rate changes of electrolyte solutions it has been found possible to classify ionic species into two major categories—the "structure makers" and the "structure breakers". Ions with a high charge/size ratio, that is relatively small ions and multivalent ions (Li^+, Na^+, H_3O^+, Ca^{++}, Ba^{++}, Mg^{++}, Al^{+++}, HO^-, F^-, etc.) have a net structure-making effect: the high electric field strengths of these ions causing an orientation of at least one layer of structured water molecules (organized through an ionic–dipolar interaction) surrounded by a less significant quantity of destructured water molecules. In contrast, large monovalent ions (K^+,

NH_4^+, Rb^+, Cs^+, Br^-, I^-, etc.) have a net structure-breaking effect, their field strength being insufficiently great to cause the ordering of a tight primary hydration layer but capable of causing a local disordering of water structure.

This classification is, however, not readily applicable to organic ionic species in which the charge can often be regarded as imbedded in a nonpolar (or relatively nonpolar) environment. Such molecules often

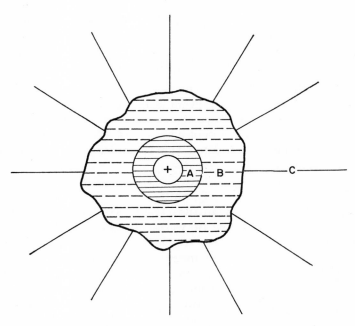

FIG. I-8. Ionic hydration layers showing "structured" (A), "destructured" (B) and bulk phase (C) water structures. Reproduced from Frank and Wen (25) with permission of the authors and The Faraday Society.

have a net structure-making effect which is, however, not related to the structured primary hydration layer formed around inorganic cations of high field strength, but is related instead largely to the formation of "icebergs" of structured water around the nonpolar areas. From several points of view, such species are best considered as organic solutes and their behaviour is discussed more fully elsewhere (see section on p. 35 and Chapter IV, section on p. 236).

It is clear that the energetics of polar group interactions will be determined in part by the reorganization of the associated water structure. Thus, the association of metal cations with ligands may be considered in three classes according to the original classification of Schwarzenbach (35):

(a) Purely electrostatic bonding predominates with the alkali, alkaline earth and other cations with the rare gas configuration. For any given ligand the association constant will increase with decreasing cationic size and increasing charge.

(b) Predominantly covalent ligand interaction occurs with cations with completely filled d-electron subshells (Cu^+, Ag^+, Zn^{++}, Cd^{++}, etc.) and electrostatic interactions are of minor importance. The association constant is determined by differences between the electronegativities of the cation and the donor ligand.

(c) Both electrostatic and covalent interactions are of importance for the transition metal cations.

Our primary concern is with the ionic interactions, but this should not obscure the important role played by other metal–ligand interactions in, for example, metalloenzyme systems (i.e., 31, 36). For cations of class (a) the association constants often lie in the order anticipated from their charge and radius,

$$Li^+ > Na^+ > K^+; \quad Mg^{++} > Ca^{++} > Sr^{++} > Ba^{++}$$

However, since the hydrated radius increases as the crystal radii decreases (Table I-1) this order may not always hold and will depend upon whether a solvent separated or contact ion pair is formed (31, 37). Information as to the role of water in the ion association process may be obtained from a study of the thermodynamic parameters involved (31): study of a large number of ion association processes reveal that most occur with a large positive change in entropy rather than the negative change

TABLE I-1. Ionic and Hydrated Radii of Alkali
and Alkaline Earth Cations (39)

Ion	Ionic radius (Å)	Effective hydrated radius (Å)
Li^+	0·60	4·5
Na^+	0·95	3·4
K^+	1·33	2·2
Rb^+	1·48	1·9
Cs^+	1·69	1·9
Mg^{++}	0·65	5·9
Ca^{++}	0·99	4·5
Sr^{++}	1·13	3·7
Ba^{++}	1·35	3·7

anticipated on the basis of the disappearance of a particle and reduction in translational and vibrational degrees of freedom. Such ion association reactions must involve the loss of coordinated, structured water molecules. Thus, George (31, 38) has demonstrated the validity of the relationship

$$\Delta S_{Assoc} = \Delta S_{Hydr} + \text{constant} \qquad (VII)$$

for the association of a series of cations with anions, the constant differing with each anion. For certain ion association reactions, the entropy change may be very small; this is noted when the product of association still has an equivalent charged structure, i.e., H^+ + glycine anion → zwitterion, and where water is merely redistributed.

TABLE I-2. Thermodynamic Parameters for the Formation of 1:1 Metal Complexes with Aminopolycarboxylate Ions (31)

Anion	Cation	ΔF kcal mole^{-1}	ΔH kcal mole^{-1}	ΔS cal deg^{-1} mole^{-1}
Iminodiacetic acid†	Mg^{++}	−3·94	2·94	23·5
	Ca^{++}	−3·47	0·3	12·7
	Sr^{++}	−2·99	0·1	10·5
	Ba^{++}	−2·24	0·1	8·0
2,2-Ethylenedioxybis [ethyliminodi(acetic)] acid	Mg^{++}	−7·20	5·49	42·6
	Ca^{++}	−14·86	−7·94	23·2
	Sr^{++}	−11·50	−5·74	19·3
	Ba^{++}	−11·32	−9·00	7·8
Nitrilotriacetic acid	Mg^{++}	−7·25	4·44	39·8
	Ca^{++}	−8·6	−1·36	24·7
	Sr^{++}	−6·68	−0·54	20·9
	Ba^{++}	−6·44	−1·44	17·1

† Ionic strength 0·1 M.

The importance of the entropy and enthalpy changes in determining the free energy change can be seen from Table I-2 giving the thermodynamic functions for 1:1 complexes with aminopolycarboxylate ions. The entropy change is invariably more positive with Mg^{++}, presumably reflecting the relatively greater disorganization of structured water but this increase is compensated by the positive enthalpy term indicative of the heat necessary to break the ion–dipole interactions of the hydration sheath.

Of particular relevance to the biological systems of greatest concern in this book, namely cell membranes, is the work of Bungdenbergh de

Jong (40) on the ability of cations to cause charge reversals of various anionic colloids from which sequences of cation affinity can be obtained (Table I-3) varying with the anion character and reflecting in part the importance of hydration. Further discussion of such ligand affinity sequences is presented in Chapter II.

In addition to the formally charged groups, other polar groups will also interact with water: their perturbing influence on water will be much less than that of the ionic species previously discussed since the electric field strength of a dipole or induced dipole will be less than that

TABLE I-3. Cation Affinity Sequences for Anionic Colloidal Systems (40)

System	Sequence
Sodium arabinate (COO⁻)	$Li < Na < K < Mg < Ca < Sr < Ba$
Ammonium oleate (COO⁻)	$K < Na < Li < Mg < Ca < Sr < Ba$
Gelatin (COO⁻)	$K < Na < Li < Mg < Ca < Sr < Ba$
Soybean phosphatide I ($-PO_3H_2^-$)	
Sphingomyelin	$K < Na < Li < Ba < Sr < Ca < Mg$
Egg lecithin	
Sodium agar (HSO_4^-)	$K < Na < Li < Sr < Ba < Mg < Ca$
Sodium carrageen (HSO_4^-)	$Li < Na \sim Mg < Ca < K < Sr < Ba$

of an ion and will probably involve the formation of single hydrogen bonds.

The interaction of ionic and polar groups in general with water has important consequences for protein (and other biological macromolecules) function. The general structure of globular proteins places the polar residues at the aqueous interface and will consequently be covered by a layer of water, the structure of which will show local variation, according to the immediate polar environment, from that of bulk water.

The fact that proteins (and other macromolecules as DNA, RNA, etc.) are extensively hydrated is well established (41), but what is not established is the state of this water of hydration. Quite recently, Bull and Breese (42, 43) have studied the binding of water by a number of solid proteins including albumin, lysozyme, hemoglobin, etc., at a relative humidity of 0·92 and have attempted to correlate the extent of hydration with the polar residues found in the various proteins. A satisfactory correlation was obtained indicating that the hydroxyls, carboxyls and basic groups contributed about 6 moles of water per mole of residue; surprisingly the amide residue were found not to contribute to the hydration (Fig. I-9) and presumably they are already involved in intermolecular hydrogen binding. The extensive studies of Hammes and co-workers (44, 45) using ultrasonic techniques also show the existence of relatively immobilized water around such molecules as dioxane, diglycine, polyethyleneglycol and polyglutamic acid. More detailed information describing the water of hydration in proteins is also available from PMR studies (46–49) in which determination of the resonance line width describes the ease and rapidity of the molecular motions of the bound water species under discussion. The adsorbed

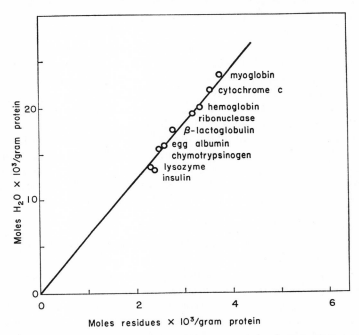

FIG. I-9. Water-binding of proteins as a function of the moles of polar residues: (o) sum of hydroxyl, carboxyl and basic residues minus amide groups. From Bull and Breese (43).

water on solid bovine serum albumin appears by this technique to exist in several states (50, 51), a primary hydration layer in which every surface polar group is hydrogen bonded to one water molecule (at very low hydration values it appears that each molecule of water may bind, on the average, to two polar groups, thus giving rise to *highly* immobilized and tightly bound water); superimposed upon this layer is a "secondary" water structure which differs in structure from bulk water, but is not as influenced by the polar surface as the primary layer of hydration. Studies on lysozyme indicate an essentially similar pattern of hydration (51). Kuntz (52) has studied frozen protein and nucleic

2*

acid solutions at $-35°$ and determined hydration values ($\sim$30% for proteins) that are in good agreement with other values. The observation of the proton signals of water and the observed activation energy for proton mobility of 4–5 kcal mole^{-1} indicates that the hydrated water is in no sense literally "ice-like" although the line widths indicate a structure more immobilized than that of liquid water. Unquestionably, similar conclusions may be drawn for more complex systems such as lipo-protein membranes: thus, from water desorption studies of hydrated keratin membranes Scheuplein and Morgan (53) conclude that about 500% of the dry weight of the membrane is "bound" water. The precise state of this water "bound" in such membranes is not yet known but it has important potential consequences for membrane structures and function (Chapter II). Furthermore, recent considerations by Ling (54, 55) and Cope (56) of the state of cell water have led them to the conclusion that substantial revision may be necessary in the general concept that cell water is essentially identical to bulk phase water and that ionic solubilities, mobilities, etc. will be those observed in aqueous solution. These workers have produced several lines of evidence indicating that cell water should be regarded as an "ice-like" matrix and that ionic solutes are to be regarded as very largely complexed to the cellular macromolecular systems.

WATER–SOLUTE (NONPOLAR) INTERACTIONS

Despite the differences amongst the various models for the structure of liquid water, all treatments agree "that a sensitive order–disorder balance within liquid water is highly significant to all its properties" (57). This statement is particularly relevant for the interaction of water and nonpolar solutes. Any discussion of such interactions must take into account the following experimental observations for the solution of nonpolar solutes in water:

(a) a large positive free energy change ($\Delta F°$) occurs, corresponding to the low aqueous solubility of hydrocarbons; this free energy change results from a negative (aliphatic hydrocarbon) or zero (aromatic hydrocarbon) enthalpy change and a large negative entropy change,

(b) there is a decrease of partial molal volume and,

(c) the partial molal heat capacity for hydrocarbon solutes in aqueous solution is much higher than in the pure solute. Some values for the thermodynamic parameters of hydrocarbon solution into water are given in Table I-4. These observations clearly indicate that the introduction of the nonpolar solute produces a change in the structure of water (58–62) and it is difficult to avoid the conclusion that nonpolar solutes have a net ordering effect on water structure (60–63). This view was formally advanced by Frank and Evans in 1945 (60) in their "iceberg" concept according to which the local ordering of water around a nonpolar solute involves the increased formation of intermolecularly hydrogen bonded water species and thus an increase in "ice-like" structure (it should be clearly noted that Frank and Evans explicitly noted that such structuring was not necessarily identical to that found in ice). Qualitatively it is clear that this proposal accommodates the negative entropy

TABLE I-4. Thermodynamic Parameters for the Transfer of Hydrocarbons from a Nonpolar Solvent to Water (63)

Process	$\Delta F°$ kcal mole^{-1}	$\Delta H°$ kcal mole^{-1}	$\Delta S_u°$† e.u.	$\Delta H°/\Delta S_u°$ (°K)
$CH_4/C_6H_6 \to CH_4/H_2O$	2·6	−2·8	−18	155
$C_2H_6/C_6H_6 \to C_2H_6/H_2O$	3·8	−2·2	−20	110
$C_3H_8 \to C_3H_8/H_2O$	5·1	−1·8	−23	78
$C_4H_{10} \to C_4H_{10}/H_2O$	5·9	−1·0	−23	44
$C_6H_6 \to C_6H_6/H_2O$	4·1	0	−14	0
$4\text{-MeC}_6H_5 \to 4\text{-MeC}_6H_5/H_2O$	4·7	0	−16	0

† The magnitude of the observed entropy change depends upon the standard states employed: for the transfer of pure solute to a solution $\Delta S_{obs} = \Delta S_u - R\ln x$, where ΔS_u, the *unitary entropy*, represents the solvent–solute interactions and $-R\ln x$, where x is the mole fraction of solute, is the *cratic* contribution to the entropy and represents the randomness of mixing with the solvent. For transfer of solute from one dilute solution to another the cratic contributions will cancel provided that differences in charge interactions do not exist (64).

(increased ordering) and negative enthalpy (increase in number of hydrogen bonds) changes observed for the hydrocarbon solution process and the increased heat capacity of aqueous hydrocarbon solutions.

This basic concept of increased ordering of water structure by nonpolar solutes is widely accepted, with quantitative variations of the degree and nature of such ordering, despite the absence of a totally acceptable model for liquid water. Based on their model of liquid water Némethy and Scheraga (11, 61) propose that the structuring arises because a tetrahedrally hydrogen bonded water molecule can bind a nonpolar solute as a fifth neighbor (Fig. I-10) to generate a structure analogous, in part, to that prevailing in clathrate gas hydrates. The analogy is limited by the fact that complete cages enclosing and stabilized by the nonpolar solute are formed in gas hydrates: for nonpolar solutes larger than n-butane such complete cages are geometrically impossible.†

† Ionic species containing large nonpolar residues (i.e., tetraalkylammonium salts) may constitute an exception: they are known to form crystalline gas hydrates in which each alkyl chain occupies a separate cage (65–67).

The fact that the partial molal volumes of nonpolar solutes are lower in water than in nonpolar solvents or the liquid state ($\Delta V° < 0$ for the solution process, Table I-5) is also accommodated in this model in which the solute molecule effectively occupies "free space" generated in the hydrogen-bonded network. The fivefold coordination shown in Fig. I-10

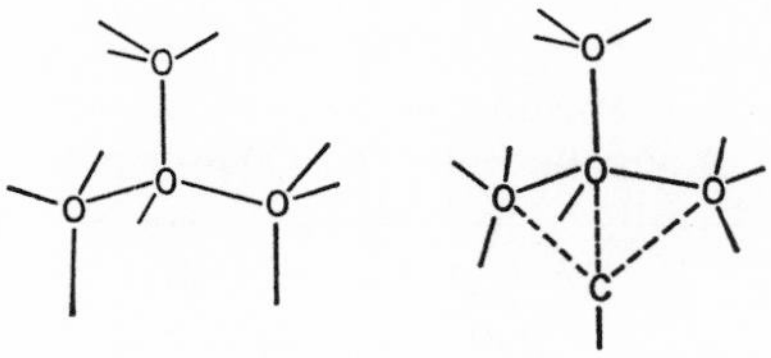

(a)   (b)

FIG. I-10. Representation of the increased coordination of a fully hydrogen-bonded water molecule (a) when adjacent to a nonpolar solute (b). Reproduced with permission from Némethy and Scheraga (61).

is stabilized by the additional van der Waals interaction energies (shown by the dotted lines) unaccompanied by significant perturbation of the hydrogen bonding; hence, the energy of the tetrahedral water species is lowered by an amount,

$$E_L = \tfrac{1}{2}E_{RW} \tag{VIII}$$

where E_{RW} is the energy of water-solute interaction. In contrast, interaction of the same solute with zero, one, two or three hydrogen bonded water molecules will result in an increase in the energy because such

TABLE I-5. Volume Changes (ΔV) for the Transfer of a Hydrocarbon from a Nonpolar Medium into Aqueous Solution (69)

Hydrocarbon	Nonpolar medium	ΔV cm³/mole
Methane	hexane	−22·7
Ethane	hexane	−18·1
Propane	gas	−22·5
Benzene	liquid	−6·4

species can only receive a solute neighbor by displacement of a water molecule, a process in which the strong water–water dipole interactions are replaced by the weaker water–solute interactions. This rise in energy is represented by

$$E_R = \tfrac{1}{2}E_{RW} - E_{dip} \tag{IX}$$

where E_{dip} is the change in water–water dipole interactions resulting from the exchange of a neighbor (Fig. I-11). Because the van der Waals interactions are inversely proportional to the sixth power of the inter-molecular distance (see section on p. 2) the effects discussed will be restricted to the first layer of water only (61). A substantial amount of

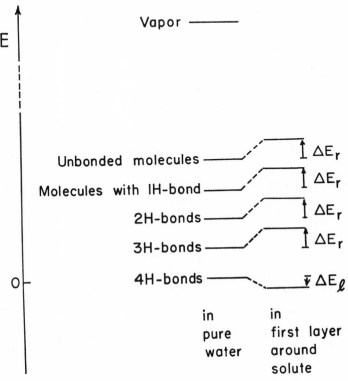

FIG. I-11. Representation of the displacement of energy levels for various states of water molecules on transfer from pure water to the layer immediately adjacent to a nonpolar solute. Reproduced with permission from Némethy and Scheraga (61).

evidence, largely indirect (viscosity, temperature coefficient of viscosity, dielectric relaxation, etc.), may be cited to support the idea of increased water structuring by nonpolar solutes (11–15, 17–20, 68). The quantita-tive success of the Némethy–Scheraga treatment is shown in Fig. I-12 which shows the agreement between the calculated and experimental thermodynamic parameters for the solution of aliphatic hydrocarbons. In particular, nuclear magnetic resonance techniques have demonstrated the relative immobilization of water around nonpolar solutes (34,

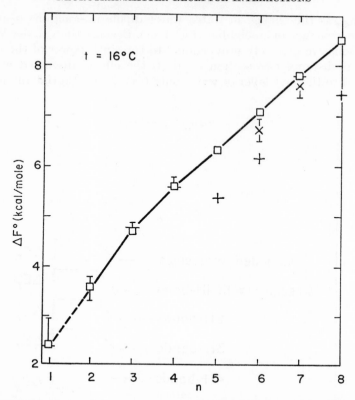

FIG. I-12. Experimental ($+$, $\times$, $\square$) and calculated (solid line) values for the free energy of solution of n-alkanes in water at $16°$ C. Reproduced with permission from Némethy and Scheraga (61).

TABLE I-6. Effect of Molecular Polarity on Proton Exchange in System (76)

$$R_3N \cdot HOH + H_2O \xrightarrow{k_H} R_3N \cdot HOH + HOH$$

Amine	$T°$ C	$10^{-10}\, k_H$ $\sec^{-1}$
NH_3	25	22
CH_3NH_2	25	6·2
$(CH_3)_3N$	25	1·0
$(C_2H_5)_3N$	25	0·38
$(PhCH_2)_2NCH_3$	30	0·27

70–75) and suggest that increased structuring has occurred. Grunwald and Ralph (76) have measured the rate constant, k_H, for breaking the R_3N—HOH hydrogen bond: k_H decreases proportionately to the size of the nonpolar R group. The substituent effect on k_H with increasing partial molal volume parallel the increase in London dispersion forces (Table I-6) suggesting that the layer of water molecules adjacent to the amino nitrogen and the nonpolar residue form a subspecies with lower free energy than that of water molecules in the bulk phase. This is,

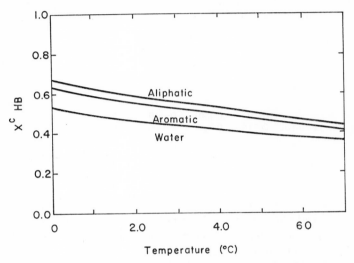

FIG. I-13. Increased hydrogen-bond formation ("ice-likeness") occurring upon introduction of nonpolar solutes into water. X_{HB} = fraction of unbroken hydrogen bonds and is 1·0 for crystalline ice. The data, refers only to the first layer of water around the nonpolar solute. Reproduced with permission from Némethy and Scheraga (61).

of course, consistent with the Némethy–Scheraga model of nonpolar solute–water interaction. Further implications of this finding are discussed in Chapter IV, p. 227.

From the quantitative Némethy–Scheraga calculations values have been obtained for the increase in "ice-likeness" occurring on introducing a nonpolar solute into water. While the change per mole of water is small the change per mole of solute is large, an effect which is reflected in the large changes in thermodynamic parameters. The increases in "ice-likeness" induced by aliphatic and aromatic hydrocarbons are shown in Fig. I-13 relative to perfectly crystalline ice having 100% unbroken hydrogen bonds. It should be noted that "ice-likeness" refers to the amount of hydrogen-bonding still existing in the solution and not to the quantity of "ice" formed: thus entropies of solution should not be interpreted in terms of any number of water molecules being frozen but only in terms of an *overall* change in water structure (61). The effects on the water structure of introducing an aliphatic hydrocarbon as calculated according to the Némethy–Scheraga treatment are shown in Table I-7. The increase in the number of water molecules making four hydrogen bonds is noteworthy.

TABLE I-7. Comparison of Hydrogen Bonded Fractions for Liquid Water Alone and in the Presence of an Aliphatic Hydrocarbon (61)

	Mole fractions of hydrogen bonded water species†					Fraction of hydrogen bonds unbroken
	x_u	x_1	x_2	x_3	x_4	
Water (20°)	0·295	0·230	0·040	0·202	0·233	0·462
Water + (20°) solute	0·213	0·120	0·176	0·059	0·430	0·593

† x_i refers to number of hydrogen bonds. The fraction of hydrogen bonds unbroken is calculated from $1/4 \sum_i x_i i$.

Comparison of the thermodynamic parameters for the freezing of water to ice and the solution of nonpolar material in an aqueous phase also reveals that the "ice-like" character of the structured water is not very great. The entropy loss in the freezing of water is 5·3 e.u. and the entropy loss (ΔS_u) for solution of a nonpolar solute is approximately 20 e.u.: thus, either four molecules of water have perfect crystallinity or, and more probably, a larger number of water molecules have much less than perfect crystallinity. Similarly the small value of ΔH upon solution of a hydrocarbon into water (1000–2000 cal mole^{-1} of hydrocarbon) relative to ΔH for the freezing of water (1440 cal mole^{-1}) also indicates that the hydrogen bonding in the structured water cannot differ very significantly from that in ordinary water. Finally, it is worth noting that $\Delta H_{fus}/\Delta S_{fus}$ for ordinary ice has the value of 273°K whereas the ratio of $\Delta H/\Delta S$ for "structured" water around nonpolar solutes is very much less (Table I-4).

HYDROPHOBIC INTERACTIONS: THE HYDROPHOBIC BOND

Following the treatment of Kauzmann (63, see also 77) hydrophobic interactions may be considered equivalent to the reversal of solution of hydrocarbons in water. Thus, the formation of a hydrophobic bond will consist of the approach to van der Waals radii of two nonpolar species with a concomitant reduction in the number of associated and "structured" water molecules. This process will be accompanied by a negative free energy change ($\Delta F° < 0$) consisting of a zero or positive enthalpy ($\Delta H° \leqslant 0$) and a large positive entropy component ($\Delta S° > 0$). The extent to which this process may be regarded as a reversal of the solution process depends upon the nature of the system under consideration: in general, it seems improbable that the thermodynamic changes associated with hydrophobic interactions will equal those for the hydrocarbon solution process. For many systems the nonpolar macromolecular areas will not be completely removed from the aqueous environment and will remain in contact with some water molecules: furthermore, as explicitly pointed out by Némethy and Scheraga (61), the nonpolar side chains of proteins and the nonpolar components of other partially polar molecules should not be considered completely equivalent to the corresponding hydrocarbon, because the presence of the peptide backbone or other polar component will alter the amount of associated "structured" water, sterically hinder the formation of the cage-like structures around the nonpolar residues and, through hydrogen bonding and dipolar interactions, alter the energy levels of the "structured" water.

According to the Némethy–Scheraga treatment the total free energy of formation of a hydrophobic bond is given by,

$$\Delta F°_{H\phi} = \Delta F°_W + \Delta F°_S \tag{X}$$

representing the contributions made by changes in water structure ($\Delta F°_W$) and the solute ($\Delta F°_S$). In the association of two nonpolar side chains of a protein a total of ΔY^s water molecules will be removed from the "structured" layer and become part of the bulk water. Thus,

$$\Delta F°_W = \Delta Y^s(F°_W - F°_W{}^c) \tag{XI}$$

where $F°_W$ represents the free energy of bulk water and $F°_W{}^c$ the free energy of water in the structured layer around the solute. Formation of the hydrophobic bond involves the breaking of ΔY^s water–hydrocarbon interactions giving an energy loss of $\Delta Y^s E_{RW}$, where E_{RW} is the energy of the water–solute interaction: simultaneously Z_R nonpolar pair interactions are introduced with a total energy gain of $Z_R E_R$. The formation of the hydrophobic bond imposes limitations upon the flexibility of the side chain with loss of internal rotations resulting in a change in free energy, ΔF_{Rot}. The magnitude of this factor may vary considerably: for the nonpolar chains of a protein it may be quite small since there already exist substantial hindering interactions and, in any event, hydrophobic association does not involve the same severe geometrical restrictions as with, for example, the formation of a hydrogen bond where the loss of configurational entropy may be −5 e.u. (This, of course, reflects a most important feature distinguishing hydrophobic interactions from other interactions—they are relatively flexible in their geometrical relationships, extent of contact, etc.) It is clear that the strength of a hydrophobic interaction may be quite variable since it is clearly dependent upon the various geometrical factors that determine the extent of contact of the nonpolar residues and thus the extent of creation of an anhydrous environment. Consequently, hydrophobic interactions can have a range of values from a minimum when the chains are barely in contact, to a maximum where all factors are operating most effectively. From the above considerations, the free energy of formation of the hydrophobic bond is given by

$$\varDelta F^{\circ}_{H\phi} = \varDelta Y^{s}(F^{\circ}_{W} - F^{c}_{W}) - 1/2\, Y^{s} E_{RW} + Z_{R} E_{R} - \sum \varDelta F_{Rot} \quad \text{(XII)}$$

For the detailed calculations, the following thermodynamic parameters were used: $E_{R} = -0.15$ kcal mole^{-1} and -0.50 kcal mole^{-1} for aliphatic and aromatic groups respectively, $1/2\, E_{RW} = -0.031$ kcal mole^{-1} and -0.16 kcal mole^{-1} for aliphatic and aromatic groups respectively, and $\varDelta F_{Rot}$ from 0–0.3 kcal mole^{-1} and $\varDelta F^{\circ}_{W} = -0.123$ kcal mole^{-1} at 25°.

From this treatment, Némethy and Scheraga calculated the upper and lower limits for $\varDelta F^{\circ}$, $\varDelta H^{\circ}$ and $\varDelta S^{\circ}$ for the interactions of the nonpolar amino acid side chains of polypeptides. A partial tabulation is presented in Table I-8: for a more comprehensive discussion reference should be made to the original paper.

For large proteins and other macromolecules it is probable that several nonpolar residues may interact simultaneously to generate a hydro-

TABLE I-8. Calculated Thermodynamic and Structural Parameters for the Formation of Hydrophobic Bonds of Minimum and Maximum Strength between Nonpolar Amino Acid Side Chains (61)

| | Thermodynamic parameters† | | | | | | Structural parameters | | | |
| | $\varDelta F^{\circ}_{H\phi}$ kcal mole^{-1} | | $\varDelta H^{\circ}_{H\phi}$ kcal mole^{-1} | | $\varDelta S^{\circ}_{H\phi}$ e.u. | | $\varDelta Y^{s}$ | | Z_{R} | |
Side chains	Min.	Max.	Min.	Max.	Min.	Max.	Min.	Max.	Min.	Max.
Ala.–Ala.	−0.3	−0.7	0.4	−0.7	2.2	4.7	2	4	1	2
Ala.–Phe.	−0.2	−0.2	0.3	0.3	1.6	1.7	2	2	1	1
Val.–Val.	−0.3	−0.9	0.4	1.1	2.2	6.7	2	6	1	3
Ileu.–Ileu.	−0.3	−1.5	0.4	1.8	2.2	11.1	2	10	1	5
Leu.–Phe.	−0.2	−0.5	0.3	0.9	1.6	4.7	2	6	1	3
Phe.–Phe.	—	−1.4	—	0.8	—	7.5	—	12	—	6

Ala. = alanine; Phe. = phenylalanine; Val. = valine; Ileu. = isoleucine; Leu. = leucine.

† 25° C.

phobic patch from some areas of which water may be totally excluded. The thermodynamic parameters may be calculated by procedures entirely analogous to those employed for two chain interactions: the energy of interaction of isoleucine chains may be calculated to be as high as $\Delta F^{\circ}_{H\phi}$, $-4 \cdot 9$ kcal mole^{-1}, $\Delta H^{\circ}_{H\phi}$, $6 \cdot 7$ kcal mole^{-1} and $\Delta S^{\circ}_{H\phi}$, 38 e.u. Higher order interactions will generate even larger thermodynamic changes. If the dimensions of the hydrophobic patch are sufficiently large, then some of the nonpolar chains will be totally excluded from the water. This will produce a hydrophobic interaction of greater strength than those previously discussed in which the calculations were specifically based upon the assumption that the number of nearest neighbor water molecules was reduced. Total exclusion of water increases the entropic contribution to $\Delta F^{\circ}_{H\phi}$ considerably. The free energy of formation of a hydrophobic bond in which an anhydrous environment is created is given by,

$$\Delta F^{\circ}_{tr} = Y^s[F^{\circ}_W - F^c_W - 1/2\,E_{RW}] + Z_R\,E_R + \Delta F_{Rot} \qquad \text{(XIII)}$$

where Y^s is the *total* number of water neighbors and $Z_R = 1/2\ Y^s$ and ΔF°_{tr} is referred to as the free energy of transfer of a side chain from water into an anhydrous environment. Some values are given in Table I-9. These figures are smaller than those calculated by Kauzmann (63)

TABLE I-9. Thermodynamic Parameters for the Transfer of a Nonpolar Side Chain into a Nonpolar Environment (61)

Nature of region	Side chain	ΔF°_{tr}†	ΔH°_{tr} kcal mole^{-1}	ΔS°_{tr} e.u.
Aliphatic	Ala.	$-1 \cdot 3$	$1 \cdot 5$	$9 \cdot 4$
	Val.	$-1 \cdot 9$	$2 \cdot 2$	$13 \cdot 7$
	Leu.	$-1 \cdot 9$	$2 \cdot 4$	$14 \cdot 3$
	Ileu.	$-1 \cdot 9$	$2 \cdot 4$	$14 \cdot 5$
	Phe.	$-0 \cdot 3$	$2 \cdot 7$	$10 \cdot 1$
Aromatic	Phe.	$-1 \cdot 8$	$1 \cdot 0$	$9 \cdot 5$

† 25° C.

for similar process: the origin of this difference presumably being that Némethy and Scheraga's calculations refer specifically to nonpolar side chains attached to a polypeptide backbone whereas the data of Kauzmann refers to the transfer of pure hydrocarbon.

EXPERIMENTAL TREATMENTS OF HYDROPHOBIC INTERACTIONS

Several experimental approaches are available that lead to estimates of the thermodynamic parameters of hydrophobic interaction for the transfer of solutes from aqueous to nonpolar media. In practice, a range of values may be obtained, with a theoretical maximum, depending upon the "completeness" (relative to the ideal nonpolar medium) of the transfer process.

Solubilities of Organic Compounds

The relative solubilities of amino acids in water and organic solvents provide a value of ΔF_{tr}° and have been intensively studied since they provide a method for estimating the hydrophobic interactions in proteins. A particularly significant observation was that of Cohn and Edsall (78) who noted that ΔF_{tr}° for amino acids could be expressed as the sum of constant constituent contributions,

$$F_{tr}^{\circ} = \sum f_{tr} \qquad\qquad (XIV)$$

Thus a —CH_2— group has $f_{tr} = 700$ cal mole^{-1} and contributes this quantity to ΔF_{tr}°. From the determined solubilities of amino acids Tanford (79) has calculated the various contributions of nonpolar amino acid residues to ΔF_{tr}° for a series of amino acids for their transfer from ethanol to water. For our purposes we report his data as though for the reverse process (Table I-10): the contribution of a methylene group to hydrophobic interactions may be estimated as, $\Delta F = -0.73$ kcal mole^{-1} (alanine–glycine; leucine–valine) in excellent agreement with the figure of -0.76 kcal mole^{-1} from the relative solubilities of methane and ethane in water and ethanol.

The differences between these values and those derived from the Némethy–Scheraga treatment may reflect differences between the side chains when present in free amino acids and when present in a protein

TABLE I-10. Free Energies of Transfer from Water to Ethanol of Amino Acids and their Nonpolar Side Chains (79)

Amino acid	ΔF_{tr} kcal mole^{-1} amino acid	Δf_{tr} kcal mole^{-1} side chain	Side chain
Glycine	4·63	0	
Alanine	3·90	−0·73	CH_3
Valine	2·94	−1·69	$(CH_3)_2CH$
Leucine	2·21	−2·42	$(CH_3)_2CHCH_2$
Isoleucine	1·69	−2·97	$CH_3CH_2CH(CH_3)$
Phenylalanine	1·98	−2·65	$PhCH_2$
Proline	2·06	−2·6	$(CH_2)_3$
Methionine	3·33	−1·3	$MeS(CH_2)_2$
Tyrosine	0·93	−2·87	$4\text{-}HOC_6H_4CH_2$

(i.e., influence of backbone and steric restrictions on water structure around the nonpolar areas). Additionally, the calculated values refer to transfer into a hydrocarbon environment whereas the data of Tanford refer to transfer into ethanol. In Fig. I-14 are plotted the solubility data for medium chain alcohols (80), medium chain hydrocarbons (81) and

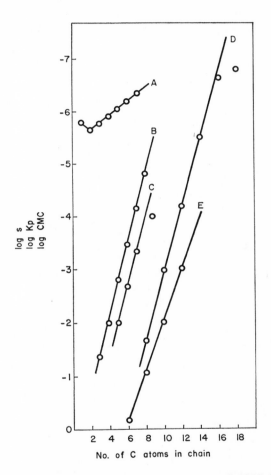

FIG. I-14. Aqueous solubilities, partition coefficients and CMC data for straight chain compounds as a function of the number of carbon atoms in the chain. A — solubilities (moles/l) of hydrocarbon gases at 1 atm. and 25°, ordinate $\log s - 3$; B — solubilities of straight chain alcohols at 25°, ordinate $\log s - 2$; C — solubilities of hydrocarbon liquids at 25°, ordinate $\log s - 1\cdot5$; D — partition coefficients (between heptane and aqueous buffer) of long chain fatty acids at 23°, ordinate $\log K_p - 1$; E — CMC data for $R(OCH_2CH_2)_6OH$ at 25°. Reproduced with permission from Mukerjee (82).

the partition coefficient data for alkane carboxylates (82). The slopes are virtually identical and correspond to a value of -825 ± 10 cal mole^{-1} CH$_2$— group for complete transfer.†

Wishnia has studied (83) the solubilities of hydrocarbon gases in a variety of protein solutions and sodium dodecyl sulfate micelles (Table I-11). This data is of great interest from two points of view: the values of the thermodynamic parameters listed in Table I-11 clearly indicate the primarily entropic determination of the binding process and ΔC_p is

TABLE I-11. Thermodynamic Parameters for Hydrocarbon Binding to Proteins and Sodium Dodecyl Sulfate (83)

System		Pentane			Butane			Neopentane		
		ΔH†	ΔS‡	ΔC_p§	ΔH	ΔS	ΔC_p	ΔH	ΔS	ΔC_p
Ideal	0°	−2·9	−33	73	−3·1	−30	61	−2·5	−30	33
	25°	−1·2	−27	64	−1·5	−25	72	−1·3	−26	64
Dodecyl sulfate	0°	−2·6	−29	73	−1·9	−23	27	−2·4	−27	82
	25°	−0·4	−21	103	−0·7	−19	67	0	−19	104
Hemoglobin	0°	1·0	−20	85	−0·8	−22	64	—	—	—
	25°	3·4	−12	106	1·0	−17	78	—	—	—
β-Lactoglobulin	0°	−0·3	−26	119	0·9	−19	61	—	—	—
monomer (pH 2·0)	25°	3·0	−15	141	2·4	−14	64	—	—	—
β-Lactoglobulin	0°	0·2	−25	103	1·4	−17	47	−2·2	−26	72
dimer (pH 5·3)	25°	3·3	−15	140	2·9	−12	71	−0·3	−19	85

† kcal mole^{-1}; ‡ e.u.; § cal deg^{-1} mole^{-1}.

essentially similar for all of the systems listed and is characteristic of hydrophobic interactions. A second extremely interesting feature of the data listed is that the heat of dissociation of butane and pentane from β-lactoglobulin and ferrihemoglobin is some 3–4 kcal mole^{-1} higher than from sodium dodecylsulfate micelles or from an ideal liquid phase: this feature accounts for the high affinity of these ligands for the protein systems. These anomalous ΔF values arise from a larger ΔH change that is only partially compensated by ΔS. The excess ΔH change cannot arise from alkane–water interactions and Wishnia considers it possible that it arises from alkane interaction at a hydrophobic site which is locally strained so that the nonpolar chains comprising the site occupy a volume larger than the normal volume of a hydrocarbon liquid

† Solubility and partition data are often quite equivalent since in the first case a self-partition process is actually being measured. Hansch (84, 85) has shown (see section on p. 35) that the aqueous solubility of a large number of neutral organic compounds may be expressed as a linear free energy relationship in terms of P (partition coefficient between octanol and water).

and the resultant interaction energy among the nonpolar chains is suboptimal. Subsequent interaction with an appropriate alkane molecule thus generates a larger than normal enthalpy change arising from the alkane-site interaction *and* some rearrangement of the nonpolar chains of the site itself leading to a more favorable intrasite interaction.†

Thermodynamics of Micelle Formation

Amphiphathic molecules containing a long hydrocarbon chain (C_8–C_{18}) to which is attached a polar head group (nonionic, zwitterionic or ionic) have the property of forming polymeric complexes (micelles) at defined concentrations of the monomer—the critical micellar concentration (CMC). Since the CMC varies with both the chain length and the nature of the polar head group, it is clear that both portions of the amphipathic molecule play a role in the determination of the monomer-micelle equilibrium (86).

However, a number of thermodynamic analyses of micelle formation have established quite clearly that the major driving force for the micellization reaction is the hydrophobic interaction of the nonpolar chains (86–89). An analysis of thermodynamic treatments of micelle formation has been given by Mukerjee (86). In the treatment used by Molyneux *et al.* (89) formation of micelles is treated as a phase separation (the basis of this treatment is discussed by Mukerjee (*loc. cit.*)) and thus,

$$\Delta F_m^\circ = -RT \ln \text{CMC} \qquad \text{(XV)}$$

Through an analysis that specifically includes the contribution of counterions (in the case of ionic micelles) to the observed free energy changes it has been found possible to analyse separately the contributions of the nonpolar chains and polar head groups to the thermodynamic parameters of the micellization process (Table I-12). The average value of ΔF (—CH_2—) for micellization is close to —0·65 kcal mole^{-1} in contrast to the —0·85 kcal mole^{-1} for the transfer of aliphatic hydrocarbons from water to the liquid state. This difference suggests that the interior of a micelle may not be anhydrous: the fluorine magnetic resonance spectra of soaps, $CF_3(CH_2)_n COONa$ ($n = 8$, 10, 11), studied by Muller and Birkhahn (90) suggest that the interior of these micelles is quite wet, having characteristics approximately half way between those of water and pure hydrocarbon. Unfortunately, little is known concerning the organization of this water. The work of Némethy and Scheraga (61) indicates that the presence of a single layer of water

† As Wishnia (83) notes this contribution to the energy of ligand binding which has obvious affinity to the "induced fit" hypothesis of Koshland (p. 63) by the "collapse" of a binding site into a less strained state may be of general significance in contributing to the specificity of enzyme–substrate interactions.

between two nonpolar chains represents a situation appropriately less thermodynamically stable than the first water layer surrounding a nonpolar solute. Thus the hydrophobic interaction is strongly favored provided, as appears likely in a micelle, that the nonpolar chains are

TABLE I-12. Thermodynamic Parameters of Micellization in Aqueous Solution (89)

Amphiphile	Head group	ΔF (—CH_2—) kcal mole^{-1}	ΔH_m° ΔS_m°† (for dodecyl chain) kcal mole^{-1}	e.u.	$\Delta H_m^\circ/\Delta S_m^\circ$
N-Alkylbetaine	—$\overset{+}{N}(Me)_2CH_2COO^-$	−0·68	−1·4	15·5	−90
C-Alkylbetaine	$Me_3\overset{+}{N}CH(R)COO^-$	−0·64	+0·6	23·0	25
K$^+$-Alkylcarboxylate	COO^-	−0·64	—	—	—
Na$^+$-Alkylsulfonate	SO_3^-	−0·65	—	—	—
Na$^+$-Alkylsulfate	$SO_4^=$	−0·60	—	—	—
Alkyldimethylamine oxide	$NMe_2 \to O$	−0·65	+1·7	26·0	65
Alkyl hexaoxyethylene glycol monoether	$(OCH_2CH_2)_6OH$	−0·68	+3·6	39·0	90

† Entropies include cratic term.

sufficiently flexible to interact. Presumably, the water is present in essentially a bulk phase at only certain areas of the micelle, thus allowing the maximum hydrophobic interactions.

HYDROPHOBIC INTERACTIONS AND PROTEIN STRUCTURE

The role played by hydrophobic interactions in determining the conformation of proteins is becoming increasingly clear. X-ray data (91) is revealing an apparently general method of construction of globular proteins (myoglobin, lysozyme, α-chymotrypsin) as having compact structures with nonpolar groups in the interior and polar groups, with few exceptions, at the aqueous interface. Those polar groups that do appear in the generally nonpolar interior are of great interest since they are often intimately involved with the catalytic function of the protein (see section on p. 52). This segregation of polar and nonpolar residues appears likely to be a general feature of macromolecular organization.

Tanford (79, 92) has approached the problem of hydrophobic stabilization of globular proteins by considering the unfolding of the native protein (Fig. I-15) subject to the assumptions that, charged groups occupy the same environment in the native and unfolded states, nonpolar groups are confined to the interior of the native protein and that polar groups may be located at the interior or exterior of globular proteins, this being a consequence of the fact that the primary structure of proteins does not involve sequential segregation of polar and nonpolar residues. The free energy of unfolding is expressed as

$$\Delta F = -T \Delta S_{conf} + \sum \Delta f_u \qquad \text{(XVI)}$$

where ΔS_{conf} is the change in conformational entropy of the unfolding process and Δf_u is the free energy change for transfer of a nonpolar residue from the native to the unfolded environment: Δf_u was calculated on the basis of additivity of the Δf_u contributions of single side chains

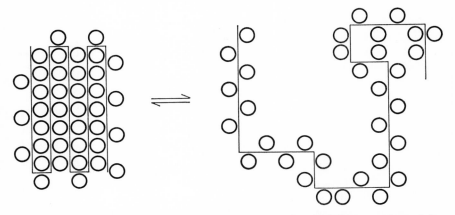

FIG. I-15. Schematic representation of the native and unfolded states of a protein. The significance is the contacts made and lost by the side chains in the native and unfolded states respectively. Reproduced with permission from Tanford (79).

and was assumed to be equatable to Δf_{tr} the free energy of transfer of the side chain from ethanol to water (see section on p. 26). For myoglobin and β-lactoglobulin, the calculated values of $-\Delta S_{conf}$ and $\sum \Delta f_u$ were found to be of the same order of magnitude suggesting, within the limitations of the calculations, that hydrophobic interactions play a major role in the determination of the native conformation.

Experimental verification of the importance of hydrophobic interactions comes from studies of the thermodynamics of denaturation of proteins (Table I-13), from which is observed that the values of ΔS_D are surprisingly small for an order–disorder transition and that they actually tend to become negative upon reduction in temperature. These entropic effects have their origin in the exposure of nonpolar side chains to solvent, and consequent ordering of solvent, as the protein is denatured. It is important to note, however, that hydrophobic interactions, being essentially nonspecific in character, determine the conformation of the native protein *only* to the extent that the nonpolar groups orient themselves in a nonpolar environment. Other specific and highly directional interactions (van der Waals, hydrogen bonds, etc.) play the determinant role in the microarchitecture (1).

TABLE I-13. Thermodynamic Parameters for some Protein Denaturation Processes (92)

Protein process	ΔF_D ΔH_D kcal mole^{-1}		ΔS_D e.u.		
			0°	25°	75°
Ribonuclease thermal transition, pH 2·5, 30° C	+0·9	+57	+31	+155	+340
Chymotrypsinogen, thermal transition, pH 3, 30° C	+7·3	+39	−80	+105	+680
Myoglobin, thermal transition, pH 9, 25° C	+13·6	+42			
β-Lactoglobulin, 5 M urea, pH 3, 25° C	+0·6	−21	−260	−72	+260

Némethy and Scheraga (61) have discussed the contributions of hydrophobic interactions to conformation stabilization in proteins. In the α-helix adjacent side chains may interact: such side chains will be adjacent along the same turn of the helix or adjacent (third and fourth in sequence) on the next turn of the helix (Fig. I-16). The magnitude of these interactions will be dependent upon the side chain character and various steric parameters. Hydrophobic interactions are also important in the pleated sheet conformations (β-forms) shown in Fig. I-17, where interactions are shown for alanine residues: here, as with the α-helix, stronger hydrophobic interactions will be anticipated with larger nonpolar chains.

The importance of hydrophobic interactions in determining the α-helix—random coil transition of synthetic polypeptides has been suggested by a number of workers (61, 79, 93–97). The studies of Klotz (97, 98) who has measured the thermodynamics of association of *N*-methylacetamide in carbon tetrachloride and in water also lends support to this conclusion. Formation of a hydrogen bonded dimer in CCl_4 solution is accompanied by $\Delta F°$, −2·4 kcal mole^{-1}, $\Delta H°$, −5·1 kcal mole^{-1} and $\Delta S°$, −9 e.u.: the same process in water has an unfavorable free energy change, $\Delta F°$, +3·1 kcal mole^{-1}, $\Delta H°$, 0 kcal mole^{-1} and $\Delta S°$, −10 e.u. The stability of α-helical poly-L-alanine, compared to poly-glycine which does not form an α-helix has been attributed to hydro-

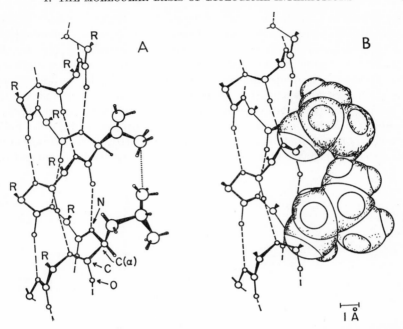

Fig. I-16. Hydrophobic interaction between a leucine and valine residue on a right-handed α-helix (– – – –, backbone hydrogen bonds; ·····, hydrophobic interaction). Reproduced with permission from Némethy and Scheraga (61).

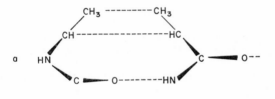

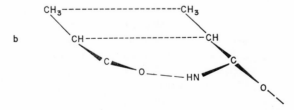

Fig. I-17. Hydrophobic interactions between alanine residues in (a) antiparallel and (b) parallel pleated sheet structures. After Némethy and Scheraga (61).

phobic interactions between the side chain methyl groups (99). While the polypeptide backbone may contribute a significant proportion of the stability of the α-helix (100), studies of mixed copolymers of L-leucine or L-alanine with DL-glutamic acid reveal an added contribution to stability by hydrophobic interactions between the bulkier leucine side chains. Studies with poly-L-ornithine and poly-L-lysine reveal that above pH 11·0 (where electrostatic repulsions will be minimized) poly-L-lysine, which has one more methylene group, is completely helical whereas poly-L-ornithine is only 20% helical (101, 102). Davidson and Fasman (103) have studied the thermally induced conformational

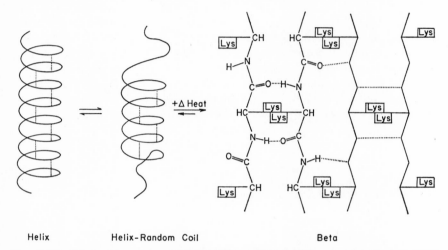

Helix   Helix-Random Coil   Beta

FIG. I-18. Schematic representation of the α-β transition of poly-L-lysine. With permission from Davidson and Fasman (103).

transition of poly-L-lysine and have shown that the β-structure (pleated form) is more stable at higher temperatures: these workers attribute this to a hydrophobic stabilization of the β-form whilst at lower temperatures the α-helical form is favored through intra-amide hydrogen bonding (Fig. I-18).

The prominent role played by hydrophobic interactions in the stabilization of the tertiary structure of proteins suggests a similar prominence in the determination of quaternary structure. The stable aggregation of protein monomers will require as a general feature hydrophobic regions on the monomer surface (104, 105): aggregation through polar interactions alone is unlikely to provide adequate stability because of the competition by water for the polar areas.

There is quite adequate experimental evidence from proteins composed of subunits that this premise is generally true. In hemoglobin

X-ray crystallographic evidence shows the contacts in the $\alpha_2\beta_2$ tetrameric species between the α and β subunits to be very largely nonpolar in character (106). A number of other subunit proteins have been studied for which various lines of evidence, including studies of the influence of ionic strengths, solvent polarity, volume changes, etc., have suggested a large component of hydrophobic interaction in the monomer association process (107). These proteins include tobacco mosaic virus protein (108), squid hemocyanin (109, 110), G actin (111), pyruvate kinase (112) and liver sulfatase (113). Some general aspects of the role of hydrophobic interactions in protein assemblage are discussed by Caspar (1, 114). As is discussed later, the subunit organization of proteins constitutes an important feature of the mediation of allosteric and cooperative regulatory effects (see section on p. 71). Since hydrophobic stabilization is of general importance to the association of subunits, it is relevant to note that the role of lipids in membrane bound and lipid dependent enzymes may be precisely that of providing an additional hydrophobic component† to the protein to permit the association of otherwise stable monomeric protein units (some further aspects of lipid dependent enzymes are discussed in Chapter II, p. 140).

Since hydrophobic interactions play an important role in the maintenance of the tertiary and quaternary structures of proteins, it is to be anticipated that modulation of these interactions by, for example, addition of nonpolar ligands, or ligands containing nonpolar functions will lead to alterations in the protein conformation. The extent and importance of any such conformational change will depend upon several factors, including the importance of hydrophobic interactions in the native structure, the nature and position of the ligand binding site, the interaction in the native structure between hydrophobic and polar interactions and the linkage between the conformational change and the catalytic site of the protein. Various aspects of this problem will be discussed from the point of view of solute–solvent interactions in the next section.

SOLUTE–SOLVENT INTERACTIONS, EXTRATHERMODYNAMIC RELATIONSHIPS AND LIGAND BINDING

The maintenance of protein conformation rests heavily on hydrophobic interactions and hence water is the key determinant to understanding protein organization and function. This is of paramount

† In the evolutionary sense, it may be presumed that subunit proteins are derived from monomeric ancestors through the incorporation of appropriately located nonpolar areas among other modifications (104, 105). Obviously this can occur through the substitution of amino acids with nonpolar side chains for polar amino acids, but might also occur through the incorporation of lipids, particularly phospholipids, to generate an associating lipid–protein complex.

importance in any consideration of the interaction and binding of small molecules with proteins.

Polyvinylpyrrolidone binds a variety of aromatic compounds both polar and nonpolar. The binding process is accompanied by an entropy gain, this being greatest for nonpolar solutes (benzene) and least for ionic solutes (sodium benzoate). These data have been rationalized by Molyneux and Frank (115) with the assumption that ΔS_u refers to the perturbation of water structure by the aromatic solute. According to their specific thermodynamic analysis, the enthalpy of binding is considered to be composed of five contributing terms: ΔH_1, enthalpy of destruction of "structured" water; ΔH_2, enthalpy of dehydration of *specifically* hydrated sites; ΔH_3, enthalpy of binding of "dehydrated" systems; ΔH_4, enthalpy of *specific* rehydration and ΔH_5, enthalpy of reforming water structure around nonpolar regions,

$$\Delta H_{tot} = \Delta H_1 + \Delta H_2 + \Delta H_3 + \Delta H_4 + \Delta H_5 \qquad \text{(XVII)}$$

By incorporating $\Delta H_2 + \Delta H_3 + \Delta H_4$ in one term, ΔH_b, then

$$\Delta H_{tot} = \Delta H_1 + \Delta H_b + \Delta H_5 = \Delta S_u(h/s) + \Delta H_b \qquad \text{(XVIII)}$$

where s is the entropy gain for the release of one mole of "structured" water and h is the corresponding enthalpy change. A plot of ΔH against ΔS_u is linear (Fig. I-19) indicating the approximate constancy of ΔH_b, at -5 kcal and principally determined by ΔH_3, with the slope indicating that the "structured" water has an apparent "melting point" of about $340°K$ ($70°C$).

The treatment offered by Molyneux and Frank is an example of an extrathermodynamic relationship (116, 117) whereby,

$$\Delta H = \beta \Delta S \qquad \text{(XIX)}$$

since,

$$\Delta F = \Delta H - T \Delta S \qquad \text{(XX)}$$

then,

$$\Delta F = (T - \beta) \Delta S \qquad \text{(XXI)}$$

$$= \left(1 - \frac{T}{\beta}\right) \Delta H \qquad \text{(XXII)}$$

so that β, the proportionality constant of eqn. XIX, has the dimensions of absolute temperature and is actually the temperature at which all differences in rate or equilibrium constants for a ligand series in a particular reaction will be eliminated,

$$F_{T=\beta} = 0 \qquad \text{(XXIII)}$$

Such relationships are actually quite common and are exhibited by diverse physical and chemical reactions including vaporization of liquids, solubilities of organic compounds, molecular complex formation, acid-base ionizations, nucleophilic displacement, esterification, hydrolytic, carbonyl addition, solvent variation and other reaction series (a more detailed listing will be found in reference 117).

Qualitatively it is easy to visualize situations under which compensating variations in ΔH and ΔS will exist. In the process of molecular association, whether this is through a covalent or reversible association,

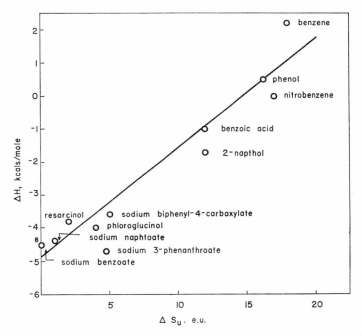

FIG. I-19. Isoequilibrium relationship (ΔH versus ΔS) for the interaction of solutes with polyvinylpyrollidone. Reproduced with permission from Molyneux and Frank (115).

a negative enthalpy change may be accompanied by a negative entropy change because of the loss of translational and rotational degrees of freedom as the molecules unite: in a structurally related series of molecules with progressively greater combining tendency the enthalpy change will become progressively more negative with increasing intermolecular interaction but this will be accompanied by a progressively negative entropy change because of the greater restrictions of the two molecules in the transition state or complex. Similarly, in reactions where solute–solvent interactions are of dominant importance a similar compensation of ΔH and ΔS is to be expected. In ionization reactions where solvation of the ion differs from the undissociated species, the ion–solvent interaction ($-\Delta H$) will increase with increasing ionization and ΔS will become progressively more negative with increasing ordering of solvent around the ionic species. In the solution of polar or nonpolar

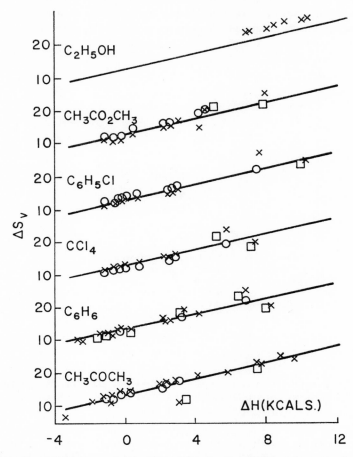

FIG. I-20. Isoequilibrium relationships (ΔH versus ΔS) for the vaporization of gases from organic solutes. Reproduced with permission from Frank and Evans (60).

solutes in solvating media, notably water which is of particular concern to biological systems, a similar compensating correlation between ΔH and ΔS is anticipated: in complex formation between polar and nonpolar solutes increased enthalpy changes will be accompanied by increasingly positive entropy changes as the ordered solvent layer surrounding the solutes is progressively converted to less ordered bulk phase solvent.

Examples of such compensating relationships have been known for over thirty years: several workers including Bell (118), Evans and Polanyi (119) and Butler (120, 121) found linear relationships between the heats and entropies of solution of gases and organic compounds in organic solutes. Barclay and Butler (122) found a wide ranging linear relationship for the vaporization of both pure liquids and dilute solutions. An extensive examination of the vaporization of low boiling solutes from nonpolar solvents has been presented by Frank and Evans (60) who

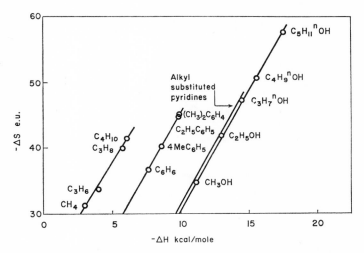

FIG. I-21. Isoequilibrium relationships (ΔH versus ΔS) for the hydration of solutes in aqueous solution. Reproduced from Anden *et al.* (125) with permission of the authors, the Chemical Society (London) and the Chemical Research Laboratory, Department of Scientific and Industrial Research, England.

observed good linearity between ΔH and ΔS for each solvent system, the relative vertical displacement of each line on the entropy axis (Fig. I-20) serving to describe the uniqueness of the solute interactions within each solvent system. Of particular interest is the data of Butler (120), Butler and Reid (123) Claussen and Polglase (124) and Anden *et al.* (125) for the entropies and enthalpies of hydration of polar and nonpolar solutes in aqueous solution (Fig. I-21). From this data it is clear that, with one exception, the slopes $\Delta H/\Delta S = \beta$, for the various series are essentially identical at $\beta = 277°K$. The exception is the inert gases, for which $\beta = 520°K$. The markedly disparate values of β for the two systems clearly suggests the existence of different solute–solvent interactions: there can be little doubt that these are "iceberg" formation

3

and clathrate inclusion for organic solutes and the rare gases respectively. Robertson *et al.* (126) have also described similar linear enthalpy–entropy relationships for the solution equilibria of alkyl halides and esters. Quite clearly, the existence of such enthalpy–entropy relationships for solubility and partition data is of very direct relevance to ligand–macromolecule interactions, where the ligand binding process may often be regarded, at least in part, as a partitioning between aqueous and macromolecular phases.

It should also be noted that such linear correlations are known for the ionization of many series of organic acids and bases: Fig. I-22 (taken

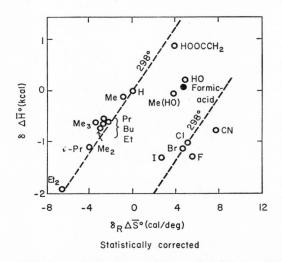

FIG. I-22. Isoequilibrium relationships (ΔH versus ΔS) for the ionization of aliphatic acids ($R_1R_2R_3CCOOH$) in water. Reproduced with permission from Leffler and Grunwald (117).

from the collection of data by Leffler and Grunwald (117)) shows the correlation for a series of aliphatic carboxylic acids. The extensive survey by Brown (127) of ionization data in aqueous solution also describes many linear enthalpy–entropy relationships with a general tendency for β to lie in the range 280–300°K. A detailed discussion of the thermodynamic parameters underlying such ionization reactions has been presented by Larson and Hepler (128).

The extent to which such enthalpy–entropy relationships will be perfectly compensatory will depend upon the extent to which the single interaction mechanism is dominant and it may be anticipated that minor fluctuations will be relatively common (129) because of the intrusion of additional interaction mechanisms specific to a particular substituent or ligand structure. Furthermore, two or more compensatory mechanisms may exist simultaneously so that the $\Delta H/\Delta S$ plot is not linear and it is also probable that compensatory mechanisms may not be evident because they are totally obscured by significant contributions from interaction mechanisms that are not compensatory.

A notable contribution to the general interpretation of ΔH–ΔS relationships was made by Hepler (128–130) in an analysis of the

TABLE I-14. Thermodynamic Parameters of Ionization of Organic Acids at 298°K (130)

Compound	K	ΔF° kcal mole^{-1}	ΔH° kcal mole^{-1}	ΔS° e.u.
Phenol	$1 \cdot 05 \times 10^{-10}$	$13 \cdot 61$	$5 \cdot 65$	$-26 \cdot 7$
m-Nitrophenol	$45 \cdot 1 \times 10^{-10}$	$11 \cdot 40$	$4 \cdot 70$	$-22 \cdot 5$
p-Nitrophenol	720×10^{-10}	$9 \cdot 75$	$4 \cdot 70$	$-16 \cdot 9$
p-Chlorophenol	$4 \cdot 18 \times 10^{-10}$	$12 \cdot 80$	$5 \cdot 80$	$-23 \cdot 5$
Chloroacetic acid	$1 \cdot 36 \times 10^{-3}$	$3 \cdot 92$	$-1 \cdot 12$	$-16 \cdot 9$
Iodoacetic acid	$0 \cdot 67 \times 10^{-3}$	$4 \cdot 33$	$-1 \cdot 42$	$-19 \cdot 3$

ionization of phenols and carboxylic acids where the greater acidity of, for example, p-nitrophenol relative to m-nitrophenol is reflected largely in the ΔS rather than the ΔH term (Table I-14). To determine the influence of solute–solvent interaction it was assumed that the observed entropy and enthalpy changes were composed of *internal* and *external* contributions,

$$\Delta S^{\circ}_{obs} = \Delta S_{ext} + \Delta S_{int} \qquad \text{(XXIV)}$$

$$\Delta H^{\circ}_{obs} = \Delta H_{ext} + \Delta H_{int} \qquad \text{(XXV)}$$

where *internal* contributions refer to the differences in enthalpy and entropy of the ionized and unionized forms and the *external* contributions refer to the differences in solvent interactions of the two species. The effect of a substituent (s) on an ionization process relative to the parent compound (u) is described by,

$$HA_s + A_u^- \rightleftharpoons A_s^- + HA_u$$

Since, according to Pitzer (131), the change in ΔS_{int} for the symmetrical reaction above is small, eqn. XXIV becomes

$$\Delta S_{obs} = \Delta S_{ext} \qquad \text{(XXVI)}$$

and since for ion-solvent interactions it may be concluded† that,

$$\Delta H_{ext} = \beta \Delta S_{ext} = \beta \Delta S^{\circ}_{obs} \qquad \text{(XXVII)}$$

then from combination of equations XXV and XXVII,

$$\Delta H^{\circ}_{obs} = \Delta H_{int} + \beta \Delta S^{\circ}_{obs} \qquad \text{(XXVIII)}$$

Since β for many ionization processes has been found to be very constant at $\sim 280°K$ it becomes possible to calculate the contributions of ΔH_{int} to ΔH°_{obs} for the ionization processes (Table I-15) thus yielding

TABLE I-15. Calculated ΔH_{int} Values
for Ionization of Organic Acids at 280°K
(130)

Compound	ΔH_{int} kcal mole^{-1}
o-Nitrophenol	$-3 \cdot 60$
m-Nitrophenol	$-2 \cdot 13$
p-Nitrophenol	$-3 \cdot 69$
p-Chlorophenol	$-1 \cdot 92$
Chloroacetic acid	$-2 \cdot 50$
Iodoacetic acid	$-2 \cdot 10$

"corrected" values for the enthalpy changes in the *absence* of solute–solvent interactions from which it is apparent that the conventional concepts of electron withdrawal and resonance stabilization in promoting electron release are indeed reflected in the ΔH_{int} values.

The value of this latter treatment is in the importance that it places upon the necessity of separating internal and external (solvation) contributions to the thermodynamic parameters of rate and equilibrium processes (132, 133). This is particularly crucial in attempts to understand the molecular basis of ligand–macromolecule complex formation in aqueous solution where the role of the solute–solvent interactions

† As pointed out by Hepler and O'Hara (129) eqn. XXVII is actually in accord with the Born equation,

$$\Delta F = \frac{-z^2 \epsilon^2}{2r} \left(1 - \frac{1}{D} \right)$$

where ΔF, the free energy of charging an ion of radius r to charge $z\epsilon$ in the gaseous phase minus the contribution made by charging the ion in a medium of dielectric constant D, is equatable to the free energy of solvation: differentiation of the medium term with respect to temperature and substitution with $\delta F/\delta T = -S$ and $F = H - T\Delta S$ gives

$$H = \left\{ \frac{1}{d\ln D/dT} + T \right\} S$$

with both the ligand and macromolecule is known to be of critical importance.

A number of such isoequilibrium relationships have been found in systems of biological interest and undoubtedly many more remain to be discovered. A large number of protein denaturation processes in water (Fig. I-23) generate a relationship of slope 282°K (135, 137) the denaturation of hemoglobin in aqueous ethanol solutions (Fig. I-24), with a very wide range of ΔH^+ and ΔS^+ values, generates a slope of 290°K (134) very similar to that found by Brandts and Hunt (136) for the denaturation of ribonuclease in aqueous ethanol solutions. Similar

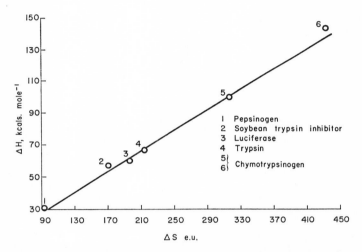

FIG. I-23. Isoequilibrium relationships for protein denaturation in aqueous solution (134).

relationships are found also with the binding of substrates and inhibitors to various enzymes including α-chymotrypsin (Fig. I-25; 135) and others cited by Likhtenshtein (137). The data depicted for α-chymotrypsin in Fig. I-25 are of particular interest since they include not only a number of inhibitors as cited but also data for the intermediates in the hydrolysis of N-acetyl-L-tryptophan ethyl ester.

Good (138, 138a) has described particularly interesting isokinetic relationships for the hemolysis of mammalian erythrocytes by hypotonic malonamide (Fig. I-26) and for the hemolysis of human erythrocytes by a variety of hypotonic solutions (Fig. I-27). It seems highly probable that the common effect of all of these agents in causing hemolysis is achieved through perturbation of the hydrated cell membrane.

It is abundantly clear that the existence of the various isoequilibrium relationships noted is a solvent-controlled phenomenon (117, 128, 132, 139). That many and diverse processes occurring in aqueous solutions have isokinetic temperatures in the range of 270–290°K is highly suggestive that they all involve the reorganization of water structure. For simple physical and chemical systems this is a matter of great interest (132), but for protein systems it is, by virtue of the fact that protein

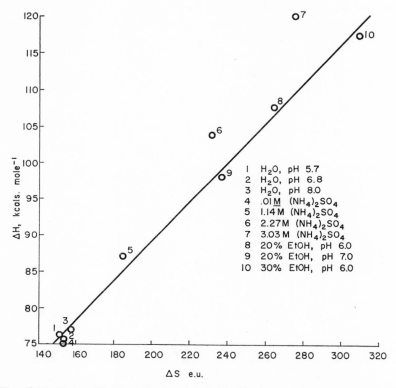

FIG. I-24. Isoequilibrium relationship for hemoglobin denaturation (134).

conformation is determined by the delicate interrelationships between water and nonpolar and polar residues, synonymous with conformational change of the protein. In turn such conformational changes, which will range in magnitude from the extremely large, associated with denaturation, to the extremely small, associated with, for example, optimum substrate or regulatory ligand binding, will regulate protein function.†

† Further developments of the importance of the concept of isoequilibrium relationships in biological regulatory phenomena, beyond the scope of the present work, are discussed by Lumry and Biltonen (135).

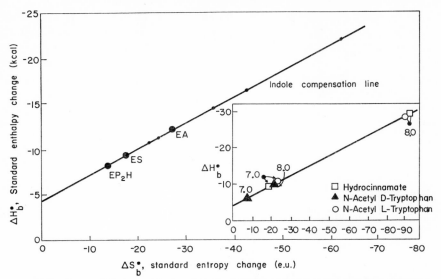

FIG. I-25. Isoequilibrium relationship for binding of substrates and inhibitors to chymotrypsin. Large figure shows the binding of indole (●) and intermediates in the hydrolysis of N-acetyl-L-tryptophan ethylester (ES → EA → EP$_2$H). Inset figure shows the binding of several inhibitors. Reproduced from Lumry and Biltonen (135) with permission of the authors and Marcel Dekker, Inc.

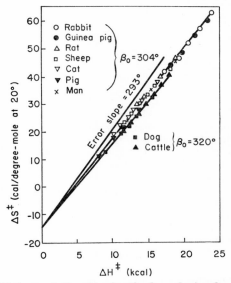

FIG. I-26. Isoequilibrium relationship for the hemolysis of mammalian erythrocytes in hypotonic malonamide solutions. Reproduced with permission from Good (138a).

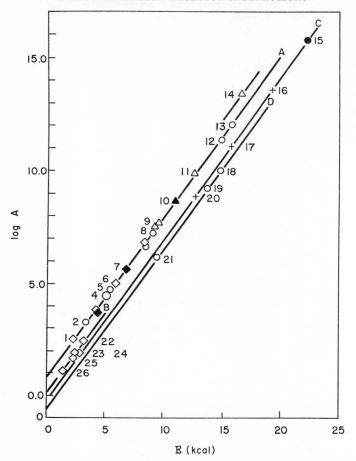

FIG. I-27. Isoequilibrium relationship for rates of hemolysis of human erythrocytes in a variety of hypotonic solutions: 1, glycine; 2, sucrose; 3, ethanol; 4, water; 5, urea; 6, methanol; 7, glucose; 8, 1,1-dimethylurea; 9, propyleneglycol; 10, trimethylene glycol; 11, methylthiourea; 12, 1,3-diethylurea; 13, ethylurea; 14, thiourea; 15, malonamide + glucose (3·5 + 1·5); 16, malonamide (6·5); 17, malonamide (5·0); 18, malonamide + sucrose (3·5 + 0·5); 19, malonamide + sodium chloride (3·5 + 1·5); 20, malonamide, (3·5); 21, malonamide + glycine (3·5 + 0·5); 22, potassium chloride; 23, rubidium chloride; 24, sodium chloride; 25, lithium chloride; 26, cesium chloride. Osmotic concentrations—Group A, 2·0 atm (glucose, malonamide, sucrose and glycine) and remainder at 6·5 atm: Group B, 2·0 atm at 20°: Groups C and D as recorded. Reproduced with permission from Good (138).

From the standpoint of regulatory mechanisms in biological macromolecules conformational changes of the latter class are obviously the more relevant although the most difficult to detect; however, to the extent that denaturation, thermal transition phenomena, etc. are regarded as representing one extreme of conformational change (140) they generate valuable and relatively easily obtained information concerning the role of bound water. von Hippel and Wong (141, 142) and Schrier and Scheraga (143) have undertaken comprehensive studies of the effects of nonpolar solutes, alcohols and tetraalkylammonium salts, on the thermal transition of ribonuclease. This transition involves the unfolding of the protein at about 60° in dilute neutral salt solution:

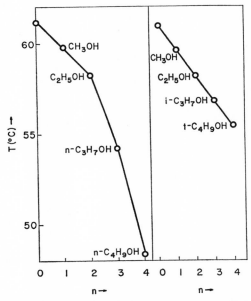

FIG. I-28. The effect of 1 M alcohol solutions on the temperature ($T°$) of thermal denaturation of ribonuclease (n = no. of carbon atoms). Reproduced with permission from Schrier, Ingwall and Scheraga (143).

the transition is demonstrated by changes in several physical parameters including catalytic activity, viscosity, ORD, changes in the environment of buried tyrosyl residues and increased susceptibility to proteolytic degradation. Thermodynamic studies of ribonuclease denaturation (136) leave little doubt that it involves the exposure of hydrophobic groups during the unfolding process and that the effects of nonpolar ligands on the temperature of thermal transition are brought about preferential binding to the exposed hydrophobic side chains. The effects of alcohols on T_m are shown in Fig. I-28. Apparently the nonpolar binding sites are limited in dimensions since it is apparent that branched chain alcohols have approximately the same effect on T_m as the next lowest straight

3*

chain alcohol. The effects of tetraalkylammonium salts (corrected for the effect of the anion) are shown in Fig. I-29 from which it is apparent that the ability to lower T_m increases with increasing length of the nonpolar chain. (A further discussion of the hydrophobic binding of quaternary ammonium ions will be presented elsewhere (Chapter IV, p. 276).) From the data of von Hippel and Wong it is apparent that the ability of alcohols or tetraalkylammonium ions to denature RNase is solely dependent upon their nonpolar character. Figure I-30 shows that the dependence of T_m of ribonuclease in 1 M solutions of alkyl chains is

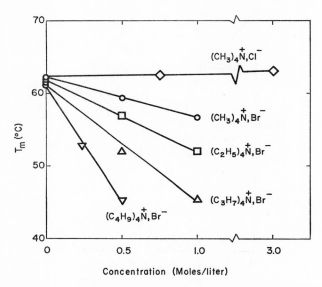

FIG. I-29. Effects of tetraalkylammonium salts on the temperature $(T_m{}^\circ)$ of thermal denaturation of ribonuclease at pH 7·0. Reproduced with permission from von Hippel and Wong (141).

dependent upon the "effective" number of methylene groups (at 1 M concentration Me_4N^+ has an effective chain length of zero since it does not lower T_m).

Finally, in considering more subtle aspects of ligand–macromolecule interactions it may be noted that the importance of the role of water structure in controlling ligand–macromolecular interactions is, without doubt, reflected in attempts to analyse, through linear free energy relationships, the effects of substituents on the ability of ligands to bind to macromolecular systems or to produce biological responses. The use of substituent constant analysis in the treatment of rates and equilibria of organic reactions by Hammett or extended Hammett theory (117,

144–150) is remarkably successful and too well documented to require additional comment. In marked contrast, application of the same treatment to systems of biological interest in terms of polar (σ) and steric (E_s) substituent constants is almost uniformly unsuccessful (147, 148), primarily because account is not taken of the several roles of hydrophobic interaction discussed previously.

This deficiency has been recognized very explicitly by Hansch and his co-workers (149–156) who have introduced the use of the partition

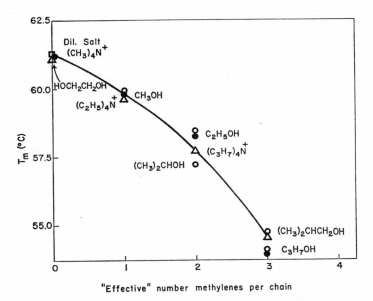

FIG. I-30. The temperature ($T_m°$) of thermal denaturation of ribonuclease as a function of the number of effective methylene units per alkyl chain. Reproduced with permission from von Hippel and Wong (141).

coefficient, P (derived from an octanol–water system), and the derived substituent constant π, where $\pi_x = \log P_x - P_H$, into linear free energy descriptions for a remarkably large range of biological processes. A similar, but much more limited finding, was that of Meyer (157) and Overton (158, 159) at the turn of this century who demonstrated the linear relationship between partition coefficient and narcotic action for a number of simple organic compounds. For a number of systems including ligand binding to some proteins and other macromolecules (Table I-16) and a number of simple biological responses (Table I-17) single parameter linear free energy relationships are found, where

$$\log K = a \log P + c \qquad \text{(XXIX)}$$

and

$$\log 1/C = a \log P + c \tag{XXX}$$

suggesting, but not proving, that the variation in binding or biological activity with variation of ligand structure is largely dependent upon the reorganization of water associated with the ligand interaction.[†]

TABLE I-16. Single Parameter (P) Linear Free Energy Relationship for Ligand–Macromolecule Binding (150)

Ligand	$\log K = a \log P + b$ Macromolecule	a	n	r
Miscellaneous organic	BSA	0·75	42	0·960
Miscellaneous organic	Hb (bovine)	0·71	17	0·950
ROH	Ribonuclease	0·50	4	0·999
Barbiturates	Liver homogenate	0·52	5	0·973
Acetanilides	Nylon	0·69	7	0·961
Penicillins	Human serum	0·49	79	0·924

TABLE I-17. Single Parameter (P) Linear Free Energy Relationships for Biological Responses (150)

Ligand	$\log \dfrac{1}{C} = a \log P + b$ Response	a	n	r
ROH	Toxicity to red spider	0·69	14	0·979
ROH	I_{50}, O_2 consumption cervical ganglion	1·16	4	0·994
Barbiturates	I_{50}, egg cell division	0·80	19	0·960
Ureas	Mice hypnosis	0·55	23	0·943
Phenylacetic acids	Inhibition of *Avena* cell elongation	0·73	18	0·972
Phenols	Inhibition of chymotrypsin	0·95	10	0·990
Barbiturates	I_{50}, Brain O_2 consumption	1·04	10	0·96

Thus, ligand binding in the systems listed in Tables I-16 and I-17 may represent partitioning into a relatively unstructured nonpolar phase in which the electronic and steric contributions of the substituted ligands

[†] This is not to imply that the binding is *solely* through hydrophobic interactions, although this may be the case for some ligand series, but rather that the polar and steric contributions to binding of the ligand series, other than those automatically reflected in P or π, remain approximately constant with substituent variation. Furthermore, Hansch and his co-workers have explicitly recognized (153), as have other workers (i.e., 160) that σ and other variables may be covariant with π for certain systems.

are either small or constant. Such single parameter relationships are limiting cases of a more generalized free energy relationship,

$$\Delta F^\circ_{Res} = \Delta F^\circ_{Hydr} + \Delta F^\circ_{Elect} + \Delta F^\circ_{Steric} \approx \ln k_{Res} \qquad \text{(XXXI)}$$

where ΔF°_{Res}, the free energy change for the determinant rate or equilibrium process involved in the production of the biological response is seen to be the sum of the hydrophobic, electronic and steric parameters of the ligand. The effect of a given substituent change is given by,

$$\delta_x \Delta F^\circ_{Res} = \delta_x \Delta F^\circ_{Hydr} + \delta_x \Delta F^\circ_{Elect} + \delta_x \Delta F^\circ_{Steric} \qquad \text{(XXXII)}$$

and the effect of a substituent x on k_{Res} is given by,

$$\log k_{Res} = \log \frac{1}{C} = k\pi_x + p\sigma_x + k' E_s + k'' \qquad \text{(XXXIII)}$$

Several examples, taken from the very large number now available of such multiparameter linear free energy relationships are presented below (others will be cited elsewhere in the text).

Toxicity of diethylphenyl phosphates ($XC_6H_4OPO(OEt)_2$) to houseflies (161)

$$\log \frac{1}{C} = 2 \cdot 42 + 0 \cdot 256\pi - 0 \cdot 600 \quad (n = 13, r = 0 \cdot 975)$$

Local anesthetic activities of diethylaminoethylbenzoates ($XC_6H_4COO(CH_2)_2NEt_2$) (152)

$$\log \frac{1}{C} = 0 \cdot 579\pi - 1 \cdot 262\sigma + 0 \cdot 961$$

Enzymatic acetylation of aromatic amines ($XC_6H_4NH_2$) (162)

$$\log A_x = 0 \cdot 252\pi - 0 \cdot 335\sigma - 0 \cdot 155 \quad (n = 6, r = 0 \cdot 998)$$

Emulsin hydrolysis of phenyl glycosides ($XC_6H_4OC_6H_{11}O_5$) (162)

$$\log K_e = 0 \cdot 358\pi + 0 \cdot 664\sigma + 1 \cdot 763 \quad (n = 13, r = 0 \cdot 917)$$

Binding of anilines to nylon (163)

$$\log K = 0 \cdot 607 \log P + 0 \cdot 174 \, \mathrm{pK}_a - 7 \cdot 033 \quad (n = 17, r = 0 \cdot 970)$$

Uncoupling of oxidative phosphorylation by phenols (164)

$$\log \frac{1}{C} = -0 \cdot 491 \, \mathrm{pK}_a + 0 \cdot 620\pi + 6 \cdot 792 \quad (n = 14, r = 0 \cdot 936)$$

Hydrolysis of p-nitrophenyl esters by human serum (162)

$$\log k = -7 \cdot 614\sigma + 0 \cdot 389\pi + 3 \cdot 808E_s + 1 \cdot 552 \quad (n = 6, r = 0 \cdot 991)$$

These relationships indicate, in marked contrast to those apparently solely dependent upon P, that the partitioning of the ligands between the aqueous and macromolecular phases is a "more structured" process involving P and electronic and steric contributions additional to those automatically included in the P term. Clearly, with the increasing importance of σ and E_s terms the specificity of the interaction process will become greater simply because the geometrical requirements for molecular interactions, other than hydrophobic interactions, are quite precise (see section on p. 2).

FUNCTIONAL ROLE OF THE NONPOLAR ENVIRONMENT AND HYDROPHOBIC INTERACTIONS

Emphasis has been placed so far on the nonpolar environment and hydrophobic interactions primarily with regard to their role as structural determinants in tertiary and quaternary structure and the provision of an appropriate binding locus for nonpolar ligands. In addition to these important roles, however, the nonpolar environment can produce rather substantial modification of the reactivities and properties of polar groups: such modifications can exert a critical role in the determination of macromolecular reactivity.

It is, of course, well known that the pK values of ionizable groups in proteins often show marked deviations from the values anticipated from studies on simple model compounds. These differences may have a variety of origins which have been discussed in detail by several workers (165–168): for the present it suffices to say that statistical and electrostatic (local and general) effects, hydrogen bonding and effects caused by a modified dielectric constant in nonpolar regions all contribute to produce modification of pK values. Phenolic groups are commonly found to have abnormally high pK values; this is not surprising since the tyrosyl residue with its hydrophobic potential would be anticipated to be readily buried in the interior of proteins. Ribonuclease, chymotrypsinogen, carbonic anhydrase, ovalbumin, and serum albumin all contain tyrosyl residues that may be considered to be buried to a greater or lesser extent. Abnormal carboxyl groups are to be found in a variety of proteins: unusually stabilized uncharged groups are found in β-lactoglobulin, pepsin, lysozyme and tobacco mosaic virus protein, etc. while unusually stabilized charged forms are to be found in lysozyme, ovalbumin, tobacco mosaic virus protein, trypsin, etc. Abnormal imidazoles are found in the heme proteins, carbonic anhydrase, etc. (For further details of these findings references 163–173 should be consulted.)

It is quite clear that the incorporation of polar groups into nonpolar areas is generally a thermodynamically unfavorable process (174) unless accompanied by an appropriately located pairing species of opposite

charge, the formation of a hydrogen bond or the production of sufficiently
compensating hydrophobic interactions (168, 175). The effects of nonpolar environment on polar functions will be generally to increase pK
values and depress ionization; this is an obvious consequence of the
unfavorable energetics of "burying" an isolated polar group. In those
cases where interactions between polar groups are possible, such interactions will be strengthened in a nonpolar environment: the exclusion
of water and the provision of an encompassing hydrophobic area will
serve to strengthen hydrogen bond, ion–ion and polar interactions quite
generally (165–168, 175). In fact, ion–ion interactions are likely to
stabilize protein structure *only* when incorporated into a nonpolar area

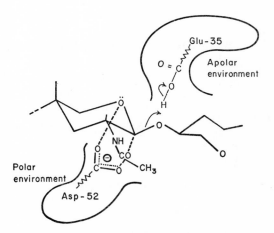

FIG. I-31. Partial mechanism of lysozyme cleavage of *N*-acetylglucosamine
hexamer.

where competition by the solvating aqueous medium is absent (176).
Additionally, it is clear that the special properties conferred upon
ionizable groups by their nonpolar environment are directly related to
the catalytic functions of some enzyme systems. Thus the mechanism
of the lysozyme catalysed hydrolysis of bacterial wall polysaccharide is
believed to involve the actions of the carboxyl groups of aspartic acid
(residue 52) and glutamic acid (residue 35). The latter residue is situated
in a relatively nonpolar environment and is anticipated to have an
abnormally high pK_a: in contrast, the aspartic acid is in a polar environment and dissociated. The glutamic residue is believed to act as a general
acid catalyst transferring hydrogen ion to a glycosidic linkage with
cleavage of the bond to C_1 to create a carbonium ion which is stabilized,
in part, by an electrostatic interaction with the ionized carboxyl group

of the aspartate (177, 178; Fig. I-31). Similarly, recent X-ray studies at 2·0 Å resolution of chymotrypsin (179) have suggested that the nonpolar residues surrounding aspartate-102 play a critical role in the catalytic events (Fig. I-32), the hydrophobic environment of the hydrogen bond between aspartate-102 and the resonating histidine-57 serving to channel electrons from the carboxylate anion to the hydroxyl of serine-195, thus converting it to a powerful nucleophile. At least two other proteases, subtilisin BPN[1] (180) and pig pancreatic elastase (181) also share this pattern of coupling a hydrophobically shielded aspartate carboxyl to histidine and serine. A similar array of hydrophobic and

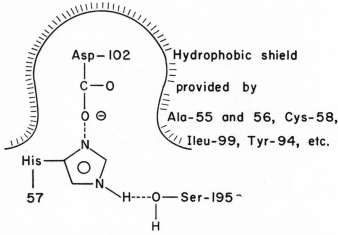

Fig. I-32. Amino acids in the active site of α-chymotrypsin showing those involved in catalysis (Asp-102, His-57 and Ser-195) and those serving as a hydrophobic shield (Ala-55, Cys-58 and Ileu-99 etc.).

polar interactions is to be found in carboxypeptidase (182), where substrate is bound between a hydrophobic tyrosine residue and a charged zinc atom; similar hydrophobic environments are found with other metalloproteins including carbonic anhydrase (183), hemoglobin (185) etc.

Such combinations of polar and nonpolar environments seem likely to provide, in a fairly general sense, considerable driving force for both ligand binding and reaction in catalytic proteins (184). Vallee and Williams (185) have discussed, in a similar context, the role of such microenvironmental effects in determining the properties of metals in metalloenzymes. It seems fairly well established that the active sites (or their immediately adjacent regions) of most functional proteins so far studied contain at least one hydrophobic region. The function of this latter region will be several fold, to produce an anhydrous or partially anhydrous environment for polar groups that will alter considerably their functional and binding† properties, to provide a binding area for the ligands and perhaps through this hydrophobic binding to promote "dehydration" of the polar functional groups involved in catalytic function and also to initiate conformational changes at the active site. Such processes seem likely to be quite general for most ligand–protein interactions.

Some further aspects of the interplay of nonpolar and polar interactions can be illustrated by a further brief reference to chymotrypsin, a system whose reactions with a large number of ligands has been widely and thoroughly studied (186–192). Chymotrypsin catalyses the hydrolysis of esters and amides of the general formula, I-1, and is well recognized

$$\text{RCONHCHR}_1\text{COR}_2$$

I-1

to show a marked preference for substrates and inhibitors possessing appropriately located nonpolar groups (R_1). The work of Niemann and his colleagues (188–190) has done much to indicate the role of nonpolar binding in determining ligand affinity and the stereoselectivity (L) of the enzyme. In a general consideration of the role of such nonpolar interactions Knowles (193–195) has compared the free energy of transfer of amino acids from water to various solvents as a function of K_o, the steady state binding constant. For the chymotrypsin catalysed reactions,

$$E + S \underset{k_{-1}}{\overset{k_1}{\rightleftharpoons}} E - S \xrightarrow{k_2} E\text{-acyl} \xrightarrow{k_3} E + \text{acyl-OH} \quad \text{(XXXIV)}$$

$$K_o = k_3(k_{-1} + k_2)/k_1(k_2 + k_3) \quad \text{(XXXV)}$$

and

$$k_o = k_2 k_3/(k_2 + k_3) \quad \text{(XXXVI)}$$

(When $k_3 \gg k_2$ and $k_{-1} \gg k_2$, K_o does, in fact, equal k_{-1}/k_1.)

For esters it appears true that in general $k_3 \gg k_2$, but the reverse may be true for amides (194, 196). With these limitations upon the significance of the experimentally determined kinetic constants in mind, the slopes of the lines in Fig. I-33, correlate the free energy of partition between water and the solvent or enzyme and indicate the competition between the enzyme active site and the solvent. The slopes are a measure of the selectivity (ability to distinguish between amino acids) of the solvents and the enzyme. A slope of unity indicates that a particular

† This may be very important in, for example, the binding of quaternary ammonium ions at the anionic sites of acetylcholinesterase and the cholinergic receptor (Chapter IV, p. 276), where a hydrophobic environment around the anionic site will strengthen the ion–ion interaction and may simultaneously cause further "dehydration" on binding leading to a conformational change in the enzyme protein.

solvent and the enzyme have equal selectivity (approximate in view of the assumptions inherent in the kinetic constants). A slope of less than unity indicates that the enzyme is more selective (less water-like).

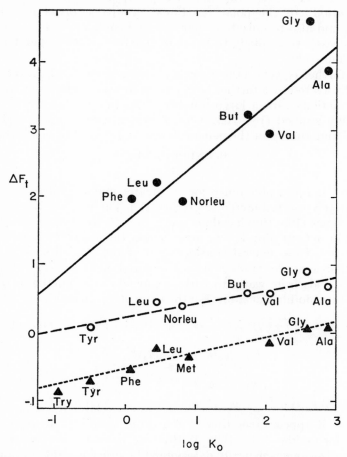

FIG. I-33. Free energies of transfer (ΔF_t) of amino acids from water to ethanol ($\bullet$), to 40% aqueous ethanol ($\circ$) and to 8 M urea ($\blacktriangle$) at 25° versus $\log K_o$ (mM) values for reactions of N-acetyl-L-amino acid methyl esters with chymotrypsin. Reproduced with permission from Knowles (193).

Clearly, the active site of chymotrypsin is relatively nonpolar. Chymotrypsin normally hydrolyses only the L-isomers, the D-isomers being inhibitors: a plot of $\log K_i$ (D-isomers) against $\log K_0$ (L-isomers) for a series of amides of N-acyl aromatic amino acids shows (Fig. I-34) the closeness of the K_i and K_o values although the slope is actually not quite

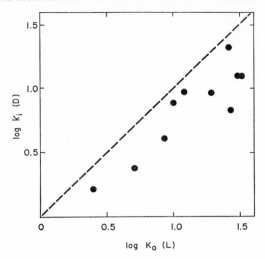

Fig. I-34. Log K_i (mM) values for D-amides of N-acyl aromatic amino acids versus log K_o (mM) values for L-substrates with chymotrypsin. Reproduced with permission from Knowles (193).

unity and indicates that the binding mechanisms of both substrates and inhibitors are very similar and that both are probably determined primarily by the nonpolar interactions. These and several other lines of

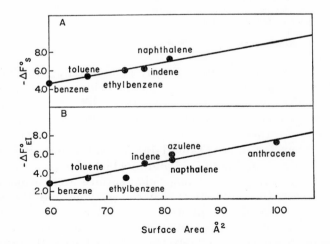

Fig. I-35. Free energy (kcals/mole^{-1}) of solution (ΔF_s°) and free energy of inhibition (ΔF_{EI}°) against molecular surface area for hydrocarbon inhibitors with chymotrypsin. Reproduced with permission from Hymes, Robinson and Canady (197).

evidence cited by Knowles leave little doubt that the binding of substrates and inhibitors to chymotrypsin is conceptually equivalent to a partitioning between polar aqueous and nonpolar enzyme phases.

Canady and his co-workers have expressed essentially the same view (197–199): these workers have demonstrated correlations between the free energy of solution (from solubility or partition (water/hydrocarbon) studies) of substrates or inhibitors and the free energy of complex formation with chymotrypsin as a function of molecular area. For hydrocarbons (benzene, toluene, etc.) a plot of ΔF_s° against molecular surface area gives a slope identical to that of ΔF_{EI}° against molecular

TABLE I-18. Correlations between Free Energies of Complex Formation and Free Energies of Partition for Series of Substrates and Inhibitors of Chymotrypsin (198)

No.	Compound series	Slope of ΔF_{Parv}° versus surface area	Slope of $\Delta F_{EI(or\ ES)}^\circ$ versus surface area
1	Hippuric acid esters	0·12*	0·02
2	Hydrocinnamic acid esters	0·12†	0·02
3	Aromatic nitro compounds	0·07‡	0·07
4	Aromatic ketones	0·12§	0·03
5	Aromatic carboxylic acids	—‖	0·12
6	Aromatic hydrocarbons	0·117¶	0·113

* Partition between xylene/water.
† Partition between pentane/water.
‡ Partition between hexane/water.
§ Partition between heptane/water.
‖ Partition data unavailable.
¶ Solubility measurements.

surface area (Fig. I-35). Quite generally plots of ΔF_{Part}° (for carboxylic acids, esters of hippuric and hydrocinnamic acids and ketones) against molecular surface area gave slopes of $\approx 0·12$ while a series of aromatic nitro compounds yielded a slope of 0·07. As inhibitors and substrates of chymotrypsin, these same series of compounds also yielded linear plots, but of varying slopes (Table I-18). From this data it is apparent that those series of inhibitors (3, 5 and 6) which give identical slopes of ΔF_{Part}° and $\Delta F_{EI(or\ ES)}^\circ$ against molecular surface area suggest a close parallel between the environment of the enzyme and the nonpolar solvent for the ligands in question. For other series, a substantial discrepancy exists between the two slopes; this may indicate a less than perfect extraction of the ligand into the enzyme. Part of the discrepancy may arise in series 1 and 2 from the ambiguity of kinetic methods in determining true affinity constants, but the fact that the aromatic ketone series yield a "normal" ΔF_{Part}°—surface area plot suggests that the gross molecular arrangement (hydrocarbon–polar–hydrocarbon) common to all three series prevents the total extraction process by the enzyme. Canady prefers to interpret these findings according to the extraction model in which the free energy change for transfer from aqueous solution to the enzyme is given by

$$\Delta F_{Part} = \frac{4\pi r^2 R}{k} (\lambda_1 - \lambda_2) \qquad (XXXVII)$$

where $4\pi r^2$ is the molecular area, λ_1 is the interfacial tension between the solute molecule and the enzyme (or nonpolar solvent) and λ_2 the interfacial tension between the solute and aqueous phase. However, hydrophobic interactions will be anticipated to be roughly proportional to molecular surface area and the data of Canady are probably to be regarded as consistent with the general theory of hydrophobic interactions previously discussed and in any case, generate substantial evidence for the generally nonpolar character of the chymotrypsin active site. As previously noted, there is an ever increasing array of evidence to substantiate the involvement of similar interactions in a large number of ligand–macromolecular systems.

It is also becoming apparent that such hydrophobic contributions to binding affinity may also be reflected in catalytic steps beyond the stage of complex formation. Thus, Hofstee has documented (200) for several esterase systems, a steady increase in V_{max} with increasing hydrophobic character of the acyl group of the ester. For chymotrypsin, Knowles (193) has pointed out an inverse relationship between K_o and k_o in the hydrolysis of L-N-acetylamino acid esters whereby k_o increases as K_o decreases. Despite the ambiguities inherent in the interpretation of K_o and k_o this finding supports the validity of the hypothesis, "better binding—better reaction"† and suggests that the same nonpolar interactions are involved in both formation of the ES complex *and* its rate determining breakdown (whether this is acylation or deacylation). From the previous comments on the active site of chymotrypsin it seems probable that the hydrophobic binding serves to insert the ester group into a relatively anhydrous nonpolar active site to facilitate formation of the acyl-enzyme intermediate and subsequently to promote deacylation. That this latter process also has its own stereospecificity has been shown by Ingles and Knowles (194) who have compared the deacylation rates of several D- and L-acyl chymotrypsins and find that with increasing size of the acyl group the L series deacylate faster and the D series deacylate slower.

† Of course, this hypothesis must not be overstated: steric and other specific interactions also contribute to the determination of ligand affinity and will upset such a simple correlation.

A similar inverse relationship between a binding constant and a catalytic constant has been noted for at least one nonenzymatic process, namely, the hydrolysis of p-nitrophenol acyl esters in the presence of mixed micelles of N^α-myristoyl-L-histidine and cetyltrimethylammonium bromide (201). A plot of the kinetic second order rate constant against the reciprocal of the apparent ester binding constant as a function of acyl chain length is presented in Fig. I-36 and shows the

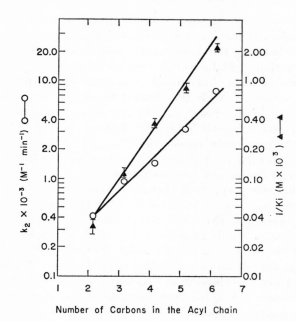

Number of Carbons in the Acyl Chain

FIG. I-36. Second order rate constants ($\log k_2$) and reciprocal of the dissociation constant ($1/K_i$) for micellar p-nitrophenylester hydrolysis as a function of the number of carbon atoms in the acyl group. Reproduced with permission from Gitler and Ochoa-Solano (201).

linear relationships between these properties. From this it may be estimated that the free energy change for the transfer of an acyl methylene group from the aqueous to the micellar phase is -630 cal mole^{-1} and the contribution per methylene group to the rate constant is -442 cal mole^{-1}. Both of these values are within the range for hydrophobic binding of a methylene group and suggest an approximately equal contribution of such interactions to both ester binding and reaction. Quite probably increased micellar binding with increasing acyl chain length serves to more effectively orient the esters in the vicinity of both the histidine and cetyltrimethylammonium bromide with the positive charge of the latter serving to stabilize the transition state of formation of the intermediate acyl-N^α-myristoyl histidine.

An extremely interesting example of the importance of hydrophobic interactions in controlling active site functionality is provided by the studies of Coletti-Previero et al. with trypsin (202). Addition of organic solvents (dioxane, 2-chloroethanol) to trypsin solutions results in complete loss of the proteolytic activity while the esterolytic activity of the enzyme remained essentially unchanged. Similarly, non-specific formylation of the enzyme also results in loss of proteolytic activity. Since both esterolytic and proteolytic activities of trypsin are presumed to be mediated through the same active site and since both formylation and addition of organic solvents will reduce hydrophobic interactions in

TABLE I-19. Free Energy Changes for Enzyme-inhibitor Complex Formation with Chymotrypsin and Modified Chymotrypsin (203)

Inhibitor	Enzyme	K	$-\Delta F^\circ$ kcal mole^{-1}
Benzene	Mod.	59	2·42
	Cont.	96	2·71
Toluene	Mod.	183	3·09
	Cont.	450	3·63
Naphthalene	Mod.	5500	5·11
	Cont.	10,500	5·50
Methylhippurate	Mod.	154	2·99
(substrate)	Cont.	328	3·44

the protein it is apparent that the two activities of the enzyme are selectively modulated by hydrophobic interactions within the native structure. A rather similar situation has been outlined for chymotrypsin by Royer and Canady (195) who found that alkylation of the protein with p-nitrophenylbromoacetyl-α-aminoisobutyrate at methionine-192 decreases the apparent affinity of the enzyme for substrate (methyl hippurate). A parallel decrease in affinity of this modified enzyme for hydrocarbon inhibitors is also observed (Table I-19) and it is suggested that a reduction in protein apolar character (together with any conformational change) caused by introduction of $-CH_2CONHC(Me)_2COO^-$ at methionine-192 may provide the basis for this loss in affinity.

Even from the brief and incomplete discussion of the role of nonpolar interactions in determining and modulating polar group functionalities and from the previous discussion of such interactions in determining protein structure, it is clear that the subtle interplay between water and nonpolar and polar functionalities provides a key to the interactions of small ligands with macromolecules. In Chapter II we shall be concerned with the role of these interactions in determining the organization and function of a supramolecular structure—the cell membrane.

From the emphasis of the preceding sections of this Chapter, it is quite clear that the fundamental control of macromolecular organization and function is exerted through the associated water structure. Perturbations of this water structure imply conformational changes and hence alterations in function of the macromolecular system. It is, therefore, to these aspects of macromolecular systems that we look for an explanation of regulation processes in biological macromolecules. Current knowledge of water structure, particularly that involved with protein and other macromolecular systems is inadequate at the present time to justify further discussion beyond that already presented. However, the role of conformational change in the control of macromolecular structure and function is fully realized even if not fully understood.

CONFORMATIONAL CHANGE AND REGULATORY PROCESSES IN PROTEINS

SUBSTRATE INDUCED CONFORMATIONAL CHANGE

In the simplest sense the specificity of interaction of small molecules with macromolecular systems may be rationalized by the assumption that the binding surface structure is complementary to that of the ligand structure and thus permits the close fit of the two systems (Fig. I-37).

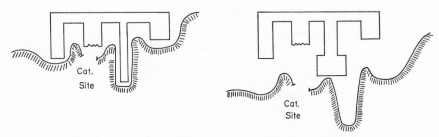

FIG. I-37. Representation of lock and key mechanism of enzyme–substrate interaction: favorable fit (left) and unfavorable fit (right).

Deviation from the optimum structure will lead to decreased binding because the same fit cannot occur (Fig. I-37). This assumption has provided the basis of the "template" or "lock and key" mechanism of enzyme action advanced by Emil Fischer (204) and which formed for many years a general basis for the discussion of the specificity of small molecule–macromolecular interactions. The existence of certain facts that did not readily accord with the above assumption led Koshland to introduce (205–208) the "induced-fit" hypothesis of enzyme action. The basic features of this hypothesis are that, (a) small molecules induce conformational changes on binding to the enzyme, (b) a precise orientation of catalytic groups is needed to cause reaction and (c) substrates induce the proper alignment of catalytic residues whereas nonsubstrates do not. This hypothesis has had far-reaching consequences in the interpretation of ligand binding and the literature on substrate-induced conformational changes is now very extensive and has been reviewed by Koshland and Neet (209). Evidence is available for such conformational changes occurring with phosphoglucomutase (210), creatine kinase (211), aldolase (212–214), luciferase (215) to cite but a few enzymes. Hammes (216–218), using relaxation spectrometry to study enzyme–substrate complex formation, has found quite generally that the formation of the complex appears as a two-step process, an initial very rapid diffusion controlled step followed by a second much slower state; the latter presumably representing a mutual reorientation of protein and substrate. Very powerful evidence for such conformational changes is of course provided by a number of X-ray studies: notably, very large conformational changes have been observed in the binding of poor substrates to carboxypeptidase (182, 219) involving residue movements as large as 15 Å. Nevertheless, it cannot be envisaged that large conformational changes are a general occurrence and indeed there is reason to believe as much more probable that very small conformational changes are more general (135).

The preceding discussion has outlined in a very general sense suggestions that substrate-induced conformational changes are important in the regulation of enzyme activity. It is important to delineate further those structural features of molecules that are important in this regulatory process: clearly, the control of active site conformation may be a function of the entire substrate molecule, of only certain molecular features of the substrate molecule or, as a logical extension of the latter, of molecules that are themselves not directly involved in the enzymatic reaction. The importance of the latter class of agents to enzymology and molecular biology is now well recognized.

Several lines of evidence are now available to suggest that substrates of some enzyme systems may be considered to contain both catalytic and regulatory functions, the latter serving to initiate perturbations in the catalytic site that lead to enhanced activity. Important work by Inagami (220) has been concerned with this aspect of trypsin catalysis. Trypsin exhibits considerable specificity towards the hydrolysis of peptides derived from L-lysine and L-arginine (Fig. I-38). The existence

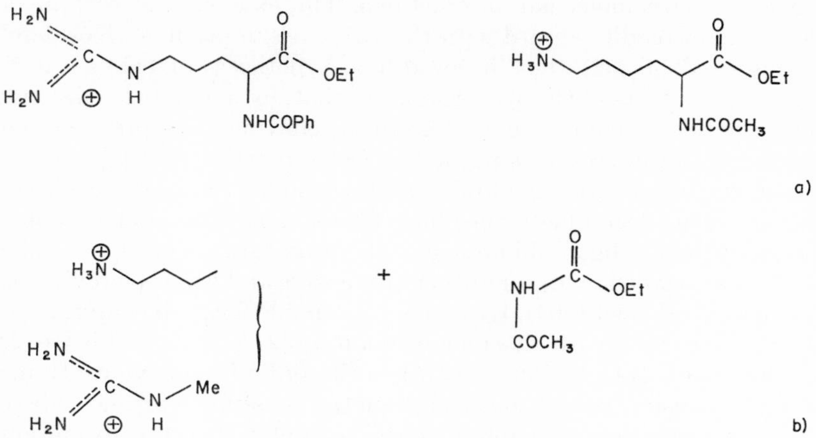

a)

b)

FIG. I-38. Lysyl and arginyl substrates (a) of trypsin and the structural analogy
to neutral substrate and exogenous ammonium salts (b).

of a positive charge located at the correct distance from the susceptible
amide bond apparently plays a determinant role in this specificity
(Fig. I-38a). Alkylammonium and alkylguanidinium ions have been
found to be competitive inhibitors of the trypsin catalysed hydrolysis
of benzoyl-L-arginine ethyl ester presumably because they compete
with the arginine side chain for its (regulatory) binding site on the
enzyme. Some inhibition parameters are presented in Table I-20.

TABLE I-20. Inhibition Constants of Alkylguanidines and Alkylamines in the
Trypsin-Catalysed Hydrolysis of Benzoyl-L-Arginine Ethyl Ester (220)

Inhibitor	K_i mM	ΔH° kcal mole^{-1}	ΔF° kcal mole^{-1}
RNH$_2$[†]			
R = Me	260	−13	−0·69
Et	62	−11	−1·6
Pr^n	8·7	−10	−2·8
Bu^n	1·7	−11	−3·8
RNHC(:NH)NH$_2$[‡]			
R = Me	11	−4·4	−2·7
Et	2·0	−4·8	−3·7
Pr^n	0·69	−4·5	−4·3
Bu^n	1·7	−4·5	−3·8

† Obtained at pH 6·6, 25° and at ionic strength 0·1.
‡ Obtained at pH 6·6, 25° and at ionic strength 0·2.

Trypsin will also catalyse, but with notably lower efficiency, the hydrolysis of neutral substrates such as acetylglycine ethyl ester (220). With this substrate alkylammonium and alkylguanidinium ions are found to accelerate the hydrolysis (Table I-21); methyl, ethyl and propylammonium and methylguanidinium ions promote hydrolysis and higher alkylammonium or guanidinium ions inhibit hydrolysis. The effects of the activating species are on k_{cat} rather than K_m, that is they increase the catalytic efficiency, rather than the affinity, of the enzyme for the neutral substrate. An obvious role for the added cationic species is to

TABLE I-21. The Effects of Alkylguanidines and Alkylamines on the Catalytic Properties of Trypsin (220)

Modifier	Conc. M	Max. rate increase	K_m† M	K_a‡ $\times 10^2$ M	K_i§ $\times 10^2$ M
RNH_3^+					
R = Me	0·85	3·2	—	38	34
Et	0·34	9·5	0·80	69	6·2
Pr^n	0·024	2·4	0·84	0·86	0·87
Bu^n	inhibitory only		—	—	—
—			0·72		
$RNH{=}C(NH_2)_2^+$					
R = Me	0·10	6·3	—	1·3	1·1
Et	0·025	2·0	—	0·2	0·2
Bu^n	inhibitory only		—	—	—

† K_m for binding of acetylglycine ethyl ester.

‡ Dissociation constant determined from the effect of alkylammonium species on hydrolysis of acetylglycine ethyl ester.

§ Dissociation constant determined from effects of alkylammonium species on hydrolysis of benzoyl-L-arginine ethyl ester.

provide interaction at an anionic site which is absent in neutral substrates such as acetylglycine ethyl ester (Fig. I-38b). Since the dissociation constants of the cationic species are the same whether acetylglycine ethyl ester or benzoyl-L-arginine ethyl ester is employed as the substrate (Table I-22, compare K_a and K_i values) it may be concluded that the ammonium or guanidinium ions occupy the same binding site whether producing inhibition or activation of hydrolysis. The mechanism by which interaction of the ammonium or guanidinium ion increases catalytic efficiency is not entirely clear: it is very important, however, that this increase is not a temperature dependent process. Thus, the increase in k_{cat} is not due to a change in the heat of activation but rather is due to an increased entropy of activation. Methylguanidine increases the rate of inactivation of trypsin by iodoacetamide (220) by the same factor as it increases the rate of hydrolysis of acetylglycine ethyl ester. In the reaction with iodoacetamide the increased reactivity is associated with an increase in reactivity of N-3 of imidazole of an active site histidine residue. A logical explanation of the accelerative effect of the lysine or arginine side chains of the cationic substrates (or of the presumably equivalent combination of neutral substrate plus guanidinium or ammonium salt) on trypsin catalysed substrate hydrolysis is that of producing the correct orientation of an active site histidine. A second and extremely relevant (in the context of the present volume) example

TABLE I-22. Acceleration of Inactivation Rates of Acetylcholinesterase by Ammonium Ions (231, 232)

Agent	Ion	Acceleration factor	K_A† M	K_I‡ M
MeSO$_2$F	Me$_2$NH$_2^+$	9·5	$3·2 \times 10^{-2}$	$2·6 \times 10^{-2}$
MeSO$_2$F	Me$_3$NH$^+$	7·5	$4·2 \times 10^{-3}$	$4·8 \times 10^{-3}$
MeSO$_2$F	Me$_4$N$^+$	6·0	7×10^{-4}	$1·2 \times 10^{-3}$
MeSO$_2$F	Et$_4$N$^+$	33·0	5×10^{-4}	$2·5 \times 10^{-4}$
Me$_2$NCOF	Me$_4$N$^+$	1·0	—	$1·2 \times 10^{-3}$
Me$_2$NCOF	Et$_4$N$^+$	14·0	3×10^{-4}	$2·5 \times 10^{-4}$
Me$_2$NCOF	Pr$_4$N$^+$	3·5	5×10^{-5}	$5·0 \times 10^{-5}$

† Dissociation constant for ion for inactivation reaction.
‡ Dissociation constant for ion for inhibition of acetylcholine hydrolysis.

of a substrate molecule that may possess an internal regulatory function is provided by acetylcholine and related substrates of acetylcholinesterase. Numerous studies of this enzyme system have established a general picture of the active site as consisting of an anionic area to which positively charged groups are bound and, some 5 Å distant, an esteratic site that catalyses the hydrolysis of the ester linkage in both cationic and neutral substrates (221–223). The general scheme of ester hydrolysis is described by equation

$$E + S \underset{k_{-1}}{\overset{k_1}{\rightleftharpoons}} ES \overset{k_2}{\longrightarrow} EA \overset{k_3}{\longrightarrow} E + A \qquad \text{(XXXVIII)}$$

With rapidly hydrolysed substrates (acetylcholine, acetylthiocholine and phenyl acetate) the rate determining step is deacetylation ($k_2 > k_3$) but with other substrates acetylation of the enzyme may be rate determining ($k_2 < k_3$, (224)). Several lines of evidence now exist to indicate that interaction of the ammonium functions at the anionic site can regulate the activity of the esteratic site. A large number of irreversible inhibitors of acetylcholinesterase are known: these include the phosphorylating agents (diisopropylfluorophosphonate, dimethylfluorophosphorylcholine, etc.), sulfonylating agents (methanesulfonyl fluoride) and carbamylating agents (dimethylcarbamyl fluoride). Several comprehensive reviews of these agents are available (222, 225–227). They differ from substrates of acetylcholinesterase in that they form a covalent bond to a serine residue of the enzyme active site that is only poorly susceptible to hydrolysis. As anticipated ammonium ions act as inhibitors to the reactions of both substrates and irreversible inhibitors of acetylcholinesterase (222, 228–230), presumably because their occupation of the anionic site offers steric hindrance to the binding of both cationic substrates and inhibitors and also to neutral substrates of sufficient bulk. However, accelerative effects of certain ammonium ions towards the irreversible inhibition of acetylcholinesterase by methanesulfonyl fluoride and dimethylcarbamyl fluoride, irreversible inhibitors of relatively small bulk, have been noted (227, 231–233) and kinetic data for these effects are presented in Table I-22. The site sulfonylated or carbamylated, in the presence or absence of the accelerating species, appears to be identical by a number of criteria. The agreement between the K_I and K_A values, which are the dissociation constants of the ammonium ions for the inhibition of acetylcholine hydrolysis and for the acceleration of mesylation (or carbamylation) respectively, is indicative of the probable identity of the cationic binding site in the two processes.

Further evidence for the role of the quaternary ammonium function in regulating activity of the esteratic site comes from a study of the irreversible actions of a number of quaternary ammonium diethylphosphoryl esters (234) in which the quaternary ammonium entity functions as the leaving group. For non-cationic diethylphosphoryl esters a correlation exists between k_2, the second order rate constant for inactivation and the pK_a of the leaving group—an increase in pK_a producing a decrease in k_2. Comparison with the data for quaternary ammonium derivatives reveals that many of the latter exhibit anomalously high k_2 values (Table I-23) and presumably the quaternary ammonium function in these compounds serves to increase the reactivity of the esteratic site.

Direct accelerative effects of quaternary ions on substrate hydrolysis have also been noted (235): a threefold enhancement of the hydrolysis of acetyl fluoride is provided by the tetramethylammonium and tetraethylammonium ions. The availability of highly purified preparations of acetylcholinesterase has made possible spectroscopic studies of the interaction with inhibitors and substrates (236). The ORD curve for acetylcholinesterase is shown in Fig. I-39 and, from the Moffitt equation,

TABLE I-23. Second Order Rate Constants for Inactivation of Acetylcholinesterase by Diethylphosphoryl Esters Containing Quaternary Ammonium Groups (234)

Compounds R = $(EtO)_2P(O)$	k_2 liter mole^{-1} min^{-1}	Enhancement factor[†] (x-fold increase)
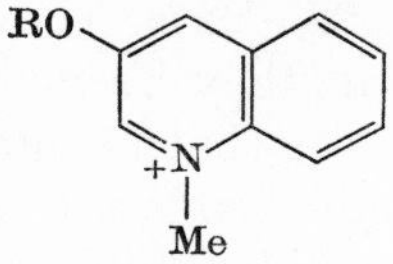 3-RO-quinolinium, N-Me (RO on quinoline, +N–Me)	$1 \cdot 2 \times 10^8$	240
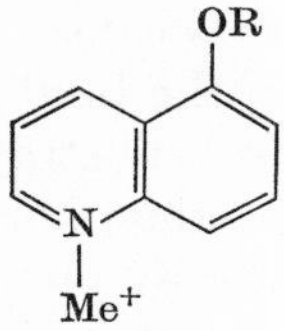 5-OR-quinoline, N-Me$^+$	$2 \cdot 4 \times 10^6$	24
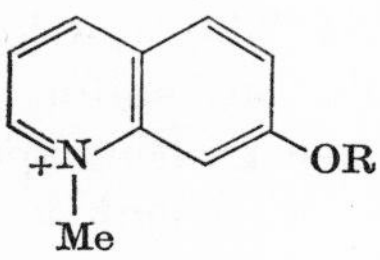 7-OR-quinolinium, +N–Me	$1 \cdot 2 \times 10^8$	400
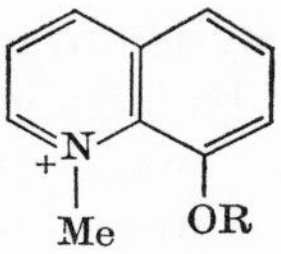 8-OR-quinolinium, +N–Me	$9 \cdot 3 \times 10^6$	230
$RSCH_2CH_2\overset{+}{N}Me_3$	$1 \cdot 6 \times 10^6$	270
$RSCH_2CH_2CH_2\overset{+}{N}Me_3$	$5 \cdot 5 \times 10^4$	220
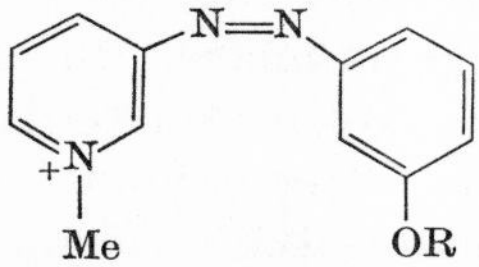 pyridinium (N-Me) –N=N– phenyl-OR	$2 \cdot 8 \times 10^6$	60

[†] Enhancement factor determined from the monotonic relationship between k_2 and pK_a for non-cationic inhibitors. It represents the increase in reactivity over that anticipated from this relationship.

the helical parameter, b_o, is approximately -600 suggesting a greater than 90% content of right handed helix. Despite the fact that changes in ORD parameters are difficult to correlate quantitatively with changes in peptide conformation it is apparent from Fig. I-40 that heat denaturation and 3-hydroxyphenyldimethylethylammonium chloride, tensilon,

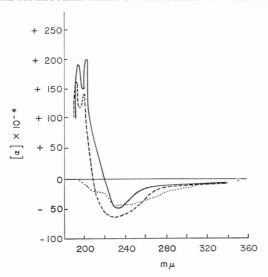

FIG. I-39. Optical rotatory dispersion of acetylcholinesterase (0·1 mg protein/ml at pH 7·0). Active enzyme (———) heat-inactivated enzyme (————), enzyme inactivated by 0·1 N KOH (······). Reproduced with permission from Kitz and Kremzner (236).

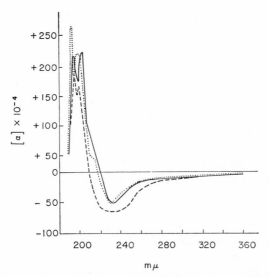

FIG. I-40. Optical rotatory dispersion of acetylcholinesterase in the presence of substrate $(CH_3CO_2(CH_2)_3N^+Me_3$, ———), inhibited by tensilon (————) and inhibited by tetraethylpyrophosphate (······). Reproduced with permission from Kitz and Kremzner (236).

a potent reversible inhibitor, $(K_i = 10^{-7}$ M) produce rather similar changes in the ORD spectrum probably suggestive of a decrease in helical content. 3-Acetyoxypropyltrimethylammonium chloride, a substrate, produced, however, only minor increases in the twin peaks of positive rotation.

Thus several lines of evidence indicate an important role for quaternary ammonium functions in the regulation of the activity of acetylcholinesterase. The extremely rapid hydrolysis of acetylcholine may thus be determined, at least in part, by a "built-in" accelerative influence of

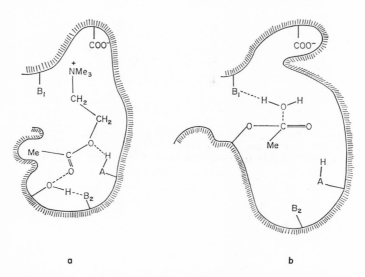

a   b

FIG. I-41. Representation of conformational change in acetylcholinesterase upon formation of the acetylenzyme (b) from the initial complex (a) B_1 and B_2 are the basic groups of pK 6·3 and 5·5 respectively and AH the acidic group of pK 9.2. Reproduced with permission from Krupka (230).

the quaternary trimethylammonium function. It is important to attempt to relate this phenomenon to the mechanism of action of acetylcholinesterase.

The detailed kinetic investigations by Krupka (224, 230, 237) and others have led to the conclusion that the active site of acetylcholinesterase contains an anionic site ($pK_a \approx 4·5$) probably the α-carboxyl of glutamic acid, two basic groups of pK_a 5·5 and 6·3, probably histidine residues, in addition to the acetylatable serine residue. The two basic residues are involved in different catalytic functions: the residue of pK_a 5·5 which, from inhibitor studies, is the more distant from the anionic site, is involved in the formation of the acetyl enzyme and the residue of pK_a 6·3, which is some 5 Å from the anionic site, is involved in deacetylation only. It is suggested that these basic residues operate sequentially through the intermediary involvement of a conformational change that serves to bring the acetylated serine residue close to the second basic residue so that deacetylation occurs. Such conformational change may well be related to the influence of the ammonium function. There exist a number of observations suggesting that the ester group in the enzyme–substrate complex is in an environment difference to that in the acetylated enzyme. Differential effects of pH on acetylation and deacetylation are observed consistent with the different pK_a's of the basic groups. Quaternary ammonium ions $(Me_4N^+$—$Bu^n_4N^+)$ block deacetylation or decarbamylation of the enzyme: however, as previously noted these ions also accelerate carbamylation and mesylation of the enzyme by irreversibly acting substrate analogs.

A possible mechanism for the influence of quaternary groups is that they maintain or produce an enzyme conformation in which interaction of the ester function and the first basic group can occur (Fig. I-41a). With formation of the acetylated enzyme and desorption of the ammonium function the conformation collapses to bring the acetyl serine into close proximity to the second basic group (Fig. I-41b). According to this mechanism quaternary ammonium groups may play the dual role of accelerating formation of the esterified enzyme and of inhibiting its subsequent hydrolysis.

ALLOSTERIC AND COOPERATIVE LIGAND BINDING

Many enzyme and protein systems shown additional complexities in ligand binding. In particular, it is often noted that the ligand saturation curve does not follow the hyperbolic relationship characteristic of Langmuir-type absorption but follows a sigmoid relationship (Fig. I-42). This sigmoid curve suggests that at least two molecules of ligand bind to the protein and that the binding of the first ligand molecule facilitates the binding of subsequent molecules. Such cooperative interactions are now known for many ligand binding processes, one of the longest known and most comprehensively investigated being the oxygen–hemoglobin system (238). A variety of lines of evidence show that the cooperativity of this process is dependent upon the polymeric structure of hemoglobin, cooperativity being absent in non-associating heme species such as myoglobin (Fig. I-43). Very early studies by Hill (239, 240) described the oxygen–hemoglobin saturation curve by the following equation:

$$y = \frac{Kp^n}{1 + Kp^n} \tag{XXXIX}$$

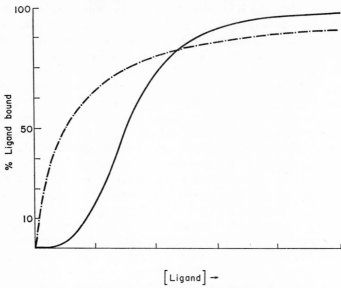

FIG. I-42. Comparison of sigmoid and hyperbolic binding curves.

where y is the fractional saturation of the hemoglobin with oxygen, p is the oxygen partial pressure and n is the number of molecules of oxygen bound per hemoglobin molecule. Since n must be an integer Hill argued that the experimentally obtained non-integral values indicate a mixture of molecules of varying degrees of polymerization. A plot of $\log p/(1 - p)$ against $\log p$, the so-called Hill plot, is found to provide a straight line, particularly for the 20–80% saturation area, with a slope

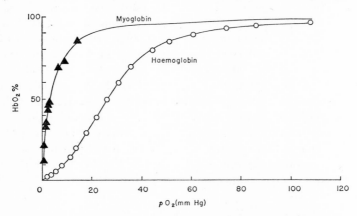

FIG. I-43. Oxygen dissociation curves of human hemoglobin and horse heart myoglobin. Reproduced with permission from Monod *et al.* (273).

of $n > 1$ (Fig. I-44). Despite the fact that the physical basis for Hill's explanation of the cooperative binding of oxygen to hemoglobin is known to be incorrect his equation still finds considerable application, particularly in the generalized form:

$$\log \frac{V}{V_{max} - V} = n \log [S] - \log K \qquad \text{(XL)}$$

where V is reaction velocity, V_{max} is maximum velocity, S is substrate concentration and K is a constant, for the plotting of kinetic data from

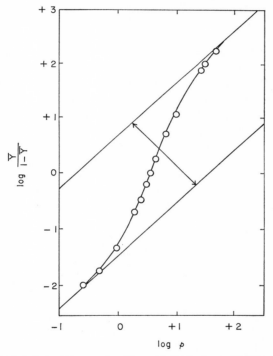

FIG. I-44. Hill plot for oxygen saturation of sheep hemoglobin: n at $\overline{Y} = 0.5$ is 3 ± 0.05. The apparent interaction energy obtained from the asymptotes according to the treatment by Wyman (260) is 3000 cal. Reproduced with permission from Wyman (260).

allosteric and regulatory enzymes. In the above form it is readily appreciated to be a form of the Michaelis–Menten equation (241). The value of n has sometimes been taken as a measure of the number of ligand binding sites: as we shall describe later, this is not generally valid although n is a parameter reflecting the number of interacting binding sites *and* the strength of their mutual interaction. However, when $n = 1$ it will be generally true that the ligand binding sites are all equivalent and that they exhibit no mutual interaction.

Despite many intensive investigations a model for ligand binding to hemoglobin completely acceptable to all workers has not yet been established. Nevertheless, the X-ray studies by Perutz and his co-workers (106, 242–246) have unambiguously delineated the role of reversible conformational changes occurring in the hemoglobin ↔ oxy-hemoglobin reaction. The mechanisms of these changes will be discussed in greater detail later; for the present it is sufficient to emphasize that such conformational changes in protein structure unquestionably provide the physical basis for the cooperative process and that the role of ligand-induced conformational change is probably one of general significance to all allosteric and regulatory phenomena.

The sigmoidal shape of the oxygen saturation curve for hemoglobin clearly confers certain important physiological characteristics. Prominent among these is that oxygen transfer between hemoglobin, oxyhemoglobin and tissues will be very sensitive to the partial pressure of oxygen: this can be readily seen from a comparison of the oxygen saturation curves of hemoglobin and myoglobin (Fig. I-43). Put more generally, it is clear that the cooperative process provides a mechanism for the amplification of low energy biological signals. As such we may expect cooperative and allied processes to play an important role in biological control processes, including neural control and information transfer mechanisms.

A further characteristic of many systems that exhibit the phenomenon of cooperative ligand binding is that the catalytic activity of the protein is susceptible to modification by agents that bear no necessary structural relationship to the substrate molecule. Obviously, this phenomenon is related to that discussed in the previous section where evidence was advanced that substrates for certain enzyme systems appear to perform the dual function of being susceptible to the catalytic function of the molecule and of providing simultaneously a built-in regulatory function. Clearly, similar regulatory function may be provided by ligands that act entirely independently of the substrate molecule: such effects are, as might be anticipated, more numerous and of greater significance. The importance of this type of regulation of enzyme activity was first realized in the phenomenon of feed back inhibition in which, in a multi-step enzyme pathway, the ultimate metabolic end product inhibits the first (or an early) step in that sequence uniquely concerned with the bio-synthesis of the end product. Many such examples of end-product inhibition are known (247–250) including L-threonine deaminase (sensitive to L-isoleucine), aspartate transcarbamylase (sensitive to cytidine triphosphate), homoserine dehydrogenase (sensitive to L-threonine) etc.

In their 1963 treatment of this phenomenon, Monod, Changeux and Jacob (251) introduced the term "allosteric" to describe a site on the enzyme, distinct from the active site at which the substrate binds, and which is complementary to the structure of the allosteric effector: one function of the allosteric effector is to modify the properties of the active site through a change (allosteric transition) in the kinetic parameters characterizing the biological activity of the protein. Since the introduction of this term its range of applicability has steadily increased to include also the phenomenon of cooperativity. Thus, *allosteric* now describes the effects of ligand binding at a non-catalytic site on catalytic efficiency *and* the effects of ligand binding at the active site upon the binding of additional molecules of the same ligand to other active sites. Because of this somewhat nonselective use of the term allosteric, it is

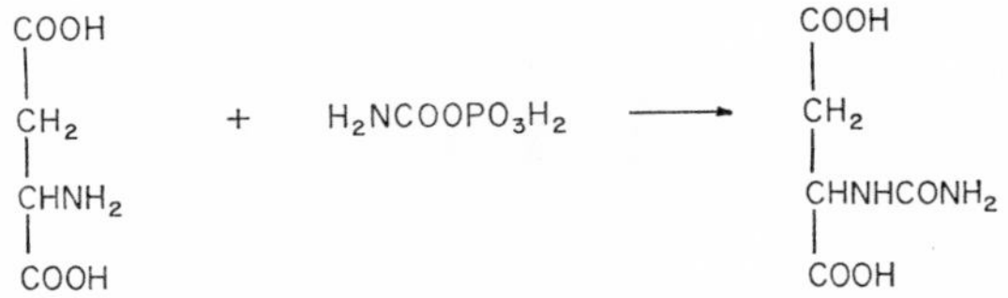

$$\begin{array}{c} \text{COOH} \\ | \\ \text{CH}_2 \\ | \\ \text{CHNH}_2 \\ | \\ \text{COOH} \end{array} \quad + \quad \text{H}_2\text{NCOOPO}_3\text{H}_2 \quad \longrightarrow \quad \begin{array}{c} \text{COOH} \\ | \\ \text{CH}_2 \\ | \\ \text{CHNHCONH}_2 \\ | \\ \text{COOH} \end{array}$$

FIG. I-45. The formation of carbamyl aspartate.

desirable to define and employ *regulatory site* as a site which binds effectors but which is topographically distinct and different in kind from the active site and which itself has no catalytic activity. As will become apparent, allosteric proteins need not possess regulatory sites and regulatory sites may function in proteins that do not exhibit allosteric (cooperative) behavior. Koshland and Neet (252) in their review of such terminology employ the term *autosteric* to define a site that is a portion of, or is immediately adjacent to, the active site and which has a regulatory function. Thus, those substrates previously described which appear to have a built-in regulatory function would be described as acting, in part, as autosteric effectors or as autosteric substrates.

The enzyme aspartate transcarbamylase which catalyses the formation of carbamylaspartate (Fig. I-45) plays an important role in the discussion of allosteric phenomena since it represents a very well investigated example of a system exhibiting both allosteric (cooperative) and regulatory behavior. Gerhart and Pardee (253) demonstrated the sigmoid character of the aspartate saturation curve (Fig. I-46). Cytidine triphosphate (CTP), an end product of the pyrimidine biosynthetic pathway, is a specific inhibitor of the enzyme, competitive with respect to aspartate, which decreases the affinity of aspartate for the enzyme

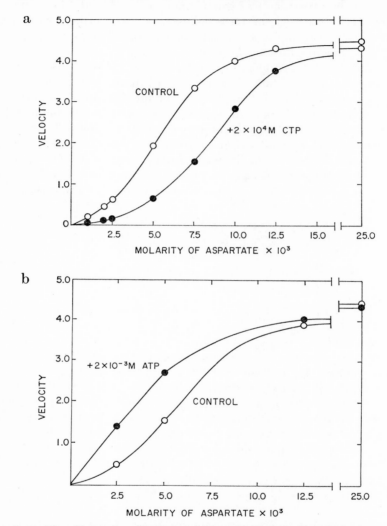

FIG. I-46. The effects of an allosteric inhibitor (CTP, a) and an allosteric activator (ATP, b) on the velocity of the aspartyl transcarbamylase reaction. Reproduced with permission from Gerhart and Pardee (253).

but produces no apparent decrease in the cooperative character of substrate binding (Fig. I-46). In contrast adenosine triphosphate activates the enzyme, producing an apparent increase in the affinity of the enzyme for aspartate and a shift from a sigmoid to a hyperbolic saturation curve (Fig. I-46): neither CTP nor ATP produce any change in V_{max} for the system. Despite the finding that CTP behaves, in a kinetic sense, competitively with regard to aspartate definitive evidence is available to demonstrate that the binding of CTP and aspartate are at topographically distinct sites.

This evidence has been obtained by several different experimental procedures. It has been found possible to selectively destroy the inhibitory actions of CTP by heat, or heavy metal ions while leaving the enzyme fully active (Table I-24). These experiments, which demonstrate the separate character of the binding sites for CTP and aspartate, also reveal their interdependence for after these treatments the maximum velocity of the reaction is increased, the pH optimum shifted from 7·0 to 8·5 and the dependence of velocity upon aspartate concentration is no

TABLE I-24. Selective Modification of Inhibitory Sites of Aspartate Trans-carbamylase

Treatment	Inhibition by CTP $(2 \times 10^{-4}$ M) %	Max. velocity units/mg protein $\times 10^{-3}$	Aspartate (M $\times 10^{-3})^{0 \cdot 5}$
None	70	4·5	6
10^{-6} M HgNO$_3$	0	10·0	12
Heat at 60°	0	9·0	12
0·8 M Urea	0	>4·5	—

longer sigmoidal (Fig. I-47). Very direct evidence for the separate location of the catalytic and the regulatory sites of ATCase has been provided by Gerhart (254–256) who dissociated the enzyme into two distinct types of protein subunits by treatment with p-hydroxy-mercuribenzoate. The subunit of higher molecular weight possesses catalytic activity some twofold greater than that of the native enzyme and its saturation curve with succinate (a non-reactive aspartate analog) is a normal hyperbolic function: the catalytic activity of this subunit, in contrast to the native enzyme, is not affected by CTP or ATP. The subunit of smaller molecular weight possesses no catalytic activity but firmly binds CTP, the binding of which is greatly reduced in the presence of the activator ATP. Finally, the recombination of the reactivated fractionated subunits provides a reconstituted enzyme with properties essentially identical to native ATCase.

X-ray, molecular weight and sequence determinations indicate (257, 258) that ATCase contains twelve amino acid chains—six with a regulatory function and six with a catalytic function. The R_6C_6 arrangement is apparently organized in a highly symmetrical fashion. That the interaction of these subunits and consequent modification of tertiary and quaternary structure is responsible for the cooperative and antagonistic effects observed in ligand binding to ATCase is strongly suggested by studies on the physical parameters of the enzyme. In the presence of carbamyl phosphate and succinate a 3·6% reduction in the enzyme sedimentation coefficient has been observed (259) suggesting a ligand induced conversion to a more "open" form of the enzyme: this effect was partially inhibited by CTP. In contrast binding of the same ligands to

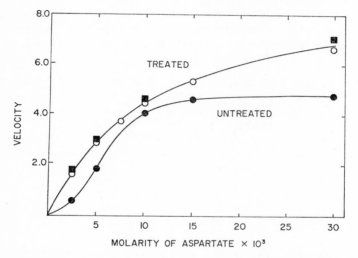

FIG. I-47. Effect of heat (o) and mercuric nitrate (■) on the velocity of the aspartate transcarbamylase reaction. Reproduced with permission from Gerhart and Pardee (253).

the catalytic subunit *alone* produced an increase in the sedimentation coefficient of about 2%. The rate of reaction of ATCase sulfhydryl groups was found to be increased sixfold (over a control lacking ligands) when both carbamyl phosphate and succinate were present: this increase in reactivity was partially inhibited by CTP or 5-bromocytidine triphosphate (a CTP analog). In the absence of carbamyl phosphate and aspartate, CTP (and 5-Br CTP) had almost no effect on the reactivity of ATCase towards the sulfhydryl reagent. The degree of partial inhibition by CTP of the aspartate and carbamyl phosphate-induced increase in sulfhydryl reactivity show a striking parallel to that observed between CTP and succinate in binding studies and between CTP and aspartate in kinetic studies of ATCase reactivity. It thus appears that the effects of ligands on sedimentation behavior, SH reactivity, substrate binding and enzyme reactivity are all mediated through a common change in protein structure.

Among noncatalytic proteins hemoglobin constitutes the example *par excellence* of cooperative ligand binding. The cooperative behavior of oxygen binding in this system has been known and studied for some fifty years: a very large amount of physical information is available, including complete X-ray data, yet complete agreement concerning the molecular basis of this, the best studied cooperative process, has not yet been reached. In the context of the present volume we shall merely present a brief discussion of some of the features of ligand-hemoglobin binding that appear most pertinent to a general interpretation of cooperative binding phenomena. (General reviews of the hemoglobins are found in references 238, 260.)

Normal adult mammalian hemoglobin is a tetrameric species consisting of four globin chains to each of which is bound a heme group. The globin chains are of two types known as α- and β-chains, normal hemoglobin having the $\alpha_2\beta_2$ structure: these differ in length and amino acid composition but their tertiary structures are remarkably similar and the tetrameric hemoglobin structure is highly compact because of the complementary configurations of the non-identical units with the heme groups located at the surface of the molecule in four widely separated pockets located at the corners of an irregular tetrahedron. The tertiary structure of the α- and β-chains of hemoglobin shows extremely close similarity to the single globin chain of myoglobin. From the 2·8 Å resolution data of horse oxyhemoglobin, Perutz and his colleagues (246, 247) have determined that, in addition to the covalent bond between iron and histidine-92, there are about sixty noncovalent interactions between the heme and globin functions; these interactions are almost exclusively nonpolar. The importance of such hydrophobic interactions has been noted elsewhere in this Chapter (p. 30). Similarly, in examinations of the contacts between the α- and β-chains it is found that of the $\alpha_1-\beta_1$ and $\alpha_1-\beta_2$ contacts the former are more extensive but are both very largely nonpolar in character and it is apparent that the stability of the tetrameric structure is largely entropic in origin. (Dissociation of the tetramer into dimers and monomers probably occurs first at the $\alpha_1-\beta_2$ and $\alpha_2-\beta_1$ contacts.) One of the most interesting features of hemoglobins is that despite extremely wide variations in primary structure in the globin chains of various hemoglobins the tertiary structure remains apparently constant (245 261–263): clearly the physiological activities of these molecules, in particular the cooperative interactions, must be relatable to this unique tertiary and quaternary structure which has been maintained through many evolutionary changes.

It has, in fact, been realized for over thirty years, since the demonstration by Haurowitz (264) that shattering of oxyhemoglobin crystals occurs upon deoxygenation, that ligand binding to hemoglobin must be related to changes in conformation. Since then a great deal of information has become available relating conformational change to the O_2–hemoglobin binding process (238, 260). Much of this information is indirect and is concerned with changes in chemical and physical properties of hemoglobin that appear to be directly related to the oxygen binding process; such properties are referred to as *linked functions* (260, 265). Direct evidence is also available, from X-ray studies, that reversible changes in the geometry of subunit packing occurs upon oxygenation (Fig. I-48).

Thus Benesch and Benesch and Guidotti (266, 267) showed that the two SH groups at β-93 are reactive towards iodoacetamide in oxyhemoglobin but are unreactive in the deoxy form. This difference in reactivity was abolished by treatment with carboxypeptidase A which removed the C-terminal residues of the β-chains and also destroys the cooperative character of the oxygen binding process. Furthermore, this difference is absent in hemoglobin H, which has four β-chains and which does not exhibit homotropic ligand binding. Similar observations have been made for the comparative reactivities of the oxygenated and deoxygenated forms towards carboxypeptidases A and B (268): in each case the oxygenated form is more reactive. Of particular interest is the additional observation that the reactivities of the two forms became identical after treatment with carboxypeptidase A, but the difference is maintained after treatment with carboxypeptidase B which removed the C-terminal peptide from the α-chain and does not alter the homotropic oxygen interactions. A further example of a linked function is provided by the work of Antonini *et al.* (269) on the binding of bromothymol blue to various liganded (O_2, CO, etc.) forms of hemoglobin. The unliganded hemoglobin is more reactive and has a higher affinity for the dye: conversely, just as oxygen reduces dye uptake, so the latter process is found to reduce oxygen uptake. In this instance also the differences in reactivity are removed by treatment with carboxypeptidase A. A further and particularly interesting example is the alkaline Bohr effect in hemoglobin in which the conversion of oxyhemoglobin to deoxyhemoglobin is accompanied by an uptake of hydrogen ions. The studies of Perutz and co-workers (269a) attribute this effect to the conformational changes produced by oxygen binding whereby the C-terminal histidines of the β-chains are free in oxyhemoglobin and are bound to carboxyl groups in deoxyhemoglobin thus raising their pK from 6·2 to 7·7.

These few examples of linked functions illustrate the effect that ligand binding at prosthetic or active centers may have on the physicochemical

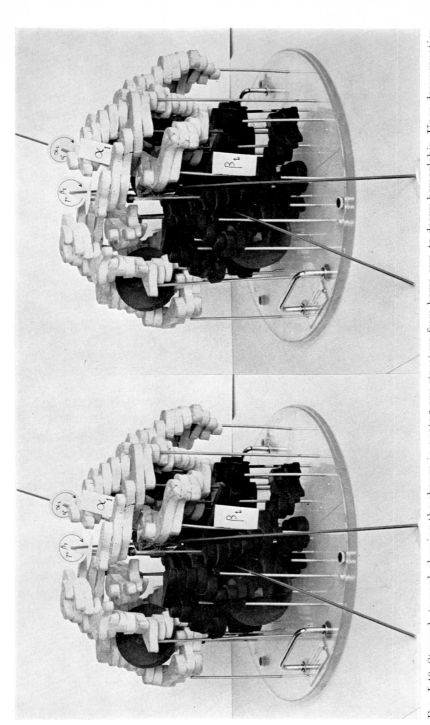

Fig. I-48. Stereophotograph showing the change in quaternary structure from horse oxy- to deoxy-hemoglobin. Upon deoxygenation α_1 turns by 9·4° and β_1 by 7·4° in a clockwise direction: α_2 and β_2 turn similarly. Reproduced with permission from Perutz (246).

properties of distal sites. Such phenomena are now realized to be of critical importance in regulatory functions and will be referred to many times elsewhere in this volume. For the case under discussion the data presented above illustrate the importance of the β-chains in determining homotropic interactions in hemoglobin; a finding in good accord with the more direct X-ray studies.

X-ray studies directly reveal the difference in conformation between oxy- and deoxy-hemoglobin (246, 261, 262). Comparative studies of horse and human hemoglobins reveal that in the transition from the oxy to the deoxy form only slight movements take place at the $\alpha_1-\beta_1$ contacts, the average displacement of contacts being about 1 Å. Greater displacements occur at the $\alpha_1-\beta_2$ contacts, the relative displacement of atoms being some 5–7 Å. To date changes in tertiary structure have not been observed; they may be found when data at higher resolution is available. From the X-ray evidence it appears that changes in the $\alpha_1-\beta_2$ subunit interactions may be of greater importance in controlling ligand binding. As was previously noted this contact is smaller in area than the $\alpha_1-\beta_1$ contact, is constructed to allow the two subunits to slide smoothly apart and involves some dozen groups that make direct contact with the heme function. Thus ligand binding at the heme function alters the quaternary structure, and variations in the quaternary structure will likewise be anticipated to alter ligand–heme binding.

Further supporting evidence comes from the studies of Simon *et al.* (270) who have used the bifunctional SH reagent, bis-(N-maleimidomethyl ether, BME), which reacts internally in each β-chain at SH-93 and a second SH group. Horse BME-hemoglobin shows no cooperative interactions upon oxygen binding and X-ray studies reveal that, whether oxygenated or deoxygenated, it remains locked in the oxy-conformation. It is thus quite clear that the conformational transition between liganded and unliganded forms is essential for the production of cooperative oxygen binding in hemoglobins containing α- and β-subunits.

However, despite this finding the detailed molecular mechanisms by which such conformational transitions actually regulate the affinity of the heme groups for ligand remains unknown. Conceivably a combination of alterations of pK_a's of various functional residues and of alterations in the hydrophobic environments of the heme groups will provide the mechanism. It is to be anticipated that qualitatively similar explanations will be found also to accommodate allosteric and regulatory phenomena in other protein systems.

THEORETICAL STUDIES ON ALLOSTERIC AND COOPERATIVE PROCESSES

There have been a number of studies designed to create models relating protein structure and binding site organization to the cooperative and allosteric processes. These various models differ substantially in their basic assumptions, yet the various mathematical formulations derived from these models are often equally, or approximately equally, consistent with the experimental data. The models of Monod, Changeux and Wyman and of Koshland, while differing substantially in their generality and basic premises, are derived from the common assumption of subunit construction; the quaternary structure of the protein being assumed to depend upon the binding of ligand at catalytic and regulatory sites. A number of other models have also been proposed which do not require subunit construction or a multicatalytic site arrangement for the existence of allosteric effects: these models simply require the existence of two substrate binding sites, one of which acts as a catalytic site and the other as a regulatory site.

The possible existence of such varying mechanisms for the production of the selectionally advantageous allosteric mechanism may appear initially to be surprising; however, as Atkinson (271) has indicated, if selection acts at the level of biological effect rather than mechanism, a number of alternative pathways may well exist for the production of a common end result.

The Monod–Wyman–Changeux (MWC) Model

The basic assumptions of the Monod–Wyman–Changeux treatment (251, 272, 273) of allosteric proteins are that the protomers (identical subunits) of an oligomeric (polymeric assembly of a small number of protomers) protein are symmetrically disposed, this symmetry also representing the symmetry of the corresponding equivalent ligand binding sites. There are presumed to be at least two conformationally distinct states of the oligomeric protein: in these states the symmetry of the oligomeric structure is conserved and hence equivalent ligand binding sites remain equivalent. Furthermore, the binding of any one ligand molecule is assumed to be independent of the binding of any other ligand. However, the microscopic dissociation constants characterizing each set of equivalent sites are different in each conformational state. Consequently, ligand binding shifts the equilibrium between the various states to that state with the highest affinity for the particular ligand. Qualitatively it is clear that this model will lead to sigmoid binding curves since the binding of ligand to the oligomer characterized by the higher affinity will result in a shift of the equilibrium to produce more of this conformational state. However, because of the postulate of conservation of symmetry the change in conformation of one subunit within an oligomer will be accompanied by equal changes in all identical subunits.

The model may be treated quantitatively in the following manner (273). Let the two accessible arrangements of protomers in the oligomer be designated R and T and let L be the equilibrium constant ("allosteric constant") for the $R \rightleftharpoons T$ transition. K_R and K_T are designated as the microscopic dissociation constants of a ligand F bound to its specific sites in the R and T states respectively. From the fundamental assumptions of the MWC model that symmetry is conserved and that the binding

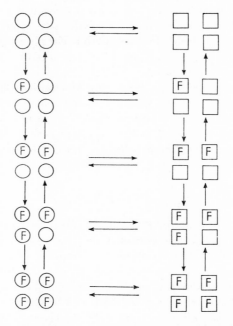

FIG. I-49. Ligand binding to a tetrameric protein existing in two states.

of a ligand is independent of the binding of other ligands, these microscopic dissociation constants are the same for all homologous sites in both accessible states. For convenience a tetrameric protein existing in two states, "round" and "square" (Fig. I-49) will be discussed. Thus the following equilibria will exist,

$$R_0 \rightleftharpoons T_0$$
$$R_0 + F \rightleftharpoons R_1 \qquad T_0 + F \rightleftharpoons T_1$$
$$R_1 + F \rightleftharpoons R_2 \qquad T_1 + F \rightleftharpoons T_2$$
$$R_2 + F \rightleftharpoons R_3 \qquad T_2 + F \rightleftharpoons T_3$$
$$R_3 + F \rightleftharpoons R_4 \qquad T_3 + F \rightleftharpoons T_4$$

The corresponding equilibrium descriptions are:

$$R_1 = R_0 \, \mathrm{n} \cdot \frac{F}{K_R} \qquad\qquad T_1 = T_0 \, \mathrm{n} \cdot \frac{F}{K_T}$$

$$R_2 = R_1 \frac{\mathrm{n}-1}{2} \cdot \frac{F}{K_R} \qquad T_2 = T_1 \frac{\mathrm{n}-1}{2} \cdot \frac{F}{K_T}$$

$$R_\mathrm{n} = R_{\mathrm{n}-1} \frac{1}{\mathrm{n}} \cdot \frac{F}{K_R} \qquad T_\mathrm{n} = T_{\mathrm{n}-1} \frac{1}{\mathrm{n}} \cdot \frac{F}{K_T} \qquad \text{(XLI)}$$

from which it follows that:

(a) the fraction of the protein in the R state, $\bar{R}$, is given by

$$\bar{R} = \frac{R_0 + R_1 + R_2 + R_3 + R_4}{(R_0 + R_1 + R_2 + R_3 + R_4) + (T_0 + T_1 + T_2 + T_3 + T_4)} \qquad \text{(XLII)}$$

and

(b) the fraction of sites actually bound by the ligand:

$$\bar{Y}_F = \frac{(R_1 + 2R_2 + 3R_3 + 4R_4) + (T_1 + 2T_2 + 3T_3 + 4T_4)}{4[(R_0 + R_1 + R_2 + R_3 + R_4) + (T_0 + T_1 + T_2 + T_3 + T_4)]} \tag*{(XLIII)}$$

From the equilibrium equations and setting

$$\frac{F}{K_R} = \alpha \quad \text{and} \quad \frac{K_r}{K_T} = c$$

the "state function", $\bar{R}$, is defined by

$$\bar{R} = \frac{(1+\alpha)^4}{L(1+c\alpha)^4 + (1+\alpha)^4} \qquad \text{(XLIV)}$$

and the "saturation function" $\bar{Y}_F$, is defined by

$$\bar{Y}_F = \frac{Lc\alpha(1+c\alpha)^3 + \alpha(1+\alpha)^3}{L(1+c\alpha)^4 + (1+\alpha)^4} \qquad \text{(XLV)}$$

In Fig. I-50 theoretical curves of $\bar{Y}_F$ are plotted as a function of ligand concentration (α) for various values of L and c. The cooperative character of the saturation process, as expressed by the curvature of the lower part of the curves, is clearly dependent upon the values assigned to L and c. The cooperativity is most marked when L is large, that is the $R_0 \rightleftharpoons T_0$ equilibrium is strongly in favor of T_0, and when c is small, that is when the ligand F shows notably preferential binding for the R state (when $c = 0$, F has zero affinity for one conformational state and exclusive ligand binding occurs).

This model, which clearly accommodates positive homotropic interactions, can be extended readily to cover heterotropic interactions also. Following the original MWC treatment, consider three ligands each binding at its own specific binding site: the substrate (S) which has significant affinity only for the R state, the inhibitor (I) which has affinity only for the T state and the activator (A) that has affinity only

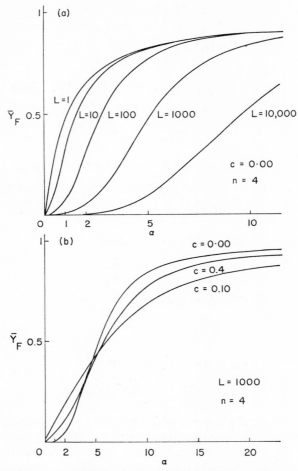

FIG. I-50. Theoretical curves for the saturation function, $\bar{Y}_F$, as a function of L and c. Reproduced with permission from Monod, Wyman and Changeux (273).

for the R state. Again it is obvious qualitatively that the inhibitor, in addition to displacing the half saturation point towards higher values of $[S]$ will increase the cooperativity of substrate binding by shifting the equilibrium to T. The activator, A, will shift the half saturation point towards lower values of S and by making more R state available will decrease the cooperativity of substrate binding. Ultimately, the effects of inhibitors and activators, through "freezing" of the conformation in the T and S states respectively will, provided that both states have equal catalytic efficiency, abolish cooperativity of substrate binding: the values of $\alpha_{0.5}$ (substrate concentration for half saturation) for the resultant hyperbola will then equal unity or $1/c$.

More formally, the saturation function for substrate in the presence of activator and inhibitor may be written as:

$$\overline{Y}_s = \frac{a(1+a)^{n-1}}{L' + (1+\alpha)^n} \qquad \text{(XLVI)}$$

where n is the number of homologous sites and L' is an "apparent" allosteric constant, defined as:

$$L' = \frac{\sum\limits_{0}^{n} T_I}{\sum\limits_{0}^{n} R_A} \qquad \text{(XLVII)}$$

then

$$L' = L\frac{(1+\beta)^n}{(1+\alpha)^n} \qquad \text{(XLVIII)}$$

where $\beta = I/K_I$ and $\alpha = A/K_A$ and K_I and K_A refer to the microscopic dissociation constants of activator and inhibitor with the R and T states respectively. From eqns. XLVI and XLVIII it follows that,

$$\overline{Y}_s = \frac{a(1+\alpha)^{n-1}}{L\dfrac{(1+\beta)^n}{(1+\alpha)^n} + (1+\alpha)^n} \qquad \text{(XLIX)}$$

This equation expresses a fundamental property of the MWC model, that the heterotropic effect of one allosteric ligand upon the saturation function for another allosteric ligand modifies the homotropic interactions of the latter. Figure I-50 describes the theoretical curves showing the effect of an allosteric activator or inhibitor upon the saturation function of a substrate ligand.

The model described so far has been specified in terms of the ligands (F and S) having differential affinities for the R and T states, and with both states having equal catalytic efficiency. The initial velocity is thus simply directly proportional to the saturation function, $\overline{Y}_F$. In the MWC terminology these systems are referred to as "K systems". Another type of effect may also be expected to operate in allosteric systems where S has the same affinity for both states, but in which R and T differ in their catalytic efficiency. Depending upon the differential affinity of F

it will behave as an activator or as an inhibitor. In the MWC terminology these are referred to as "V systems". These latter systems are described by the "state function" ($\bar{R}$) which will indicate that fraction of the oligomer in the active (or inactive) state in the presence of F. The properties of "V systems" have not been developed extensively, although as will be discussed later they may provide an interesting basis for the discussion of neurotransmitter and other hormone actions (Chapter V, p. 413).

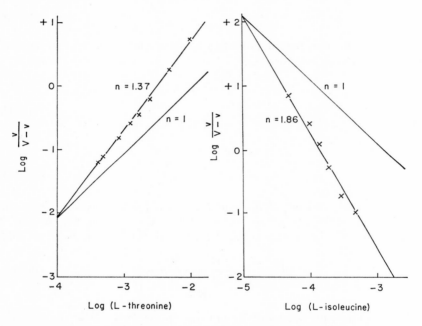

Fig. I-51. Hill plots for interaction of substrate (L-threonine, left) and substrate and inhibitor (L-isoleucine, right). Reproduced with permission from Monod *et al.* (273).

Heterotropic effects in K systems may, as noted previously, be described by the alterations of the homotropic cooperativity of one ligand when in the presence of another. A number of predictions that follow from this model have been experimentally tested. For threonine deaminase (273–275) the saturation curve for substrate is sigmoid and remains sigmoid in the presence of the inhibitor, isoleucine, as shown by the Hill plots (Fig. I-51). Interpreted by the MWC model these observations indicate that the favored state of the enzyme, in the absence of ligands, is that which has minimum affinity for threonine and maximum affinity for isoleucine. Furthermore, the saturation curve for the inhibitor alone is hyperbolic and exhibits no cooperativity and the activator, L-norleucine, reduces cooperativity of binding. Further specific predictions of the model, that substrate analogs that are *true* competitive inhibitors (i.e., allothreonine) and bind at the same site as the substrate, should exert the same effect as the substrate itself in antagonizing the allosteric inhibitor (L-isoleucine) and that low concentrations of the substrate analog should activate, rather than inhibit, the enzyme at very low substrate concentrations have also been confirmed.

Estimation of Homotropic Interactions

Heterotropic effects produced by the ligand are, in the MWC model, derived from their effects on the homotropic binding of a second ligand. The Hill equation (239–241) has proved to be very useful in providing a measure of these homotropic interactions. The Hill coefficient n, does

TABLE I-25. Variations in Hill Coefficients of Homotropic Interactions

System	n	Ref.
Phosphofructokinase +		276
fructose-6-phosphate (substrate)	3·8	
ADP (activator)	1·1	
phosphoenolpyruvate (inhibitor)	1·4	
L-Threonine deaminase +		274, 275
L-threonine (substrate)	1·37	
L-isoleucine (inhibitor)	1.86	
heat desensitized prep^n	1·0	
Fructose-1,6-diphosphatase	2·3	277
papain treatment	1·1	
Hemoglobin (horse)	2·9	278
bis(N-maleimidomethyl)ether treated	1·0	
Deoxycytidine deaminase +		279, 280
deoxycytidine monophosphate (substrate)	2·0	
deoxythymidine triphosphate (inhibitor)	4·1	
deoxycytidine triphosphate (activator)	1·0	
Phosphofructokinase		281
substrate (fructose-6-phosphate)	3·8	
ADP 2×10^{-3} M	1·1	
phosphoenolpyruvate ($3·5 \times 10^{-2}$ M)	1·4	
L-Threonine deaminase		253
substrate (L-threonine)	1·37	
inhibitor (L-isoleucine)	1·86	
heat desensitized	1·0	

not generally represent the number of interacting ligand binding sites but rather is a measure of the interaction between these sites. In a qualitative sense n provides a useful guide to the changes in cooperativity of ligand binding induced by other ligands. Table I-25 gives some representative examples.

Consider the interaction of a ligand X with a macromolecule and denote by $\bar{X}$ the amount of this ligand bound per mole of macromolecule and the activity of X by x. A graphical representation of this equilibrium is obtained by plotting $\bar{X}$ against $\log x$ and for a macromolecule containing only a single binding site or a number of identical non-interacting sites a simple titration curve is obtained. The value of $x = x_{0.5}$ at the

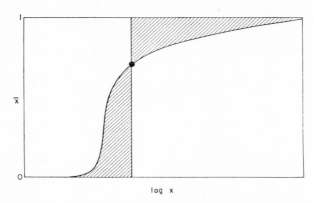

FIG. I-52. Ligand binding curve demonstrating the median ligand activity, x_m (●).
Reproduced with permission from Wyman (260).

midpoint ($\bar{X} = 0.5$) is equal to $1/K_x$ where K_x is the equilibrium constant for the ligand: macromolecule interaction: thus, ΔF, the free energy for saturation of the macromolecule is,

$$\Delta F = 2.303 \, RT \log x_{0.5} \tag{L}$$

If $\bar{X}/t = \bar{x}$, the amount of ligand bound per site (fractional saturation), is plotted against $\log x$, the free energy for saturation per site is obtained. For macromolecular systems where mutual interaction of the binding sites occurs the simple titration curve is generally found to become asymmetric (Fig. I-52). For such curves Wyman (260, 282, 283) has demonstrated that the free energy for ligand saturation per site is given by,

$$\Delta F = 2.303 \, RT \log x_m \tag{LI}$$

where x_m is the median ligand activity and is that value of the ligand activity for which the two shaded areas in Fig. I-52 are equal. The deviation from a simple titration curve of the ligand binding curve means that there are positive homotropic interactions between the binding sites. The nature of these interactions may be investigated further through the use of a Hill plot in which $\log \overline{X}/n - \overline{X} = \log \overline{x}/(1 - x)$ is plotted against $\log x$. For the simplest case corresponding to a simple titration curve the plot gives a straight line of unit slope, $n = 1$. For systems with interacting sites the Hill plot will show deviations from unit slope (Fig. I-53) but will, unless intersite interactions are infinitely strong, approach unit slope at either end of the plot. Wyman has shown, for the case where the interacting sites are identical, that the perpendicular distance between the final asymptotes multiplied by

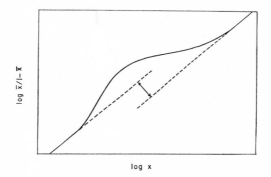

FIG. I-53. Hypothetical Hill plot. The perpendicular distance between the asymptotes ($\leftrightarrow$) is a measure of the interaction energy. Reproduced with permission from Wyman (283).

$RT\sqrt{2}$ gives an averaged value of the free energy of interaction between sites. Additionally, the Hill plot provides information concerning the minimum free energy of interaction (ΔF_I) between sites at any degree of saturation of the system through the relationship,

$$\Delta F_I = \frac{RT}{\overline{x}(1 - \overline{x})} \cdot \left(1 - \frac{1}{\overline{n}}\right). \tag{LII}$$

where $\overline{n}$ is the slope at saturation $\overline{x}$. Despite the many factors that will disturb this simple treatment, and which are discussed more fully by Wyman (260, 282–283) it is clear that $\overline{n}$ provides a useful measure of the free energy of interaction between the binding sites of an allosteric macromolecule that is realized during the ligand saturation process. For the limiting case, in which all n sites interact with the ligand simultaneously (very strong inter-site interactions) it is clear that $\overline{n} = n$, but of course $\overline{n} \not> n$.

5

Interpretation of $\bar{n}$ is further complicated by the possibility of non-exclusive ligand binding. For the limiting case of the MWC model, previously discussed, exclusive ligand binding to one or other of the

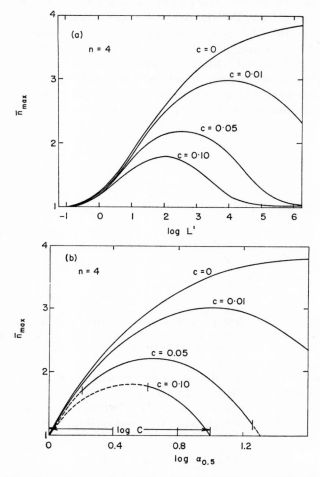

FIG. I-54. The effect of nonexclusive ligand binding on slope of Hill plot. (a) Variation as a function of the apparent allosteric constant. (b) Variation as a function of $\alpha_{0.5}$. Reproduced with permission from Rubin and Changeux (284).

conformational states $(c = K_R/K_T = 0)$ is assumed to occur. Non-exclusive ligand binding $(c > 0)$, where ligands have a preferential but not exclusive affinity for one conformational state, may significantly modify the general conclusions and predictions drawn from the limiting MWC model. Qualitatively, it is apparent that the finite affinity of a ligand for *both* states of a protein will impose limitations upon the extent to which the ligand can shift the equilibrium between the states. These limitations will be determined by c, the non-exclusive binding coefficient, and by L', the apparent allosteric constant, which is a measure of heterotropic interactions. Rubin and Changeux (284) have computed the relationships between $\bar{n}_{max}$, a measure of homotropic interactions, L' and $\alpha_{0.5}$, the substrate concentration for half saturation; this latter parameter, being directly experimentally determinable is a more convenient measure of the effects of heterotropic ligands than is L'. From their results (Fig. I-54a,b) it is clear that non-exclusive binding ($c \neq 0$) produces qualitatively different results than exclusive binding ($c = 0$). Thus, the values of $\bar{n}_{max}$ as a function of L' or $\alpha_{0.5}$, are bell shaped, reach a maximum ($\bar{n}_{max}^{max}$) and tend at *both* extremes to unity. The values of $\bar{n}_{max}^{max}$ are relatively insensitive to changes in L' and $\alpha_{0.5}$ and, hence with appropriate values of L' and c, allosteric effectors may produce changes in $\alpha_{0.5}$ unaccompanied by changes in $\bar{n}_{max}^{max}$.

The Subunit Association–Dissociation Model

Macromolecular systems that are composed of subunits capable of participating in an association–dissociation interaction are also capable of showing abnormal sensitivity of macromolecular function to changes in ligand concentration. Frieden (285) has proposed a broad division of this system into two subclasses:

1. Those in which the association–dissociation reaction is rapid compared to the overall rate of the catalytic reaction and
2. Those in which the association–dissociation reaction is slow compared to the rate of the catalytic reaction.

Bovine liver glutamate dehydrogenase appears to fall into the first subclass. This enzyme can exert in a range of molecular weight forms from 400,000 to 2,000,000, all of which have essentially the same intrinsic activity (285, 286). Studies of GTP (an inhibitor) binding to the enzyme in the presence of NADH showed an increasingly sigmoid dependence of the fractional saturation of GTP sites on GTP concentration, indicating that increasing association of the enzyme to higher molecular weight forms is responsible for the cooperative behavior (Fig. I-55). Studies with a chemically modified enzyme of normal catalytic activity but which cannot associate revealed only a hyperbolic saturation. GTP binds preferentially to the 400,000 molecular weight enzyme and at high enzyme levels cooperativity of binding is observed because the ligand can, by virtue of the rapid character of the association–dissociation reaction, promote conversion of the high molecular weight to the low molecular weight form. The resemblance of this statement to the formalism of the MWC model is obvious with the clear difference that in the present case the two conformational forms represent different molecular weight species. The association–dissociation interaction probably also contributes to the cooperative ligand binding behavior of hemoglobin where the α,β-dimer shows a high Hill coefficient (n = 2·7).

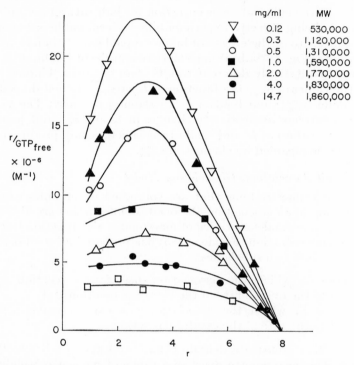

FIG. I-55. Scatchard plot of GTP binding to glutamate dehydrogenase as a function of enzyme concentration r = moles GTP bound: mole enzyme (M.W. = 400,000). The enzyme concentration and molecular weights given in figure. Reproduced with permission from Frieden (285).

In contrast, polymeric systems that undergo slow association–dissociation reactions may serve a different control function. If the slow equilibrium is between active and inactive forms (i.e., phosphorylase a, (287) the assocation–dissociation does not alter the kinetic characteristics of the system but does regulate the total amount of enzyme activity. Freiden notes that such slowly equilibrating systems may serve to prevent violent metabolic alterations that might otherwise be caused by sudden increases in ligand concentrations under, for example, conditions of stress.

The Koshland–Némethy–Filmer (KNF) Model

In contrast to the MWC model which rationalizes cooperativity of ligand binding on the basis of an allosteric preequilibrium between two conformations of the oligomeric protein and which is shifted by preferred binding of ligands to one conformation or another, Koshland, Némethy and Filmer have proposed (288) a model for cooperativity based upon the "induced fit" hypothesis, in which *sequential* changes of subunit structure *induced* by the ligand are presumed to be of dominant importance.

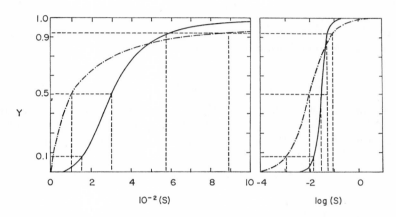

FIG. I-56. Comparison of sigmoid (———) and hyperbolic (–·–·–) saturation curves on linear (left) and log (right) scales. On both plots the saturation levels (Y) are indicated at the 10, 50 and 90% levels. Reproduced with permission from Koshland, Némethy and Filmer (288).

In this latter model cooperativity is defined in terms of the ratio of ligand concentration at Y (fraction of binding sites occupied) $= 0.9$ to ligand concentration at $Y = 0.1$,

$$R_s = (S)_{0.9}/(S)_{0.1} \qquad \text{(LIII)}$$

Since, for any system obeying simple adsorption kinetics with noninteracting binding sites $R_s = 81$, a value of less than 81 indicates a saturation curve steeper than that predicted from independent binding at noninteracting sites. A comparison of such curves is presented in Fig. I-56.

As in the MWC model, it is assumed that the individual subunits of the protein can exist in two conformational states, A and B, and that only B can bind S in significant quantities. However, unlike the MWC model, the KNF model retains neither the concertedness of transition of A to B subunits nor the symmetry restrictions for the binding sites, but proposed hybrid conformational states of the protein can exist, i.e., that one subunit can change conformation without necessarily causing an equal change in all other subunits. It is further assumed that a change in conformation of one subunit may change the relative stabilities of the conformations of neighboring subunits through subunit interactions.

The substrate binding constant, K_s, describes the affinity of S for an individual subunit,

$$K_s = \frac{[BS]}{[B][S]} \tag{LIV}$$

K_t, the transformation constant, represents the equilibrium constant for the conversion of subunit A to subunit B,

$$K_t = \frac{[B]}{[A]} \tag{LV}$$

The constants, K_{AA}, K_{AB} and K_{BB} are employed to define subunit interactions: it is assumed (as a standard state) that $K_{AA} = 1$. When, for example, $K_{AB} > 1$ the AB interaction is stabilized relative to the AA

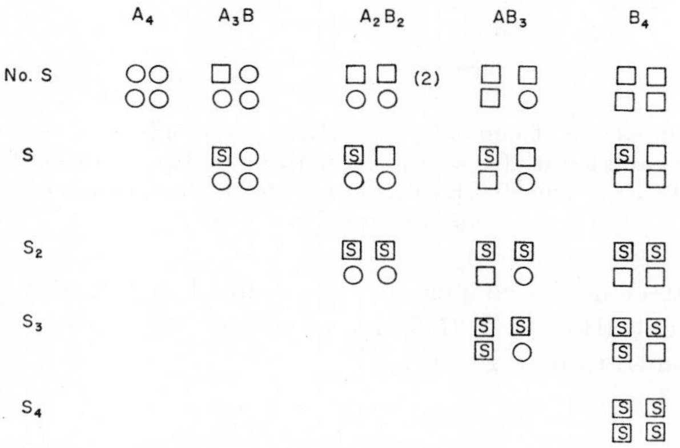

	A_4	A_3B	A_2B_2	AB_3	B_4
No. S	OO OO	□O OO	□□ (2) O O	□□ □O	□□ □□
S		⑤O OO	⑤□ O O	⑤□ □O	⑤□ □□
S_2			⑤⑤ O O	⑤⑤ □O	⑤⑤ □□
S_3				⑤⑤ ⑤O	⑤⑤ ⑤□
S_4					⑤⑤ ⑤⑤

Fig. I-57. Ligand (S) binding to a tetrameric protein capable of existing in A and B subunits and hybrid forms. Reproduced with permission from Haber and Koshland (290).

interaction. Figure I-57 represents a generalized and simplified scheme for ligand binding to a tetrameric protein capable of existing with A and B subunits. The relative amounts of the various tetrameric species of Fig. I-57 for selected values of the constants K_S, K_T, K_{AB} and K_{BB} are shown in Table I-26. For the first three examples the protein exists

TABLE I-26. Ligand Binding and Distribution of Molecular Species in a Tetrameric Protein† (289, 290)

No.	K_T	K_{BB}	Distribution of conformational states in absence of A					Distribution of conformational states at $\bar{Y} = 0.5$					R_s
			A_4	$A_3 B$	$A_2 B_2$	$A B_3$	B_4	A_4	$A_3 B$	$A_2 B_2$	$A B_2$	B_4	
1	10^{-2}	10	96	4	0	0	0	25	11	13	13	27	7
2	10^{-3}	10	99.6	0.4	0	0	0	30	12	13	12	31	6
3	10^{-4}	10	100	0	0	0	0	31	12	13	12	31	5
4	10^{-2}	10^3	0	0	0	0.04	99.9	0	0	0	0	100	81
5	10^{-3}	10^3	50	0.2	0.2	0.2	50	6	0	0	0	94	49
6	10^{-4}	10^3	100	0	0	0	0	40	0	0	0	60	4

† $K_s = 10^3$: $K_{AA} = K_{AB} = 1$. S is assumed to bind only to B conformation.

essentially in the A_4 form in the absence of substrate. When $K_{BB} \gg K_{AA}$ appreciable amounts of the B_4 form appear even in the absence of substrate (examples 4 and 5, Table I-27) and, dependent upon the energy of interconversion, the protein may exist almost entirely (example 4, $K_T = 10^{-2}$) or less completely (example 5, $K_T = 10^{-3}$) in the B_4 form. Table I-26 also includes data for the relative amounts of these species present when the fractional saturation by substrate is 0.5: the first three examples clearly show the hybrid conformational states and correspond to the KNF model and examples 5 and 6 in which only the A_4 and B_4 subunits are found correspond to the concerted MWC model. From such simple considerations it is apparent that, other things being equal, very strong subunit interactions will lead to the concerted model and weak subunit interactions will lead to the sequential model.

Koshland has calculated ligand binding curves for various geometries ("square", tetrahedral'', "linear") of the tetrameric assembly and for various values of the constants K_S, K_{AB}, K_{BB}, etc., and have presented nomograms correlating the experimental parameters ($S_{0.5}$ and R_S) with

TABLE I-27. Constants of O_2–Hemoglobin Binding Curves derived from Koshland–Némethy–Filmer model (288)

Geometry	$K_s K_t$ (mm^{-1})	K_{BB}
"Square"	8.8×10^{-3}	12.5
"Tetrahedral"	8.3×10^{-3}	5.6
"Linear"	5.8×10^{-3}	50.0

$K_S K_t$ (full details of these procedures and the format of the ligand binding equations may be obtained from their original paper (288)). The applicability of this approach was tested for the O_2–hemoglobin equilibrium by taking the experimental values of $S_{0.5}$ and R_S and determining the theoretical saturation curve: models based upon the square and tetrahedral arrangement of subunits were found to give the

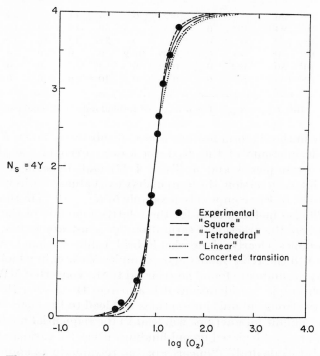

FIG. I-58. The agreement between theory and experiment for O_2 binding to hemoglobin. The terms "square", "tetrahedral" and "linear" refer to the geometries of the subunit arrangements and the concerted transition represents the MWC model. Reproduced with permission from Koshland, Némethy and Filmer (288).

best agreement with experiment. Figure I-58 presents a comparison between the "square sequential" model of Koshland, Némethy and Filmer and the concerted model of Monod, Wyman and Changeux. It is apparent that, despite their fundamentally different characteristics, both models give equally good agreement with the experimental data. Clearly, the shape of ligand saturation curves cannot necessarily be used to distinguish mechanisms. This is evident also from the data of Table I-26 in which examples 3 and 6 are of closely similar cooperativity and hence will give very similar saturation curves, but exhibit quite distinct distributions of molecular species.

From the data of Table I-27 it is clear, that the fit to the experimental data for hemoglobin which can be obtained by both the "square", "tetrahedral" and "linear" models of the KNF mechanism are characterized by rather different values of the intrinsic constants. More generally, very similar ligand saturation curves can often be derived for the various subunit geometries by appropriate manipulation of these constants. It is clear that the information contained within a given saturation curve does not indicate, *per se*, a unique mechanism. However, saturation curves may limit the number of models that have to be considered and also indicate the information required to distinguish between them. Nevertheless, it is pertinent that many combinations of subunit interactions (K_{BB}, K_{AB}, etc.), conformational transitions (K_t) and ligand affinity (K_S) lead to the two simplest and extreme models— the symmetrical concerted and the sequential models.

The Koshland–Némethy–Filmer treatment has also been extended to cover two ligand binding (substrate–activator, substrate–inhibitor) by Kirtley and Koshland (291). Because of the complexity of this treatment when it is applied to the many possibilities of subunit geometry and interactions and modes of ligand binding (competitive, independent, ordered, etc.) this extension will not be discussed here in detail. However, as with the treatment of the single ligand case, the sequential model is capable of explaining a wide range of data including the effects of activators and inhibitors upon substrate binding predicted by the MWC model.

A particularly interesting consequence predictable from the sequential model of Koshland, Némethy and Filmer, but not from the MWC model, is that of negative cooperativity in which binding of each ligand molecule progressively hinders the interaction of subsequent molecules of ligand (292, 293): there are apparently several such examples of negative

TABLE I-28. Dissociation Constants (Averaged) for NAD Dissociation from Rabbit Muscle Glyceraldehyde-3-phosphate Dehydrogenase (292)

Step	K (average)
$ED \rightarrow E + D$	10^{-11}
$ED_2 \rightarrow ED + D$	10^{-9}
$ED_3 \rightarrow ED_2 + D$	3×10^{-7}
$ED_4 \rightarrow ED_3 + D$	$2 \cdot 6 \times 10^{-5}$

cooperativity known, i.e., phosphoenolpyruvate carboxylase, rabbit muscle glyceraldehyde-3-phosphate dehydrogenase, cytidine triphosphate synthetase and several other enzymes for which reasonable indirect evidence can be derived. The effect of such negative cooperativity on ligand binding is seen rather clearly in the data of Table I-28, for the dissociation of NAD from rabbit muscle glyceraldehyde 3-phosphate dehydrogenase: the dissociation of the NAD molecules becomes progressively more difficult with successive removal of NAD. This points, perhaps, to the significance of negative cooperativity since it is clear that this phenomenon can "insulate" enzymes against large fluctuations in metabolite concentrations and hence ensure enzyme function even under unfavorable conditions (292).

"Two Site" Models for Allosteric Proteins

Both the Monod-Wyman-Changeux and the Koshland-Némethy-Kilmer (KNK) models have as a basic premise the existence of multiple substrate binding sites with a subunit construction of the protein. Certainly, many allosteric enzymes are known to be composed of discrete subunits with catalytic or regulatory functions. However, as Atkinson and Stadtman have indicated (249, 294, 295) sigmoid rate curves that generate formal orders of reaction >1 do not necessarily require subunit construction or even the existence of more than one catalytic site. Thus a system that contains one catalytically active substrate binding site and n substrate binding sites that serve a regulatory function to affect substrate binding at the catalytic site can, in principle, lead to kinetics of nth order with respect to substrate. Such systems clearly relate to the concept of ligand-induced conformational change as proposed by Koshland. Systems for which the existence of this very simple cooperative ligand binding mechanism has been unequivocally demonstrated do not appear to be known. However, at least one enzyme system is known whose complex kinetic behavior can be predicted on the basis of this assumption.

The kinetics of the yeast NAD–isocitrate dehydrogenase reaction (Fig. I-59) are fourth order with respect to isocitrate in the presence or absence of the positive effector AMP, second order with respect to NAD,

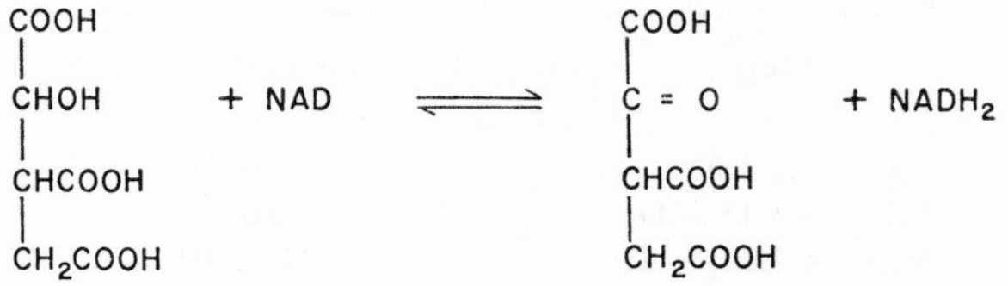

$$
\begin{array}{ccc}
\text{COOH} & & \text{COOH} \\
| & & | \\
\text{CHOH} & + \text{ NAD} \rightleftharpoons & \text{C = O} \quad + \text{ NADH}_2 \\
| & & | \\
\text{CHCOOH} & & \text{CHCOOH} \\
| & & | \\
\text{CH}_2\text{COOH} & & \text{CH}_2\text{COOH}
\end{array}
$$

FIG. I-59. Isocitrate dehydrogenase-catalysed reaction of isocitric acid.

Mg^{++} and AMP and first order with respect to enzyme. The overall reaction follows eleventh order kinetics (241). The kinetic data indicate that at least 4 molecules of isocitrate and 2 molecules each of NAD, AMP and Mg^{++} function in the rate determining step(s). If these represent the actual number of binding sites then an obvious possibility is that there are two catalytic sites each binding isocitrate, NAD and Mg^{++}, two regulatory isocitrate sites and two regulatory AMP sites. According to the model advanced to fit the kinetic data by Atkinson, Hathaway and Smith (241) the isocitrate binding sites have identical intrinsic dissociation constants and binding of isocitrate at one site decreases by a twenty-fold factor the effective dissociation constant for the subsequent binding of a second isocitrate molecule (this corresponds to a ratio of 8000 for the dissociation constants at the first and fourth sites), and thus isocitrate binding is extremely cooperative. The effects of the activator AMP which produces an increase in affinity for isocitrate without affecting the order of the reaction suggests that AMP has no effect on the interactions between isocitrate binding sites. The co-operative binding of isocitrate might be rationalized on the basis of ligand-induced association–dissociation of subunits; however, the existence of discrete subunits has not been demonstrated and, further-more, the reaction rate is clearly first order with respect to enzyme. The association of subunits would necessarily be at least a bimolecular reaction.

The effect of low concentrations of the substrate analog, citrate, present with subsaturation concentrations of isocitrate, is to increase reaction rate and, at higher concentrations, to reduce the reaction rate. Presumably citrate binds at the regulatory isocitrate sites and thus promotes substrate binding at catalytic sites: at higher concentrations citrate will, however, function as a classical competitive inhibitor. In conformity with the model proposed by Atkinson *et al.*, it is found that a given level of citrate increases the reaction rate at low isocitrate levels and inhibits at higher isocitrate levels and that citrate, unlike AMP, changes the order of reaction with respect to isocitrate. The excellent agreement between the experimental and calculated values for these effects may be seen in Fig. I-60.

The NAD–isocitrate dehydrogenase from *Neurospora crassa* (296) appears to be similar to the yeast enzyme but to possess only half the number of ligand binding sites. However, the nature of the two isocitrate binding sites appears to be different as judged by the behavior of sub-strate analogs: citrate and erythro-L_s-isocitrate are both catalytically inactive and strongly activate the enzyme at low isocitrate concentra-tions. However, these analogs function only as activators and do not, at high concentrations, inhibit the enzyme: clearly, these analogs do not bind at the catalytic site but at a separate allosteric site which is, however, also capable of binding isocitrate. This is an important point in the general consideration of whether cooperative phenomena occur through substrate or substrate analog binding at *identical* interacting catalytic sites as proposed in its simplest form in the MWC model.

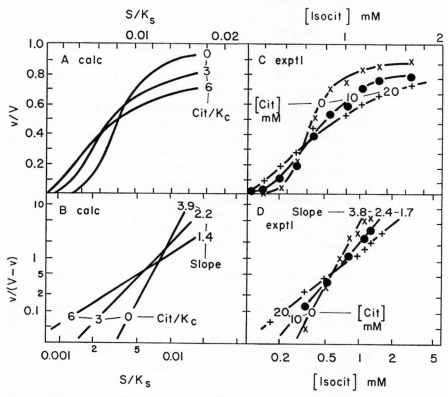

FIG. I-60. Comparison of the calculated (A and B) and experimental (C and D) effects of citrate on the isocitrate dehydrogenase reaction. In the calculated figures the concentrations of citrate are expressed as intrinsic dissociation constants (S/K).
Reproduced with permission from Atkinson, Hathaway and Smith (241).

Sanwal, Stachow and Cook (296) propose that the two isocitrate sites in the neurospora enzyme function via an obligatory sequential two-step binding such that binding of isocitrate at the allosteric site must precede binding at the catalytic site.

While physicochemical evidence is not yet available to describe the mechanisms of interaction between the proposed regulatory and catalytic isocitrate binding sites it seems difficult to avoid the conclusion that it resides within the overall framework of the Koshland induced fit theory of ligand interaction, conformational changes induced by the binding of citrate or isocitrate at the regulatory site being transmitted to the catalytic site to facilitate subsequent binding.

Differentiation Between the Various Models of Cooperative Processes

Despite the basic differences in the fundamental premises of the several models for cooperative ligand binding it is clear from the preceding discussion and particularly from Koshland's highly generalized model that they may not be distinguishable by equilibrium studies. Differentiation may, however, prove possible by techniques in which the extent of ligand binding can be correlated with the conformational change(s) assumed to occur in all models. In the MWC model the number of subunit transitions does not, in general equal the number of molecules of substrate bound; in other words, there will not be a strict linear relationship $\bar{Y}$ and $\bar{R}$, whereas in the simplest sequential KNF model one subunit conformational change occurs for every molecule of ligand bound. Differentiation from the more complex extensions of the KNF model, in which subunit interactions are strong, appears to require extremely sensitive techniques. From the few studies currently available it appears that examples of both the symmetry and sequential models exist although it is too early to say whether either model will encompass the majority of systems (297–305) and, indeed it seems most probable that neither model has any exclusive claim to the generation of cooperative binding processes.

Kirschner, Eigen and their co-workers (297, 298) have applied the technique of relaxation spectroscopy to the study of NAD binding to yeast D-glyceraldehyde-3-phosphate dehydrogenase and have shown the binding process to be characterized by three discrete relaxation processes with time constants, $1/\tau_1 = 10^{-3}$–10^{-4}, $1/\tau_2 = 10^{-2}$–10^{-3} and $1/\tau_3 = 0{\cdot}1$–$1{\cdot}0$ sec^{-1} which have been interpreted as describing binding to the R states, the T states and the first order conformational transition between the R and T states. These findings are consistent with predictions of the MWC model.

As previously noted, however, rabbit muscle D-glyceraldehyde-3-phosphate dehydrogenase exhibits negative cooperativity, a finding which is not easy to reconcile with the MWC model of ligand binding.

In a penetrating application of NMR and EPR techniques Sulman and co-workers (305) have analysed the structural changes occurring in hemoglobin and myoglobin upon ligand binding; their evidence indicates very strongly that direct heme–heme interactions play no significant role in the cooperative binding process. Myoglobin and oxymyoglobin show substantial differences in their NMR spectra consistent with extensive structural changes taking place in this non-associating system under oxygenation. The spectra of the α- and β-chains of hemoglobin differ significantly from one another and from the tetrameric deoxyhemoglobin: these differences arise from differences in the heme environment of the monomeric and tetrameric species. In contrast the spectral differences between hemoglobin and oxyhemoglobin are attributable, not to changes in the heme group environment, but to conformational changes in the protein structure arising from oxygen binding. NMR and EPR spectra of mixed state hemoglobins (α^{III}, β^{II}) reveal that the environments of the heme groups in the α-chains are unaffected by ligand binding in the β-chains and vice versa. Furthermore, the heme spectra of the mixed tetramers did not differ from the homogeneous tetramers. It seems clear that the portion of the free energy change of the Hb $\rightarrow$ HbO$_2$ transition attributable to cooperativity and which Wyman has calculated as approximately 3 kcal is contributed by protein conformational change and not by heme–heme interactions. This is quite consistent with findings that this free energy change is quite independent of the nature of the ligand attached (O$_2$, cyanides, CO, etc.) despite their differences in binding energies. These findings are not consistent with the MWC model which requires the affinity, and hence environment, of the ligand binding site to change since they indicate that the source of the cooperative lies in conformational changes outside the ligand binding site. Several lines of evidence including the spin-label studies of Ogawa (306) which indicate that a maleimide label attached at β 93-SH is sensitive principally to the state of oxygenation of the β-chain and the findings of Antonini and Brunori (307) that the reactivity of the β 93-SH group is sensitive only to ligand binding at the β-chain support the idea that the conformational changes induced by ligand binding are propagated only as far as the subunit interface. These changes in tertiary structure cause the quaternary changes, revealed by the X-ray studies of Perutz, in which the α- and β-chains rotate around the α_1, β_2 interfaces.

General Comments on Cooperative and Allosteric Effects

Even from the brief survey of existing data given in the preceding pages it is clear that there is no general theoretical or experimental agreement on the mechanism for cooperative ligand binding. As noted previously it seems quite probable that there are many individual mechanisms in existence and Atkinson has pointed out that sigmoid ligand binding curves presumably offer specific selectional advantage and that if selection acts at the level of effect, rather than mechanism, there is no reason to assume a single mechanism. However, it may well be that the KNF model of sequential ligand-induced conformational change has wider applicability. This is perhaps not surprising in view of the fewer limitations placed on this model relative to the highly restrictive MWC model which probably reflects the limiting case where subunit interactions are extremely strong. It should also be emphasized that it is possible to set up models for enzyme–substrate interactions that do not involve more than one single and independent ligand binding site but where alternate binding pathways exist so that with appropriate manipulation of the various kinetic constants sigmoid curves can be generated (308, 309).

The increased sensitivity of the enzyme to small changes in ligand concentration that is characteristic of positive homotropic systems may clearly be of biochemical and physiological significance. The recent discovery of at least one negative homotropic system in which the enzyme will be of decreased sensitivity to changes in ligand concentration indicates that two regulatory systems of opposing function may exist: in the most general sense we may regard the positive homotropic systems as biological and biochemical amplifiers designed to increase response to small changes in the level of information input. In contrast negative homotropic systems will function to maintain the constancy of a given biological or biochemical output despite large variations in the information input. The potential importance of this latter mechanism to those biological functions that must be kept operating at a constant level seems quite clear.

Thus far allosteric and regulatory proteins have been considered primarily as isolated components although the importance of the allosteric mechanism as a means of response to alterations in the cellular environment does not require further comment. A number of workers (i.e., 104, 105) have commented that proteins composed of subunits appear to have a higher nonpolar:polar residue ratio than monomeric proteins: nonpolar areas on the protein surface will, of course, favor subunit association although more specific interactions are doubtless also employed in such associating systems (310). Since, a large number of biologically active proteins appear to function as part of the cell membrane, one of the most important regulatory areas of the cell, it may well be that hydrophobic association between these proteins and other nonpolar constituents such as phospholipids and "structural" protein forms the basis for the generation of linked protein systems in the cell membrane such that conformational changes initiated through ligand interaction at one protein can be transmitted and serve as regulatory signals in other proteins. The general problem of membrane cooperativity and function is discussed in Chapter II.

Finally, it is pertinent to note that while the preceding discussion has related cooperative and allosteric effects almost entirely to proteins of defined structure and function, it should be realized that these properties are probably fundamental to all macromolecular structure: they simply arise from the fact that the design of macromolecular systems involves a dominant role of coordinated weak interactions. In turn this renders the molecule or molecular system highly susceptible to small changes in the local environment.

REFERENCES

1. D. L. D. Caspar, *in*: "Principles of Biomolecular Organization", Ciba Foundation Symposium (eds. G. E. W. Wolstenholme and M. O'Connor) (1965). Little, Brown, Boston.
2. J. L. Webb, "Enzyme and Metabolic Inhibitors", Vol. I, p. 193 (1963). Academic Press, New York and London.
3. R. W. Gurney, "Ionic Processes in Solution" (1953). Wiley, New York.
4. R. A. Robinson and R. H. Stokes, "Electrolyte Solutions", p. 559 (1959). Butterworths, London.
5. J. G. Kirkwood and F. H. Westheimer, *J. Chem. Phys.* (1938) **6**, 506, 513.
6. D. Pressman, A. L. Grossberg, L. H. Pence and L. Pauling, *J. Amer. Chem. Soc.* (1946) **68**, 250.
7. B. E. Conway, J. O'M. Bockris and I. A. Ammar, *Trans. Faraday Soc.* (1951) **47**, 756.
8. L. Salem, *Can. J. Biochem. Physiol.* (1962) **40**, 1287.
9. H. Jehle, *Proc. Nat. Acad. Sci. U.S.A.* (1963) **50**, 516.
10. A. Szent-Gyorgi, "Bioenergetics" (1957) p. 38, Academic Press, New York and London.
11. G. Némethy and H. A. Scheraga, *J. Chem. Phys.* (1962) **36**, 3382.
12. H. S. Frank, *Fed. Proc. Fed. Amer. Soc. Exp. Biol.* (1965) **24** (5), 3.
13. G. Némethy, *Fed. Proc. Fed. Amer. Soc. Exp. Biol.* (1965) **24** (5), 38.
14. E. Wicke, *Angew. Chem. Int. Ed. Engl.* (1966) **5**, 106.
15. J. L. Kavanau, "Water and Solute–Water Interactions" (1964). Holden-Day, San Francisco.
16. R. A. Horne, *Surv. Prog. Chem.* (1968) **4**, 1.
17. B. E. Conway, *Annu. Rev. Phys. Chem.* (1966) **17**, 481.
18. D. Eisenberg and W. Kauzmann, "The Structure and Properties of Water" (1969). Oxford University Press, Oxford.
19. W. Drost-Hansen, *in*: "Equilibrium Concepts in Natural Water Systems" (1967). American Chemical Society Special Publications No. 67. Washington, D.C.
20. O. Y. Samoilov, "The Structure of Aqueous Electrolyte Solutions and the Hydration of Ions" (1965). Consultants Bureau, New York.
21. E. Forslind, *Acta Polytech.* (1952) **155**, 9.
22. L. Pauling, *Science, N.Y.* (1961) **134**, 15.
23. R. P. Marchi and H. Eyring, *J. Phys. Chem.* (1964) **68**, 221.
24. H. S. Frank and A. S. Quist, *J. Chem. Phys.* (1961) **34**, 604.
25. H. S. Frank and W-Y. Wen, *Discuss. Faraday Soc.* (1957) **24**, 133.
26. B. V. Derjaguin, N. N. Fedyakin and M. V. Talaev, *Dokl. Akad. Nauk. SSSR* (1966) **167**, 376.
27. E. R. Lippincott, R. R. Stromberg, W. H. Grant and G. L. Cessac, *Science, N.Y.* (1969) **164**, 1482.

28. R. W. Bolander, J. L. Kassrer, Jr. and J. T. Zing, *Nature (London)* (1969) **221**, 1233.
29. L. C. Allen and P. A. Kollman, *Science, N.Y.* (1970) **167**, 1443.
30. D. L. Rousseau and S. P. S. Porto, *Science, N.Y.* (1970) **167**, 1715.
31. G. H. Nancollas, "Interactions in Electrolyte Solutions" (1966). Elsevier, Amsterdam.
32. J. O'M. Bockris, *Quart. Rev. Chem. Soc.* (1949) **3**, 179.
33. J. E. Desnoyers and C. Jolicoeur, "Modern Aspects of Electrochemistry" Vol. 5, (eds. J. O'M. Bockris and B. E. Conway) (1968). Butterworth, London.
34. "Hydrogen-bonded Solvent Systems" (eds. A. K. Covington and P. Jones) (1968). Taylor and Francis, London.
35. G. Schwarzenbach, *Experientia* (1956) (Suppl. 5) 162.
36. A. E. Dennard and R. J. P. Williams, *in*: "Transition Metal Chemistry", Vol. 2 (ed. R. L. Carlin) (1966). Dekker, New York.
37. M. Swarc, *Accounts Chem. Res.* (1969) **2**, 87.
38. J. H. B. George, *J. Amer. Chem. Soc.* (1959) **81**, 5530.
39. L. Pauling, "The Nature of the Chemical Bond" (1960). Cornell University Press, Ithaca, New York.
40. H. G. Bungdenburg de Jong, *in*: "Colloid Science", Vol. II (ed. H. R. Kruyt) (1949). Elsevier, New York.
41. H. F. Fisher, *Biochim. Biophys. Acta* (1965) **109**, 544.
42. H. B. Bull, *J. Amer. Chem. Soc.* (1944) **66**, 1499.
43. H. B. Bull and K. Breese, *Arch. Biochem. Biophys.* (1968) **128**, 488.
44. G. G. Hammes and T. B. Lewis, *J. Phys. Chem.* (1966) **70**, 1648.
45. G. G. Hammes and W. Knoche, *J. Chem. Phys.* (1966) **45**, 4041.
46. A. Odajima, J. Sohma and S. Watanabe, *J. Chem. Phys.* (1959) **31**, 276.
47. J. A. Glasel, *Proc. Nat. Acad. Sci. U.S.A.* (1967) **58**, 27.
48. F. W. Cope, *Biophys. J.* (1969) **9**, 303.
49. T. J. Swift and O. G. Fritz, Jr., *Biophys. J.* (1969) **9**, 54.
50. M. E. Fuller, II and W. S. Brey, Jr., *J. Biol. Chem.* (1968) **243**, 274.
51. W. S. Brey, Jr., T. G. Evans and L. H. Hitzrot, *J. Colloid. Interface Sci.* (1968) **26**, 306.
52. I. D. Kuntz, Jr., T. S. Brassfield, G. D. Law and G. V. Purcell, *Science, N.Y.* (1969) **163**, 1329.
53. R. J. Scheuplein and L. J. Morgan, *Nature (London)* (1967) **214**, 456.
54. G. N. Ling, *Ann. N.Y. Acad. Sci.* (1965) **125**, 401.
55. G. N. Ling, *Int. Rev. Cytol.* (1969) **26**, 1.
56. F. W. Cope, *Biophys. J.* (1969) **9**, 303.
57. F. Franks and D. J. G. Ives, *Quart. Rev. Chem. Soc.* (1966) **20**, 1.
58. J. A. V. Butler, *Trans. Faraday Soc.* (1937) **33**, 229.
59. D. D. Eley, *Trans. Faraday Soc.* (1939) **35**, 1281, 1421.
60. H. S. Frank and M. W. Evans, *J. Chem. Phys.* (1945) **13**, 507.
61. G. Némethy and H. A. Scheraga, *J. Chem. Phys.* (1962) **36**, 3382, 3401; *J. Phys. Chem.* (1962) **66**, 1773.
62. H. A. Scheraga, *in*: "The Proteins", Vol. I, 477, (ed. H. Neurath) (1963). Academic Press, New York and London.
63. W. Kauzmann, *Advan. Protein Chem.* (1959) **14**, 1.
64. R. W. Gurney, "Ionic Processes in Solution", p. 90 (1953). Wiley, New York.
65. D. L. Fowler, W. V. Loebenstein, D. B. Pall and C. A. Kraus, *J. Amer. Chem. Soc.* (1940) **62**, 1140.

66. G. Beurskens, G. A. Jeffrey and R. K. McMullan, *J. Chem. Phys.* (1963) **39**, 3311.
67. G. A. Jeffrey, *Accounts. Chem. Res.* (1969) **2**, 344.
68. W-Y. Wen and J. H. Hung, *J. Phys. Chem.* (1970) **74**, 170.
69. W. L. Masterton, *J. Chem. Phys.* (1954) **22**, 1830.
70. S. S. Danyluk and E. S. Gore, *Nature (London)* (1964) **203**, 748.
71. J. Clifford and B. A. Pethica, *Trans. Faraday Soc.* (1964) **60**, 1483.
72. H. G. Hertz and M. D. Zeidler, *Ber. Bunsenges. Phys. Chem.* (1964) **68**, 821.
73. H. G. Hertz and M. D. Zeidler, *Ber. Bunsenges. Phys. Chem.* (1964) **68**, 824.
74. H. G. Hertz, *Ber. Bunsenges. Phys. Chem.* (1964) **68**, 907.
75. J. Cerbon, *Biochim. Biophys. Acta* (1967) **144**, 1.
76. E. Grunwald and E. K. Ralph, III, *J. Amer. Chem. Soc.* (1967) **89**, 4405.
77. J. J. Kozak, W. S. Knight and W. Kauzmann, *J. Chem. Phys.* (1968) **48**, 675.
78. E. J. Cohn and J. T. Edsall, "Proteins, Amino Acids and Peptides", Ch. 9 (1943). Reinhold Publishing Corp., New York.
79. C. Tanford, *J. Amer. Chem. Soc.* (1962) **84**, 4240.
80. K. Kinoshita, H. Ishikawa and K. Shinoda, *Bull. Chem. Soc. Jap.* (1958) **31**, 1081.
81. C. McAuliffe, *Nature (London)* (1963) **200**, 1092.
82. P. Mukerjee, *J. Phys. Chem.* (1965) **69**, 2821.
83. A. Wishnia, *Biochemistry* (1969) **8**, 5064, 5070.
84. C. Hansch and S. M. Anderson, *J. Org. Chem.* (1969) **32**, 2583.
85. C. Hansch, J. E. Quinlan and G. L. Lawrence, *J. Org. Chem.* (1968) **33**, 347.
86. P. Mukerjee, *Advan. Colloid Interface Sci.* (1967) **1**, 241.
87. E. D. Goddard, C. A. J. Hoeve and G. C. Benson, *J. Phys. Chem.* (1957) **61**, 593.
88. J. M. Corkill, J. F. Goodman and S. P. Harrold, *Trans. Faraday Soc.* (1963) **60**, 202.
89. P. Molyneux, C. T. Rhodes and J. Swarbrick, *Trans. Faraday Soc.* (1964) **61**, 1043.
90. N. Muller and R. H. Birkhahn, *J. Phys. Chem.* (1967) **71**, 957.
91. L. Stryer, *Annu. Rev. Biochem.* (1968) **37**, 25.
92. C. Tanford, *Advan. Protein Chem.* (1968) **23**, 121.
93. C. Tanford, P. K. De and V. G. Taggart, *J. Amer. Chem. Soc.* (1960) **82**, 6028.
94. D. Kotelchuck and H. A. Scheraga, *Proc. Nat. Acad. Sci. U.S.A.* (1969) **62**, 14.
95. G. N. Ramachandran and V. Sasisekharan, *Advan. Protein Chem.* (1968) **23**, 283.
96. H. A. Scheraga, *Advan. Phys. Org. Chem.* (1968) **6**, 103.
97. I. M. Klotz and J. S. Franzen, *J. Amer. Chem. Soc.* (1962) **84**, 3461.
98. G. C. Kresheck and I. M. Klotz, *Biochemistry* (1969) **8**, 8.
99. M. Bixon, H. A. Scheraga and S. Lifson, *Biopolymers* (1963) **1**, 419.
100. H. E. Auer and P. Doty, *Biochemistry* (1966) **5**, 1716.
101. S. R. Chaudhuri and J. T. Yang, *Biochemistry* (1968) **5**, 1379.
102. G. Blauer and Z. B. Alfassi, *Biochim. Biophys. Acta* (1967) **133**, 206.
103. B. Davidson and G. D. Fasman, *Biochemistry* (1967) **6**, 1616.
104. J. T. Edsall, *in*: "Structural Chemistry and Biology" (eds. A. Rich and N. Davidson) (1968). W. H. Freeman, San Francisco.
105. H. F. Fisher, *Proc. Nat. Acad. Sci. U.S.A.* (1964) **51**, 1285.
106. M. F. Perutz, H. Muirhead, J. M. Cox and L. C. G. Goamann, *Nature (London)* (1968) **219**, 131.

107. F. J. Reithel, *Advan. Protein Chem.* (1963) **18**, 123.
108. C. L. Stevens and M. A. Lauffer, *Biochemistry* (1965) **4**, 37.
109. K. E. Van Holde and L. B. Cohen, *Biochemistry* (1964) **3**, 1803.
110. D. Kotelchuck and H. A. Scheraga, *Proc. Nat. Acad. Sci. U.S.A.* (1969) **62**, 14.
111. T. Ikkai and T. Ooi, *Biochemistry* (1966) **5**, 1551.
112. M. A. Stein and W. C. Deal, Jr., *Biochemistry* (1966) **5**, 1399.
113. L. W. Nichol and A. B. Ray, *Biochemistry* (1966) **5**, 1379.
114. D. L. D. Caspar, *Advan. Protein Chem.* (1963) **18**, 37.
115. P. Molyneux and H. P. Frank, *J. Amer. Chem. Soc.* (1961) **83**, 3169.
116. J. E. Leffler, *J. Org. Chem.* (1955) **20**, 1202.
117. J. E. Leffler and E. Grunwald, "Rates and Equilibria of Organic Reactions" (1963). Wiley, New York.
118. R. P. Bell, *Trans. Faraday Soc.* (1937) **33**, 496.
119. M. G. Evans and M. Polanyi, *Trans. Faraday Soc.* (1936) **32**, 1333.
120. J. A. V. Butler, *Trans. Faraday Soc.* (1937) **33**, 229.
121. J. A. V. Butler, "Chemical Thermodynamics", Fifth Edition (1962). Macmillan, London.
122. I. M. Barclay and J. A. V. Butler, *Trans. Faraday Soc.* (1938) **34**, 1445.
123. J. A. V. Butler and W. S. Reid, *J. Chem. Soc.* (1936) 1171.
124. W. F. Claussen and M. F. Polglase, *J. Amer. Chem. Soc.* (1952) **74**, 4817.
125. R. J. L. Andon, J. D. Cox and E. F. G. Herington, *J. Chem. Soc.* (1954) 3188.
126. R. E. Robertson, R. L. Heppolette and J. M. W. Scott, *Can. J. Chem.* (1959) **37**, 803.
127. R. F. Brown, *J. Org. Chem.* (1962) **27**, 3015.
128. J. W. Larson and L. G. Hepler, *in*: "Solute–Solvent Interactions", (eds. J. F. Coetzee and C. D. Ritchie) (1969). Dekker, New York.
129. L. G. Hepler and W. F. O'Hara, *J. Amer. Chem. Soc.* (1961) **65**, 811.
130. L. G. Hepler, *J. Amer. Chem. Soc.* (1963) **85**, 3089.
131. K. S. Pitzer, *J. Amer. Chem. Soc.* (1937) **59**, 2365.
132. D. J. G. Ives and P. D. Marsden, *J. Chem. Soc.* (1965) 649.
133. R. L. Schowen, *J. Pharm. Soc.* (1967) **56**, 931.
134. R. Lumry and H. Eyring, *J. Phys. Chem.* (1954) **58**, 110.
135. R. Lumry and R. Biltonen, *in*: "Structure and Stability of Biological Macromolecules" (eds. S. N. Timasheff and G. D. Fasman) (1969). Dekker, New York.
136. J. F. Brandts and L. Hunt, *J. Amer. Chem. Soc.* (1967) **89**, 4826.
137. G. Likhtenshtein, *Biofizika* (1966) **11**, 24.
138. W. Good, *Nature (London)* (1967) **214**, 1250.
138a. M. F. Goldman and W. Good, *Biochim. Biophys. Acta* (1968) **150**, 194, 206.
139. B. Belleau and J. L. Lavoie, *Can. J. Biochem.* (1968) **46**, 1397.
140. J. F. Brandts, *in*: "Structure and Stability of Biological Macromolecules" (eds. S. N. Timasheff and G. D. Fasman) (1969). Dekker, New York.
141. P. H. von Hippel and K-Y. Wong, *J. Biol. Chem.* (1965) **240**, 3909.
142. P. H. von Hippel and K-Y. Wong, *in*: "Structure and Stability of Biological Macromolecules" (eds. S. N. Timasheff and G. D. Fasman) (1969). Dekker, New York.
143. E. E. Schrier, R. T. Ingwall and H. A. Scheraga, *J. Phys. Chem.* (1965) **69**, 298.
144. H. H. Jaffé, *Chem. Rev.* (1953) **53**, 191.

145. R. W. Taft, *in*: "Steric Effects in Organic Chemistry" (ed. M. S. Newman) (1956). Wiley, New York, N.Y.

146. C. D. Ritchie and W. F. Sagar, *Phys. Org. Chem.* (1964) **2**, 323.

147. P. R. Wells, "Linear Free Energy Relationships" (1969). Academic Press, New York and London.

148. J. Shorter, *Chem. Brit.* (1969) 269.

149. M. Charton, *J. Amer. Chem. Soc.* (1969) **91**, 624.

150. C. Hansch, *Accounts, Chem. Res.* (1969) **2**, 232.

151. C. Hansch, *in*: "Drug Design" (ed. E. J. Ariens) Vol. I (1970). Academic Press, New York and London.

152. C. Hansch and T. Fujita, *J. Amer. Chem. Soc.* (1964) **86**, 1616.

153. T. Fujita, J. Iwasa and C. Hansch, *J. Amer. Chem. Soc.* (1964) **86**, 5175.

154. C. Hansch, *Annu. Rep. Med. Chem.* (1966) 347; *Annu. Rep. Med. Chem.* (1967) 348.

155. C. Hansch, *Il Farmaco, Ed. Sci.* (1968) **23**, 293.

156. C. Hansch, *in*: "Proceedings Third International Pharmacological Meeting", Vol. 7 (ed. E. J. Ariëns) (1968). Pergamon Press, London.

157. H. Meyer, *Arch. Exp. Pathol. Pharmakol.* (1899) **42**, 109.

158. E. Overton, *Vierteljahrsschr. Naturforsch. Ges. Zürich* (1899) **44**, 88.

159. E. Overton, "Studien uber die Narkose" (1901) Fischer, Jena, Germany.

160. R. B. Hermann, H. W. Culp, R. E. McMahon and M. M. Marsh, *J. Med. Chem.* (1969) **12**, 749.

161. C. Hansch and E. W. Deutsch, *Biochim. Biophys. Acta* (1966) **126**, 117.

162. C. Hansch, E. W. Deutsch and R. N. Smith, *J. Amer. Chem. Soc.* (1965) **87**, 2738.

163. C. Hansch and F. Helmer, *J. Polym. Sci.* (1968) **6A**, 3295.

164. C. Hansch, K. Kiehs and G. Lawrence, *J. Amer. Chem. Soc.* (1965) **87**, 5770.

165. C. Tanford, *Advan. Protein Chem.* (1962) **17**, 69.

166. C. Tanford, "The Physical Chemistry of Macromolecules" (1961). Wiley, New York.

167. J. Steinhardt and S. Beychok, *in*: "Protein Chemistry", Vol. II, p. 139 (ed. H. Neurath) (1963). Academic Press, New York and London.

168. G. Némethy, I. Z. Steinberg and H. A. Scheraga, *Biopolymers* (1963) **1**, 43.

169. J. T. Edsall, *in*: "Aspects of Protein Structure", p. 179 (ed. G. N. Ramachandran) (1963). Academic Press, New York and London.

170. M. Laskowski, Jr., *Fed. Proc. Fed. Amer. Soc. Exp. Biol.* (1966) **25**, 20.

171. M. J. Gorbinoff, *Biochemistry* (1968) **7**, 2547.

172. R. B. Scheele and M. A. Lauffer, *Biochemistry* (1967) **6**, 3076.

173. E. Mihalyi, *Biochemistry* (1968) **7**, 208.

174. C. Tanford and J. G. Kirkwood, *J. Amer. Chem. Soc.* (1957) **79**, 5333.

175. H. A. Scheraga, *J. Phys. Chem.* (1961) **65**, 1071.

176. J. A. Schellman, *J. Phys. Chem.* (1953) **57**, 472.

177. C. C. F. Blake, L. N. Johnson, G. A. Mair, A. C. T. North, D. C. Phillips and V. R. Sarma, *Proc. Roy. Soc. London B* (1967) **167**, 378.

178. C. A. Vernon, *Proc. Roy. Soc. London B* (1967) **167**, 389.

179. D. M. Blow, J. J. Birktoft and B. S. Hartley, *Nature (London)* (1969) **221**, 337.

180. C. S. Wright, R. A. Alden and J. Kraut, *Nature (London)* (1969) **221**, 235.

181. B. S. Hartley and D. M. Shotton, quoted in Ref. 179.

182. M. L. Ludwig, J. A. Hartsuck, T. A. Steitz, H. Muirhead, J. C. Coppola, G. N. Reeke and W. N. Lipscomb, *Proc. Nat. Acad. Sci. U.S.A.* (1967) **57**, 511.
183. M. E. Riepe and J. H. Wang, *J. Amer. Chem. Soc.* (1967) **89**, 4229; *J. Biol. Chem.* (1968) **243**, 2779.
184. R. L. Snell, W.-K. Kwok and Y. Kim, *J. Amer. Chem. Soc.* (1967) **89**, 6728.
185. B. L. Vallee and R. J. P. Williams, *Chem. Brit.* (1968) 397.
186. M. Dixon and E. C. Webb, "Enzymes", pp. 226, 243. Second Ed. (1964). Academic Press, New York and London.
187. J. L. Webb, "Enzymes and Metabolic Inhibitors", Vol. II, p. 368 (1966). Academic Press, New York and London.
188. G. E. Hein and C. Niemann, *J. Amer. Chem. Soc.* (1962) **84**, 4495.
189. J. B. Jones, C. Niemann and G. E. Hein, *Biochemistry* (1965) **4**, 1735.
190. G. E. Hein and C. Niemann, *Proc. Nat. Acad. Sci. U.S.A.* (1962) **47**, 1341.
191. B. R. Baker, "Design of Active Site Directed Irreversible Inhibitors", p. 48 (1968). Wiley, New York.
192. Y. Hayashi and W. B. Lawson, *J. Biol. Chem.* (1969) **244**, 4158.
193. J. R. Knowles, *J. Theor. Biol.* (1965) **9**, 213.
194. D. W. Ingles and J. R. Knowles, *Biochem. J.* (1967) **104**, 369.
195. D. W. Ingles and J. R. Knowles, *Biochem. J.* (1968) **108**, 561.
196. K. G. Brandt, A. Himoe and G. P. Hess, *J. Biol. Chem.* (1967) **242**, 3973.
197. A. J. Hymes, D. A. Robinson and W. J. Canady, *J. Biol. Chem.* (1965) **240**, 134.
198. R. Wildnauer and W. J. Canady, *Biochemistry* (1966) **5**, 2885.
199. A. J. Hymes, C. C. Coppett and W. J. Canady, *J. Biol. Chem.* (1969) **244**, 637.
200. B. H. J. Hofstee, *Nature (London)* (1967) **213**, 42.
201. C. Gitler and A. Ochoa-Solano, *J. Amer. Chem. Soc.* (1968) **90**, 5004.
202. M.-A. Coletti-Previero, A. Previero and E. Zuckerkandl, *J. Mol. Biol.* (1969) **39**, 493.
203. G. Royer and W. J. Canady, *Arch. Biochem. Biophys.* (1968) **124**, 530.
204. E. Fischer, *Chem. Ber.* (1894) **27**, 2985.
205. D. E. Koshland, *Proc. Nat. Acad. Sci. U.S.A.* (1958) **44**, 98.
206. D. E. Koshland, *J. Cell. Comp. Physiol.* (1959) **54**, Suppl. 1, 245.
207. D. E. Koshland, *Fed. Proc. Fed. Amer. Soc. Exp. Biol.* (1964) **23**, 719.
208. D. E. Koshland, *Proc. 1st Int. Pharmacol. Meet.* (1964) **7**, Pergamon, New York.
209. D. E. Koshland and K. E. Neet, *Annu. Rev. Biochem.* (1968) **37**, 359.
210. J. A. Yankeelov and D. E. Koshland, *J. Biol. Chem.* (1965) **240**, 1593.
211. W. J. O'Sullivan and M. Cohn, *J. Biol. Chem.* (1966) **241**, 3116.
212. A. H. Mehler and M. E. Cusic, *Science, N.Y.* (1967) **155**, 1101.
213. R. C. Adelman, D. E. Morse, W. Chan and B. L. Horecker, *Arch. Biochem. Biophys.* (1968) **126**, 343.
214. D. E. Morse and B. L. Horecker, *Advan. Enzymol.* (1968) **31**, 125.
215. M. DeLuca and M. Marsh, *Arch. Biochem. Biophys.* (1967) **121**, 233.
216. M. Eigen and G. G. Hammes, *Advan. Enzymol.* (1963) **25**, 1.
217. G. G. Hammes, *Advan. Protein Chem.* (1968) **23**, 1.
218. G. G. Hammes, *Accounts Chem. Res.* (1968) **1**, 321.
219. T. A. Steitz, M. L. Ludwig, F. A. Quiocho and W. N. Lipscomb, *J. Biol. Chem.* (1967) **242**, 4662.

220. T. Inagami, *J. Biol. Chem.* (1964) **239**, 787, 1395; (1965) **240**, 3435; *Biochemistry* (1968) **7**, 4045.

221. I. B. Wilson, *in*: "The Enzymes", Vol. I (1960). Academic Press, New York and London.

222. J. A. Cohen and R. A. Oosterbaan, *in*: "Handbuch Der Experimentellen Pharmakologie", Vol. 15, Ch. 7 (ed. G. B. Koelle) (1963). Springer-Verlag, Berlin.

223. N. Engelhard, K. Prchal and M. Nenner, *Angew Chem. Int. Ed. Engl.* (1967) **6**, 615.

224. R. M. Krupka, *Biochemistry* (1964) **3**, 1749.

225. B. Holmstedt, *in*: "Handbuch Der Experimentellen Pharmakologie", Vol. 15, Ch. 9 (ed. G. B. Koelle) (1963). Springer-Verlag, Berlin.

226. R. D. O'Brien, *in*: "Molecular Pharmacology", Vol. 3 (ed. E. J. Ariëns) (1970). Academic Press, New York and London.

227. I. B. Wilson, *in*: "Drugs Affecting the Peripheral Nervous System", Vol. I, Ch. 7 (ed. A. Burger) (1967). Dekker, New York.

228. R. J. Kitz and I. B. Wilson, *J. Biol. Chem.* (1962) **237**, 3245.

229. J. Alexander, I. B. Wilson and R. J. Kitz, *J. Biol. Chem.* (1963) **238**, 741.

230. R. M. Krupka, *Biochemistry* (1966) **5**, 1988.

231. R. J. Kitz and I. B. Wilson, *J. Biol. Chem.* (1963) **238**, 745.

232. H. P. Metzger and I. B. Wilson, *J. Biol. Chem.* (1963) **238**, 3432.

233. I. B. Wilson, *Ann. N.Y. Acad. Sci.* (1967) **144**, 664.

234. R. J. Kitz, S. Ginsburg and I. B. Wilson, *Mol. Pharmacol.* (1967) **3**, 225.

235. H. P. Metzger and I. B. Wilson, *Biochem. Biophys. Res. Commun.* (1967) **28**, 263.

236. R. J. Kitz and L. T. Kremzner, *Mol. Pharmacol.* (1968) **4**, 104.

237. R. M. Krupka, *Biochemistry* (1967) **6**, 1183.

238. *Advan. Protein Chem.* (1964) **19**.

239. A. V. Hill, *J. Physiol.* (1910) **40**, IV.

240. W. E. L. Brown and A. V. Hill, *Proc. Roy. Soc. London* B (1922) **XCIV**, 297.

241. D. E. Atkinson, J. A. Hathaway and E. C. Smith, *J. Biol. Chem.* (1965) **240**, 2682.

242. H. Muirhead and M. F. Perutz, *Nature (London)* (1963) **199**, 633.

243. M. F. Perutz, W. Bolton, R. Diamond, H. Muirhead and H. C. Watson, *Nature (London)* (1964) **203**, 687.

244. H. Muirhead, J. M. Cox, L. Mazzarella and M. F. Perutz, *J. Mol. Biol.* (1967) **28**, 117.

245. W. Bolton, J. M. Cox and M. F. Perutz, *J. Mol. Biol.* (1968) **33**, 283.

246. M. F. Perutz, *Proc. Roy. Soc. London* B (1969) **173**, 113.

247. W. A. Wood, *Curr. Top. Cell. Reg.* (1969) **I**, 161.

248. D. E. Atkinson, *Ann. Rev. Biochem.* (1966) **35**, 85.

249. E. R. Stadtman, *Advan. Enzymol.* (1966) **28**, 41.

250. H. R. Mahler and E. H. Cordes, "Biological Chemistry" (1966). Harper and Row, New York.

251. J. Monod, J. P. Changeux and F. Jacob, *J. Mol. Biol.* (1963) **6**, 306.

252. D. E. Koshland, and K. E. Neet, *Ann. Rev. Biochem.* (1968) **37**, 362.

253. J. C. Gerhart and A. B. Pardee, *J. Biol. Chem.* (1962) **237**, 891.

254. J. C. Gerhart and H. K. Schachman, *Biochemistry* (1965) **4**, 1054.

255. J. C. Gerhart and H. Holoubek, *J. Biol. Chem.* (1967) **242**, 2886.

256. J.-P. Changeux, J. C. Gerhart and H. K. Schachman, *Biochemistry* (1968) **7**, 531.

257. D. C. Wiley and W. N. Lipscomb, *Nature (London)* (1968) **218**, 1119.

258. K. Weber, *Nature (London)* (1968) **218**, 1116.
259. J. C. Gerhart and H. K. Schachman, *Biochemistry* (1968) **7**, 538.
260. J. Wyman, *Quart. Rev. Biophys.* (1968) **1**, 35.
261. M. F. Perutz, J. C. Kendrew and H. C. Watson, *J. Mol. Biol.* (1965) **13**, 669.
262. M. F. Perutz and H. Lehmanin, *Nature (London)* (1968) **219**, 902.
263. C. Nolan and E. Margoliash, *Ann. Rev. Biochem.* (1968) **37**, 727.
264. F. Haurowitz, *Z. Physiol. Chem.* (1938) **254**, 266.
265. J. Wyman, *Advan. Protein Chem.* (1964) **19**, 224.
266. R. E. Benesch and R. Benesch, *Biochemistry* (1962) **1**, 735.
267. G. Guidotti, *J. Biol. Chem.* (1967) **242**, 3673.
268. R. Zito, E. Antonini and J. Wyman, *J. Biol. Chem.* (1964) **239**, 1804.
269. E. Antonini, J. Wyman, R. Moretti and A. Rossi-Fanelli, *Biochim. Biophys. Acta* (1963) **71**, 124.
269a. M. F. Perutz, H. Muirhead, L. Mazzarella, R. A. Crowther, J. Greer and J. V. Kilmartin, *Nature (London)* (1969) **222**, 1240.
270. S. R. Simon, W. H. Konigsberg, W. Bolton and M. F. Perutz, *J. Mol. Biol.* (1967) **28**, 451.
271. D. E. Atkinson, *Ann. Rev. Biochem.* (1966) **35**, 85.
272. J.-P. Changeux, *Brookhaven Symp. Biol.* (1964) **17**, 232.
273. J. Monod, J. Wyman and J.-P. Changeux, *J. Mol. Biol.* (1965) **12**, 88.
274. J.-P. Changeux, *Cold Spring Harbor Symp. Quant. Biol.* (1963) **28**, 497.
275. J.-P. Changeux, *J. Mol. Biol.* (1962) **4**, 220.
276. D. Blangy, H. Buc and J. Monod, *J. Mol. Biol.* (1968) **31**, 13.
277. K. Taketa and B. M. Pogell, *J. Biol. Chem.* (1965) **240**, 651.
278. S. R. Simon, W. H. Konigsberg, W. Bolton and M. F. Perutz, *J. Mol. Biol.* (1967) **28**, 451.
279. E. Scarano, G. Geraci, A. Polzella and E. Campanile, *J. Biol. Chem.* (1963) **238**, 1556.
280. E. Scarano, G. Geraci and M. Rossi, *Biochem. Biophys. Res. Commun.* (1964) **16**, 239.
281. D. Blangy, H. Buc and J. Monod, *J. Mol. Biol.* (1968) **31**, 13.
282. J. Wyman, *Advan. Protein Chem.* (1964) **19**, 223.
283. J. Wyman, *J. Amer. Chem. Soc.* (1967) **89**, 2202.
284. M. M. Rubin and J. P. Changeux, *J. Mol. Biol.* (1966) **21**, 265.
285. C. Frieden, *in*: "Regulation of Enzyme Activity and Allosteric Interactions", p. 59, Proceedings of Fourth Federation of European Biochemical Societies, Oslo, July, 1967 (1968). Academic Press, New York and London.
286. C. Frieden and R. Colman, *J. Biol. Chem.* (1967) **242**, 1705.
287. B. Metzger, E. Helmreich and L. Glaser, *Proc. Nat. Acad. Sci. U.S.A.* (1967) **57**, 994.
288. D. E. Koshland, G. Némethy and D. Filmer, *Biochemistry* (1966) **5**, 365.
289. D. E. Koshland, and M. E. Kirtley, *in*: "International Symposium Enzymatic Aspects of Metabolic Regulation" (ed. M. P. Stulberg) (1967). National Cancer Institute Monograph. No. 27. U.S. Dept. of Health, Education and Welfare.
290. J. E. Haber and D. E. Koshland, *Proc. Nat. Acad. Sci. U.S.A.* (1967) **58**, 2087.
291. M. E. Kirtley and D. E. Koshland, *J. Biol. Chem.* (1967) **242**, 4192.
292. A. Conway and D. E. Koshland, *Biochemistry* (1968) **7**, 4011.
293. A. Levitzki and D. E. Koshland, *Proc. Nat. Acad. Sci. U.S.A.* (1969) **62**, 1121.

294. D. E. Atkinson and G. M. Walton, *J. Biol. Chem.* (1965) **240**, 757.
295. D. E. Atkinson, *Biochemistry* (1968) **7**, 4030.
296. B. D. Sanwal, C. S. Stachow and R. A. Cook, *Biochemistry* (1965) **4**, 410.
297. K. Kirschner, M. Eigen, R. Bittman and B. Voigt, *Proc. Nat. Acad. Sci. U.S.A.* (1966) **56**, 1661.
298. M. Eigen, *Quart. Rev. Biophys.* (1968) **1**, 1.
299. S. Ogawa and H. M. McConnell, *Proc. Nat. Acad. Sci. U.S.A.* (1967) **58**, 19.
300. C. L. Hamilton and H. M. McConnell *in*: "Structural Chemistry and Molecular Biology" (eds. A. Rich and N. Davidson) (1968). Freeman, San Francisco.
301. D. K. McClintock and G. Markus, *J. Biol. Chem.* (1968) **243**, 2855.
302. J. P. Changeux and M. M. Rubin, *Biochemistry* (1968) **7**, 553.
303. D. K. McClintock and G. Markus, *J. Biol. Chem.* (1969) **244**, 36.
304. R. W. Noble, *J. Mol. Biol.* (1969) **39**, 479.
305. R. G. Shulman, S. Ogawa, K. Wüthrich, T. Yamane, J. Peisach and W. E. Blumberg, *Science N.Y.* (1969) **165**, 251.
306. S. Ogawa, H. M. McConnell and A. Horwitz, *Proc. Nat. Acad. Sci. U.S.A.* (1968) **61**, 401.
307. E. Antonini and M. Brunori, *Fed. Proc. Fed. Amer. Soc. Exp. Biol.* (1969) **28**, 603.
308. K. Dalziel, *Acta Chem. Scand.* (1957) **11**, 1706.
309. W. Ferdinand, *Biochem. J.* (1966) **98**, 278.
310. R. A. Cook and D. E. Koshland, *Proc. Nat. Acad. Sci. U.S.A.* (1969) **64**, 247.

Chapter II

THE CELL MEMBRANE

Introduction

From the previous discussion of molecular interactions and regulatory phenomena existing in isolated macromolecules attention must now be turned to a consideration of their role in a complex macromolecular assembly—the excitable cell membrane—that represents the primary site of action at which the physiological effects of neurotransmitter molecules (and many related agents) are initiated. Unfortunately attempts to elucidate the structure(s) of cell membranes have not, despite considerable effort, yielded any totally satisfactory general concept. Similarly, the elucidation of the structure, function and mechanisms of integration with the general cell machinery of those highly specialized areas involved in transport, chemical excitation, etc. remains in general to be achieved. Nevertheless, because the regulatory properties of macromolecular assemblies are themselves intrinsic properties of the structure and organization of the component macromolecules (Chapter I) significant discussion of such events as neurotransmitter action must relate inevitably to membrane organization.

The General Structure and Composition of Cell Membranes

The most widely accepted concept of membrane structure has been essentially that proposed by Danielli and Davson (1, 2) in which cell membranes are conceived to be a thin film of lipid molecules with their polar heads directed outwards and covered by a layer of protein (Fig. II-1). Danielli and Davson were not able originally to specify the number of lipid layers present in this structure although Gorter and Grendel (3), some ten years previously, had provided some evidence from a determination of the extracted lipid film area : cell area of red blood cells that these membranes contained a single bimolecular lipid leaflet. However, the heuristic value of the Danielli–Davson model lies in its recognition of the properties of the lipid bimolecular leaflet and the prediction of the important role played by protein at the cell membrane surface.

This concept of the cell membrane has formed the foundation of the unit membrane hypothesis as elaborated by Robertson (4–7) in which membranes are supposed to share a basic structural design, that of the lipid bilayer. The unit membrane hypothesis is supported primarily by X-ray and electron microscopic data. The unit membrane is proposed to consist of a single bimolecular lipid leaflet covered with protein or other non-lipid layers: as in the Danielli–Davson model it is implicit that the lipid bimolecular leaflet determines the essential structural characteristics of the membrane and that the lipid and protein layers

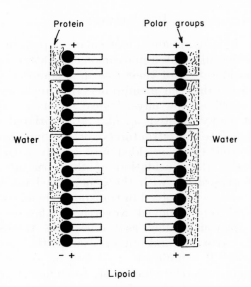

FIG. II-1. The Danielli–Davson lipid bilayer representation of the cell membrane. Reproduced with permission from "Permeability of Natural Membranes", Cambridge University Press.

are essentially distinct entities although the possibility of a certain amount of lipid–protein intercalation at specialized areas is not ignored in this model.

Much of the experimental evidence adduced in favor of the unit membrane hypothesis is derived from studies on myelin, the primarily lipid multilayered material that envelops many nerves. As depicted in Fig. II-2, the myelin sheath is formed from a repetitive envelopment of the axon by the Schwann cell membrane (8), the repeating pattern so formed being highly amenable to X-ray diffraction analysis. The original X-ray data of Schmitt (9, 10), confirmed and extended by Finean (11–13), demonstrated the presence in mammalian peripheral nerve of a radially oriented 180–185 Å repeating unit: this was interpreted as two bi-molecular lipid leaflets and associated protein structures—the basic repeat pattern being that of one lipid leaflet. By the early 1950's EM studies of OsO_4 and $KMnO_4$ fixed nerve myelin (6, 14–16) had revealed a series of dense lines of 25 Å thickness separated by a gap of some 100–120 Å with a major density line occurring in the latter gap. The compound membrane of the myelin sheath is thus related to the 75 Å triple layered structure of the Schwann cell plasma membrane (Fig. II-3), the major dense line being formed by the fusion of two internal surfaces of the Schwann cell membrane. Since many systems, including plasma, mitochondrial and nuclear membranes reveal a general approximation to the structure observed with myelin it has been proposed that

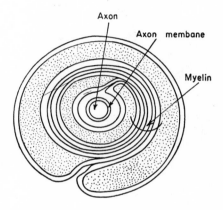

FIG. II-2. The formation of the myelin sheath of the Schwann cell membrane.

this represents a unit structure common to most membranes. The unit membrane basically identical to the structure proposed originally by Danielli and Davson, restricts the lipids to a single bimolecular leaflet and requires that the lipid be considered as a basic structural determinant of the membrane (4–7, 17–21).

Further support for this structure comes from the X-ray diffraction analysis of frog retinal rod outer segments by Blaurock and Wilkins (22). Their data suggest an unhydrated membrane of 55 Å thickness with a central core, 26 Å thick, of phospholipid covered by protein layers.

The state of the proposed central lipid bilayer is probably not that of a closely packed array, but rather that of the liquid state (23, 24) and the hydrocarbon chains must be considerably curled or interdigitated. Hence, the area occupied by one lipid molecule is likely to exceed considerably that occupied in a close packed array (24, 25). In general, little can be said about the surface layers of protein save that their configuration cannot be fully extended and it may be that, because of the relatively loose packing of the lipid molecules, considerable insertion of protein can occur between the hydrophilic head groups (21, 27).

The concept of cell membrane structure as expressed in the Danielli–Davson model has not been universally accepted, particularly in recent years and there now exists a body of evidence to indicate that some cell membranes, or perhaps even substantial areas of all cell membranes, may be constructed on an alternative basis, through the assemblage of discrete lipoprotein repeating units. Assembly according to this principal

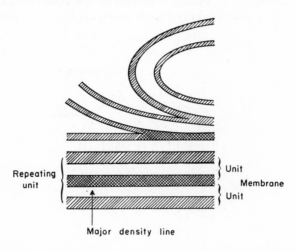

FIG. II-3. Representation of the formation of the triple layered unit membrane of myelin.

will confer upon the resultant membrane two important features—subunit construction and interactions and lipid–protein hydrophobic interactions—that are absent or minimized in the simplest Danielli–Davson model.

This modular construction hypothesis receives support from several lines of evidence including direct observations of repeating unit structure, reinterpretation of existing EM and X-ray evidence, composition and enzymatic activities of membranes, studies of lipid–protein interaction and consideration of the general principles of biological aggregation and organization. These various lines of evidence will be briefly reviewed, within the limitations of the subject matter of the present volume, in an attempt to view their relationship to current models of cell membrane structure.

Some evidence for the existence of membrane substructure is derived from EM studies on mitochondrial membranes. Fernandez-Moran, Green and Smith (28–30) described the existence of a repeating unit on the inner membrane of the mitochondrion: this was originally termed the "elementary particle" but, since it does not contain all of the components of the inner membrane electron transport chain is better referred to as an "inner membrane particle" (21). As originally described this was a tripartite structure (Fig. II-4) with the dimensions indicated: the appearance of the head piece is well documented and has been identified as the mitochondrial ATPase and is a component of the oxidative phosphorylation mechanism but not of the electron transport chain (31).

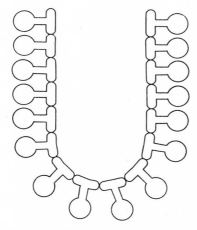

Fig. II-4. Diagrammatic representation of the proposed tripartite elementary particle of the inner mitochondrial membrane.

However, considerable controversy exists about the separate existence of the basepiece unit: according to Green and his co-workers (32–34) the basepieces are lipoprotein complexes which can be dissociated to four complexes of the electron chain (see section on p. 136) and recombined to form a catalytically active membrane as shown in Fig. II-5. Green has proposed that this mode of subunit membrane construction may, in fact, be quite general for the majority of membranes (31–33). For membranes other than those of mitochondria the evidence is, however, substantially more controversial (21).

Sjöstrand has presented EM evidence (17, 35–37) for inner mitochondrial membranes which reveal a distinctly globular appearance to the characteristic dense lines of the unit membrane structure. Similar globular construction has also been observed by Sjöstrand in plasma and endoplasmic reticular membranes, although it cannot be excluded that this apparent evidence for subunit construction is an artifact of the EM technique (21, 38). EM evidence for globular substructure in chloroplast lamellae has been advanced by several workers (40–42) and Moor and Branton (43–46), employing the freeze-etching technique, have described the occurrence of particles averaging *ca.* 85 Å in diameter on many freeze-etched membrane surfaces. Structural units closely resembling those of the inner mitochondrial membrane have also been observed in the membranes of thermopilic bacteria (47): these observations are

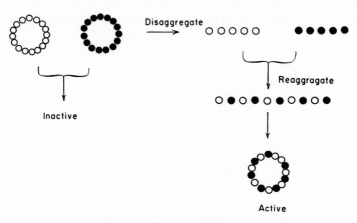

FIG. II-5. Representation of dispersion, mixing and reconstitution of subunits of inner mitochondrial membrane to give functionally active material (○, ● represent two types of subunits).

consistent with findings that the enzyme systems localized on the inner mitochondrial membrane are also those localized on the bacterial cell membrane.

It must, of course, be recognized that evidence for substructure obtained by EM techniques is not accepted by many workers, who prefer to regard such structures as essentially artifactual and produced through the various treatments necessary to prepare specimens for EM examination (48, 49). In this connection the statement by Finean (50) assumes considerable relevance,

Electron microscopy . . . suffers the disadvantage of complex preparative procedures which diffraction studies of myelin show leads to a marked increase in disorder so that the finer detail revealed (or not revealed) becomes of doubtful significance. For instance, the decrease in the number of diffraction orders of the layer spacing that occurs when the myelin sheath is fixed and embedded must reflect either a decrease in the regularity of repetition of the layers or a marked increase in disorder within the individual units. Electron microscopy reveals that the layering remains very orderly and one must therefore suspect that the most significant increases in disorder have occurred within the structural unit.

Criticism has also been offered of the interpretation of the experimental techniques upon which the unit membrane hypothesis is founded. Korn (49) has pointed out that comparatively little is known about the chemistry of the various fixative and staining techniques used in EM. Using evidence from model studies of unsaturated compounds with osmium tetroxide Korn questions whether the dense lines in membranes fixed with this reagent reveal anything about the orientation of the phospholipids in the original membrane. It is most interesting that the triple-layered structure characteristic of the unit membrane is revealed in osmium-fixed mitochondria from which all lipids had previously been removed (50).

It is generally accepted that the width of the triple-layered unit membrane is about 75 Å; nevertheless, it is apparent that there may be very substantial variations in the reported thicknesses of membranes (37, 47) with values of 50–150 Å available (35, 51). Part of this variation may be due to experimental techniques but the possibility of fundamental structural differences is very apparent. It is also to be noted that the use of mild preparative techniques such as negative staining and particularly freeze-etching (43) in which frozen cells are fractured along membrane surfaces and then shadowed has also revealed the existence of the substructures visualized less perfectly in preparations made by more vigorous techniques.

It is quite apparent that the structural studies reported to date have not succeeded in generating a totally satisfactory representation of membrane structure, and it is clear that the original Danielli–Davson model remains, at least from considerations of gross structure, quite consistent with much available data from EM and X-ray studies. However, a number of other approaches are available to complement the direct structural analyses outlined in this section.

COMPOSITION OF CELL MEMBRANES

At the present time, knowledge of the detailed molecular composition of cell membranes cannot serve to describe the corresponding molecular architecture although appropriate comparative studies, currently few in number, may serve to indicate some general features of membrane structure (53–57). One basic problem is that of obtaining pure membrane fractions; progress is being made and membranes have now been obtained from smooth and skeletal muscle, erythrocytes, mitochondria, Ehrlich ascites cells, etc. In the analyses of their composition major emphasis has been placed upon the two principal constituents, lipids and proteins, with comparatively little attention having been paid to the minor constituents. A second problem is that membranes are most unlikely to be homogeneous and thus gross analyses of membrane composition will not reflect local variations in composition that will, insofar as molecular composition determines membrane structure, be of critical significance in determining the activities of enzymatic, permease and receptor functions. Thus, Murphy has shown that the distribution of cholesterol over the erythrocyte membrane is not uniform (58). Nevertheless, within these defined limitations these studies are of value insofar as they may yield information on the *general* organization of membranes.

TABLE II-1. Lipid and Protein Ratios in some Cell Membranes

Species and Tissue		Protein %	Lipid %	Reference
Human	CNS myelin	20	79	53, 59
Bovine	PNS myelin	23	76	53
Rat	Muscle (Skeletal)	65	15	60
Rat	Liver	60	40	61
Human	Erythrocyte	40	40–50	53, 62, 63
Rat	Liver mitochondrion	70	27–29	53, 64, 65

		Molar ratio		Area ratio	
	Amino acid	Phospholipid	Cholesterol	Protein : lipid	Ref.
Myelin	264	111	75	0·43	48, 59
Erythrocyte	500	31	31	2·5	48, 66

In Table II-1 are presented data for the relative amounts of lipid and protein in some cell membranes. Even from this limited data it is apparent that wide variations exist in the lipid : protein ratio. The bottom half of this table presents data which show the relative molar compositions of two cell membranes together with calculated values of the area ratios of protein and lipid. These latter values show that there is insufficient protein in myelin to permit the lipids to be covered with a monomolecular film. This calculation is in good accord with recent X-ray data (67). In contrast there is more than sufficient protein in the erythrocyte membrane to cover a bimolecular lipid leaflet with a protein film. From this type of evidence it appears that myelin may not be characteristic of cell membranes in general, a point that has been explicitly made by Korn (48).

STRUCTURES OF MEMBRANE LIPIDS

Fairly complete lipid analyses are available for a number of membranes and a selection of this data is presented in Table II-2 from which it is apparent that large differences do exist between various membranes (69): this difference is particularly marked between myelin and the mitochondrial membrane and seems clearly related to the marked differences in function of these two membranes. Analyses of other membrane lipids

TABLE II-2. Lipid Composition of Cell Membranes

	Molar % of total lipids			% of total lipids	
	Human CNS myelin (56, 59)	Bovine PNS myelin (53)	Human erythrocyte (53, 62, 63)	Rat liver mitochondria (53, 64, 65)	Rat liver (68)
Phosphatidyl-ethanolamine	13·5	12·5	14·0	27·4	6·0
Phosphatidylserine	5·0	7·0	4·8	trace	3·2
Phosphatidylcholine	11·0	10·0	15·0	43·4	14·3
Phosphatidylinositol	2·0	2·0	3·8	6·7	2·8
Diphosphatidyl-glycerol(cardiolipin)	trace	trace	—	8·5	2·9
Sphingomyelin	4·5	13·0	9·5	4·4	7·2
Other sphingolipids	1·5	—	6·0	—	—
Cerebroside	15·5	11·5	—	—	—
Cerebroside sulfate	4·0	2·0	—	—	—
Phosphatidylglycerol	trace	trace	—	2·6	4·7
Minor lipids	3·1	3·0	5·2	1·1	4·7
Cholesterol	40·0	39·0	42·0	6·0	18·9
Total glycerolipids	34·6	34·5	42·8	89·6	—
Total sphingolipids	25·5	26·5	15·5	4·4	7·2

(Fig. II-6) have been less extensive: the cholesterol:phospholipid molar ratio has been reported as 0·5 in rat uterine membranes (70) and 0·9, 0·46, 0·26, 0·51 and 0·11 for rat erythrocyte, intestinal microvilli, liver cell, brain mitochondria and liver mitochondria respectively (71).

Some consideration of the composition of the lipid acyl moieties is also of general relevance. Myelin lipids are rich in long and medium chain length fatty acids (53, 59); erythrocyte lipids from various species contain as dominant materials the C_{16} and C_{18} saturated, the C_{18} with one and two double bonds and the C_{20} acid with four double bonds (53, 57), although their distribution is not constant among the various classes

6

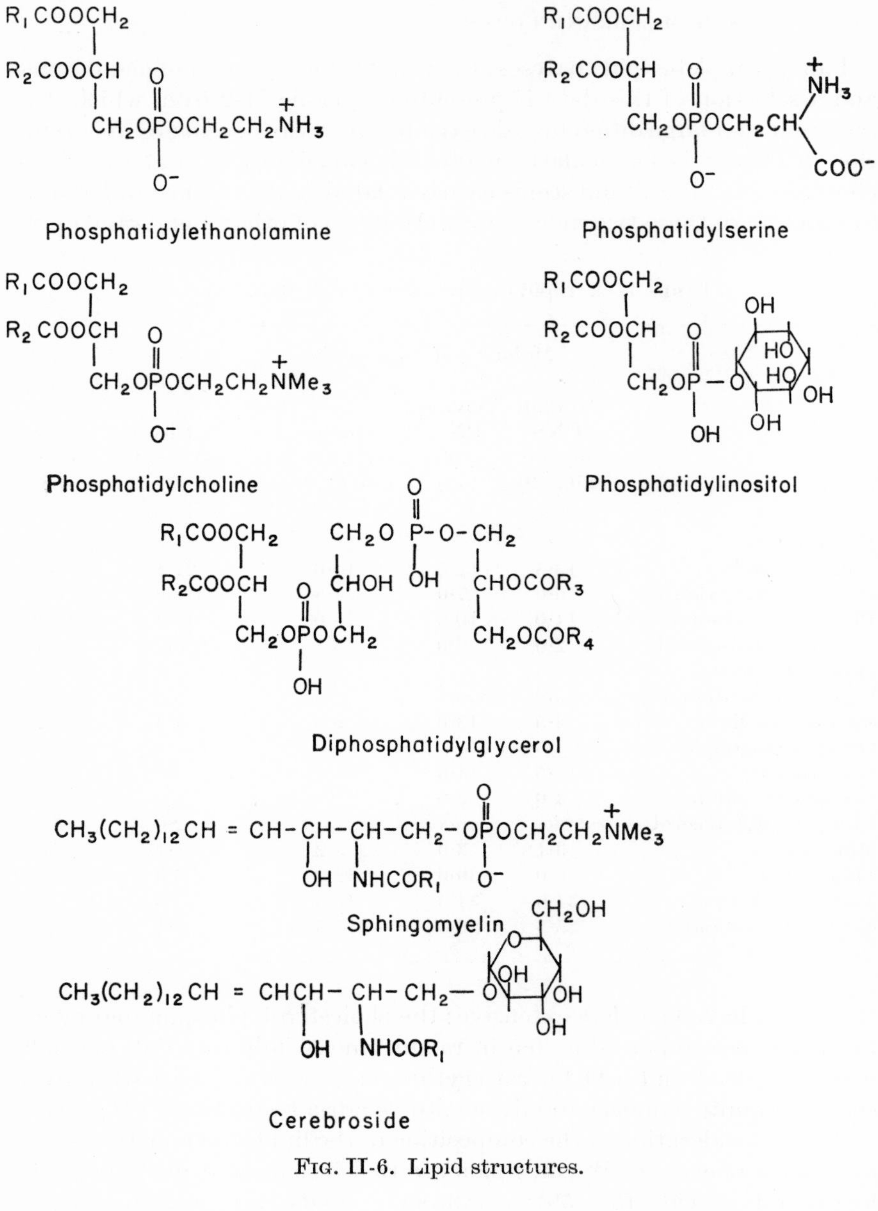

R_1COOCH_2

R_2COOCH

$CH_2OPOCH_2CH_2\overset{+}{N}H_3$

Phosphatidylethanolamine

R_1COOCH_2

R_2COOCH

$CH_2OPOCH_2\overset{+}{C}H$

Phosphatidylserine

R_1COOCH_2

R_2COOCH

$CH_2OPOCH_2CH_2\overset{+}{N}Me_3$

Phosphatidylcholine

R_1COOCH_2

R_2COOCH

CH_2OP-O

Phosphatidylinositol

$R_1COOCH_2 \quad CH_2O \quad P-O-CH_2$

$R_2COOCH \quad CHOH \quad CHOCOR_3$

$CH_2OPOCH_2 \quad CH_2OCOR_4$

Diphosphatidylglycerol

$CH_3(CH_2)_{12}CH = CH-CH-CH-CH_2-OPOCH_2CH_2\overset{+}{N}Me_3$

OH NHCOR$_1$

Sphingomyelin

$CH_3(CH_2)_{12}CH = CHCH-CH-CH_2-O$

OH NHCOR$_1$

Cerebroside

FIG. II-6. Lipid structures.

of phospholipids or from phospholipids from different species. Mitochondrial lipids are particularly rich in polyunsaturated acids (53, 72). The above findings together with the overall phospholipid:cholesterol ratios have some bearing on the potential structural role of lipids in cell membranes. Studies of surface pressure–surface area relationships in monolayers of fatty acids and phospholipids reveal quite generally that the tightness of packing in the film decreases with decreasing chain length, increasing unsaturation and increasing chain branching (Table II-3). Cholesterol has an important effect on the packing of lipids in monolayers, producing a compacting effect (74–79), the extent of which depends upon the amount of cholesterol and the state of expansion of the film (Table II-3). A discussion is given by Cadenhead (79). Similar

TABLE II-3. Effects of Chain Length, Branching, Unsaturation and Cholesterol on Packing of Fatty Acids and Lipids

Compound	Surface pressure dynes/cm	$t°$ C	$Å^2$ molecule	Reduction in area after cholesterol	Ref.
Myristic acid	5	25	37	—	73
Pentadecylic acid	5	25	37	—	73
Palmitic acid	5	25	24	—	73
Stearic acid	5	25	23·5	—	73
Oleic acid	5	15–20	48	—	73
3,7,11,15-Tetramethyl-hexadecanoic acid	24	20	36	—	73
1,2-Didecanoyl-lecithin	12		79·5	0	74
1,2-Dimyristoyl-lecithin	12		72	11	74
1,2-Distearoyl-lecithin	12		45·5	0	74
1-Stearoyl-2-lauroyl-lecithin	12		77	7	74
1-Stearoyl-2-oleoyl-lecithin	12		75	11	74
1-Stearoyl-2-oleoyl-phosphatidylethanolamine	12		72·5	9·5	74
Egg lecithin	—		96	40	81

effects of cholesterol have been noted in lipid bilayers (80). A direct extrapolation of these findings to cell membrane structure cannot be made at the present time, but it seems probable that, in the absence of other controlling features, the presence of long chain saturated acyl entities and a high cholesterol content will promote the formation of a condensed lipid phase and that the presence of highly unsaturated acyl entities and a low cholesterol content will favor an expanded lipid phase (53, 75, 77). The condensed lipid phase is most reasonably equated with the bimolecular lipid leaflet but a number of structural possibilities are available for an expanded phase.

The net charge existing on the head group of each phospholipid is also of interest. The choline-containing phospholipids (lecithin, sphingomyelin, etc.) will be electrically neutral because the zwitterionic charges are balanced. Such lipids will thus be able to pack tightly because of lack of electrostatic repulsion. The "acidic" phospholipids (phosphatidylserine, phosphatidylethanolamine) bear a net negative charge which will be anticipated to hinder such close packing unless the excess negative charge is neutralized by a cation (82). Clearly, the presence or absence of such a cation could have an important bearing on the degree of "tightness of lipid organization" in the membrane: this will be discussed more fully later (see section on p. 164).

Despite the obvious impossibility at the present time of relating membrane composition to membrane structure and function, certain generalizations do appear to be forthcoming. The high lipid content of myelin together with the approximately 1:1 ratio of phospholipids and cholesterol reinforces those arguments based on physical measurements and which indicate a condensed lipid bilayer as the fundamental structural unit. The same situation may hold true for the erythrocyte membrane although the significantly higher protein content may cause substantial structural modification of the bilayer. The mitochondrial and chloroplast membranes have the least cholesterol and the highest content of lipids with unsaturated acyl groups and it is, of course, for these membranes that the direct evidence is strongest for the occurrence of structures other than the lipid bimolecular leaflet. We may also note that there appears to be some correlation between protein and lipid contents and composition and biochemical activities of the respective membranes—in general the greatest and most highly organized biochemical activities being associated with membranes of high protein content and low cholesterol content. It is, therefore, important to consider also the structural aspects of lipids in relation to their interactions with proteins (see section on p. 136).

Most views of membrane structure and function are framed largely with reference to the predominating lipid and protein constituents. Nevertheless, attention must be directed also to the role of other membrane materials, notably the glycoproteins, that are present in small quantities and whose role is but poorly defined.

Glycoproteins (Fig. II-7) characteristically contain N-acylneuraminic acids (sialic acid) in common with the gangliosides. The evidence for glycoproteins in membranes has been summarized by Cook (83) and discussions of their functions are given by Cook (loc. cit.) and Kent (84). An important function, discussion of which lies outside the scope of this book, is the conferral of antigenic specificities on the cell surface (83, 85). Additionally, the carboxyl group of the sialic acid undoubtedly confers negative charge upon the cell surface (83, 86–88) and may also function in specific cation binding. Sialic acid-containing materials have also been postulated to play a role in cell recognition phenomena (83,

89). It is noteworthy that sialic acid residues are also found in ganglio-sides: the demonstration that gangliosides are associated with neuronal membranes of the central nervous system has led to considerable speculation (90, 91) that they are involved in neuronal transmission processes. While the properties of neither the glycolipids nor the glyco-proteins are currently well integrated into cell membrane structure, it is

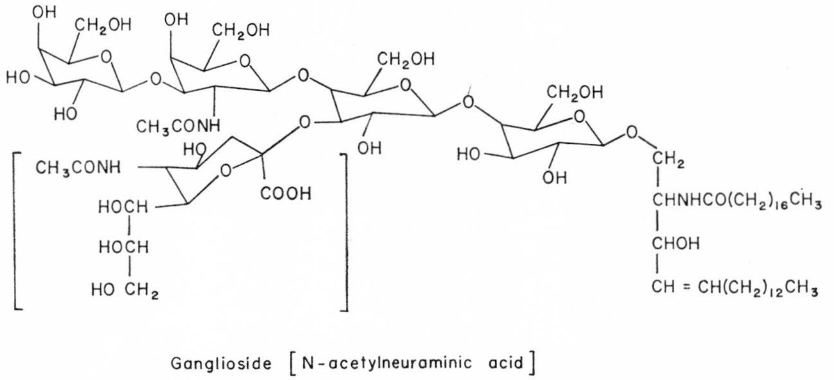

Ganglioside [N-acetylneuraminic acid]

FIG. II-7. Glycoprotein structure.

apparent that this will need rectification and that considerations of such agents may play an important role in ligand recognition phenomena at the cell surface.

THE PROPERTIES AND ORGANIZATION OF PHOSPHOLIPIDS

The continuing work of Chapman, Luzatti and their respective collaborators continues to emphasize the potential dynamic role that phospholipids may play in cell membranes. With increasing temperature phospholipids exhibit thermotropic mesomorphism (75, 92–96) and the hydrocarbon chains are actually in a liquid state at temperatures considerably below their formal melting point. The transition tempera-ture at which this endothermic phase change occurs is critically dependent upon the nature of the hydrocarbon chain and is progressively lowered with decreasing chain length or increasing unsaturation of the fatty acids. For appropriate lipids, the transition temperature is approximately that of the biological environment, and for mixtures of lipids such as are normally found in membranes, the transition tem-perature will cover a broad range (Fig. II-8). Of equal interest is the observation that water has a marked influence on this transition, small quantities of water producing a lowering of the temperature (Fig. II-9). Thus, most lipids in biological systems will be in a liquid form under physiological conditions. The role of the water bound to lipid is of some interest since some of it appears to be "structured", 1,2-dipalmitoyl-DL-phosphatidylcholine binding about 20 per cent water in this way. This water may be of particular significance in two ways: (a) as possessing those various properties of structured water previously considered and

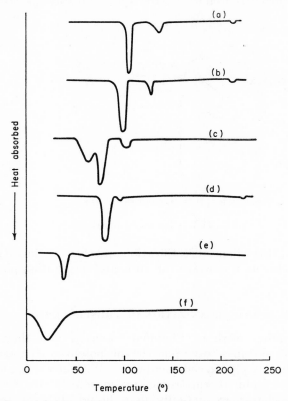

FIG. II-8. Differential thermal analysis heating curves for phospholipids: (a) 2.3-dimyristoyl-DL-1-phosphatidylethanolamine; (b) 2,3-dielaidoyl-DL-1-phosphatidylethanolamine; (c) 2-oleoyl-3-stearoyl-1-phosphatidylethanolamine; (d) 2,3-distearoyl-DL-1-phosphatidylcholine; (e) 2-oleoyl-3-stearoyl-DL-1-phosphatidylcholine; (f) egg yolk lecithin. Reproduced with permission from Chapman (93).

(b) as exerting control over the physical state of lipid areas. Clearly, removal or addition of water to an appropriate lipid (presumably in association with protein) could have profound effects on the mobility of the hydrocarbon chains of the lipid.

In studies of thermal phase transitions of membranes and membrane lipids from *Mycoplasma laidlawii* it has been observed (24) that the transition temperatures are lowered by increasing lipid unsaturation (Fig. II-10). However, the transition temperatures for both membranes and isolated lipids are identical suggesting that the organization of lipids within the membrane is that of the bilayer found in the water dispersions.

In their studies of the lyotropic mesomorphism of lipids, Luzatti and his colleagues (23, 80, 97, 98) have demonstrated that different liquid crystalline organizations are adopted with changing temperature and

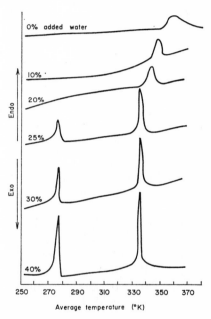

FIG. II-9. Effect of water on thermal transition temperatures of 1,2-distearoyl-phosphatidylcholine. Reproduced with permission from Chapman (96).

water concentration. The important liquid crystalline structures are shown in Fig. II-11 and it is clearly to be anticipated that the properties (permeability, conductivity, etc.) of the hexagonal-II phase will be substantially different from the lamellar phase. The ability to exist in the arrangements pictured above is dependent in part, upon lipid concentration; high concentrations favoring the hexagonal phase (generally II, but hexagonal-I for lysolecithin) and in part, upon lipid structure; a high hydrophilic:hydrophobic molecular ratio favoring those states with a high surface:volume ratio. Significantly, lamellar phase stability is greatly extended in mixtures of phospholipids such as mitochondrial and brain lipids.

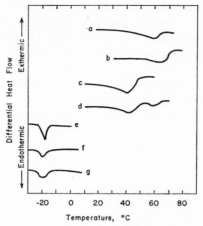

FIG. II-10. Thermal transitions of *Mycoplasma laidlawii* lipids, membranes and whole cells. (a) Total membrane lipids from cells grown in tryptose with added stearate; (b) membranes from stearate-supplemented tryptose; (c) total membrane lipids from cells grown in unsupplemented tryptose; (d) membranes from cells grown in unsupplemented tryptose; (e) total membrane lipids from cells grown in tryptose with added oleate; (f) membranes from cells grown in tryptose with added oleate and (g) whole cells grown in tryptose with added oleate. Reproduced with permission from Steim *et al.* (24).

Valuable information concerning lipid organization in both phospholipid dispersions and cell membranes is being derived from spin-label studies (99–100a) in which advantage is taken of the sensitivity of the electron spin resonance (ESR) spectrum of an incorporated radical to the relative viscosity and polarity of the environment and the orientation relative to an external magnetic field. In their original studies Hubbell

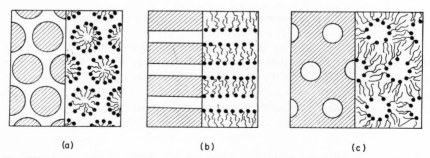

FIG. II-11. Liquid crystalline structures ($\bullet$ = polar head group, $\sim$, nonpolar chain): (a) Hexagonal I, water outside; (b) lamellar, an alternate array of planar layers of lipid and water; (c) Hexagonal II, water inside. Reproduced with permission from Luzatti (97).

and McConnell (101) used 2,2,6,6-tetramethylpiperidine-N-oxide (II-1):
in aqueous solution this radical gives rise to a simple triplet but when
incorporated into vagus nerve (rabbit), skeletal muscle (frog) or walking
leg nerve of the lobster the high field component is split to give a spectrum
that is essentially duplicable by the superimposition of spectra obtained

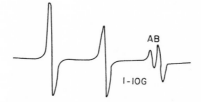

II-1

from aqueous and dodecane solutions (Fig. II-12). Lipid extraction of
the vagus nerve abolishes the binding capacity for II-1 which is also
absent in glycerinated muscle fibers. Apparently II-1 is incorporated
into membranes and its signals emanate from an essentially fluid hydrocarbon region. Essentially similar spectra to those of Fig. II-12 are

AB

I-10G

FIG. II-12. The electron spin resonance of 2,2,6,6-tetramethyl-N-oxide (TEMPO)
in the rabbit vagus nerve (A) and in surrounding aqueous solution and axoplasm
(B). This spectrum can be duplicated by dual recording from TEMPO in water and
TEMPO in dodecane. Reproduced with permission from Hubbell and McConnell
(101).

obtained from II-1 incorporated into phospholipid vesicles: in this
system binding of the label is strongly decreased by cholesterol, a
finding confirmed by Barratt *et al.* (102) for the lecithin–water system
and consistent with monolayer and prior evidence (103) for the "tighten-
ing" effect of cholesterol in decreasing the fluidity of the hydrocarbon
environment.

Me

Me

O   N→O

$CH_3(CH_2)_m$ $(CH_2)_nCOOH$

II-2

6*

More direct evidence for the organization of phospholipids in membranes and multilayers have been obtained through the use of the fatty acid analogs (II-2; 104–106). The labels II-2 ($m = 17$, $n = 3$; $m = 12$, $n = 3$ and $m = 5$, $n = 10$) have a preferred orientation in the walking leg nerve fiber of the lobster which is perpendicular to the local membrane surface and show spectra which are essentially identical to those obtained in sonicated phospholipids. Hubbell and McConnell conclude (105) that the neural membrane contains at least substantial areas of a lipid bilayer structure. Similar results were obtained with erythrocytes save that the labels were more strongly immobilized than the phospholipid dispersions so that the lipid organization in the erythrocyte membrane may be much tighter than in the neural membrane.

THE CONFORMATION AND ORGANIZATION OF MEMBRANE PROTEINS

A number of cell membrane preparations have been examined by ORD and CD techniques (75, 107–112) and all show basically the same features namely a spectral shape characteristic of the α-helical structure but of low amplitude and showing a red shift (Fig. II-13). From the data currently available it is difficult to estimate the amounts of the various conformations present but Wallach and Gordon (112) have suggested 50–60 per cent α-helix, no more than 15 per cent β-form and the remainder random coil: the low value for the β-form is supported by infra-red measurements (113–115).

The feature of greatest interest in the ORD and CD spectra of membranes is their displacement to longer wavelength with retention of general α-helical characteristics thus suggesting that the spectra observed are those of the α-helix in a modified environment. Such modification of the environment of the amide chromophores is most likely to arise from adjacent or partially intercalated lipid or protein (75, 107–111). Wallach and his co-workers (*loc. cit.*) consider the shift to originate from hydrophobic interactions between membrane lipids and proteins, a view that is supported by the work of Urry and co-workers on the mitochondrial membrane (109). This conclusion is strengthened by several distinct lines of evidence: theoretical studies on the effect of decreasing medium polarity and increasing polarizability on the electronic transitions involved in the optical activity of the peptide link indicate (107, 109, 116–118) that shifts to longer wavelengths will be anticipated. The ORD and CD spectra of membranes show "blue" shifts back to the "normal" polypeptide spectra upon treatment with lysolecithin and 2-chloroethanol which induce dissociations of the lipids and proteins (107, 108, 111) and with phospholipase A (112) which converts lecithin to lysolecithin and fatty acid but not with phospholipase C (119). Membrane spectra are quite different from those of ionic lipid–

protein complexes such as those of cytochrome c (120) or soluble serum lipoproteins (121) which exhibit normal, unperturbed, ORD spectra.

Thus, the ORD and CD spectra indicate a role for membrane proteins in which substantial hydrophobic association with lipids may occur. This contrasts with the predictions of the simplest Danielli–Davson model in which lipid–protein association is primarily through ionic interactions, but accords with the general experience of the usefulness of organic solvents and detergents in the separation and solubilization of membrane lipids and proteins. It is of some interest to note that

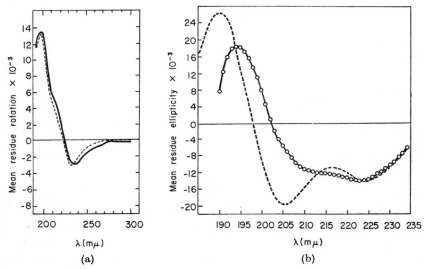

FIG. II-13. (a) ORD spectrum of ascites membrane in aqueous suspension: —— membrane, ———— poly-L-glutamic acid. (b) CD spectrum of ascites membrane: ○——○, membrane, ———— poly-L-glutamic acid (40% α-helix). Reproduced with permission from Wallach and Zahler (107) and Wallach and Gordon (110).

sodium dodecyl sulfate converts random coil poly-L-ornithine to α-helix and causes a simultaneous red shift and reduction in intensity of the ORD spectrum (122): this may constitute a model system of some relevance to the lipid–protein organization of cell membranes.

This view of hydrophobic lipid–protein interactions in membranes is strengthened by the PMR measurements of Chapman and his colleagues (75, 103) on erythrocyte membranes. Ultrasonically dispersed membrane fragments reveal several well-defined peaks for the protons of the choline group, sugar and sialic acid residues; however, the methylene and ethylene group signals of the fatty acid chains are absent or indistinct but become sharper with increasing temperature. Treatment of membranes with detergents or denaturants results in the appearance of signals from the phospholipids: the inhibition of these signals in the untreated membrane dispersion is indicative of a high environmental viscosity for the alkyl chains which is not due to lipid complexing with cholesterol and may be due to the formation of hydrophobic associations of proteins and lipids, such association decreasing the intensity and increasing the line width of the signals.

TABLE II-4. Amino Acid Composition of Soluble and Membrane Lipoproteins (123)

Class (Number)	Hydrophilic mole %	Nonpolar mole %	H/N ratio	Charged mole %
Soluble lipoproteins (8)	49·8 ± 0·8 (SEM)	27·3 ± 0·9	1·8 ± 0·1	33·8 ± 1·4
Membrane lipoproteins (12)	42·7 ± 1·6	29·9 ± 0·8	1·4 ± 0·1	28·8 ± 1·7
Soluble proteins (27)	49·1 ± 0·6	23·9 ± 0·7	2·1 ± 0·1	33·3 ± 0·8
Soluble oligomeric proteins (31)	45·1 ± 0·6	27·5 ± 0·5	1·7 ± 0·1	31·0 ± 0·6

Studies of the amino acid composition of membrane lipoproteins also reveal very clearly the importance of nonpolar association. Hatch and Bruce (123) have compared the amino acid composition of soluble and membranous lipoproteins (Table II-4) and have found significant differences. Soluble proteins have a higher content of hydrophilic amino acids and any affinity for lipids must be generated from special amino acid sequences (Table II-5). In contrast membranous lipoproteins have the highest content of nonpolar residues and the lowest content of charged residues and are thus better adapted for cross linking in membrane protein.

TABLE II-5. Comparison of Two Soluble Lipoproteins and Lipid Binding Capacity (123)

	Lipid content wt %	Hydrophilic amino acids mole %	Nonpolar amino acids mole %
Human plasma high density	50	53·2	24·8
Bovine plasma albumin	0·2	50·3	24·5

In addition to those proteins of the cell membrane that have well-defined catalytic functions there is present another protein (actually a class of proteins) which appears to be essentially noncatalytic in function and for which has been proposed a role in the maintenance of the molecular integrity of the cell membrane (34).

This class of proteins was first obtained from mitochondria where it contributes some 30 per cent of the total protein (124–126), but essentially similar proteins have now been obtained from a variety of cell membranes including mitochondria of diverse sources, red blood cells (127, 128), microsomes (127), muscle sarcolemma (129), sarcoplasmic reticulum (126) and synaptic plasma membranes (130). The apparently very general occurrence of such protein has led to speculations that it plays some common role in membrane organization (124, 127, 128, 130) but this question is still very much undecided (31). These proteins, whatever their source, have a number of chemical and physical properties in common: their chemical properties (amino acid composition) indicate that they form a distinct structural class, they show a great tendency to polymerize by hydrophobic association, they are quite insoluble in aqueous media, they have generally similar molecular weights of 20,000–50,000 and require pH extremes, detergents or strongly protic solvents for solubilization and they show quantitatively similar abilities to bind phospholipids. Additionally, these proteins show a remarkable tendency to exist in varying degrees of order, according to their treatment and mode of preparation (126). Circular dichroism studies have revealed that these proteins can exist in the random coil, β-conformation and the α-helical conformations (131). The unique properties of structural protein are, in part, to be found in the hydrophobic character of the monomer units (123) and in its ability to exist in a variety of conformational states (126). Such properties are consistent with, but do not prove, the proposed role of structural protein in the organization of the catalytic protein and phospholipid macromolecular systems into a functional continuum.

The possibility of such involvement is demonstrated by several findings that the presence of structural protein can significantly modify enzymatic activities. Structural protein has been shown to combine with cytochromes a, b and c, and with cytochrome lipids to form stable complexes (125, 132) and, when so combined to modify the redox potential of the cytochrome (133, 134). In this connection the studies of Woodward and Menkres (135) assume considerable importance: they found that alterations in the structural protein by a single amino acid replacement in mutants of *Neurospora crassa* were relatable to the much lower affinity of the complex between malate dehydrogenase and structural protein from the mutant for malate.

Whether the structural protein from a given source is homogeneous is a vexed question (136) and the answer depends very much upon the probing technique. Despite the obvious need for much further work on the role of these presumed structural proteins the very real possibility exists that they indeed represent a unique genetically controlled structural determinant for the functional lipid and protein organization of cell membranes. Lehninger suggests (137) that membranes may contain a variety of closely related structural proteins each one binding selectively a single type of membrane phospholipid and so generating a specific phospholipid mosaic at the cell surface. The apparent importance of structural protein in the activity of the highly organized mitochondrial enzyme systems suggests that it may also play an important role in such systems as the neuronal cell membrane where the organization of the macromolecular systems also appears to be critical for integrated activity.

LIPID–PROTEIN INTERACTIONS

It is clear that an understanding of lipid–protein interactions is of vital importance to the interpretation both of the general organization of membranes and the various biochemical functions of membranes. According to the Danielli–Davson model of the plasma membrane the role of membrane lipids is considered primarily to be that of providing a permeability barrier while the membrane proteins retain essential responsibility for the various enzymatic, transport, regulatory and ligand-recognition properties. Recent developments have begun to emphasize the *functional* role of membrane lipids and this in turn has led to reinterpretations of the structural roles of membrane lipids and proteins.

In the bimolecular lipid leaflet representation of the cell membrane, the binding of the external protein layers and the phospholipids is assumed to be primarily polar. This, however, imposes somewhat severe restrictions on the structure of the protein: if the protein is entirely unfolded then a large fraction of nonpolar amino acids will be exposed to the aqueous environments. Those portions of the proteins that may be helical will require an amino acid of sufficient polarity to interact with the aqueous environment on one surface of the helix and the polar head groups of the lipids on the other surface. Such helical structures are unlikely to be stable (108, 137).

It is evident, however, from the discussion of the preceding chapter that hydrophobic interactions play a major role in the determination of protein conformation, catalytic activity, etc. It is to be anticipated that hydrophobic interactions will play a similarly important role in the lipid–protein interactions of cell membranes (139, 140). Several lines of evidence (p. 132) favor this possibility and indicate a deep penetration of the lipid by protein or, through a more extreme interaction, complete association of the lipids and proteins as lipoprotein complexes or hydrophobic associations of separate lipid and protein subunits (Fig. II-14).

Some support for the occurrence of lipoprotein complexes may be derived from observations that some membranes can be solubilized by detergents to give "lipoprotein" complexes: this has been observed with

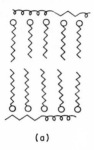

(a)

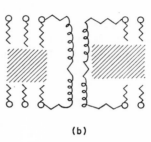

(b)

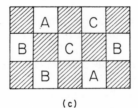

(c)

FIG. II-14. Representations of cell membrane structure (a) Danielli–Davson lipid leaflet; (b) model according to Lenard and Singer (108) showing an exterior composed of polar head groups and polar proteins and a hydrophobic (crosshatched) interior; (c) association of lipids and proteins (surface view) in which various protein subunits (A, B, C) are shown associated with lipid subunits: this could also represent the association of discrete lipoprotein subunits.

erythrocytes (141), liver cells (142), bacterial (143–148) and mitochondrial (32–34, 149, 150) membranes. However, it has not been conclusively demonstrated that the observed complexes are genuinely homogeneous or that they are actually found as such in the cell membrane.

Morowitz and co-workers have investigated in detail the solubilization of the plasma membranes of *Mycoplasma laidlawii* (143–145). The sodium dodecyl sulfate solubilized material was shown to be a mixture of SDS–lipid and SDS–protein complexes. Removal of the detergent by dialysis in the absence of Mg^{++} led to the formation of a small lipoprotein aggregate which upon treatment with Mg^{++} leads to a reaggregated structure with membrane-like properties (Fig. II-15). The physical properties, composition and structure of the original membrane and the reaggregated forms show few differences, although the functional properties do not seem to have been investigated. However, the important point is that separated membrane components can interact spontaneously to form membrane-like material in *the absence of pre-existing membrane*. Nevertheless, caution must be exercised before such findings are interpreted as evidence for the subunit construction of membranes for, as noted by Engelman, "...the possibility of a distinction between units of assembly and subunits must be recognized. The unit of assembly may be altered upon incorporation by the membrane in such a fashion as to remove it from consideration as a subunit in the membrane

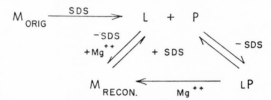

FIG. II-15. Solubilization and reaggregation of *Mycoplasma Laidlawii* membranes (M, membrane; L, lipid; P, protein).

structure, and the subunit need not necessarily be assembled prior to appearance in the membrane" (151).

According to Green and his colleagues mitochondrial membranes can be dispersed through the action of bile salts or other detergents to give four distinct complexes of the electron-transport chain that will form vesicular membranes after removal of the dispersing agent (149, 150, 152, 153). The four individual complexes of the electron transport chain of bovine heart mitochondria catalyse the sequence:

$$NADH + H^+ + CoQ \xrightarrow{\text{Complex I}} NAD + CoQH_2$$

$$\text{Succinate} + CoQ \xrightarrow{\text{Complex II}} \text{fumarate} + CoQH_2$$

$$CoQH_2 + 2\,cyt\,c\,(Fe^{+++}) \xrightarrow{\text{Complex III}} CoQ + 2\,cyt\,c\,(Fe^{++})$$

$$4\,cyt\,c\,(Fe^{++}) + O_2 \xrightarrow{\text{Complex IV}} 4\,cyt\,c\,(Fe^{+++}) + 2H_2O$$

These individual complexes can be reassembled into a functional system, although mere mixing of complexes I and III does not produce a system in which oxidation of NADH by $cyt\,c\,(Fe^{+++})$ occurs: functional reassembly requires dispersion, mixing and reconstitution (Fig. II-5) and there is an absolute dependence on phospholipids both for the processes of membrane reconstitution and biochemical activity in the inner mitochondrial membrane (149, 150, 154–156). These conclusions have been challenged by Stoeckenius (21), amongst others, who has argued that complete disaggregation of the inner mitochondrial membrane has not been clearly demonstrated.

The association of lipids with the membrane proteins of the chloroplast has been studied by Benson and his colleagues (157, 158). The extent of lipid association with chloroplast lamellar protein is independent of the character of the hydrophilic lipid head group and is determined essentially by the number of hydrocarbon chains per lipid molecule. Similarly, the competitive inhibition of chlorophyll or monogalactosyl diglyceride association with the membrane proteins is dependent only upon the hydrophobic character of the competing species (fatty acids, phytol, fatty acid esters) indicating that lipid–protein association in the chloroplast membrane is hydrophobically determined.

The several lines of evidence thus far outlined are suggestive of a significant hydrophobic contribution to membrane lipid–protein associations. That treatment of erythrocytes with phospholipase C (119) or mitochondria with acetone (154, 159) to remove 70–95% of the phospholipids leaves the structure virtually unaffected indicates that some modification of the simple Danielli–Davson model may be required: at the least it is necessary to postulate protein-cross bridges across the bilayer but more drastic reconsideration could also be required in which the bilayer is no longer a structural determinant.

According to Green and his colleagues the process of membrane assembly is to be regarded as the association of lipoprotein "subunits", the function of the phospholipid being to provide a hydrophilic surface that restricts combination to the remaining hydrophobic faces of the subunit (Fig. II-16) and thus generates a laminar sheet—the cell membrane. Such a method of membrane construction (or some variant, i.e., 160) is clearly compatible with current thinking on protein organization, provides an appropriate mechanism of membrane formation through the delivery of preformed lipoprotein "subunits" and provides a satisfactory explanation of the structural role of permeases, translocases, receptors in the cell membrane since such entities may be regarded as comprising individual subunits of the membrane. The concept does not necessarily restrict the subunits to being lipoprotein in character; it is perfectly appropriate that the membrane contain separate protein and lipid subunits although it would be anticipated that the latter would not be common. This type of modular construction would obviously account for the occurrence of readily dissociable permeases etc. from bacterial cell membranes (160–163). Nevertheless, it seems clear from the preceding discussion that much experimental work is still required to clarify the possible role of subunit membrane construction.

Because of these arguments it is clearly desirable to obtain more information about the relative functions of phospholipids and proteins in cell membranes. Among the important questions to be solved is the following: do phospholipids function merely to provide hydrophilic surfaces for membrane subunits or do they have other and more functional roles to play? An answer to this and many related questions is not presently forthcoming from cell membrane studies, but it is appropriate

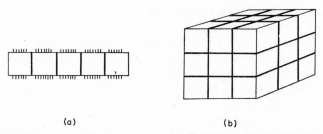

(a)   (b)

FIG. II-16. A representation of how the presence of phospholipid head groups at a membrane subunit surface prevents (a) the three-dimensional aggregation shown in (b).

at this stage to consider lipid–protein interactions in terms of lipid-dependent enzymes, the role of which in membranes is well documented and which appear to represent a simpler experimental system.

LIPID-DEPENDENT ENZYME SYSTEMS

A partial listing of enzyme systems, the activity of which is dependent upon phospholipid is given in Table II-6. A number of investigations have been concerned with mitochondrial D(−)-β-hydroxybutyric acid dehydrogenase which catalyses the oxidation of β-hydroxybutyric acid by NAD and is in most respects a rather typical pyridinoprotein save in its absolute requirement for lecithin: the apodehydrogenase cannot be reactivated by lysolecithin, sphingomyelin etc. Furthermore, maximum reactivation requires unsaturated fatty acids in the lecithin and saturated lecithins such as L-α-dimyristoyl-lecithin can only *partially* activate the enzyme. The lecithin has to be supplied to the apodehydrogenase in dispersed form and it can be calculated that at maximum activity the molar ratio of lipid:protein is ∼100:1. However, lecithin present (30 per cent) in a mixed micelle with individually inactive phospholipids produces maximal reactivation of the enzyme at the same phospholipid:protein molar ratio. Thus the requirement for phospholipid is partly specific and partly non-specific, the specificity relating no doubt to the binding of the choline entity of lecithin to the protein. Since β-hydroxybutyrate dehydrogenase actually oxidizes a series of β-hydroxy acids,

TABLE II-6. Lipid Dependent Enzymes

Enzyme	Lipid specificity	References
D(−)-β-Hydroxybutyrate dehydrogenase	Lecithin (absolute)	155, 164–167
Electron transport chain of mitochondria	No absolute specificity	152, 155, 168–170
Na$^+$/K$^+$ ATPase (rat brain)	Phosphatidyl serine	171
Stearyl-Coenzyme A desaturase	Lecithin and triglycerides + fatty acids required	172
Glucose-6-phosphatase (rat liver microsomes)	Phosphatidyl ethanolamine > other single lipids but < total microsomal lipid	173
Phosphatidic acid phosphatase (pig kidney microsomes)	—	174
Phosphorylcholine cytidyltransferase (rat liver)	Lysolecithin ≫ lecithin. Individual lipids less effective than mixed liver lipids	175
Na$^+$/K$^+$ ATPase (beef brain)†	Lecithin > lysolecithin > phosphatidic acid, mono- and dialkyl phosphates	176, 177
K$^+$/Mg^{++} Phosphatase (beef brain)	Dialkyl phosphates	177
Nicotinamide-adenine dinucleotide (phosphate) transhydrogenase	Lecithin—but other lipids not tested	178
ATPase Ca^{++} transport (skeletal muscle microsomes)	Lecithin, lysolecithin and anionic or neutral detergents for ATPase: lecithin lysolecithin or phosphatidic acid for Ca^{++} transport	179
UDP galactose: lipopolysaccharide α, 3-galactosyl transferase (bacterial)	Phosphatidylethanolamine	180, 181
Deoxycorticosterone 11β-hydroxylase (bovine adrenal mitochondria)	General mitochondrial lipid	182

† The interesting observation was made by Tanaka and Strickland (176) that sensitivity of this enzyme to ouabain was noted *only* in the presence of lecithin.

from C_4–C_9, with equal ease (183) it is quite probable that a non-specific function of the phospholipid is the provision of an appropriate hydrophobic substrate binding surface and a further non-specific function in the provision of the micellar environment: it is noteworthy that increases in K_m and V_{max} for both β-hydroxybutyrate and NAD occur with increasing lipid concentration (184). In this connection it is of interest that Gotterer (185) has found competitive inhibition of β-hydroxybutyrate binding to the enzyme by a varied series of local anesthetics and that a good correlation exists between the inhibition of the enzyme and the local anesthetic potency.

Among the other enzymes listed in Table II-6 particular interest also attaches to nicotinamide-adenine dinucleotide (phosphate) transhydrogenase which is capable of catalysing reactions 1 and 2 (178).

$$NADH_2 + 3\text{-}APAD\dagger \rightarrow NAD + 3\text{-}APADH_2 \qquad (1)$$

$$NADPH_2 + 3\text{-}APAD \rightarrow NADP + 3\text{-}APADH_2 \qquad (2)$$

Treatment with phospholipase A or phospholipid solvents abolishes activity (2) but leaves activity (1) unchanged, thus indicating that the lecithin–protein interaction directs substrate specificity. The ATPase/ Ca^{++} transport activities of skeletal muscle microsomes (179) are both phospholipid dependent processes which are abolished by treatment with phospholipase C: the decline in the ATPase and Ca^{++} transport activities is approximately the same and is paralleled closely by the decline in lecithin content. Activities can be restored by the addition of phospholipids but the structural requirements for the restoration of the two activities are quite different: ATPase activities are restored by phospholipids *and* various anionic or nonionic detergents (Triton X-45, X-100, Tween-80 etc.) but not by cationic detergents. In contrast, restoration of Ca^{++} transport activity has a much more specific requirement for lecithin, lysolecithin or phosphatidic acid and detergents only served to inhibit the Ca^{++} transport activity. In contrast to D(–)-β-hydroxybutyrate dehydrogenase the degree of unsaturation of the added lecithin or lysolecithin for the activation of the ATPase Ca^{++} transport system is unimportant.

A particularly interesting example of a lipid dependent enzyme system is provided by UDP-galactose:lipopolysaccharide-α,3-galactosyl transferase (180, 181, 186) found in the cell walls of gram-negative bacteria and involved in the synthesis of the complex cell wall lipopolysaccharide (Fig. II-17) by catalysing the transfer of galactose to lipopolysaccharide. Transfer does not take place to purified lipopolysaccharide or to lipid-extracted cell wall preparations and phosphatidylethanolamine containing unsaturated acyl chains is an essential component of the reaction:

† 3-Acetylpyridine-adenine dinucleotide.

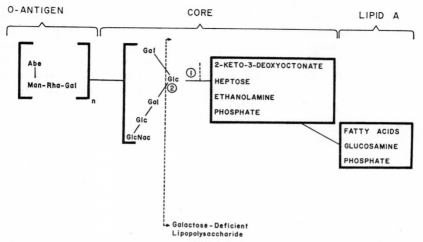

FIG. II-17. Structure of lipopolysaccharide from *S. typhimurium* indicating (2) the site of action of UDP-galactose, lipopolysaccharide α, 3 galactosyl transferase. Reproduced from Rothfield, Wesser and Endo (181) with permission of the authors, the New York Heart Association, Inc. and Little Brown and Company.

phosphatidylcholine is completely ineffective in restoring activity indicating the specificity residing in the polar head group of the molecule. Rothfield and his co-workers (180, 181, 186) have been able to isolate

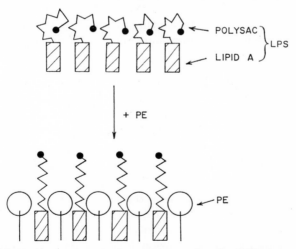

FIG. II-18. Schematic representation of how phosphatidylethanolamine (PE) could orient the polysaccharide chain to make it available for the transfer of galactose. Reproduced from Rothfield, Weiser and Endo (181) with permission of the authors, the New York Heart Association, Inc. and Little Brown and Company.

binary and ternary complexes of lipopolysaccharide–enzyme and lipopolysaccharide–enzyme–phosphatidylethanolamine respectively and have suggested that for effective catalysis to occur an ordered sequence of the three constituents must occur in the cell membrane and that the function of the phosphatidylethanolamine may be to provide the matrix in which the terminal polysaccharide is made accessible to the enzyme (Fig. II-18).

A number of potential roles may be ascribed to the lipids in lipid-dependent enzymes:

a. Cofactor requirement: this is rather improbable because of the large quantities of phospholipid that are required.

b. Determination of the tertiary and quaternary structure of proteins: there appears to be insufficient information currently available to determine the significance of this effect.

c. Provision of hydrophobic binding sites for ligands: this is clearly an important function not only for binding but also for the provision of a nonpolar environment that may drastically alter the rates and specificities of polar interactions.

d. Provision of an orienting matrix: this may be of particular importance for sequential reactions (such as the mitochondrial electron transport chain) where it may be anticipated that precise alignment of the several enzymes and efficient mechanisms for stepwise transfer of substrates and cofactors will be operative.

e. Provision of ionic interfaces: this will be of significance in providing locally perturbed ion concentrations and in stabilizing ionic transition states.

It is not easy to define the importance of any of the above roles for a given lipid-dependent enzyme system or to extend the considerations to membranes. However, some further clarification may be obtained through considerations of reactions taking place in micelles.

REACTIONS IN MICELLAR SYSTEMS

Over the past few years it has been realized that reactions occurring at micellar surfaces bear a substantial similarity to enzyme catalysed processes. Both processes occur at interfaces, the relative disposition of hydrophilic and hydrophobic groups are similar, both enzymatic and micellar systems exhibit saturation kinetics and substrate specificity and micellar functional groups can also exhibit enhanced reactivity as in proteins. Further discussion of these points is to be found in references 187–189. In the present context the major emphasis is that the micellar disposition of amphipathic molecules represents one approximation to lipid orientation within cell membranes and that reactions in micelles, particularly mixed micelles of two or more types of amphipathic molecules, may represent a convenient approach to the study of some aspects of lipid–protein interactions.

Because of the presence of fixed charges at a micellar surface an electrical double layer is set up. This electrical double layer is actually composed of two parts (190–192) (Fig. II-19) the innermost or Stern layer and the outer or Gouy–Chapman layer. The Stern layer, which is

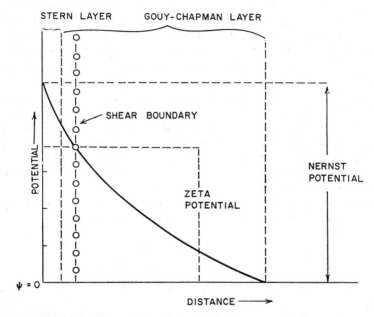

FIG. II-19. Representation of charged layers at a micellar surface.

comparable in thickness to the dimensions of single ions and solvent molecules contains a number of tightly bound counterions and solvent molecules inside this shear layer, while the Gouy–Chapman layer is much more diffuse and contains the remaining associated counterions. The microscopic properties of the Stern layer are of substantial interest in any attempt to describe the environment of a ligand species bound at a micellar surface. Mukerjee (193) has studied the charge-transfer bands of dodecylpyridinium iodides as micelles and as ion-pairs in various solvents; this technique leads to an "effective" dielectric constant of 36 for the micellar surface.

That the pH at the surface of a charged interface (pH$_s$) is different from the bulk pH (pH_b) has long been known (194–196), the relationship between the two being described by,

$$pH_s = pH_b + \frac{\epsilon\psi}{2\cdot3kT}$$

where ψ is the electric potential of the micellar surface relative to the bulk environment, ϵ is the electronic charge and k is the Boltzmann constant. Thus a micelle (or a polyelectrolyte) with a negative surface charge will tend to have an increased concentration of hydrogen counterions at the interface and the opposite will be true for a positively charged interface. This will modify the rates of reactions in which H_3O^+ or OH^- are involved and will also produce shifts in the apparent pK_a values of functional groups. Thus, the apparent pK_a values of the conjugate acid of p-chlorobenzylidene-1,1-dimethylethylamine have been determined as 6·55 in water, 7·02 in 0·02 M sodium lauryl sulfate and 4·96 in 0·05 M cetyltrimethylammonium bromide (197). Similarly the apparent pK_a of the —SH group in N-dodecanoyl-DL-cysteine changes from 10·01 in water to 9·07 in a cetyltrimethylammonium bromide micelle (187). The effect of the interfacial surface charge will not, of course, be confined to producing local variations in hydrogen and hydroxyl ions but will, quite generally, produce increases in the local concentrations of oppositely charged counterions.

Duynstee and Grunwald (198) observed that the rate of fading of triphenylmethane dyes is described by the equations,

$$Ar_3\overset{+}{C} \rightleftharpoons Ar_3COH$$

$$Rate = k_1[R^+] + k_2[R^+][OH^-]$$

In micelles k_1 is found to be decreased but k_2 is increased in cationic micelles (cetyltrimethylammonium bromide) and decreased in anionic micelles (sodium lauryl sulfate). From the data of Table II-7 the ratio k_1^+/k_1^- is small (2–25) but k_2^+/k_2^- is large ($\sim$700–4000). The effect of the micellar surface charge on the overall rate is primarily attributable to changes in $[OH^-]$ and will obviously lead to an increase in k_2 with cationic micelles and, to a lesser extent, to a "medium" effect reflected in k_1; this latter effect is small as is clear from the ratios k_1/k_1^+ and k_1/k_1^-.

Similar conclusions were drawn by Dunlap and Cordes (199) in their investigation of the catalysis of the acid hydrolysis of methyl ortho-benzoate by sodium alkysulfate micelles. Below the cmc the second

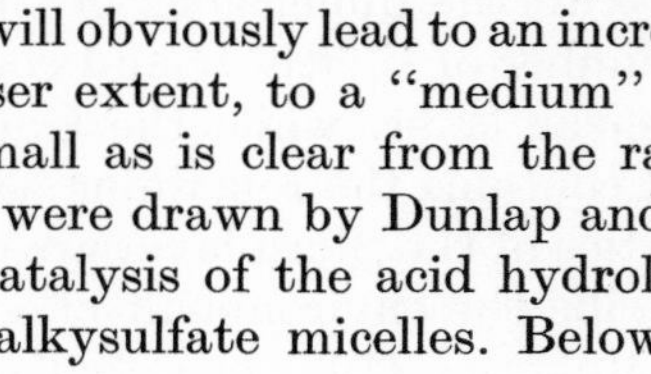

II-3

TABLE II-7. Rate Constants for Fading of Triphenylmethane Dyes at Micellar Surfaces (198)

Dye	10^4 k_1 sec^{-1}	10^4 k_1^+†‡ sec^{-1}	10^4 k_1^-†§ sec^{-1}	10^4 k_2 sec^{-1}	10^4 k_2^+†‡ sec^{-1}	10^4 k_2^-†§ sec^{-1}
Crystal violet	0·65	<0·03	0·05	0·16	8·0	<0·002
Malachite green	3·8	3·0	1·4	1·36	27·4	~0·0
Rosaniline	9·0	4·8	0·18	1·21	4·8	<0·006

† 0·05 M boric acid–sodium borate buffer and 0·01 M detergent.
‡ Cetyltrimethylammonium bromide.
§ Sodium lauryl sulfate.

order rate constants for this reaction, formulated as II-3 are independent of the surfactant concentration, increase rapidly above the cmc and subsequently decline (Fig. II-20). This behavior obviously indicates the necessity of a micellar phase for catalysis, the inhibition at high surfactant concentration being due to counterion (Na$^+$) binding. The medium (surface polarity) effect is unlikely to contribute significantly to the observed catalysis since it is known that decreasing solvent polarity

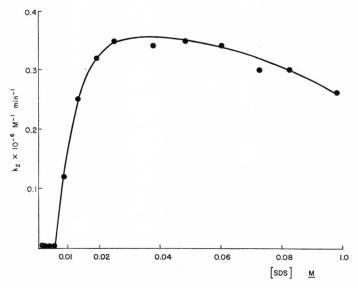

FIG. II-20. Rate profile for the acid catalysed hydrolysis of methyl orthobenzoate in the presence of sodium dodecyl sulfate. Reproduced with permission from Dunlap and Cordes (199).

decreases the hydrolysis rate of orthoesters. The principal catalytic effect is probably the electrostatic stabilization by the anionic micelle of the developing positive charge in the hydrolysis transition state (hydrophobic interactions which probably account for the incorporation of the orthoester into the micelle are almost certainly the same in the ground and transition states). Such stabilization probably invoves both increased protonation of the substrate and stabilization of the transition state. The counterion effects observed in this study are of some interest because of their magnitude (Table II-8): an explanation of these effects

TABLE II-8. Salt Effects on Second-order Rate Constants for the Hydrolysis of Methyl Orthobenzoate in 0·01 M Sodium Dodecylsulfate (199)

Salt	T°C	Conc. M	$k_2 \times 10^{-5}$† $M^{-1} min^{-1}$
NaCl	(25°)	0·00	2·13
		0·02	1·27
		0·12	0·49
KCl	(40°)	0·00	4·25
		0·01	3·16
		0·06	1·07
NH_4Cl	(25°)	0·03	0·84
$MeNH_3Cl$	(25°)	0·03	0·522
Me_2NH_2Cl	(25°)	0·03	0·395
Me_3NHCl	(25°)	0·03	0·301
Me_4NCl	(25°)	0·03	0·36
Et_4NCl	(25°)	0·03	0·158
Pr_4NCl	(25°)	0·03	0·060

† Initial concentration of methyl orthobenzoate, $5·0 \times 10^{-5}$ M.

being available decreasing in their micellar surface field strength and thus reducing the surface concentration of protons and the electrostatic stabilizing ability of the interface. Substituted ammonium ions act as effective counterions, their effect increasing with increasing hydrophobic character.

The effects of charge stabilization have also been noted by Heitmann (187) who studied the alkylation of N-dodecanoyl-DL-cysteine with iodoacetamide, chloroacetamide and p-nitrophenylacetate as an ionic micelle (alone) or when incorporated into a cationic micelle (hexadecyltrimethylammonium bromide). Incorporation into the cationic micelle produced marked second-order rate increases of some 100–200-fold with iodoacetamide and p-nitrophenyl acetate with respect to the bulk phase rates. The catalytic effect of the micelle is probably due to the stabilization of the negatively charged transition state by the positive charge of the micellar surface (Fig. II-21). In contrast, rates in the anionic micelle are sharply decreased probably because of a direct destabilizing effect of the negative micellar charge and also because of the decreased surface $[OH^-]$.

Nonpolar binding of the substrate in the micelle can also make a significant contribution to the reaction rate. This is apparent from the

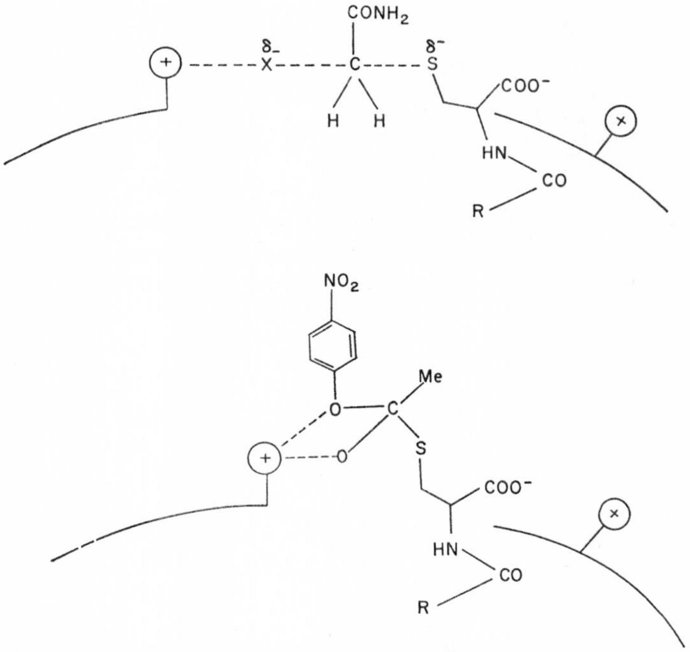

FIG. II-21. Representation of stabilization by positively charged micellar surface (hexadecyltrimethylammonium) of alkylation of N-dodecanoyl-DL-cysteine by (a) haloacetamide, (b) p-nitrophenylacetate.

study by Gitler and Ochoa-Solano (200) of the hydrolysis of p-nitrophenyl esters in mixed micelles of N^α-myristoyl-L-histidine and cetyltrimethylammonium bromide compared to the corresponding reaction with N-acetyl-L-histidine in the presence or absence of cetyltrimethylammonium bromide (Table II-9). Since in the micellar reaction [cetyltrimethylammonium bromide] > [myristoylhistidine] the micellar surface must consist of regions containing myristoylhistidine and nearest neighbor cetyltrimethylammonium ("catalytic" regions) and regions

TABLE II-9. Kinetic Data for the Hydrolysis of p-Nitrophenyl Esters Catalysed by N^{α}-Acetylhistidine and by Mixed Micelles of N^{α}-Myristoylhistidine and Cetyltrimethylammonium Bromide (200)†

p-Nitrophenyl ester‡	N-Ac-His§ $k_2\|$, M^{-1} min^{-1}	N-Ac-His§ + CTABr $k_2\|$, M^{-1} min^{-1}	Micelles of Mir-His + CTABr¶	
			$K_2\|$, M^{-1} min^{-1}	K_i, $\mathrm{M} \times 10^3$
Acetate	$12 \cdot 6 \pm 0 \cdot 50$	$9 \cdot 6 \pm 0 \cdot 42$	$377 \pm 8 \cdot 0$	$33 \cdot 2 \pm 6 \cdot 50$
Propionate	$16 \cdot 2 \pm 0 \cdot 02$	$9 \cdot 6 \pm 0 \cdot 72$	$871 \pm 3 \cdot 4$	$9 \cdot 3 \pm 1 \cdot 0$
Butyrate	$9 \cdot 8 \pm 0 \cdot 60$	$4 \cdot 0 \pm 0 \cdot 24$	1350 ± 32	$2 \cdot 9 \pm 0 \cdot 19$
Valerate	$11 \cdot 6 \pm 0 \cdot 36$	$3 \cdot 0 \pm 0 \cdot 16$	3025 ± 110	$1 \cdot 3 \pm 0 \cdot 13$
Hexanoate	$9 \cdot 0 \pm 0 \cdot 24$	$2 \cdot 2 \pm 0 \cdot 04$	7310 ± 290	$0 \cdot 5 \pm 0 \cdot 04$

† [CTABr] > [Mir-His] > [PNPX].
‡ Concentration from $0 \cdot 34$–$1 \cdot 0 \times 10^{-5}$ M.
§ [N-Ac-His] from $0 \cdot 02$–$0 \cdot 20$ M.
¶ [Mir-His] from $0 \cdot 1$–$0 \cdot 8 \times 10^{-3}$ M.
‖ Corrected for basic form of imidazolyl group.

containing cetyltrimethylammonium only ("nonproductive" binding regions); this accords with the decrease in the second order rates (k_2) of acylation of the imidazolyl moiety observed with increasing cetyltri-

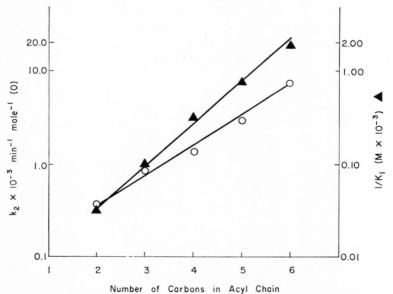

FIG. II-22. The dependence of hydrolytic rate constants ($\circ$) and binding constants ($\blacktriangle$) of p-nitrophenylesters in mixed micelles of N^{α}-myristoyl-L-histidine and cetyltrimethylammonium bromide on acyl group chain length. Reproduced with permission from Gitler and Ochoa-Solano (200).

methylammonium concentration. A most pertinent observation from this study is the marked acceleration in the rate of ester hydrolysis in mixed micelles containing N-myristoylhistidine relative to N-acetylhistidine. Furthermore there is a linear increase of $\log k_2$ with the number of carbon atoms in the acyl group of the substrate for hydrolysis in the cetyltrimethylammonium-N-myristoyl-L-histidine micelle (Fig. II-22) which yields a value of 442 cal mole^{-1} CH$_2$ group free energy contribution. This value is comparable to that obtained (Fig. II-22) for the free energy of transfer of an acyl methylene group from the aqueous environment to the mixed micelle. The close correspondence of these values to those previously discussed for various hydrophobic interactions (Chapter 1, Section on p. 25), suggests that, in addition to the probable contribution of the positive charge of cetyltrimethylammonium to transition state stabilization, the hydrophobic bonding energy contributed by the acyl chain is utilized at the micellar surface in the stabilization of the activated complex.

The micellar reactions just discussed are proposed to serve as partial models of lipid–protein interactions in membranes. It is clear that the polar and nonpolar functionalities of amphipathic molecules can serve to substantially modify binding and catalytic events through the various mechanisms outlined and, together with the discussion of lipid-dependent enzymes, it is abundantly clear that any discussion of ligand binding and catalysis at the cell membrane must ascribe a functional role to the lipids in addition to, and quite distinct from, any role that they play as determinants of cell membrane structure.

MEMBRANE STRUCTURE AND MEMBRANE MODELS

From the preceding discussion no totally satisfactory general structural representation is apparent. It may well be, however, that no single structure is satisfactory and that we should perceive a spectra of membrane organizations ranging from the essential Danielli–Davson lipid bilayer for those membrane systems best regarded as generating impermeable, insulating barriers (notably myelin) to very highly modified structure, in which the bilayer component may be very much reduced or even absent, for those membranes (inner mitochondrial membrane) known to be the seat of complex and highly organized biochemical sequences.

Because of the obvious complexities in studying natural membranes considerable attention is now being paid to membrane models that will reproduce, in systems that are hopefully simplified, the structures and properties of biological membranes. A number of reviews of such membrane models are available (201–206).

The two most widely employed systems are the lipid bilayers introduced by Mueller, Rudin, Tien and Wescott in 1961 (207, 208) and the liposomes, dispersed smectic mesophases of phospholipids arranged in concentric bimolecular lamellae and extensively studied by Bangham, Papahadjopoulos and their co-workers (204, 209–213). Both of these membrane systems demonstrate, in their unmodified state, a number of substantial similarities to biological membranes and most importantly, can, through the addition of various modifying substances, reproduce a number of the dynamic features, including electrical excitability, associated with biological membranes.

Bimolecular lipid membranes, separating two aqueous phases, are prepared by painting lipid solutions of varying degrees of complexity across small holes in teflon or polythene discs. The simplest systems

TABLE II-10. Comparison of Bilayers and Biological Membranes

Property	Biological Membranes (20–25° C)	Bilayers (36° C)
EM image	trilaminar	trilaminar
Thickness, Å	60–100	60–75
Capacitance, $\mu F\ cm^2$	0·5–1·3	0·38–1·0
Resistance, $\Omega\ cm^2$	10^2–10^5	10^6–10^9
Surface tension, dynes/cm	0·03–1	0·5–2
Water permeability, μ/sec	0·37–400	31·7 (25°)
Activation energy for water permeation, kcal/mole	9·6	12·7 (25°)

Data taken from the compilation by Thompson and Henn (206).

are those containing an amphiphathic lipid dissolved in a neutral hydrocarbon such as decane, but other and far more complex mixtures of partially oxidized lipids, cholesterol and solvents have been employed (201, 206, 208): inevitably a number of important questions concerning the precise composition of such membranes may be raised. However, it is generally agreed that such membranes are essentially bimolecular and are of the same order of thickness as biological membranes. A number of comparisons between bimolecular lipid and biological membranes are presented in Table II-10. The most serious discrepancies between the two systems are the higher electrical resistance of the bilayers and, most notably, their inability, in the unmodified state, to permit selective permeation of alkali metal cations. Biological membranes show marked discrimination between alkali metal cations and furthermore Cl^- is much more permeable than Na^+ or K^+ in biological membranes whereas in unmodified bimolecular lipid membranes Cl^- is less permeable than Na^+ or K^+.

It is, therefore, quite apparent that lipids alone do not confer upon membranes the ion-selective and related properties so characteristic of biological membranes. This is well demonstrated by the work of Tosteson and his co-workers (214, 215) on the membrane properties of high potassium (HK) and low potassium (LK) red cells of the sheep. In these two genetically determined red cell types the permeabilities and intracellular concentrations of potassium and sodium are markedly different; however, bimolecular lipid membranes prepared from the membrane phospholipids of the two cell types were found to have essentially identical electrical properties to other membranes, to be equally permeable to Na^+ and K^+ and both were found to be some four to five times less permeable to chloride ion.

THE EXCITABLE MEMBRANE

The previous discusion of membranes was deliberately confined almost exclusively to general aspects of structure and function. From these basic considerations attention is now directed towards the electrically and chemically excitable membranes of nerve and muscle since events initiated at these membranes will form the basis of much of the remainder of the book. Primary emphasis will be placed in future chapters on chemically excitable membranes, those that respond with characteristic electrical, mechanical and biochemical responses to the binding of certain ligands.

ELECTRICALLY EXCITABLE MEMBRANES

In general,† nerve and muscle cells maintain a potential difference across their surface caused by the unequal distributions of ions; the cell interior is rich in potassium and the extracellular fluid is rich in sodium and chloride ions and the interior of the cell is maintained negative with respect to the exterior. The steady state of the excitable cell is maintained through the utilization of metabolic energy in driving a Na^+-K^+ ATPase that serves to expel accumulated Na^+ from the interior and accumulate K^+ from the exterior (Fig. II-23). Because the K^+ (and Cl^-) conductances are larger than the Na^+ conductance, a potential difference is built up and maintained across the cell membrane. These ionic conductances are represented in the equivalent circuit diagram shown in Fig. II-24 which is concerned solely with the various "leakage" pathways open to these ions and which become dramatically more important during impulse conduction. Figure II-24 indicates that

† Limitations to this general treatment will be noted later in this section and in subsequent chapters.

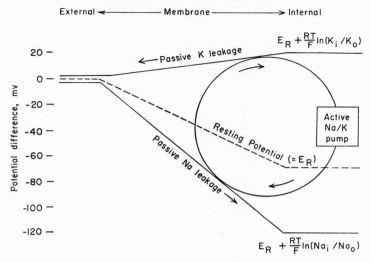

FIG. II-23. The role of the Na/K pump in maintaining the resting potential across the cell membrane by reversing the inward and outward leakages of Na$^+$ and K$^+$ ions respectively. Reproduced from "Nerve, Muscle and Synapse" by B. Katz. Copyright 1966, McGraw-Hill, Inc. Used with permission of the author and the McGraw-Hill Book Company.

the membrane acts as a leaky resistance to the three ions depicted and that each of these resistances is subject to independent control. Each pathway is defined by a characteristic equilibrium potential that

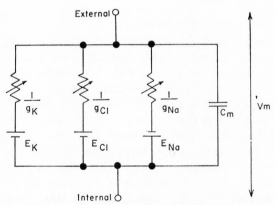

FIG. II-24. Equivalent circuit diagram for excitable membrane showing three separate channels, each with a leakage resistance, for Na$^+$ ($E_{Na^+} = +50$ to $+65$ mV), K$^+$ ($E_{K^+} = -70$ to -100 mV) and Cl$^-$ ($E_{Cl^-} = -45$ to -90 mV). Reproduced from "Nerve, Muscle and Synapse" by B. Katz. Copyright, 1966, McGraw-Hill, Inc. Used with permission of the author and the McGraw-Hill Book Company.

represents that potential difference across the membrane necessary to balance the tendency of the ion to diffuse down its activity gradient. The observed membrane potential will lie between the values for Na^+ and K^+ and, because of the greater K^+ conductance, will be closer to the equilibrium potential for K^+.[†]

Despite the fact that Fig. II-24 stresses only the electrical analogy of the excitable membrane and not the molecular events underlying excitation, it nevertheless indicates that the rapid changes of membrane potential occurring during conduction arise from changes in ionic conductance and *not* from alterations of equilibrium potentials since the latter depend upon the internal/external ratio of ionic concentrations and these do not change sufficiently rapidly.

Turning now to the mechanism of impulse conduction, the impulse may be initiated by a transient depolarization of the membrane.[‡] Below a certain level of depolarizing stimulus the membrane potential is simply depressed and then returns to the original value (Fig. II-25); however, a depolarization of some 10–15 mV produces a displacement of the membrane potential that is distinctly greater than the input stimulus and the recovery is somewhat delayed. Finally, with slightly higher input stimuli a critical depolarization is reached upon which the change in membrane potential becomes converted to the propagating spike (Fig. II-25).

A treatment of this process whereby a partial membrane depolarization becomes amplified has been provided by Hodgkin and Huxley (223) and has resulted in the widely accepted Hodgkin–Huxley axonal conduction model and which is based very largely on studies with the giant axons of squid. In this description, the sodium conductance (g_{Na^+}) is a function of membrane potential and increases as the potential is lowered, thus setting up a reinforcing process (Fig. II-26). In the absence of other ionic currents, the membrane potential should thus displace towards and equal the sodium equilibrium potential. This does not occur because the Na^+ conductance increase is only transient and is rapidly followed by an opposing increase in K^+ conductance which drives the system back to the resting state.

The dependence of the sodium conductance upon membrane potential is shown in Fig. II-27 and may be seen to be sigmoid with a steep dependence of g_{Na^+} upon the extent of depolarization induced suggesting the operation of a highly cooperative process.

[†] Only the briefest possible outline of ionic equilibria in nerve and muscle can be presented here. For further detail, the books of Hodgkin (216, 217), Katz (218) and Cole (219) should be consulted as well as standard texts of physiology.

[‡] Again, only a very short outline of some salient points of the conduction process will be mentioned. For further details references (216–219) should be consulted as well as the original papers of Hodgkin, Huxley and others (220–228).

7

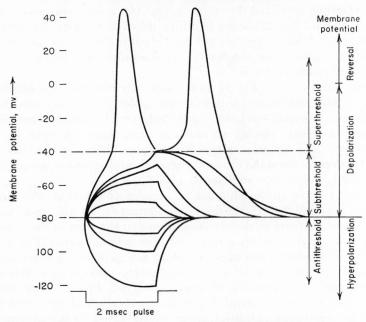

FIG. II-25. The initiation of a spike potential by a local depolarization. Note that only pulses that depolarize beyond a critical threshold level produce a spike potential. Reproduced from "Nerve, Muscle and Synapse" by B. Katz. Copyright 1966, McGraw-Hill, Inc. Used with permission of the author and the McGraw-Hill Book Company.

The voltage-clamp technique which permits the membrane potential to be held at any predetermined level has enabled a complete analysis to be made of the ionic events occurring during the spike potential.

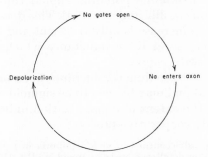

FIG. II-26. Representation of the regenerative Na^+ current depolarization phase of the spike potential. Reproduced from "Nerve, Muscle and Synapse by B. Katz. Copyright 1966, McGraw-Hill, Inc. Used with permission of the author and the McGraw-Hill Book Company.

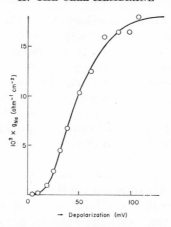

FIG. II-27. Relationship between Na$^+$ current magnitude and membrane potential in squid giant axon. Reproduced from "Nerve, Muscle and Synapse" by B. Katz. Copyright 1966, McGraw-Hill, Inc. Used with permission of the author and the McGraw-Hill Book Company.

The ionic contributions to this potential are an initial rapid increase in the Na$^+$ conductance that is converted within a few msec into an increased and opposing K$^+$ conductance (Fig. II-28). Major emphasis is

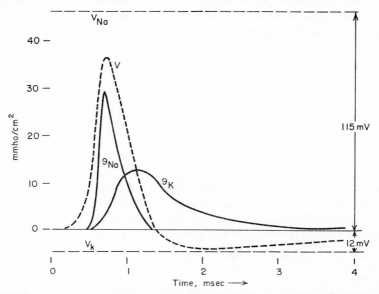

FIG. II-28. Representation of the time and potential courses of the sodium (g_{Na^+}) and potassium (g_{K^+}) components of the action potential (V). Reproduced with permission from Hodgkin and Huxley (220).

to be placed on the asynchronous character of the Na^+ and K^+ currents and the fact that the membrane, although depolarized, continues to discriminate between Na^+ and K^+ despite the reversal of conductances from those in the resting membrane.†

The mechanism of propagation along the excitable membrane is thus based upon the regenerative increase in Na^+ permeability producing an all or none response: a threshold change of ~ 20 mV is automatically amplified by a fivefold factor and can thus propagate without decrease in amplitude; a simple depolarization would, of course, be attenuated quite rapidly.‡

The permeability changes involve only a small fraction of the membrane surface. The specific resistance of the membrane is $\sim 10^{10}$ ohm cm^{-1} (about 10^8 times larger than the bulk medium) and falls during excitation to about 10^8 ohm cm^{-1} with little change in the capacitance of some 1 μF/cm^2. Thus the bulk of the membrane serves to act as a highly effective high resistance barrier and very much less than 1% of the cell surface is involved during these changes (231). From the values of Na^+ and K^+ transferred per impulse (3–4×10^{-12} mole/cm^2 in squid axons), an *average* transfer of one ion per 70 Å^2 takes place. The actual ion transfer process is probably concentrated at a much smaller number of sites, however, with each site being responsible for the transfer of several ions. This is revealed from studies with tetrodotoxin (II-4) an agent which appears to block specifically the Na^+ channel responsible for the inward current leaving the potassium channel unaffected (232–235).

II-4

Moore, Narahashi and Shaw (236) calculated from studies of tetrodotoxin uptake in lobster axon, that there is no more than one Na^+ channel/ 700 Å^2 and each channel must therefore pass at least 10 Na^+ ions per impulse. Clearly, the sites of ion permeation are relatively rare entities

† Some emphasis is necessary that this is in original reference to the squid axon and it must not be assumed that an *exactly* identical mechanism will automatically apply to all tissues (216–219).

‡ In almost all respects, the preceding discussion has been considerably oversimplified. The scope of the present work makes this unavoidable. As will be noted later, other ions (notably Ca^{++}) may play an important current carrying role; in smooth muscle impulse propagation and the ionic events are rather different from those outlined here.

on the membrane surface, yet the kinetics of the spike process indicate a highly cooperative interaction that must be relatable to the interactions between the various ion channels.

The Hodgkin–Huxley treatment of ionic conduction has been extremely successful and yet, in some respects, it does not offer any detailed physicochemical description of the molecular basis for the various ionic events. This, of course, may constitute one of the main reasons for its continued success, since it does not claim to rest on any highly specified description of the excitable membrane.

Nevertheless, attempts are being made to provide specific physicochemical descriptions of these ionic events, one of the most notable being that due to Tasaki and his co-workers (237–240). These workers have adopted the procedure of internal and external perfusion of squid axons with a variety of ionic media to determine the effects of various ions on the ability of the axon to remain excitable and to generate action potentials.

Substitution of internal anions (as K salts) led to the following order of ability to maintain or restore excitability,

$$F > HPO_4 > \text{glutamate, aspartate} > SO_4 > Cl > NO_3 > Br > I > SCN$$

This sequence is of considerable interest since it parallels exactly the sequence described by Bungenburg de Jong (240a) for charge reversal (i.e., binding) of positively charged colloids, i.e., $SCN > I > Br - - - F$. Substitution of internal cations led to the sequence $Cs > Rb > K > NH_4 > Na > Li$ for maintaining excitability which is in partial agreement with the order of affinity, $Li > Na > K$, noted by Bungenburg de Jong for charge reversal of phosphate colloids.

In contrast to the effects of internal perfusion, the effects of external anion substitution appear to be of little consequence. This is in accord with most current thought that the external membrane surface contains a high density of negative charge (241–244) and will tend to serve as a cationic exchanger for which anions will have little affinity. In contrast, the internal surface must contain significant positive charge and the effects of intracellular anions in modifying excitability have been ascribed to their modifying intermolecular ionic linkages of the inner membrane surface. The effectiveness of external cations in maintaining or restoring excitability lies in the order (238, 245–247) suggesting that the

$$K < Rb < Cs < Na < Li$$

external cation binding site is carboxylate since the sequence $K < Na < Li$, has been well documented by Bungenburg de Jong (*loc. cit.*) as the order of effectiveness for charge reversal of carboxyl colloids. The study of ammonium ions revealed the following sequences,

(a) $RNH_3^+ < NH_4^+ < NH_2NH_3^+$

(b) $R_4N^+ < R_3NH^+ < R_2NH_2^+ < RNH_3^+ < NH_4^+$
   $(R = Me, Et, Pr^n, Bu^n)$

(c) $(C_4H_9)_nNH_m^+ < (C_3H_7)_nNH_m^+ < (C_2H_5)_nNH_m^+ < (CH_3)_nNH_m^+$
   $(n + m = 4)$

Quite clearly, the presence of alkyl groups and increasing size of alkyl substitution reduces the ability of the molecule to substitute for Na^+ in the maintenance of excitability of the squid axon and the most favorable substitutes for Na^+ are the ammonium, hydrazine and guanidinium cations. It is noteworthy that tetrodotoxin (II-4) contains a guanidinium group.

Under certain conditions action potentials can be obtained from the squid axon in the total absence of external Na^+ provided that an appropriate substitute is present (NH_4^+, $N_2H_5^+$, etc.); these potential changes do not seem to be significantly different from those obtained in the normal sodium-containing media and, moreover, in this case also, the inward current is abolished by tetrodotoxin. Furthermore, under appropriate conditions (internal perfusion with Cs^+) the requirement for external univalent cations can be abolished entirely and Ca^{++} can substitute to give the normal all-or-none action potentials in response to electrical stimulation (238, 239, 248, 249). Voltage clamp studies reveal that the current components of the action potential in this highly modified system are apparently analogous to the normal system and involve an initial inward current rapidly followed by an outward current. From experiments in which Na^+ or K^+ was added to the external Ca^{++} medium, it was found that at critical M^+/M^{++} ratios, the axon responds with a large and abrupt depolarization (238, 249).

Tasaki has interpreted this work according to proposals which differ quite substantially from the widely accepted Hodgkin–Huxley treatment. A full account of the Tasaki proposals are to be found in references 238 and 239 and are, in brief, that the membrane acts as a cation exchanger and that changes in the cation concentration at the membrane result in its conversion from a relatively impermeable state to a highly permeable state. Whether it is necessary to assume, as Tasaki does, that the cations do not move through separate channels, seems open to question (250). The fact that a variety of ions can substitute for Na^+ and K^+ is not, however, inconsistent with the Hodgkin–Huxley treatment since it may readily be assumed that the "sodium channels" do not have absolute specificity for sodium. Similarly, the fact that tetrodotoxin blocks the inward current due to hydrazine, guanidinium, etc., is certainly consistent with the assumption that it blocks the channel concerned with ion influx—the fact that tetrodotoxin possesses a guanidinium function is particularly worthy of note in this connection. Furthermore, the observations made on the perfused axon all indicate the importance of the biphasic, asynchronous current components of the action potential which form such a prominent part of the Hodgkin–Huxley treatment. It is important to note that the Hodgkin–Huxley treatment does not make any particular assumption as to the current carrying species other than they are Na^+ and K^+ under physiological conditions: the experiments of Tasaki reveal very clearly that a number of other cations can substitute for Na^+ and K^+. The great strength and, at the same time a weakness, of the Hodgkin–Huxley treatment is that it makes the minimum number of assumptions concerning the under-lying molecular basis of excitation; the concept of conformational change of the membrane is, however, certainly implicit in their treatment. In contrast, the approach put forward by Tasaki does offer a fairly detailed picture of the molecular basis of excitation and his treatment of the membrane conformational change will be further discussed in a later section. Whatever the ultimate merit of the Tasaki hypothesis as a model for impulse conduction, his experimental data seem certain to shed further light on this process; in particular, the observed role of the bivalent/univalent cation ratio is consistent with much accumulated data on Ca^{++} and membrane function. However, before proceeding to further discussions of Ca^{++} function and membrane conformational change, it is desirable to complete this brief introductory review of electrical events at excitable membranes by introducing some general comments on chemically excitable membranes.

CHEMICALLY EXCITABLE MEMBRANES

The subject matter of this section properly belongs to subsequent chapters; nonetheless, a brief review may assist at this point to complete a perspective of excitable membrane phenomena and facilitate a general discussion of the membrane conformational changes as they may relate to membrane excitability.

There is general acceptance of the concept that at many synapses continuous electrical transmission is unlikely (218, 230) and that impulse transmission is achieved through the intermediary actions of specific chemical agents liberated from the presynaptic terminal (Chapter III). Direct evidence for the occurrence of such a transmitter was first obtained by Loewi in his discovery of the "vagustoffe" liberated in stimulation of the vagal nerve to the frog heart (251). It cannot be assumed automatically, however, that chemical transmission occurs at all synapses and there is some evidence for direct electrical transmission at certain tightly coupled and highly contiguous synapses (218, 252).

In many respects, one of the most straightforward instances of chemical transmission is at the vertebrate skeletal neuromuscular junction (Fig. II-29) which has been studied very intensively (218, 229,

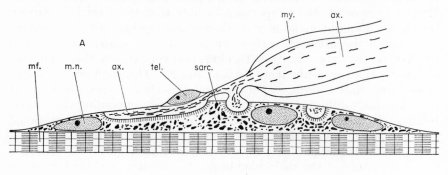

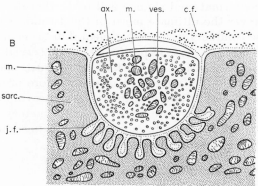

FIG. II-29. A. Drawing of a motor end plate; ax., axoplasm; my., myelin sheath; tel., teloglia (terminal Schwann cells); sarc., sarcoplasm; m.n., muscle nuclei; mf., myofibrils. B. Cross section through synaptic gutter; ves, vesicles; j.f., junctional fold; c.f., collagen fibers. Reproduced with permission from Couteaux (*Exp. Cell. Res.* (1958) Suppl. 5, 294).

253–260) and where an extracellular gap of some 500 Å exists between the nerve terminal and the muscle end plate region. Ionophoretic application of acetylcholine reveals that only a small area, the end plate region, is chemically sensitive with the remaining area of the muscle cell being electrically sensitive. Fast skeletal muscle fibers respond to electrical stimulation by initiation of a propagated impulse provided that the stimulus is above a threshold level. This suprathreshold stimulus is normally initiated by the interaction of presynaptically liberated acetylcholine at the end plate to produce a local depolarization, the end plate potential, which then triggers the spike potential (Fig. II-30). The end plate potential arises as a graded response to acetylcholine; the graded response is a general characteristic of the action of ligands at chemically sensitive membranes. Analysis of the ionic events of the epp reveals (254, 255, 261, 262) that the reversal point is (approximately) −15 mV, so that unlike the subsequently generated action potential there is no actual reversal of membrane polarities. The null point (maximum depolarization) does not correspond to the equilibrium potentials of Na^+, K^+ or Cl^-, but, in fact, represents the Na^+ and K^+

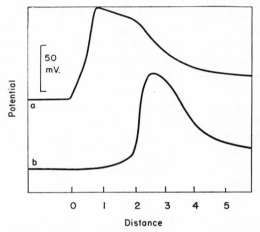

FIG. II-30. Potential changes at the skeletal neuromuscular junction; (a) at the end plate showing the end plate potential "hump" during generation of the action potential; (b) 2·5 mm away showing the absence of the epp. Reproduced with permission from Fatt and Katz (253).

channels opening simultaneously. Thus, in this instance the response of the chemically excitable membrane differs from the response of the electrically excitable membrane in at least two important aspects, graded responsiveness and synchrony of alteration of Na^+ and K^+ conductances. A third important distinction is that, unlike the electrically excitable membrane, the conductance change produced by acetylcholine is independent of the membrane potential (253, 261, 262): thus the action of acetylcholine will not become regenerative as in axonal conduction and acetylcholine will produce a current flow across the end plate region proportional to $(E - 15)$ mV, where E is the membrane potential. Thus the AP and epp are molecularly distinct processes that occur in physically separate areas of the cell membrane.

7*

Attention has thus far been confined to two examples of electrical phenomena—giant axon conduction and skeletal neuromuscular transmission. This was a deliberate selection presenting two well-investigated examples demonstrating rather clear cut differences between events at chemically and electrically excitable cell membranes that must form part of subsequent discussions of conformational changes in excitable membranes. It is to be emphasized, however, that attention cannot be focused solely upon Na^+ and K^+ as current carrying species and, depolarizations, all-or-none and graded responses in giant axons and skeletal neuromuscular junctions even though they are representative of a large number of electrical and chemical events. Other processes are known to be important; hyperpolarization at inhibitory neuronal synapses (263) and smooth muscle junctions (264), Ca^{++} as a current carrying species in invertebrate muscle (265, 266) and mammalian smooth muscle (267–269), the geometry of the latter being very poorly defined compared to skeletal muscle junctions and the occurrence of graded responses in some electrically excitable membranes (230, 270), where the conductile function of the spike is taken care of by diffuse innervation, are but a few examples of variations upon the theme of changing ionic permeabilities as a basis for membrane excitability. However, before any discussion of the general molecular basis of membrane excitability it is necessary to discuss the role of calcium, an ion that appears to play a rather central role in the control of many membrane functions.

THE ROLE OF CALCIUM IN EXCITABLE MEMBRANES

While the major emphasis has rested with Na^+ and K^+ as the cationic current carrying species across excitable membranes it is clear that other ions, most notably Ca^{++}, play a critical role in the maintenance of cell excitability and of the integrity of the cell membrane in general (271–279) as well as, in certain systems, serving as a charge carrier. Calcium is known to be important in the maintenance of cellular adhesion (277, 280), the mechanical integrity (277) and permeability control of membranes (*inter alia*, 278, 279, 281–285), the release of neurotransmitters (286–289) and hormones generally (290) and, as will be discussed in Chapter VII, plays a critical role in the initiation and maintenance of contractile processes.

The influence of Ca^{++} on cell excitability has been known since the work of Ringer in 1883 (291) and the classification of Ca^{++} as a membrane stabilizer in excitable systems has gradually developed since then (271–279). Thus, in elevated concentrations Ca^{++}_{EXT} will maintain or increase the resting potential (*inter alia*, 274, 275, 278, 279, 292–298), raise the threshold and increase membrane resistance (278, 279, 299). Conversely, reduction of Ca_{EXT}^{++} levels may lead quite generally to a lowering of membrane potential and increased spontaneous excitability (*inter alia*, 224, 274, 275, 278, 279, 292, 297, 298, 300–304) in nerve and muscle preparations. It appears that the stabilizing effects of increased Ca_{EXT}^{++} and the destabilizing effects of lowered Ca_{EXT}^{++} are essentially similar to the effects produced by increased and reduced membrane potential respectively (302).

Voltage-clamp studies with squid axons reveals (244, 279, 302) that the primary effect of increased Ca_{EXT}^{++} is a displacement along the voltage axis of the curves that relate the activation of the sodium conductance to the membrane potential: a fivefold reduction in Ca_{EXT}^{++} shifts the curve by about 15 mV so that a smaller initial depolarization suffices to raise the sodium conductance to a given level (Fig. II-27) while elevation of Ca_{EXT}^{++} produces the opposite effect. A similar effect has been observed with frog medullated nerves (244) and frog skeletal muscle fibers and spinal ganglion cells (279). The rates of rise and fall of the sodium conductance are also affected by variations in Ca_{EXT}^{++}, a reduction in Ca_{EXT}^{++} increasing the rate of rise and decreasing the rate of decline of sodium conductance (279, 292, 302, 305, 306).†

The situation in smooth muscle appears to be more complex and in any event is less well understood. In general, reduction of Ca_{EXT}^{++} causes depolarization and a decreased rate of rise of the action potential (268, 297, 298, 308–313) suggesting a contribution by Ca^{++} to the inward current flow. Thus, in the guinea-pig vas deferens a tenfold reduction of Ca_{EXT}^{++} reduces the resting potential by some 25 mV and decreases the action potential overshoot by 22 mV (Fig. II-31). Further support for the role of Ca^{++} as a partial or dominant current carrying species in smooth muscle comes from the many observations documenting the occurrence of spikes in the absence of Na_{EXT}^{++} (*inter alia*, 297, 311–314),‡ by spike generation in Ca^{++} free media containing Ba^{++} as a Ca^{++} substitute (298) and the ineffectiveness of tetrodoxin, presumed to act specifically at sodium channels, on smooth muscle spikes (265, 316–318). These lines of evidence are basically similar to those advanced for crayfish and barnacle muscle fibers and mollusc giant nerve cells (265, 266, 319–321) where Ca^{++}-action potentials have also been observed

---

† It is not certain that Na^+ and Ca^{++} share the same binding site. Ca^{++} is known to bind tightly to phospholipids but Na^+ does not. Tetrodotoxin, which does not affect Ca^{++} currents but does abolish Na^+ currents, does not bind to the polar phospholipids of squid axons, but does produce expansion of monolayers of the nonpolar lipids (307).

‡ However, it should be noted that Kao (315) has offered particularly pertinent criticism of experiments purporting to show independence of spikes from Na^+ primarily on the grounds that adequate time may not have been allowed to ensure complete removal of Na_{INT}^+.

and for the plateau phase of the frog heart ventricular action potential (320, 322).

From this very abbreviated review of the effects of Ca^{++} on the nerve and muscle membrane it is clear that the binding to and displacement of Ca^{++} from the membrane is a critical step in the excitation process (further discussion of this point will be presented in Chapters V and VII). It seems most profitable to consider the Ca^{++}-membrane equilibrium as almost certainly related to competition between Na^+, K^+ and Ca^{++} for fixed negative charges on the cell membrane (*inter alia*, 217, 238, 272, 279, 244, 323–328) and an analysis of such potential binding sites should, therefore be directly relevant to an understanding of excitation processes.

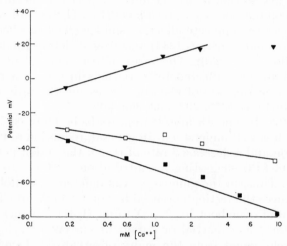

FIG. II-31. Effect of Ca^{++} concentration on the characteristics of the action potential in the guinea-pig vas deferens. ■, resting potential; □, initiation threshold; ▲, overshoot of the AP. Reproduced with permission from Bennett (268).

A variety of studies, encompassing tissue and model preparations, indicate very strongly that lipids, notably phospholipids and gangliosides, play an important role in the binding of cationic species, both inorganic and organic. That phospholipids bind inorganic cations and facilitate their transport from aqueous into non-aqueous environments has been known for some time (329–333). In a series of investigations Schulman and his collaborators have shown (334–336) that cephalin (phosphatidylserine plus some phosphatidylethanolamine) facilitates the transport of Na^+ and K^+ across an aqueous layer separated by an organic phase: of particular interest is the observation that this transport was inhibited by low concentrations of Ca^{++} (336). Wooley and Campbell

(337) have demonstrated that Ca^{++} is the most tightly bound cation (of Na^+, K^+ and Ca^{++}) to crude lipid extracts of hog stomach and spinal cord (containing phospholipids, cerebrosides and gangliosides).

In a study of the interactions of phospholipids and Ca^{++} (to which more detailed reference will be made later), Feinstein (338) showed that Ca^{++} is transported into $CHCl_3$ from an $H_2O/MeOH$ phase. Some results are presented in Table II-11 from which it is evident that phosphatidyl-serine is particularly effective in Ca^{++} transport—these results are of physiological relevance since they were carried out with a Na^+/Ca^{++}

TABLE II-11. Calcium Transport into Chloroform from a Water:Methanol Phase (338)

Lipid† (2mg/ml)	Ca^{++} in $CHCl_3$ phase μ moles
None	0
Cholesterol	0
Tripalmitin	0
Lecithin (animal)	0·327
Lecithin (synthetic) (β,γ-dipalmitoyl-L-α-lecithin)	0·284
Cephalin (animal)	0·746
Phosphatidylserine	0·804

† Experimental conditions: 2 ml aliquots of $CHCl_3$:MeOH (2:1) containing 1 mg/ml of lipid, or extracted lipids from nerve or muscle, were shaken for 10 min with 1·0 ml aq. solution containing NaCl (110 mM), KCl (2·5 mM), $CaCl_2$ (1·0 mM) and 1 μC/ml Ca^{45} at pH 6·0.

ratio of 100:1. Similar studies by Blaustein and Goldman (339) have revealed that synthetic phosphatidylethanolamine is very much less effective than phosphatidylserine in facilitating Ca^{++} transport. Studies of the pH changes produced on the addition of cationic species to phospholipid dispersions reveal that a fall in pH occurs, polyvalent cations being more effective in this regard (338, 340–342; Fig. II-32). The interaction of calcium with cephalin has a stoichiometry of 2 moles cephalin: 1 mole Ca^{++} and presumably calcium binds two molecules of phospholipid through the phosphate group. It seems probable that phosphatidylserine binds Na^+ and K^+ at both the carboxyl and phosphate groups (340, 341).

As anticipated the phospholipid–cation interaction is also markedly dependent upon the lipid structure: Dervichian showed (341) that neither Na^+ nor Ca^{++} produces any significant pH change with phosphatidylcholine. This is undoubtedly due to the fact that between pH 3–11 phosphatidylcholine is zwitterionic.

Studies on the relative abilities of inorganic cations to coagulate phospholipid sols (338, 342, 343) have also led to similar conclusions. Robins and Thomas (343) reported that Ca^{++} concentrations of $0{\cdot}5{-}1{\cdot}0$ mM coagulate phosphatidylserine and phosphatidylethanolamine sols and that Ca^{++} is some 1000 times more effective in this regard than either Na^+ or K^+. Feinstein showed (338) that Ca^{++} has no effect on phosphatidylcholine sols and that Na^+ and K^+ inhibited the coagulative

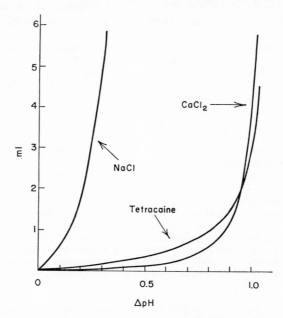

FIG. II-32. Titration of aqueous cephalin dispersion by $0{\cdot}05$ M NaCl, $CaCl_2$ and tetracaine HCl. ΔpH—fall in pH. Reproduced with permission from Feinstein (338).

ability of Ca^{++} on cephalin, phosphatidylserine and phosphatidylethanolamine sols.

In studies that are somewhat more directly relatable to physiological conditions Rojas and Tobias (344) have studied the interaction of cationic species with phospholipid monolayers. Surface pressure-area studies with phosphatidylcholine revealed that Na^+, K^+ and Ca^{++} exerted no significant effect: Ca^{++} had a slight condensing effect on phosphatidylethanolamine and exerted a fairly marked condensing effect on phosphatidylserine monolayers (Fig. II-33) which was antagonized with equal effectiveness by Na^+ and K^+. The condensing effect of Ca^{++} is probably due to its forming an ionic link between two phospholipid heads diminishing their repulsion and permitting a closer arrangement of the lipids. Papahadjopoulos (213) has also demonstrated the binding of Ca^{++} to acidic phospholipids to give rise to a decrease in surface pressure and has suggested the formation of linear polymeric Ca^{++}-complexes (Fig. II-34). In similar studies Hauser and Dawson (345) found no adsorption of Ca^{++} on phosphatidylcholine and in a

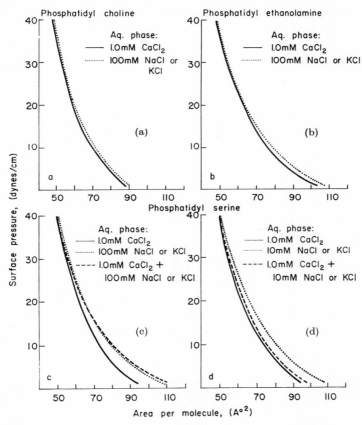

FIG. II-33. Surface pressure–area diagrams for (a) phosphatidylcholine, (b) phosphatidylethanolamine and (c, d) phosphatidylserine monolayers ($t° = 24 \pm 2$, pH $5·6 \pm 0·25$). Reproduced with permission from Rojas and Tobias (344).

variety of other phospholipids including phosphatidylserine, phosphatidylinositol, phosphatidic acid, triphosphoinositide, etc., Ca^{++} binding was found to be dependent primarily upon the excess negative charge of the lipid and to be relatively independent of lipid structure. Na^+ and K^+ were again found to be equally effective in displacing bound Ca^{++} but were themselves bound some 5000–10,000 times less effectively than calcium. In a further extension of their work on monolayers Tobias and his colleagues (346, 347) have studied the effects of Na^+, K^+ and Ca^{++} on phospholipid : cholesterol membranes formed in a Millipore filter impregnated with cephalin (mainly phosphatidylserine) and cholesterol and separated by two aqueous phases : the resistance of such membranes in 0·1 M NaCl and KCl is approximately 100 ohms and is reversibly increased by a sixfold factor on addition of 0·05 M $CaCl_2$.

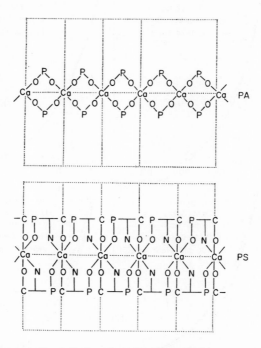

FIG. II-34. Representation of phosphatidic acid—Ca^{++} (PA) and phosphatidyl-serine—Ca^{++} complexes. Dotted lines represent the carbon chains. Reproduced with permission from Papahadjopoulos (213).

Interesting effects of Ca^{++} on the permeability of phospholipid liposomes have also been noted by Papahadjopoulos and Watkins (212) : elevated Ca^{++} concentrations increased the self diffusion rate of K^+ through the lamellae (Fig. II-35). These results are somewhat surprising in view of the previous studies indicating the stabilizing effects of Ca^{++} on biological membranes and phospholipid monolayers. However, later studies (348) with phosphatidylserine bimolecular lipid films have revealed that Ca^{++} stabilizes and increases the resistance of the membrane when symmetrically distributed on both sides of the membrane but when present on only one side of the membrane produces a drastic decrease in film stability and resistance. Quite probably the decrease in membrane stability arises from the asymmetric distribution of charges across the bilayer resulting in a difference in surface energy between the two sides and producing an initially localized membrane breakdown (349). This conclusion is of very considerable importance to a possible understanding of molecular events in electrically and chemically excitable membranes where it is becoming increasingly obvious that a key role is played by the displacement of membrane-bound calcium.

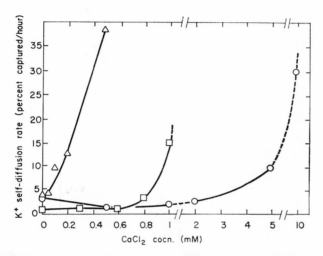

FIG. II-35. Effect of Ca^{++} on K^+ diffusion through phosphatidic acid ($\triangle$), phosphatidylserine ($\square$), and phosphatidylinositol ($\bigcirc$) liquid crystals (pH 7·4, room temp.). Reproduced with permission from Papahadjopoulos and Watkins (212).

As anticipated, polyvalent cations are able to compete much more effectively than Na^+ or K^+ for the Ca^{++} binding sites on phospholipids. Blaustein (350) has studied the effects of a group of such polyvalent cations on the binding of Ca^{++} to phosphatidylserine by determining their effects on the transfer of $^{45}Ca^{++}$ from an aqueous media to a $CHCl_3$–MeOH phase; La^{+++}, Al^{+++} and Ce^{+++} were found to be particularly effective in this regard.

In a refined study Barton (351) has investigated the influence of the surface charge density of phospholipids on cation binding. The concentrations of cationic species to induce charge reversal in dispersions of phospholipids,

$$(R_3N^+\sim PO_3H_2^-)_n + M^{(+)n} \rightleftharpoons (R_3N^+\sim PO_3H_2M)$$

were determined and used to evaluate approximate dissociation constants. These have been plotted in Fig. II-36 against the relative inhibition of binding of Ca^{++} to phosphatidylserine as determined by Blaustein, the correlation is good, save for one important exception, the UO_2^{++} cation which binds very much more effectively to phosphatidylserine than Blaustein's data would indicate. This is a very important finding which suggests that the UO_2^{++} species has a much higher affinity

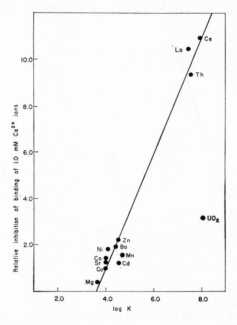

FIG. II-36. Relative inhibition of binding of Ca^{++} to phosphatidylserine as a function of $\log K$ (calculated from the charge-reversal data of polyvalent cations determined by Blaustein (350)). Reproduced with permission from Barton (351).

for the aggregated species (Barton experiments) than for the monomolecular film (Blaustein experiments) of phosphatidylserine. As suggested by Barton, this may be related to the fact that in the uranyl phosphate lattice of the mineral autonite the phosphate groups of the tetragonal lattice occupy an area of 58·5 Å which is very close to the limiting area for many phosphatides. Thus the adsorption of the UO_2^{++} onto a phosphate surface will be greatly facilitated for the aggregated form of phosphatides.†

† The extreme potency of UO_2^{++} in producing charge reversal of lecithin colloid was noted by Kruyt (352).

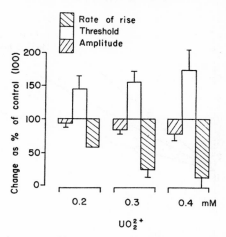

FIG. II-37. The effects of UO_2^{++} on the characteristics of the action potential in skeletal muscle. Reproduced with permission from Sokoll and Thesleff (356).

This finding is of direct relevance to membrane phenomena since the UO_2^{++} cation has been shown to exert a profound effect on several membrane mediated processes. In a series of studies of sugar transport in yeast Rothstein and Van Steveninck have presented good evidence that UO_2^{++} complexes with phosphate residues (possibly polyphosphates or phospholipids) and inhibits glucose transport. The binding of UO_2^{++} is a saturable process, is confined to the cell membrane and a number of other cations, including Ca^{++}, compete for the membrane binding site.

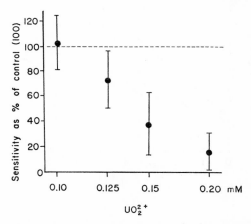

FIG. II-38. The effects of UO_2^{++} on the ACh sensitivity of the chronically denervated muscle membrane. Reproduced with permission from Sokoll and Thesleff (356).

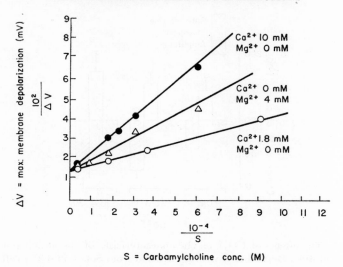

Fig. II-39. Competitive inhibition (Lineweaver-Burk plot) by Ca^{++} of the membrane depolarization produced by carbamylcholine in skeletal muscle. Reproduced with permission from Nastuk (358).

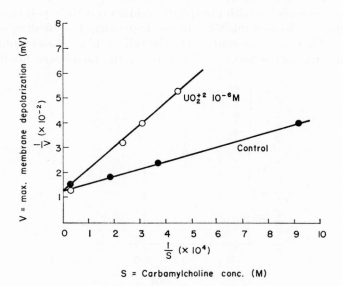

Fig. II-40. Competitive inhibition by UO_2^{++} of the membrane depolarization produced by carbamylcholine in skeletal muscle. Reproduced with permission from Nastuk (358).

Schulman (335) has also shown that UO_2^{++} inhibits Ca^{++} transport by cephalin.

In excitable systems Sokoll and Thesleff (356) have shown that UO_2^{++} decreases the rate of rise and increases the threshold for action potential generation with little effect on the amplitude in skeletal muscle (Fig. II-37), and decreases the sensitivity to acetylcholine (Fig. II-38). These results may suggest some basic similarity between electrically and chemically excitable membranes. Nastuk (357, 358) has demonstrated the competitive interaction of Ca^{++} and carbamylcholine (H_2NCOO $(CH_2)_2N^+Me_3$) at the chemosensitive postjunctional membrane of skeletal muscle (Fig. II-39) and a similar competitive interaction with UO_2^{++} (Fig. II-40) suggesting very strongly an involvement of phospholipids in the acetylcholine receptor and a basic similarity of the molecular events involved in action potential generation and acetylcholine-induced depolarization involving, perhaps, the displacement of Ca^{++} from a cation binding site.

CALCIUM AND LOCAL ANESTHETIC ACTION

The relationship between Ca^{++}, phospholipids and excitable membranes may also be demonstrated from studies of local anesthetics such as procaine (II-5), butacaine (II-6) and a large number of related compounds (359) which, like Ca^{++}, are also known as membrane

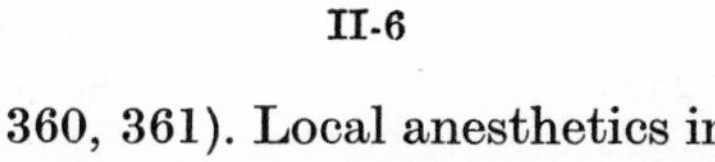

$$H_2N-\langle\bigcirc\rangle-COOCH_2CH_2NEt_2$$

II-5

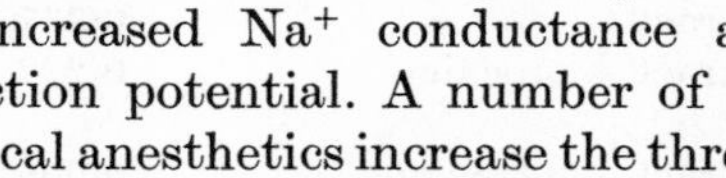

$$H_2N-\langle\bigcirc\rangle-COOCH_2CH_2NBu_2$$

II-6

stabilizers (274, 276, 360, 361). Local anesthetics interfere with impulse conduction in nerve and muscle through a probable primary action (361–365) on the increased Na^+ conductance associated with the generation of the action potential. A number of studies have clearly demonstrated that local anesthetics increase the threshold for excitation, slow propagation of the impulse and reduce the rate of rise of the action potential in both nerve and muscle fibers (274, 362, 364, 366–368). The similar stabilizing effects of Ca^{++} and local anesthetics led to the suggestion (292) that they share a common site of action and in agreement with this suggestion Blaustein and Goldman have shown (369), in voltage clamp studies in the lobster axon, that procaine decreases the sodium conductance and the action potential overshoot and that these effects of procaine are antagonized by increased Ca^{++}_{EXT} and potentiated by reduced Ca^{++}_{EXT}. Similar conclusions have been drawn from studies on the squid giant axon (365). In a later chapter (Chapter VII) the powerful effects of local anesthetics in modifying the role of Ca^{++} in excitation-contraction coupling will be discussed.

Nevertheless, certain differences between the actions of Ca^{++} and local anesthetics have also led to the view that they act at different sites. Thus elevated Ca^{++}_{EXT} and local anesthetics both increase the threshold of excitation but Ca^{++} increases the rate of rise and height of the action potential while local anesthetics produce the opposite effect. Local anesthetics decrease Na^+ conductance whereas elevated Ca^{++}_{EXT} maintains and increases the sodium conductance of the rising phase of the action-potential although shifting it along the potential axis. Aceves and Machne (295) have shown that the effects of local anesthetics in increasing the threshold of frog spinal ganglion cells are potentiated by elevated Ca^{++}_{EXT}, but that the depressant effects of the anesthetics on the amplitude and rate of rise of the action potential are antagonized by elevated Ca^{++}_{EXT}. These and related findings (364) led them to suggest that Ca^{++}

TABLE II-12. Inhibition of Ca^{++} Uptake into Lipids by Local Anesthetics (338)

Lipid	Ca^{++} in $CHCl_3$ phase moles	% Inhibition of Ca^{++} uptake
None	0	—
Lecithin (animal)	0·327	—
Lecithin + procaine (4·4 mM)	0·080	76
Lecithin (synthetic)	0·284	—
Lecithin + procaine (4·4 mM)	0·046	84
Cephalin (animal)	0·746	—
Cephalin + procaine (4·4 mM)	0·417	44
Cephalin (animal)	0·485†	—
Cephalin + tetracaine (2·2 mM)	0·095	79
Phosphatidylserine	0·804	—
Phosphatidylserine + procaine (4·4 mM)	0·539	33
Rabbit sciatic nerve extract	0·337	—
Rabbit sciatic nerve extract + procaine (4·4 mM)	0·222	34
Rabbit sciatic nerve extract + tetracaine (4·4 mM)	0·006	98

Two ml aliquots of $CHCl_3$:MeOH (2:1) containing 1 mg/ml of lipid material were shaken for 10 min with 1·0 ml of aqueous solution containing NaCl 116 mM, KCl 2·5 mM, $CaCl_2$ 1·0 mM and 1 μc/ml Ca^{45} at pH 6·0.

† Contained lipid at 0·5 mg/ml.

TABLE II-13. Effects of Local Anesthetics on Calcium Binding
to Phosphatidylserine (338)

Drug	Relative inhibition of Ca^{++} binding[†]	Relative anesthetic potency[‡]
Procaine§	1·0	1·0
Mepivacaine¶	1·6	2·1
Lidocaine‖	3·5	3·8
Hexylcaine††	4·4	2·7
Piperocaine‡‡	4·7	3·5
Tetracaine§§	8·7	36·5
Dibucaine¶¶	10·1	53·8

† The relative inhibition of Ca^{++} binding reflects the amount of
agent necessary to inhibit Ca^{++} binding by 20%.
‡ Determined on frog sciatic nerve trunk at pH 7·18–7·20.
§ $4\text{-}H_2NC_6H_4COOCH_2CH_2NEt_2$.

¶ $2,6\text{-}Me_2C_6H_3NHCO-$

‖ $2,6\text{-}Me_2C_6H_3NHCOCH_2NEt_2$.
†† $C_6H_4COOCH(Me)CH_2NHC_6H_{11}$.

†† $C_6H_4COOCH_2CH_2CH_2N$

§§ $4\text{-}C_4H_9NHC_6H_4COOCH_2CH_2NMe_2$.
¶¶ $CONHCH_2CH_2NEt_2$

OBu^7

and local anesthetics, while undoubtedly involved in a mutually interacting system, do not compete for an identical binding site. An alternative explanation is, however, at least equally plausible since it is probable
that Ca^{++} has the dual function of both stabilizing the resting membrane
and of supporting generation of the action potential. Local anesthetics
almost certainly lack the ability to substitute for Ca^{++} in its second role.

Of obvious relevance to the competitive behavior of Ca^{++} and local
anesthetics in excitable systems are the increasingly well-documented
findings that local anesthetics, as well as Ca^{++}, are bound significantly
by phospholipids and also compete with Ca^{++} in such binding phenomena. Feinstein (338) has shown that (Table II-12) procaine and tetracaine inhibit the uptake of Ca^{++} by cephalin, tetracaine being more
potent in this regard. Blaustein (339, 370) has also determined the
ability of a number of local anesthetics to inhibit Ca^{++} binding to
phospholipids and noted that those agents that most effectively inhibit
Ca^{++} uptake by phospholipids are also the most effective local anesthetics
(Tables II-13, II-14).

TABLE II-14. Inhibition by Local Anesthetics of Ca^{++} Binding to Phospholipids (370)

Agent	Conc mM	Ca^{++} bound to phosphatidylserine (μmole)	Inhibition %	Ca^{++} bound to phosphatidylethanolamine (μmole)	Inhibition %	Anesthetic effect
Control	—	0·776	—	0·056	—	—
A	1·25	0·742	4	0·050	11	0
B	1·25	0·503	35	0·004	93	+++
C	1·25	0·471	39	0·002	96	+++
D	1·25	0·427	45	0·004	93	+
Control	—	0·848	—	0·058	—	—
E (xylocaine)	0·5	0·771	9	0·037	36	—
	2·0	0·503	41	0·013	78	—
F	0·5	0·804	5	0·056	3	+
	2·0	0·630	26	0·052	10	0

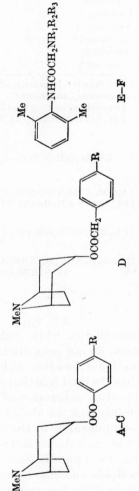

A, R = Cl (tropine-p-chlorophenyl acetate).
B, R = H (tropine phenylacetate).
C, R = Me (tropine p-tolylacetate).
D, R = Me (tropine p-tolylacetate, methiodide).
E, R$_1$ = R$_2$ = Et, R$_3$ = H.
F, R$_1$ = R$_2$ = R$_3$ = Et.

The ability of Ca^{++} to coagulate phospholipid sols has previously been noted (p. 168): local anesthetics share this property (338). For phosphatidylethanolamine the order of effectiveness is tetracaine > butacaine > procaine, corresponding to their anesthetic activity *in vivo*. An identical pH change is noted when a phosphatidylethanolamine sol is titrated with either Ca^{++} or tetracaine suggesting (p. 168) that the stoichiometry of the reaction is local anesthetic: (lipid)$_2$ and that binding occurs to the phosphate group (371).

At the present time the binding orientation of local anesthetics to phospholipids (and other acidic molecules) of the cell membrane is not entirely clear although it is obvious that ionic interactions are of very considerable importance and there appears to be little doubt that the

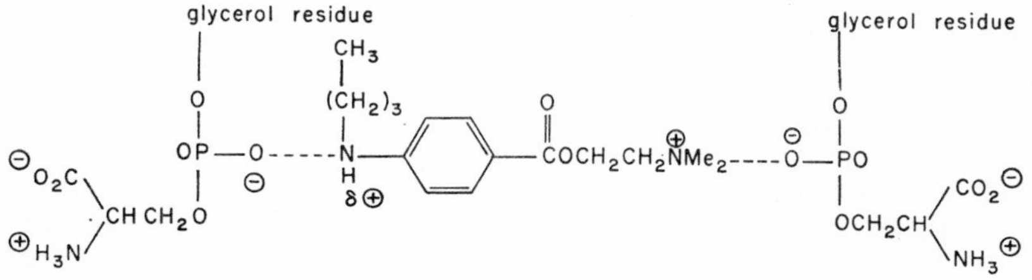

FIG. II-41. Model for the mechanism of complex formation between local anesthetics and acidic phospholipids. After Feinstein (338).

protonated form of local anesthetics is the pharmacologically active species (361, 372, 373). Feinstein (338, 371) visualizes an interaction as shown in Fig. II-41: at physiological pH the tertiary alkylamino group will bear a positive charge and binds through an ion–ion interaction. The aromatic amino group is uncharged but is presumed to find efficiently through the induced partial charge interaction shown. However, not all local anesthetics can bind in this way and for those without two basic functions a 1:1 interaction with phospholipid must occur.

MEMBRANE MODELS AND MEMBRANE EXCITABILITY

Despite the obviously important roles of phospholipids and calcium in controlling membrane properties it is quite clear that these constituents alone do not generate the unique ion-selective and related properties of biological membranes and that these latter properties depend very largely upon the proteins of the membrane. Valuable information in this area is now being accumulated through the incorporation into model membranes of agents that confer ion selectivity and, in two instances, confer excitability. Among the agents of the former class are included a number of macrocyclic compounds including valinomycin (II-7), nonactin (II-8), cyclic polyethers (II-9), enniatin (II-10) and other agents (374). In their original investigation of the modifying effects of these agents on bimolecular lipid membranes Mueller and Rudin (375) demonstrated that they reduced membrane

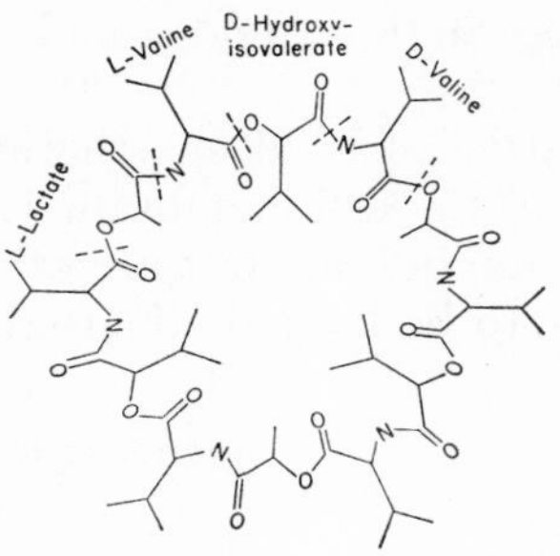

II-7 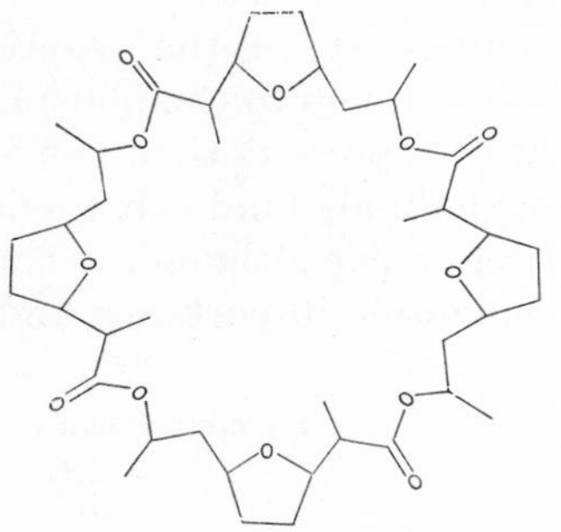　　　　　　　　　　　　　　　　　　II-8

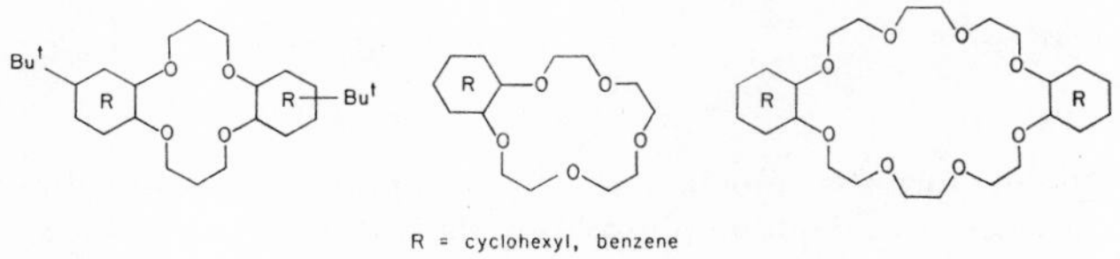

R = cyclohexyl, benzene

II-9

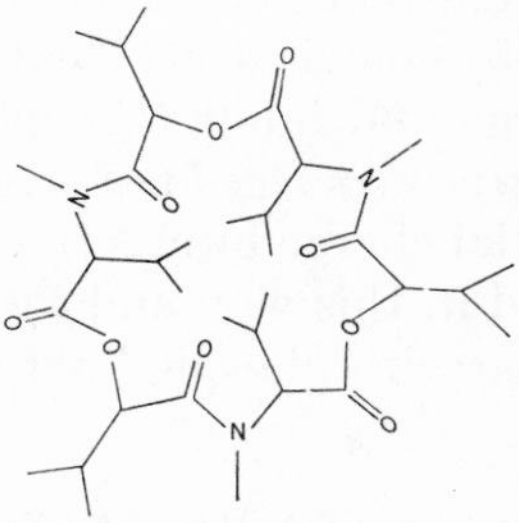

II-10

resistance and selectively increased potassium permeability (Table II-15). The order of ion permeabilities was found to be Li $\leqslant$ Na $<$ Cs $<$ K $<$ Rb corresponding to the order normally found for biological membranes. Detailed studies of the effect of valinomycin on bimolecular lipid membranes under a variety of conditions have been reported by Lev and Buzhinski (376) and Tosteson and his colleagues (374, 377, 378). It is noteworthy that the actions of valinomycin and related macrocycles are relatively independent of the composition of the lipid bilayer but that cation selectivity is markedly dependent upon the structure of the macrocycle (205, 206, 375). Since it seems quite well established that these macrocyclic agents probably function through cation binding into their central hydrophilic cavity (various discussions in ref. 374) with their outer nonpolar structure permitting them to traverse nonpolar media it is probable that their functions in membranes are to act as ion

TABLE II-15. Effects of Valinomycin, Dinactin and Enniatin B on Ionic Selectivity of Bimolecular Lipid Membranes (375)

		Li	Na	Cs	K	Rb
Biionic potential	Val	0	8	135	151	172
$E_{AB}(mV)$	Enn		0	21	90	
	Din	0	5	35	85	110
Selectivity coefficient	Val	1	1·4	210	395	920
$K_{AB} = p_A/p_B$	Enn		1	2·3	37	
	Din	1	1·2	4·1	30	82
Single ion conductance	Val	1	1·2	50	>200	>300
Ratio g_A/g_B						

Val, 10^{-6} g/ml; Din = Dinactin, 10^{-6} g/ml; Enn = Enniatin B, 10^{-5} g/ml. Observed biionic potentials at 0·05 M. Selectivity coefficients are derived from E_{AB} from $K_{AB} = p_A/p_B = [A_0]/[B_i] \exp E_{AB} F/RT$ where p_A and p_B are permeability coefficients for ions A and B; $[A_0]$ and $[B_i]$ are activities in the outside and inside compartment—B_i is always Li^+.

"shuttles" or to provide stacked arrays that function as ion-selective pores. These agents also produce remarkable changes in ion permeability in biological membranes including mitochondria (379–381), red cells (382, 383) and electroplax (384).

Undoubtedly, the most remarkable modifications of bimolecular lipid membranes have been achieved through the use of excitability inducing material (EIM), first reported by Mueller, Rudin, Tien and Wescott (207) as a material of unidentified composition but possibly ribonucleo-protein (385) extractable from *Aerobacter cloacae*, and alamethicin (II-11) a cyclic polypeptide (386). Either of these agents, under carefully

(glutamine)$_2$, (glutamate)$_2$, (proline)$_2$, (glycine)$_2$, (alanine)$_2$, (2-methylalanine)$_{7 \text{ or } 8}$, (valine)$_2$, (leucine)$_1$.

II-11

controlled conditions will permit the generation of action potentials in bimolecular lipid membranes.

Thus addition of EIM to the bilayer membrane causes a fall in membrane resistance (from 10^8 ohm/cm^2 to 10^3–10^5 ohm/cm^2 or lower) and, in the presence of an ion gradient, the development of a membrane

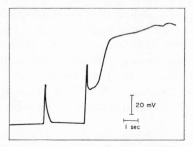

Fig. II-42. Potential changes in bilayer membrane containing EIM. A subthreshold pulse produced no change but the second suprathreshold pulse initiated a regenerative resistance change. Reproduced with permission from Mueller and Rudin (387).

potential (207, 387–389). Additionally the membrane is now excitable in the sense that an applied suprathreshold stimulus causes a reversible regenerative change between two resistance states (Fig. II-42). According to Mueller and Rudin this regenerative phenomenon may represent a potential-dependent rearrangement of a transmembrane EIM structure responsible for the resting cationic conductance. In the presence of protamine the membrane responds to suprathreshold stimuli by the generation of single or rhythmic action potentials (Fig. II-43). Since very careful titration by protamine is necessary to see these effects it is probable, as originally suggested by Mueller and Rudin (loc. cit.), that the protamine converts a fraction of the cationic channels (which are capable of existing in two resistance states) into anion selective channels also capable of existing in two resistance states.

Alamethicin behaves in many ways very similarly to EIM (386): addition in concentrations as low as 10^{-7} g/ml causes the development

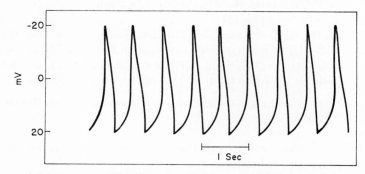

Fig. II-43. Rhythmic action potentials in bilayer membrane of purified sphingomyelin with EIM and protamine. Maintained with a steady depolarization. Reproduced with permission from Mueller and Rudin (388).

of a concentration-dependent cationic conductance (Fig. II-44) which is dependent upon the sixth power of the alamethicin concentration. This has been suggested to represent the formation of intramembrane alamethicin hexamers that will serve as cation transporting systems. In the presence of protamine, histone or spermine the alamethicin— BLM system develops a second resting potential but of negative sign and with careful regulation of the protein *and* membrane composition it is possible to generate both single and rhythmic action potentials.

The molecular basis of these remarkable changes remains unknown: the highly cooperative kinetics shown by EIM and alamethicin would

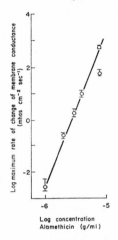

FIG. II-44. Dependence of rate of change of membrane conductance in bilayer following displacement of membrane potential by 100 mV as a function of alamethicin concentration. Reproduced with permission from Mueller and Rudin (386).

appear to rule out a single univalent carrier mechanism. There is some possibility that both alamethicin and EIM may interact rather specifically with the phospholipids of the membrane for the extent to which these agents modify the properties of BLM is very dependent upon the lipid composition of the latter. There is, in fact, some evidence from PMR, X-ray diffraction and differential scanning calorimetry that alamethicin and phospholipids form complexes in which the mobility of the phospholipid chains is greatly reduced (390).

MEMBRANES AND CONFORMATIONAL CHANGE

Implicit in current molecular considerations of electrically and chemically excitable membranes is the concept that conformational changes of part or all of the membrane are involved in the excitatory events. The role of conformational change in determining the unique properties of allosteric and regulatory protein systems is now well established (Chapter I, p. 62) and a number of attempts have been made to extend such considerations to biological and artificial membranes.

From the limited experimental evidence so far available it appears that ligand-induced conformational change is a phenomenon of general importance in cellular membranes and is not confined to excitable membranes of neural tissues. Among the techniques being applied in these studies are the "spin-label" and "fluorescent-label" molecular probes, changes in optical properties and electron microscopy.

Changes in light scattering and birefringence have been observed (391) to accompany the action potential from nonmyelinated nerve

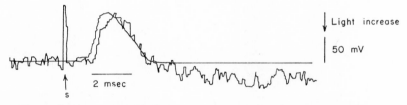

Fig. II-45. Light scattering (thick trace) at 45° from a squid giant axon and a simultaneous record of the action potential (thin smooth trace). Reproduced with permission from Cohen, Keynes and Hille (391).

fibers of the crab (walking leg) and squid (giant axons). These changes are very small but do correlate well with the time course of the action potential (Fig. II-45). Voltage clamp studies (391) reveal that the birefringence changes depend very closely upon the membrane potential and are thus associated with the axon membrane although the precise macromolecular basis of the changes remains to be established. Tasaki et al. have reported similar experiments (392, 393) and have noted very small fluorescent changes (using acridine orange and 8-anilino naphthalene-1-sulfonate) in squid and spider crab axons which appear to correlate with the time course of the action potential.

Fluorescent probe studies (394, 395) have been reported for mitochondrial membranes (396, 397): 8-anilino-1-naphthalene sulfonic acid (ANS) has been shown (396) to bind to bovine heart mitochondrial membrane fragments at sites significantly more hydrophobic (equivalent to 80% aqueous ethanol) than the aqueous medium. Kinetic studies of NAD reduction and ANS fluorescence in reversed electron transport indicate the fluorescent changes to precede initiation of the NAD reduction, suggesting that energy conservation may be linked to the mitochondrial membrane conformation.

The concept that mitochondrial membrane conformation is related to the mitochondrial energy state has been explored vigorously by Green and his colleagues (150, 398–400) who argue that the membrane conformation as revealed by EM techniques reflects the conformations of the repeating subunits, proposed by Green to be the basic construction unit of the membrane, and that the conformation may be changed to the energized state by treatment with ATP; uncoupling agents (2,4-DNP, etc.) prevent the appearance of the energized conformation.

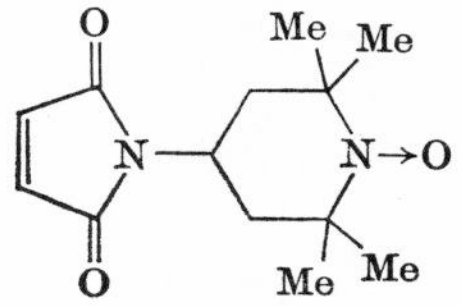

II-12

Landgraf and Inesi (401) have employed vesicular sarcoplasmic reticulum spin-labelled with II-12 which itself did not produce any significant alteration in the Ca^{++}-transporting or ATP-hydrolysing ability of the preparation. The EPR spectrum revealed the existence of both weakly and tightly immobilized labels. Addition of the substrate, ATP, to the system demonstrated a reversible increase in the ratio of weakly:tightly immobilized label ratio. Evidence for a conformational change in sarcoplasmic vesicles occurring during Ca^{++} transport has been obtained by Francois (402) who observed that a small fraction of exchangeable hydrogen atoms, normally immediately lost when the membrane was at rest, were protected from exchange during Ca^{++} transport.

Sandberg and Piette (403, 404) have employed the maleimide derivative (II-13) to spin-label erythrocyte ghosts: both weakly and tightly

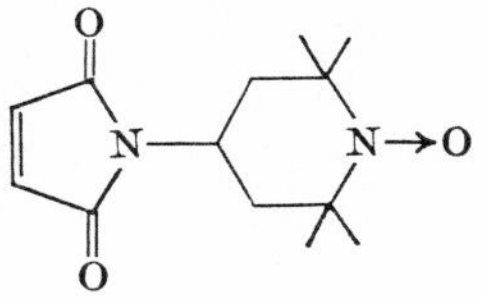

II-13

immobilized labels are found indicating two different environments for the label. Subsequent treatment with phenothiazines, including chlorpromazine, results in a reversible disappearance of the weakly immobilized label: this may be indicative of a membrane conformational change induced by the phenothiazines.

Sonenberg has documented (405) an extremely interesting example of an induced conformational change in cell membranes. Interaction of human growth hormone in concentrations as low 5×10^{-11} M with human erythrocyte membranes revealed a significant change in the CD spectra (Fig. II-46) suggestive of an approximately 25% reduction in α-helical content of the cell membrane under the influence of human

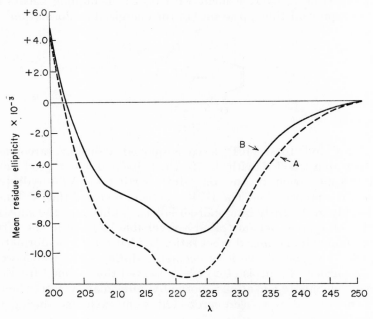

FIG. II-46. CD spectra of human erythrocyte membranes and human growth hormone ($4 \cdot 8 \times 10^{-7}$ M). A, control (membranes and hormone noninteracting); B, interacting system. Reproduced with permission from Sonenberg (405).

growth hormone. Since bovine growth hormone, bovine serum albumin, insulin and cortisol were without effect on the human erythrocyte membrane, this interaction is of unquestioned specificity and may relate to the physiological effects of the hormone.

"TWO STATES" HYPOTHESIS OF MEMBRANE EXCITABILITY

The obviously important role of calcium in controlling membrane stability and excitability forms a prominent feature of the "two stable states" hypothesis of neural excitability offered by Tasaki (238, 240, 406, 407) and Koketsu (408, 409).

In brief, the hypothesis offered by Tasaki proposes that, at rest, a large fraction of the negative sites on the external membrane surface are occupied by Ca^{++} and that in the excited state these same sites are occupied by univalent cations. The resting and excited states represent two (interconvertible) configurations of membrane macromolecules that differ in such properties as ionic selectivity, mobility and water content. The interconversion from resting to excited state is presumed to occur by the outward directed (stimulating) current driving internal univalent cations across the cell membrane to displace Ca^{++}_{EXT}; at a critical ratio of $M^{+}_{EXT}/Ca^{++}_{EXT}$ the membrane (Ca^{++}-associated) undergoes an abrupt conformational change to the excited (Ca^{++}-dissociated) highly permeable state and triggering the massive ion fluxes of the action potential†

Koketsu (*loc. cit.*) has also proposed a concept of two membrane states controlled by Ca^{++}_{EXT} and interpreted according to the Hodgkin–Huxley treatment so that during the action potential phase of increased Na^+ conductance the Ca^{++}_{EXT} is displaced from the membrane in regenerative fashion and is restored to the membrane during the falling phase (repolarization) of the action potential.

Quite generally, it is of course well known that ions have an important controlling influence on macromolecular conformation as has been well documented in the extensive studies of von Hippel (410–413).

The critical influence of the M^+/M^{++} ratio on macromolecular properties is also well documented. Thus, soaps of bivalent metals tend to form water-in-oil emulsions and soaps of univalent metals tend to form oil-in-water emulsions; these emulsions will "invert" if critical M^+/M^{++} ratios are attained (414–417). The generally low water solubility of the Ca^{++} salts and high water solubility of the Na^+ or K^+ salts indicate that Ca^{++}-carboxylate or phosphate layers will present a largely hydrophobic and that the Na^+/K^+ salts will present a largely hydrophilic ion permeation barrier respectively (418). Furthermore such inversion effects occur very dramatically as was pointed out by Clowes in 1916 (419) and shown in Fig. II-47 depicting the abrupt change in resistance of sodium oleate with increasing concentration of Ca^{++} (420), a finding cited by Tasaki in support of the proposed role of the M^+/Ca^{++} ratio in determining the relative stability of two stable states. Similar effects of the Na^+/Ca^{++} ratio have been described for a variety of systems including polyacrylic, polymethacrylic, alginic and pectinic acids (421–423).

The rapidity of the transition process may be considered by viewing the membrane as a lattice array containing binding sites for Na^+ or Ca^{++} (240). Because of the different properties of the Na^+ and the Ca^{++}

† The full implications of the Tasaki model and the details of how it differs from the Hodgkin–Huxley model cannot be dealt with here but have been touched on earlier (p. 153) to which section reference should be made for further details and original citations.

8

states, caused primarily by the higher charge density and polarizing ability of the Ca^{++} ions producing closer packing of carboxylate or phosphate anionic structures, it may be energetically more favorable to have "unmixed" rather than "mixed" areas of bound uni- and di-valent cations. These small "unmixed" sites may serve as initiators (407, 424) for phase transitions (Fig. II-48).

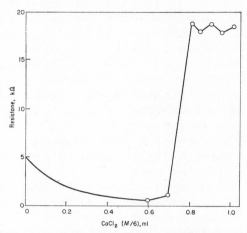

FIG. II-47. Change in resistance of sodium oleate dispersion as a function of Ca^{++} concentration. Reproduced with permission from Lerman, Watanabe and Tasaki (240).

In this connection the previously noted observations of Papahadjo-poulos and Ohki (348) that phosphatidylserine bimolecular lipid films are stable with Ca^{++} on both sides of the membrane but unstable with Ca^{++} on one side of the membrane only appear of obvious importance.

EXCITABLE MEMBRANES AS COOPERATIVE ASSEMBLIES

To this point, consideration of electrical events at the excitable membranes of nerve and muscle cells indicates both the graded and all-or-none character of these events. Several lines of experimental evidence indicate that discretely observable conformational changes occur during neural excitation and an interpretation of the latter process as a Ca^{++} controlled phase change between two distinct membrane states has been offered.

Changeux *et al.* (425–427) have advanced a formalized model of membranes and cooperative behavior in which they make the following assumptions:

a) membranes are an ordered collection of repeating lipoprotein units or protomers organized into a lattice structure;

b) at least two conformational states are available to each protomer;

c) each protomer possesses specific ligand binding sites the affinities of which are dependent upon the conformational state of the protomer;

d) the conformation adopted by any protomer depends upon its interactions with neighboring protomers. These interactions may vary considerably in strength.

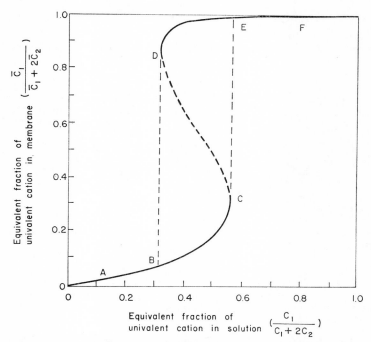

FIG. II-48. Theoretical ion exchange isotherm for a cation exchanger exposed to univalent and divalent cations based on the assumption that neighboring occupancy of anionic sites by unlike cations is energetically unfavorable. C_1 and C_2 represent the concentrations of monovalent and divalent cations respectively; $\bar{C}_1$ and $\bar{C}_2$ represent the concentrations within the membrane. The C---D line represents an experimentally unrealizable state. Reproduced with permission from Lerman, Watanabe and Tasaki (240).

The behavior of such a system in which only two conformational states ($R \rightleftharpoons S$) are accessible to each protomer and in which a single receptor site (specific for ligand F) is present per protomer can be described, as in the MWC model of cooperative proteins (Chapter I, p. 83), by a state function, $\bar{R}$, and a saturation function, $\bar{Y}$, that correspond to the fraction of the membrane protomers in the R state and the fraction of sites to which the ligand is bound respectively. In Fig. II-49 are plotted the state and saturation functions for the interaction of a single ligand with the protomer system as a function of ligand concentration (α), c, the ratio of dissociation constants of the ligand to the R and S protomers, 1, the isomerization constant of an $R \rightarrow S$ transition in an all R environment and Λ, a measure of the constraint imposed on such transition by the nearest protomer neighbors. When $\Lambda = 1$, there is no lattice constraint and all protomers are independent (Fig. II-49) and as the lattice constraints become more and more severe ($\Lambda \rightarrow 0$) the cooperativity of the ligand binding becomes very apparent. Figure II-50 shows that at critical values of 1 and Λ the state and binding curves become discontinu-

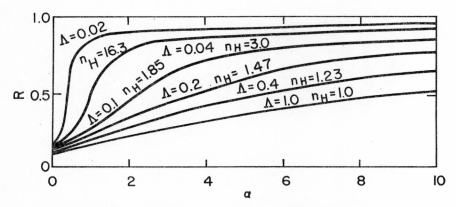

Fig. II-49. State function curves for various values of Λ with $1 = 10$ and $c = 0$. With decreasing values of Λ the Hill coefficient (n_H) becomes progressively larger. Reproduced with permission from Changeux, Thiery, Tung and Kittel (425).

ous so that the effects of added ligand are to generate an all-or-none response whereby a transition occurs between two stable states of the membrane.[†], [‡], [§]. Whether the graded or all-or-none response occurs is presumed to be essentially dependent upon the strength of the interprotomer interactions. Clearly the all-or-none response permits the occurrence of very large biological amplifications and there are a

[†] This is equivalent to the transition between two stable states of the membrane explicitly proposed by Tasaki (p. 186) to arise from fluctuations in Ca^{++} binding.

[‡] Phase transitions in macromolecules under the influence of an electric field have been discussed by Hill (428, 429); Hill noted that an electric field could shift the equilibrium between two states to favor the state with greatest polarizability and that a likely application of this effect would be to changes in state and properties of biological membranes resulting from changes in membrane potential; such change in potential presumably altering the distribution of membrane bound ions.

[§] Other aspects of the Changeux–Thiery treatment, particularly in reference to the stereospecific ligand binding phenomena at chemically excitable membranes will be discussed in later chapters.

number of systems known for which the operation of such a system would seem appropriate. The extremely high specificity and sensitivity of a number of insect pheromones (430) where a very small number of molecules ($\sim 10^3$–10^5 molecules) can induce behavioral responses may reflect an all-or-none membrane reorganization. The "taste-modifying"

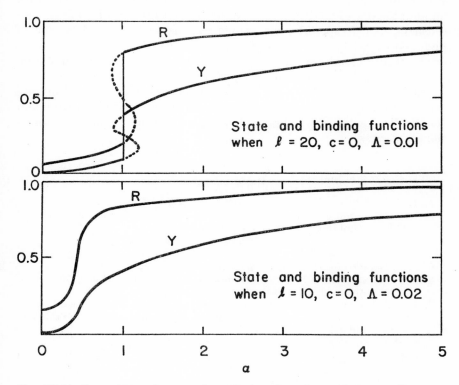

FIG. II-50. State (R) and saturation (Y) functions for graded response (lower figure) and all-or-none response (upper figure): in the upper figure the metastable states are indicated by dotted lines. Reproduced with permission from Changeux, Thiery, Tung and Kittel (425).

protein isolated from miracle fruit which modifies taste so that sour substances taste sweet (431) may constitute an example of an agent that modifies membrane organization or conformational susceptibility through its incorporation into the membrane.

Wyman has recently considered (432, 433) cooperative effects in the giant respiratory pigments found in certain invertebrates; these pigments contain many O_2 binding sites (of the order of 100) and show large Hill numbers (Chapter I, p. 89) coupled with relatively low interaction energies. The treatment offered by Wyman is essentially analogous to that offered by Changeux *et al.*, save that the number of protomers is finite. The important features of Wyman's studies are that the assumption of simultaneous existence of several protomer conformations permits the occurrence of high n values *and* low F_I values, that very high n values can occur with relatively small (by comparison with an infinite lattice) binding arrays so that the occurrence of small chemosensitive areas (responding via graded responses which are, however, of high cooperativity) set in the much larger electrically sensitive nerve or muscle cell membrane and serving as a primary stage of amplification required to initiate the all-or-none phase transitions becomes conceptually clear. That the same treatment serves both finite and infinite arrays can, furthermore, only reinforce conclusions that electrically and chemically excitable membranes may share certain common organizational features.

REFERENCES

1. J. F. Danielli and H. Davson, *J. Cell. Comp. Physiol.* (1935) **5**, 495.
2. H. Davson and J. F. Danielli, "The Permeability of Natural Membranes" (1943). Cambridge University Press, Cambridge.
3. E. Gorter and R. Grendel, *J. Exp. Med.* (1925) **41**, 439.
4. J. D. Robertson, *Biochem. Soc. Symp.* (1959) **16**, 3.
5. J. D. Robertson, *Ann. N.Y. Acad. Sci.* (1966) **137**, 421.
6. J. D. Robertson, *in* "Cellular Membranes in Development" (ed. M. Locke) (1964). Academic Press, New York and London.
7. J. D. Robertson, *in* "Principles of Biomolecular Organization", Ciba Foundation Symposium (eds G. E. W. Wolstenholme and C. M. O'Connor) (1966). Little Brown, Boston.
8. B. B. Geren, *Exp. Cell Res.* (1954) **7**, 558.
9. F. O. Schmitt, R. S. Bear and G. L. Clark, *Radiology* (1935) **25**, 131.
10. F. O. Schmitt, R. S. Bear and K. J. Palmer, *J. Cell. Comp. Physiol.* (1941) **18**, 31.
11. J. B. Finean, *Exp. Cell Res.* (1953) **5**, 202.
12. J. B. Finean, *Exp. Cell Res.* (1954) **6**, 283.
13. J. B. Finean, "Biological Ultrastructure", Ch. VI, 2nd Ed. (1967). Academic Press, London and New York.
14. H. Fernandez-Moran, *Exp. Cell Res.* (1949) **1**, 309.
15. F. S. Sjöstrand, *Experentia* (1953) **11**, 68.
16. J. D. Robertson, *J. Biophys. Biochem. Cytol.* (1957) **3**, 1043.
17. F. S. Sjöstrand, *in* "The Membranes" (eds. A. J. Dalton and F. Haguenau) (1968). Academic Press, London and New York.
18. E. D. Korn, *Science, N.Y.* (1966) **153**, 1491.
19. R. W. Hendler, "Protein Biosynthesis and Membrane Biochemistry", Ch. 5 (1968). Wiley, New York.
20. W. Stoeckenius and D. M. Engelman, *J. Cell Biol.* (1969) **42**, 613.
21. W. Stoeckenius, *in* "Membranes of Mitochondria and Chloroplasts", (ed. E. Racker) (1970). Van Nostrand Reinhold, New York.

22. A. E. Blaurock and M. H. F. Wilkins, *Nature (London)* (1969) **223**, 906.
23. V. Luzzati and F. Husson, *J. Cell Biol.* (1962) **12**, 207.
24. J. M. Steim, M. E. Tourtellotte, J. C. Reinert, R. N. McElhaney and R. L. Rader, *Proc. Nat. Acad. Sci. U.S.A.* (1969) **63**, 104.
25. T. Gulik-Krzywicki, E. Rivas and V. Luzzati, *J. Mol. Biol.* (1967) **27**, 303.
26. J. Rojers and P. A. Winsor, *Nature (London)* (1967) **216**, 477.
27. D. M. Engelman, *Nature (London)* (1969) **223**, 1279.
28. H. Fernandez-Moran, *Circulation* (1962) **26**, 1039.
29. H. Fernandez-Moran, T. Oda, P. V. Blair and D. E. Green, *J. Cell Biol.* (1964) **22**, 63.
30. D. S. Smith, *J. Cell Biol.* (1963) **19**, 115.
31. E. Racker, *in* "Membranes of Mitochondria and Chloroplasts" (ed. E. Racker) (1970). Van Nostrand Reinhold, New York.
32. D. E. Green and O. Hechter, *Proc. Nat. Acad. Sci. U.S.A.* (1965) **53**, 318.
33. D. E. Green and J. F. Perdue, *Proc. Nat. Acad. Sci. U.S.A.* (1966) **55**, 1295.
34. D. E. Green and R. F. Goldberger, "Molecular Insights Into The Living Process", Ch. 10, (1967). Academic Press, New York and London.
35. F. S. Sjöstrand, *J. Ultrastruct Res.* (1963) **9**, 340.
36. F. S. Sjöstrand, Conference on Membrane Structure and Function, St. Marguerite, P. Q., Canada. *Science, N.Y.* (1967) **158**, 146.
37. F. S. Sjöstrand, *J. Ultrastruct. Res.* (1963) **9**, 340.
38. W. Stoeckenius, *in* "Principles of Biomolecular Organization" (eds G. E. W. Wolstenholme and C. M. O'Connor) (1966). Little Brown, Boston.
39. R. B. Park and N. G. Pon, *J. Mol. Biol.* (1961) **3**, 1.
40. E. Kreutz, *Z. Naturforsch.* (1964) **196**, 441.
41. R. B. Park, *J. Cell Biol.* (1965) **27**, 151.
42. A. A. Benson, *J. Amer. Oil. Chem. Soc.* (1966) **43**, 265.
43. H. Moor and K. Muhlethaler, *J. Cell Biol.* (1963) **17**, 609.
44. H. Moor, C. Ruska and H. Ruska, *Z. Zellforsch. Mikrosk. Anat.* (1964) **62**, 581.
45. D. Branton and H. Moor, *J. Ultrastruct. Res.* (1965) **11**, 401.
46. D. Branton, *Proc. Nat. Acad. Sci. U.S.A.* (1966) **55**, 1048.
47. D. Abram, *J. Bacteriol.* (1965) **89**, 855.
48. E. D. Korn, *Science, N.Y.* (1966) **153**, 1491.
49. E. D. Korn, *Annu. Rev. Biochem.* (1969) **38**, 263.
50. J. B. Finean, *Ann. N.Y. Acad. Sci.* (1965) **122**, 51.
51. S. Fleischer, B. Fleischer and W. Stoeckenius, *Fed. Proc. Fed. Amer. Soc. Exp. Biol.* (1965) **24**, 296.
52. J. C. Hampton and B. Rosario, *Anat. Rec.* (1966) **156**, 369.
53. J. S. O'Brien, *J. Theor. Biol.* (1967) **15**, 307.
54. J. B. Finean, "Biological Ultrastructure", p. 283, 2nd Ed. (1967). Academic Press, London and New York.
55. W. D. Stein, "The Movement of Molecules Across Cell Membranes", Ch. I (1967). Academic Press, London and New York.
56. A. Kuksis, L. Marai, W. C. Breckenridge, D. A. Gornall and O. Stachnyk, *Can. J. Physiol. Pharmacol.* (1968) **46**, 511.
57. G. Rouser, G. J. Nelson, S. Fleischer and G. Simon, *in* "Biological Membranes—Physical Fact and Function" (ed. D. Chapman) (1968). Academic Press, London and New York.
58. J. R. Murphy, *J. Lab. Clin. Med.* (1965) **65**, 756.
59. J. S. O'Brien and L. Sampson, *J. Lipid Res.* (1965) **6**, 537.

60. T. Kono and S. P. Colowick, *Arch. Biochem. Biophys.* (1961) **93**, 520.
61. P. Emmelot, C. J. Bos, E. L. Benedetti and P. L. Rumke, *Biochim. Biophys. Acta* (1964) **90**, 126.
62. J. N. Farquar, *Biochim. Biophys. Acta* (1962) **60**, 80.
63. J. T. Dodge, C. Mitchell and D. J. Hanahan, *Arch. Biochem. Biophys.* (1965) **100**, 119.
64. H. P. Schwarz, L. Driesbach, M. Barrionuevo, A. Kleschick and I. Kostyk, *Arch. Biochem. Biophys.* (1961) **92**, 133.
65. A. L. Lehninger, "The Mitochondrion" (1964). Benjamin, New York.
66. A. H. Maddy and B. R. Malcolm, *Science, N.Y.* (1965) **150**, 1616.
67. C. R. Worthington and A. E. Blaurock, *Nature (London)* (1968) **218**, 87.
68. V. P. Skipski, M. Barclay, F. M. Archibald, O. Terebus-Kekish, E. S. Reichman and J. H. Good, *Life Sci.* (1965) **4**, 1673.
69. G. Rouser, G. J. Nelson, S. Fleischer and G. Simon, in "Biological Membranes, Physical Fact and Function" (ed. D. Chapman) (1968). Academic Press, London and New York.
70. P. M. Carrol and D. D. Sereda, *Nature (London)* (1968) **217**, 666.
71. L. A. E. Ashworth and C. Green, *Science, N.Y.* (1966) **151**, 211.
72. L. A. Witting, C. C. Harvey, B. Century and M. K. Horwitt, *J. Lipid Res.* (1961) **2**, 412.
73. G. L. Gaines, "Insoluble Monolayers at Liquid-Gas Interfaces", Chs. 5 and 6 (1966). Interscience, New York.
74. L. L. M. van Deenen, *Ann. N.Y. Acad. Sci.* (1966) **137**, 717.
75. D. Chapman and D. F. H. Wallach, in "Biological Membranes—Physical Fact and Function" (ed. D. Chapman) Ch. 4, (1968). Academic Press, London and New York.
76. D. O. Shah and J. H. Schulman, *J. Lipid Res.* (1967) **8**, 215.
77. D. Chapman, N. F. Owens and D. A. Walker, *Biochim. Biophys. Acta* (1966) **120**, 148.
78. R. A. Demel, L. L. M. van Deenen and B. A. Pethica, *Biochim. Biophys. Acta* (1967) **135**, 11.
79. D. A. Cadenhead, *Rec. Prog. Surf. Sci.* (1970) **3**, 169.
80. R. P. Rand and V. Luzzati, *Biophys. J.* (1968) **8**, 125.
81. D. G. Dervichian, in "Surface Phenomena in Chemistry and Biology" (eds J. F. Danielli, K. G. A. Pankhurst and A. C. Riddiford) (1958). Pergamon Press, New York.
82. R. M. C. Dawson, *Essays Biochem.* (1966) **2**, 69.
83. G. M. W. Cook, *Biol. Rev.* (1968) **43**, 363.
84. P. W. Kent, *Essays Biochem.* (1967) **3**, 105.
85. W. M. Watkins, *Science, N.Y.* (1966) **152**, 172.
86. G. M. W. Cook, D. H. Heard and G. V. F. Seaman, *Nature (London)* (1960) **188**, 1011.
87. G. M. W. Cook, D. H. Heard and G. V. F. Seaman, *Nature (London)* (1961) **191**, 44.
88. D. F. H. Wallach and V. B. Kamat, *J. Cell Biol.* (1966) **30**, 660.
89. L. Weiss, *J. Cell Biol.* (1965) **26**, 735.
90. D. W. Wooley and B. W. Gommi, *Nature (London)* (1964) **202**, 1074.
91. H. Wiegandt, *Angew. Chem. Int. Ed. Engl.* (1968) **7**, 87.
92. D. Chapman, P. Byrne and G. G. Shipley, *Proc. Roy. Soc. Ser. A* (1966) **290**, 115.
93. D. Chapman, in "Thermobiology" (ed. A. H. Rose) (1967). Academic Press, London and New York.

94. D. Chapman, R. M. Williams and B. D. Ladbrooke, *Chem. Phys. Lipids* (1967) **1**, 445.

95. D. Chapman, *in* "Membrane Models and the Formation of Biological Membranes" (eds. L. Bolis and B. A. Pethica) (1968). John Wiley, New York.

96. D. Chapman, *Lipids* (1969) **4**, 251.

97. V. Luzzati, F. Reiss-Husson, E. Rivas and T. Gulik-Kryzwicki, *Ann. N.Y. Acad. Sci.* (1966) **137**, 409.

98. V. Luzzati, *in* "Biological Membranes—Physical Fact and Function" (ed. D. Chapman) (1968). Academic Press, London and New York.

99. C. L. Hamilton and H. M. McConnell, *in* "Structural Chemistry and Molecular Biology" (eds. A. Rich and N. Davidson) (1968). Freeman, San Francisco.

100. O. H. Griffith and A. S. Waggoner, *Accounts Chem. Res.* (1969) **2**, 17.

100a. H. M. McConnell and B. G. McFarland, *Quart. Rev. Biophys.* (1970) **3**, 91.

101. W. L. Hubbell and H. M. McConnell, *Proc. Nat. Acad. Sci. U.S.A.* (1968) **61**, 12.

102. M. D. Barratt, D. K. Green and D. Chapman, *Chem. Phys. Lipids* (1969) **3**, 140.

103. D. Chapman, V. B. Kamat, J. de Gier and S. A. Penkett, *J. Mol. Biol.* (1968) **31**, 101.

104. A. D. Keith, A. S. Waggoner and O. H. Griffith, *Proc. Nat. Acad. Sci. U.S.A.* (1968) **61**, 819.

105. L. J. Libertini, A. S. Waggoner, P. C. Jost and O. H. Griffith, *Proc. Nat. Acad. Sci. U.S.A.* (1969) **64**, 13.

106. W. L. Hubbell and H. M. McConnell, *Proc. Nat. Acad. Sci. U.S.A.* (1969) **64**, 20.

107. D. F. H. Wallach and P. H. Zahler, *Proc. Nat. Acad. Sci. U.S.A.* (1966) **56**, 1552.

108. J. Lenard and S. J. Singer, *Proc. Nat. Acad. Sci. U.S.A.* (1966) **56**, 1828.

109. D. W. Urry, M. Mednieks and E. Bejnarowicz, *Proc. Nat. Acad. Sci. U.S.A.* (1967) **57**, 1043.

110. D. F. H. Wallach and A. Gordon, *in* "Regulatory Functions of Biological Membranes" (ed. J. Järnefelt) (1968). Elsevier, Amsterdam.

111. D. F. H. Wallach, *in* "Membrane Proteins", Proceedings of Symposium Sponsored by New York Heart Association (1969). Little, Brown, Boston.

112. D. F. H. Wallach and A. Gordon, *in* "Protides of Biological Fluids", Proc. 15th Symposium (ed. H. Peeters) (1968). Elsevier, Amsterdam.

113. A. H. Maddy, *Int. Rev. Cytol.* (1966) **20**, 1.

114. D. F. H. Wallach and P. H. Zahler, *Biochim. Biophys. Acta* (1968) **150**, 186.

115. D. Chapman, V. B. Kamat and R. J. Levene, *Science, N.Y.* (1968) **160**, 314.

116. N. S. Bayliss and E. G. McRea, *J. Phys. Chem.* (1954) **58**, 1002.

117. J. Y. Cassim and E. W. Taylor, *Biophys. J.* (1965) **5**, 553.

118. J. P. Carver, G. Schechter and E. R. Blout, *J. Amer. Chem. Soc.* (1966) **88**, 2550, 2562.

119. J. Lenard and S. J. Singer, *Science, N.Y.* (1968) **159**, 738.

120. D. D. Ulmer, B. L. Vallee, A. Gorcheim and A. Neuberger, *Nature (London)* (1965) **206**, 825.

121. A. Scanu, *Proc. Nat. Acad. Sci. U.S.A.* (1965) **54**, 1699.

122. M. J. Grourke and J. H. Gibbs, *Biopolymers* (1967) **5**, 586.

123. F. T. Hatch and A. L. Bruce, *Nature (London)* (1968) **218**, 1166.

124. D. E. Green, H. D. Tisdale, R. S. Criddle, P. T. Chen and R. M. Bock, *Biochem. Biophys. Res. Commun.* (1961) **5**, 109.

125. R. S. Criddle, R. M. Bock, D. E. Green and H. D. Tisdale, *Biochemistry* (1962) **1**, 827.

126. D. E. Green, N. F. Haard, G. Lenaz and H. I. Silman, *Proc. Nat. Acad. Sci. U.S.A.* (1968) **60**, 277.

127. S. H. Richardson, H. O. Hultin and D. E. Green, *Proc. Nat. Acad. Sci. U.S.A.* (1963) **50**, 821.

128. L. J. Scheiderman and I. G. Junga, *Biochemistry* (1968) **7**, 2281.

129. H. O. Hultin, quoted in reference 126.

130. C. W. Cotman, H. R. Mahler and T. E. Hugli, *Arch. Biochem. Biophys.* (1968) **126**, 821.

131. D. W. Urry, O. Hechter, G. Lenaz, N. F. Haard and D. E. Green, *Abstracts,* 154th National Meeting, American Chemical Society, Chicago, September 1967, abs. 183.

132. D. E. Green, H. D. Tisdale, R. S. Criddle and R. M. Bock, *Biochim. Biophys. Res. Commun.* (1961) **5**, 81.

133. R. F. Goldberger, A. Pumphrey and A. Smith, *Biochim. Biophys. Acta* (1962) **58**, 307.

134. S. S. Deeb and L. P. Hager, *J. Biol. Chem.* (1964) **239**, 1025.

135. D. O. Woodward and R. D. Menkres, *Proc. Nat. Acad. Sci. U.S.A.* (1960) **55**, 872.

136. R. S. Criddle, D. L. Edwards and T. G. Petersen, *Biochemistry,* (1966) **5**, 578.

137. A. L. Lehninger, *Naturwissenschaften* (1966) **53**, 57.

138. M. F. Perutz, J. C. Kendrew and H. C. Watson, *J. Mol. Biol.* (1965) **13**, 669.

139. D. E. Green and A. Tzagoloff, *J. Lipid Res.* (1966) **7**, 587.

140. D. E. Green, *Is. J. Med. Sci.* (1965) **1**, 1187.

141. S. Bakerman, *Fed. Proc. Fed. Amer. Soc. Exp. Biol.* (1965) **24**, 224.

142. M. Barclay, R. K. Barclay, E. S. Essner, V. P. Skipski and O. Terebus-Kekish, *Science, N.Y.* (1967) **156**, 665.

143. S. Razin, H. J. Morowitz and T. M. Terry, *Proc. Nat. Acad. Sci. U.S.A.* (1965) **54**, 219.

144. T. M. Terry, D. M. Engelman and H. J. Morowitz, *Biochim. Biophys. Acta* (1967) **135**, 391.

145. D. M. Engelman and H. J. Morowitz, *Biochim. Biophys. Acta* (1968) **150**, 376, 385.

146. S. Rottem, O. Stein and S. Razin, *Arch. Biochem. Biophys.* (1968) **125**, 46.

147. R. D. Brown, *J. Mol. Biol.* (1965) **12**, 491.

148. M. R. J. Salton and A. Netschea, *Biochim. Biophys. Acta* (1965) **107**, 539.

149. D. G. McConnell, A. Tzagoloff, D. H. MacLennan and D. E. Green, *J. Biol. Chem.* (1966) **241**, 2373.

150. D. E. Green and D. H. MacLennan, *Bioscience* (1969) **19**, 213.

151. D. M. Engelman, *in* "Membrane Models and the Formation of Biological Membranes" (eds L. Bolis and B. A. Pethica (1968). Wiley, New York.

152. D. E. Green, D. W. Allmann, E. Bachmann, H. Baum, K. Kopaczyk, E. F. Korman, S. H. Lipton, D. H. MacLennan, D. G. McConnell, J. F. Perdue, J. S. Rieske, and A. Tzagoloff, *Arch. Biochem. Biophys.* (1967) **119**, 312.

153. D. E. Green and A. Tzagoloff, *Arch. Biochem. Biophys.* (1966) **116**, 293.

154. S. Fleischer, G. Brierley, H. Klouwen and D. B. Slauterback, *J. Biol. Chem.* (1962) **237**, 3264.

155. D. E. Green and S. Fleischer, *Biochim. Biophys. Acta* (1963) **70**, 554.

156. A. Tzagoloff and D. H. MacLennan, *Biochim. Biophys. Acta* (1965) **99**, 476.

157. T. H. Ji and A. A. Benson, *Biochim. Biophys. Acta* (1968) **150**, 686.

158. A. A. Benson, *in* "Membrane Models and the Formation of Biological Membranes" (eds L. Bolis and B. A. Pethica) (1968). Wiley, New York.

159. S. Fleischer, B. Fleischer and W. Stoeckenius, *J. Cell Biol.* (1967) **32**, 193.

160. C. A. Homewood, L. R. Smith and W. D. Stein, *in* "Fundamental Concepts in Drug-Receptor Interactions" (eds J. F. Danielli, J. F. Moran and D. J. Triggle) (1970). Academic Press, New York and London.

161. A. B. Pardee, *J. Biol. Chem.* (1966) **241**, 3962.

162. J. R. Piperno and D. L. O. Oxender, *J. Biol. Chem.* (1966) **241**, 5732.

163. A. B. Pardee, *Science, N.Y.* (1969) **162**, 632.

164. I. Sekuzu, P. Jurtshuk, Jr. and D. E. Green, *Biochem. Biophys. Res. Commun.* (1961) **6**, 71.

165. P. Jurtshuk, Jr., I. Sekuzu and D. E. Green, *Biochem. Biophys. Res. Commun.* (1961) **6**, 76.

166. I. Sekuzu, P. Jurtshuk, Jr. and D. E. Green, *J. Biol. Chem.* (1963) **238**, 975.

167. P. Jurtshuk, Jr., I. Sekuzu and D. E. Green, *J. Biol. Chem.* (1963) **238**, 3595.

168. S. Fleischer and H. Klouwen, *Biochem. Biophys. Res. Commun.* (1961) **5**, 378.

169. G. P. Brierly, A. J. Merola and S. Fleischer, *Biochim. Biophys. Acta* (1962) **64**, 218.

170. E. Racker and A. Bruni, *in* "Membrane Models and the Formation of Biological Membranes" (eds L. Bolis and B. A. Pethica) (1968). Wiley, New York.

171. L. J. Fenster and J. H. Copenhauer, Jr., *Biochim. Biophys. Acta* (1967) **137**, 406.

172. P. D. Jones, P. W. Holloway, R. O. Peluffo and S. J. Wakil, *J. Biol. Chem.* (1969) **244**, 744.

173. S. M. Duttera, W. L. Byrne and M. C. Ganoza, *J. Biol. Chem.* (1968) **243**, 2216.

174. R. Colman and G. Hübscher, *Biochim. Biophys. Acta* (1963) **73**, 257.

175. W. G. Fiscus and W. C. Schneider, *J. Biol. Chem.* (1966) **241**, 3324.

176. R. Tanaka and K. P. Strickland, *Arch. Biochem. Biophys.* (1965) **111**, 583.

177. R. Tanaka and T. Sakamoto, *Biochim. Biophys. Acta* (1969) **193**, 384.

178. L. A. Pesch and J. Peterson, *Biochim. Biophys. Acta* (1965) **96**, 390.

179. A. Martonosi, J. Donley and R. A. Halpin, *J. Biol. Chem.* (1968) **243**, 61.

180. M. Weiser and L. Rothfield, *in* "Membrane Models and the Formation of Biological Membranes" (eds. L. Bolis and B. A. Pethica) (1968). Wiley, New York.

181. L. Rothfield, M. Weiser and A. Endo, *in* "Membrane Proteins: Proceedings of a Symposium Sponsored by the New York Heart Association" (1969). Little Brown, Boston.

182. D. G. Williamson and V. J. O'Donnell, *Biochemistry* (1969) **8**, 1289.

183. K. Lang, *Hoppe-Seyler's Z. Physiol. Chem.* (1943) **227**, 114.

184. G. S. Gotterer, *Biochemistry* (1967) **6**, 2147.

185. G. S. Gotterer, *Biochemistry* (1969) **8**, 641.

186. M. M. Weiser and L. Rothfield, *J. Biol. Chem.* (1968) **243**, 1320.

187. P. Heitmann, *Eur. J. Biochem.* (1968) **5**, 305.

188. W. P. Jencks, "Catalysis in Chemistry and Enzymology", p. 403 (1969). McGraw-Hill, New York.

189. E. H. Cordes and R. B. Dunlap, *Accounts. Chem. Res.* (1969) **2**, 329.

190. N. K. Adam, "The Physics and Chemistry of Surfaces", Chapter VIII, 3rd Ed. (1941). Oxford University Press, London.

191. J. Th. G. Overbek, *in* "Colloid Science", Vol. I (ed. H. R. Kruyt) (1949). Elsevier, New York.

192. D. Stigter, *J. Colloid Interface Sci.* (1967) **23**, 379.

193. P. Mukerjee and A. Ray, *J. Phys. Chem.* (1966) **70**, 2144.

194. G. S. Hartley and J. W. Roe, *Trans. Faraday Soc.* (1939) **35**, 101.

195. P. Mukerjee and K. Banerjee, *J. Phys. Chem.* (1964) **68**, 3567.

196. D. Stigter, *J. Phys. Chem.* (1964) **68**, 3603.
197. M. T. A. Behme and E. H. Cordes, *J. Amer. Chem. Soc.* (1965) **87**, 260.
198. E. F. J. Duynstee and E. Grunwald, *J. Amer. Chem. Soc.* (1959) **81**, 4540, 4542.
199. R. B. Dunlap and E. H. Cordes, *J. Amer. Chem. Soc.* (1968) **90**, 4395.
200. C. Gitler and A. Ochoa-Solano, *J. Amer. Chem. Soc.* (1968) **90**, 5004.
201. H. T. Tien and A. L. Diana, *Chem. Phys. Lipids* (1968) **2**, 55.
202. G. Sessa and G. Weissmann, *J. Lipid Res.* (1968) **9**, 310.
203. J. A. Castleden, *J. Pharm. Sci.* (1969) **58**, 149.
204. A. D. Bangham, *Progr. Biophys. Biophys. Chem.* (1969) **18**, 29.
205. F. A. Henn and T. E. Thompson, *Annu. Rev. Biochem.* (1969) **38**, 241.
206. T. E. Thompson and F. A. Henn, *in* "Membranes of Mitochondria and Chloroplasts" (ed. E. Racker) (1970). Van Nostrand Reinhold, New York.
207. P. Mueller, D. O. Rudin, H. T. Tien and W. C. Wescott, *Nature (London)* **194**, 979.
208. P. Mueller, D. O. Rudin, H. T. Tien and W. C. Wescott, *in* "Recent Progress in Surface Science", Vol. I, p. 379 (eds J. F. Danielli, K. G. A. Pankhurst and A. C. Riddiford) (1964). Academic Press, New York and London.
209. A. D. Bangham, M. M. Standish and J. C. Watkins, *J. Mol. Biol.* (1965) **13**, 238.
210. A. D. Bangham, M. M. Standish, J. C. Watkins and G. Weissmann, *Protoplasma* (1967) **63**, 183.
211. D. Papahadjopoulos and A. D. Bangham, *Biochim. Biophys. Acta* (1966) **126**, 185.
212. D. Papahadjopoulos and J. C. Watkins, *Biochim. Biophys. Acta* (1967) **135**, 639.
213. D. Papahadjopoulos, *Biochim. Biophys. Acta* (1968) **163**, 240.
214. D. C. Tosteson and J. F. Hoffman, *J. Gen. Physiol.* (1960) **44**, 169.
215. T. E. Andreoli, J. A. Bangham and D. C. Tosteson, *J. Gen. Physiol.* (1967) **50**, 1729.
216. A. L. Hodgkin, *Proc. Roy. Soc. Ser. B* (1958) **148**, 1.
217. A. L. Hodgkin, "The Conduction of the Nervous Impulse" (1964). Liverpool University Press, Liverpool.
218. B. Katz, "Nerve, Muscle and Synapse" (1966). McGraw-Hill, New York.
219. K. S. Cole, "Membranes, Ions and Impulses" (1968). University of California Press, Berkeley, California.
220. A. L. Hodgkin and A. F. Huxley, *J. Physiol. (London)* (1952) **116**, 449.
221. A. L. Hodgkin and A. F. Huxley, *J. Physiol. (London)* (1952) **116**, 473.
222. A. L. Hodgkin and A. F. Huxley, *J. Physiol. (London)* (1952) **116**, 497.
223. A. L. Hodgkin and A. F. Huxley, *J. Physiol. (London)* (1952) **117**, 500.
224. A. L. Hodgkin, A. F. Huxley and B. Katz, *J. Physiol. (London)* (1952) **116**, 424.
225. R. D. Keynes, *Proc. Roy. Soc. Ser. B* (1954) **142**, 359.
226. K. S. Cole, *Physiol. Rev.* (1965) **45**, 340.
227. R. D. Keynes and P. R. Lewis, *J. Physiol. (London)* (1951) **114**, 151.
228. J. A. M. Hinke, *J. Physiol. (London)* (1961) **156**, 314.
229. B. Katz, *Proc. Roy. Soc. Ser. B* (1962) **155**, 455.
230. H. Grundfest, *Advan. Comp. Physiol. Biochem.* (1966) **2**, 1.
231. A. M. Shanes, *Pharmacol. Rev.* (1958) **10**, 165.
232. T. Narahashi, J. W. Moore and W. R. Scott, *J. Gen. Physiol.* (1964) **47**, 965.
233. Y. Nakamura, S. Nakajima and H. Grundfest, *J. Gen. Physiol.* (1965) **48**, 985.
234. M. Takata, J. W. Moore, C. Y. Kao and F. A. Fuhrman, *J. Gen. Physiol.* (1966) **49**, 977.

235. B. Hille, *J. Gen. Physiol.* (1968) **51**, 199.
236. J. W. Moore, T. Narahashi and T. I. Shaw, *J. Physiol.* (*London*) (1967) **188**, 99.
237. I. Tasaki, I. Singer and T. Takenaka, *J. Gen. Physiol.* (1965) **48**, 1095.
238. I. Tasaki, "Nerve Excitation: A Macromolecular Approach" (1968). Thomas, Springfield, Illinois.
239. I. Singer and I. Tasaki, *in* "Biological Membranes, Physical Fact and Function" (ed. D. Chapman) (1968). Academic Press, London and New York.
240. L. Lerman, A. Watanabe and I. Tasaki, *Neurosci. Res.* (1969) **2**, 72.
240a. J. H. Bungenburg de Jong, *in* "Colloid Science", Vol. 2 (ed. H. R. Kruyt) (1949). Elsevier, Amsterdam.
241. T. Teorell, *Progr. Biophys. Biophys. Chem.* (1953) **3**, 305.
242. T. Teorell, *J. Gen. Physiol.* (1959) **42**, 847.
243. R. Elul, *J. Physiol.* (*London*) (1967) **189**, 351.
244. B. Hille, *J. Gen. Physiol.* (1968) **51**, 221.
245. I. Tasaki, I. Singer and A. Watanabe, *Amer. J. Physiol.* (1966) **211**, 746.
246. I. Tasaki, I. Singer and A. Watanabe, *J. Gen. Physiol.* (1966) **50**, 989.
247. I. Tasaki, A. Watanabe and I. Singer, *Proc. Nat. Acad. Sci. U.S.A.* (1966) **56**, 1116.
248. I. Tasaki, A. Watanabe and L. Lerman, *Amer. J. Physiol.* (1969) **213**, 1465.
249. I. Tasaki, A. Watanabe and S. Yamagishi, *Amer. J. Physiol.* (1968) **215**, 152.
250. D. Noble, *Nature* (*London*) (1968) **219**, 767.
251. O. Löewi, *Pflügers Arch. Physiol.* (1921) **189**, 239.
252. E. J. Furshpan and D. D. Potter, *J. Physiol.* (*London*) (1959) **145**, 289.
253. P. Fatt and B. Katz, *J. Physiol.* (*London*) (1951) **115**, 320.
254. J. Del Castillo and B. Katz, *J. Physiol.* (*London*) (1954) **124**, 586.
255. J. Del Castillo and B. Katz, *J. Physiol.* (*London*) (1954) **125**, 546.
256. J. Del Castillo and B. Katz, *J. Physiol.* (*London*) (1955) **128**, 157.
257. J. Del Castillo and B. Katz, *Progr. Biophys. Biophys. Chem.* (1956) **6**, 126.
258. B. Katz and R. Miledi, *Proc. Roy. Soc. Ser. B* (1965) **161**, 453.
259. B. Katz and R. Miledi, *Proc. Roy. Soc. Ser. B* (1965) **161**, 483.
260. B. Katz and S. Thesleff, *J. Physiol.* (*London*) (1957) **137**, 267.
261. A. Takeuchi and N. Takeuchi, *J. Physiol.* (*London*) (1960) **154**, 52.
262. A. Takeuchi and N. Takeuchi, *J. Neurophysiol.* (1960) **23**, 397.
263. J. C. Eccles, "Physiology of Synapses" (1964). Academic Press, New York and London.
264. B. L. Ginsborg, *Pharmacol. Rev.* (1967) **19**, 289.
265. P. Fatt and B. L. Ginsborg, *J. Physiol.* (*London*) (1958) **142**, 516.
266. S. Hagiwara and K. Naka, *J. Gen. Physiol.* (1964) **48**, 141.
267. E. Bülbring and H. Kuriyama, *J. Physiol.* (*London*) (1963) **166**, 29.
268. M. R. Bennett, *J. Physiol.* (*London*) (1967) **190**, 465.
269. E. Bülbring and T. Tomita, *Proc. Roy. Soc. Ser. B* (1969) **172**, 121.
270. R. Werman and H. Grundfest, *J. Gen. Physiol.* (1961) **64**, 997.
271. R. Guttman, *J. Gen. Physiol.* (1940) **23**, 346.
272. A. M. Shanes, *J. Cell. Comp. Physiol.* (1942) **19**, 249.
273. F. Brink, *Pharmacol. Rev.* (1954) **6**, 243.
274. A. M. Shanes, *Pharmacol. Rev.* (1958) **10**, 59.
275. J. A. Cerf, *in* "Handbuch der Experimentellen Pharmakologie" Vol. 17, Ch. 8 (eds O. Eichlor and A. Farah) (1963). Springer-Verlag, Berlin.
276. P. M. Seeman, *Int. Rev. Neurobiol.* (1966) **9**, 145.
277. J. F. Manery, *Fed. Proc. Fed. Amer. Soc. Exp. Biol.* (1966) **25**, 1804.
278. C. P. Bianchi, "Cell Calcium" (1968). Butterworth, London.

279. K. Koketsu, *Neurosci. Res.* (1969) **2**, 1.

280. S. Ringer, *J. Physiol. (London)* (1888) **11**, 79.

281. V. Bolingbroke and M. Marels, *J. Physiol. (London)* (1959) **149**, 563.

282. A. K. Solomon, *J. Gen. Physiol.* (1960) Suppl. **43**, pt. 2,1.

283. H. Davson, "A Textbook of General Physiology", 3rd Ed., pp. 321, 381, (1964). Little Brown, Boston.

284. K.-E. Berntsson, B. Haglund and S. Lutrop, *J. Cell. Comp. Physiol.* (1965) **65**, 101.

285. A. Brading, E. Bülbring and T. Tomita, *J. Physiol. (London)* (1969) **200**, 621.

286. J. Del Castillo and B. Katz, *J. Physiol. (London)* (1954) **124**, 553.

287. B. Katz and R. Miledi, *J. Physiol. (London)* (1968) **195**, 481.

288. F. A. Dodge, Jr. and R. Rahamimoff, *J. Physiol. (London)* (1967) **193**, 419.

289. R. I. Birks, P. G. R. Burstyn and D. R. Firth, *J. Gen. Physiol.* (1968) **52**, 887.

290. L. L. Simpson, *J. Pharm. Pharmacol.* (1968) **20**, 889.

291. S. Ringer, *J. Physiol. (London)* (1883) **4**, 29.

292. S. Weidmann, *J. Physiol. (London)* (1955) **129**, 568.

293. H. P. Jenerick, *J. Gen. Physiol.* (1956) **39**, 773.

294. B. A. Curtis, *J. Physiol. (London)* (1963) **166**, 75.

295. J. Aceves and X. Machne, *J. Pharmacol. Exp. Ther.* (1963) **140**, 138.

296. L. Levine, *J. Cell. Comp. Physiol.* (1966) **67**, 107.

297. A. Brading, E. Bülbring and T. Tomita, *J. Physiol. (London)* (1969) **200**, 637.

298. E. Bülbring, *Proc. Roy. Soc. Ser. B* (1969) **172**, 121.

299. K. S. Cole, *Arch. Sci. Physiol.* (1949) **3**, 253.

300. R. Stampfli and K. Nishie, *Helv. Physiol. Acta* (1956) **14**, 93.

301. R. Straub, *Helv. Physiol. Acta* (1956) **14**, 1.

302. B. Frankenhaeuser and A. L. Hodgkin, *J. Physiol. (London)* (1957) **137**, 218.

303. R. Niedergerke, *J. Physiol. (London)* (1963) **167**, 515.

304. A. P. Somlyo and A. V. Somlyo, *Pharmacol. Rev.* (1968) **20**, 197.

305. N. Ishiko and M. Sato, *Jap. J. Physiol.* (1957) **137**, 245.

306. B. Frankenhaeuser, *J. Physiol. (London)* (1957) **137**, 245.

307. R. Villegas and G. Camejo, *Biochim. Biophys. Acta* (1968) **163**, 421.

308. G. Burnstock, M. E. Holman and C. L. Prosser, *Physiol. Rev.* (1963) **43**, 482.

309. R. Casteels and H. Kuriyama, *J. Physiol. (London)* (1965) **177**, 263.

310. H. Kuriyama, *J. Physiol. (London)* (1964) **175**, 211.

311. G. Burnstock and M. E. Holman, *Annu. Rev. Pharmacol.* (1966) **6**, 129.

312. E. Bülbring and H. Kuriyama, *J. Physiol. (London)* (1963) **166**, 29.

313. J. M. Marshall, *Amer. J. Physiol.* (1963) **204**, 723.

314. D. F. Bohr, *Pharmacol. Rev.* (1964) **16**, 93.

315. C. Y. Kao, *in* "Cellular Biology of the Uterus" (ed. R. M. Wynn) (1967). Appleton-Century-Crofts, New York.

316. H. Kuriyama, T. Osa and N. Toida, *Brit. J. Pharmacol.* (1966) **27**, 366.

317. Y. Nonomura, Y. Hotta and H. Ohashi, *Science, N.Y.* (1966) **152**, 97.

318. E. Bülbring and T. Tomita, *J. Physiol. (London)* (1967) **189**, 299.

319. S. Hagiwara and S. Nakajima, *J. Gen. Physiol.* (1966) **49**, 807.

320. S. Hagiwara and S. Nakajima, *J. Gen. Physiol.* (1966) **49**, 793.

321. S. G. Chamberlain and G. Kerkut, *Nature (London)* (1967) **216**, 89.

322. R. K. Orkand and R. Niedergerke, *Science N.Y.* (1964) **146**, 1176.

323. R. Niedergerke and H. C. Lüttgau, *Nature (London)* (1957) **179**, 1066.

324. G. Schaechtelin, *Pflügers Arch. Physiol.* (1961) **273**, 164.

325. J. M. Tobias, *Nature (London)* (1964) **203**, 13.

326. D. E. Goldman, *Biophys. J.* (1964) **4**, 167.

327. P. J. Goodford, *J. Physiol. (London)* (1966) **186**, 11; (1967) **192**, 145.

328. J. R. Segal, *Biophys. J.* (1968) **8**, 470.
329. H. N. Christensen and A. B. Hastings, *J. Biol. Chem.* (1940) **136**, 387.
330. A. K. Solomon, F. Lionetti and P. Curran, *Nature (London)* (1956) **178**, 582.
331. L. B. Kirschner, *J. Gen. Physiol.* (1948) **42**, 231.
332. H. A. Ward and P. Fantl, *Arch. Biochem. Biophys.* (1963) **100**, 338.
333. E. Baer and D. Buchnea, *Arch. Biochem. Biophys.* (1958) **78**, 294.
334. H. L. Rosano, P. Duby and J. H. Schulman, *J. Phys. Chem.* (1961) **65**, 1704.
335. H. L. Rosano, J. H. Schulman and J. B. Weisbuch, *Ann. N.Y. Acad. Sci.* (1961) **92**, 457.
336. H. L. Rosano, H. Schiff and J. H. Schulman, *J. Phys. Chem.* (1962) **66**, 1928.
337. D. W. Wooley and N. K. Campbell, *Biochim. Biophys. Acta* (1962) **57**, 384.
338. M. B. Feinstein, *J. Gen. Physiol.* (1964) **48**, 357.
339. M. P. Blaustein and D. E. Goldman, *Science, N.Y.* (1966) **153**, 429.
340. M. B. Abramson, R. Katzman and B. Gregor, *J. Biol. Chem.* (1964) **239**, 70.
341. D. G. Dervichian, *in* "Biochemical Problems of Lipids" (eds G. Popjak and E. LeBreton) (1955). Interscience, New York.
342. M. B. Abramson, R. Katzman, C. F. Wilson and H. P. Gregor, *J. Biol. Chem.* (1964) **239**, 4066.
343. D. C. Robins and J. L. Thomas, *J. Pharm. Pharmacol.* (1963) **15**, 157.
344. E. Rojas and J. M. Tobias, *Biochim. Biophys. Acta* (1965) **94**, 394.
345. H. Hauser and R. M. C. Dawson, *Eur. J. Biochem.* (1967) **1**, 61.
346. J. M. Tobias, D. P. Agin and R. Pawlowski, *J. Gen. Physiol.* (1962) **45**, 989.
347. G. J. Leitch and J. M. Tobias, *J. Cell. Comp. Physiol.* (1964) **63**, 225.
348. D. Papahadjopoulos and S. Ohki, *Science, N.Y.* (1969) **164**, 1075.
349. S. Ohki, *in* "Physical Principles of Biological Membranes" (ed. F. M. Snell) (1969). Gordon and Breach, New York.
350. M. P. Blaustein, *Biochim. Biophys. Acta* (1967) **135**, 653.
351. P. G. Barton, *J. Biol. Chem.* (1968) **243**, 3884.
352. H. R. Kruyt, *in* "Colloid Science" Vol. 2 (ed. H. R. Kruyt) (1949). Elsevier, New York.
353. J. Van Steveninck and A. Rothstein, *J. Gen. Physiol.* (1965) **49**, 235.
354. J. Van Steveninck and H. L. Booij, *J. Gen. Physiol.* (1964) **48**, 43.
355. A. Rothstein, *Annu. Rev. Physiol.* (1968) **30**, 15.
356. M. D. Sokoll and S. Thesleff, *Eur. J. Pharmacol.* (1968) **4**, 71.
357. J. H. Liu and W. L. Nastuk, *Fed. Proc. Fed. Amer. Soc. Exp. Biol.* (1966) **25**, 570.
358. W. L. Nastuk, *Fed. Proc. Fed. Amer. Soc. Exp. Biol.* (1967) **26**, 1639.
359. S. Wiedling and C. Tegner, *Progr. Med. Chem.* (1963) **3**, 332.
360. A. M. Shanes, *Pharmacol. Rev.* (1958) **10**, 165.
361. J. M. Ritchie and P. Greengard, *Annu. Rev. Pharmacol.* (1966) **6**, 405.
362. G. A. Condouris, *J. Pharmacol. Expt. Ther.* (1961) **131**, 243.
363. G. A. Condouris, *J. Pharmacol. Expt. Ther.* (1963) **141**, 253.
364. A. M. Shanes, W. H. Freygang, H. Grundfest and E. Amatnieck, *J. Gen. Physiol.* (1959) **42**, 793.
365. R. E. Taylor, *Amer. J. Physiol.* (1959) **196**, 1071.
366. S. Thesleff, *Acta Physiol. Scand.* (1956) **37**, 335.
367. F. Inoue and G. B. Frank, *J. Pharmacol. Expt. Ther.* (1952) **136**, 190.
368. K. Karpel, M. H. Draper and H. Friebel, *Arch. Exp. Pathol. Pharmakol.* (1965) **250**, 405.
369. M. P. Blaustein and D. E. Goldman, *J. Gen. Physiol.* (1966) **49**, 1043.
370. M. P. Blaustein, *Biochim. Biophys. Acta* (1967) **135**, 653.
371. M. B. Feinstein and M. Paimre, *Biochim. Biophys. Acta* (1966) **115**, 33.

372. T. Narahashi, D. T. Frazier and M. Yamada, *J. Pharmacol. Exp. Ther.* (1970) **171**, 32.
373. D. T. Frazier, T. Narahashi and M. Yamada, *J. Pharmacol. Exp. Ther.* (1970) **171**, 45.
374. Symposium on Biological and Artificial Membranes, *Fed. Proc. Fed. Amer. Soc. Exp. Biol.* (1968) **27**, 1249–1309.
375. P. Mueller and D. O. Rudin, *Biochem. Biophys. Res. Commun.* (1967) **26**, 398.
376. A. A. Lev and E. P. Buzhinsky, *Tsitologiya* (1967) **9**, 102.
377. T. E. Andreoli, M. Tieffenberg and D. C. Tosteson, *J. Gen. Physiol.* (1967) **50**, 2527.
378. D. C. Tosteson, T. E. Andreoli, M. Tieffenberg and P. Cook, *J. Gen. Physiol.* (1968) **51**, 373S.
379. C. Moore and B. C. Pressman, *Biochem. Biophys. Res. Commun.* (1964) **15**, 562.
380. B. C. Pressman, *Proc. Nat. Acad. Sci. U.S.A.* (1965) **53**, 1076.
381. B. C. Pressman, *Ann. N.Y. Acad. Sci.* (1969) **147**, 829.
382. J. P. Chapell and A. R. Crufts, *in* "Ion Transport and Reversible Volume Changes of Isolated Mitochondria" (eds T. M. Tager, S. Papa, E. Quagliariello and E. C. Slater) (1966). Elsevier, Amsterdam.
383. D. C. Tosteson, P. Cook, T. E. Andreoli and M. Tieffenberg, *J. Gen. Physiol.* (1967) **50**, 2513.
384. T. R. Podleski and J.-P. Changeux, *Nature (London)* (1969) **221**, 541.
385. L. D. Kushnir, *Biochim. Biophys. Acta* (1968) **150**, 285.
386. P. Mueller and D. O. Rudin, *Nature (London)* (1968) **217**, 713.
387. P. Mueller and D. O. Rudin, *J. Theor. Biol.* (1963) **4**, 268.
388. P. Mueller and D. O. Rudin, *Nature (London)* (1967) **213**, 603.
389. P. Mueller and D. O. Rudin, *J. Theor. Biol.* (1968) **18**, 222.
390. D. Chapman, R. J. Cherry, E. G. Finer, H. Hauser, M. C. Phillips, G. G. Shipley and A. I. McMullen, *Nature (London)* (1969) **224**, 692.
391. L. B. Cohen, R. D. Keynes and B. Hille, *Nature (London)* (1968) **218**, 438.
392. I. Tasaki, A. Watanabe, R. Sandlin and L. Carnay, *Proc. Nat. Acad. Sci. U.S.A.* (1968) **61**, 883.
393. I. Tasaki, L. Carnay, R. Sandlin and A. Watanabe, *Science, N.Y.* (1969) **163**, 683.
394. G. M. Edelman and W. O. McClure, *Accounts. Chem. Res.* (1968) **1**, 65.
395. L. Stryer, *Science, N.Y.* (1968) **162**, 526.
396. A. Azzi, B. Chance, G. K. Radda and C. P. Lee, *Proc. Nat. Acad. Sci. U.S.A.* (1969) **62**, 612.
397. B. Chance, A. Azzi, L. Mela, G. K. Radda and H. Vainio, *FEBS Lett.* (1969) **3**, 10.
398. D. E. Green, J. Asai, R. A. Harris and J. T. Penniston, *Arch. Biochem. Biophys.* (1968) **125**, 684.
399. J. T. Penniston and D. E. Green, *Arch. Biochem. Biophys.* (1968) **128**, 339.
400. R. A. Harris, M. A. Asbell, J. Asai, W. W. Jolly and D. E. Green, *Arch. Biochem. Biophys.* (1969) **132**, 545.
401. W. C. Landgraf and G. Inesi, *Arch. Biochem. Biophys.* (1969) **130**, 111.
402. C. Francois, *Biochim. Biophys. Acta* (1969) **173**, 86.
403. H. E. Sandberg and L. H. Piette, *Agressologie* (1968) IX, 59.
404. H. E. Sandberg and L. H. Piette, *Biophys. J. Abstract Issue* (1969) **9**, A-178.
405. M. Sonenberg, *Biochem. Biophys. Res. Commun.* (1969) **36**, 450.
406. I. Tasaki and S. Hagiwara, *J. Gen. Physiol.* (1957) **40**, 859.
407. I. Tasaki, *J. Gen. Physiol.* (1963) **46**, 755.
408. K. Koketsu, *Neurosci. Res.* (1969) **2**, 1.

409. K. Koketsu, *Proc. 23rd Int. Congr. Physiol. Sci.* Tokyo (1965) **87**, 521.
410. P. H. von Hippel and K.-Y. Wong, *Science, N.Y.* (1964) **145**, 577.
411. P. H. von Hippel and K.-Y. Wong, *J. Biol. Chem.* (1965) **240**, 3909.
412. P. H. von Hippel and T. Schleich, *in* "Biological Macromolecules", Vol. II (eds S. Timasheff and G. Fasman) (1969). Dekker, New York.
413. P. H. von Hippel and T. Schleich, *Accounts Chem. Res.* (1969) **2**, 257.
414. N. K. Adam, "The Physics and Chemistry of Surfaces", 3rd Ed., pp. 146–152 (1941). Oxford University Press.
415. A. E. Alexander and P. Johnson, "Colloid Science", p. 653 (1950). Oxford University Press.
416. C. G. Sumner, "Clayton's the Theory of Emulsions and Their Technical Treatment" (1954). Chemical Publishing Co. New York.
417. J. L. Kavanau, "Structure and Function in Biological Membranes", Vol. I, Ch. 2 (1965). Holden-Day, San Francisco.
418. W. D. Bancroft, *J. Phys. Chem.* (1913) **17**, 501.
419. G. H. A. Clowes, *J. Phys. Chem.* (1916) **20**, 407.
420. N. Waterman, *in* "Colloid Chemistry", Vol. II (ed. J. Alexander) (1928). Reinhold, New York.
421. I. Michaeli, *J. Polym. Sci.* (1960) **48**, 291.
422. J. L. Mongar and A. Wassermann, *Nature (London)* (1947) **159**, 746.
423. R. Speiser, M. J. Copley and G. C. Nutting, *J. Phys. Colloid Sci.* (1947) **51**, 117.
424. R. M. Barrer and J. D. Falconer, *Proc. Roy. Soc. Ser. A*, (1956) **236**, 227.
425. J.-P. Changeux, J. Thiéry, Y. Tung and C. Kittel, *Proc. Nat. Acad. Sci. U.S.A.* (1967) **57**, 335.
426. J.-P. Changeux and J. Thiéry, *in* "Regulatory Functions of Biological Membranes" (ed. J. Järnefelt) (1968). Elsevier, New York.
427. J.-P. Changeux and T. R. Podleski, *in* "Fundamental Concepts in Drug-Receptor Interactions" (eds J. F. Moran, J. F. Danielli and D. J. Triggle) (1970). Academic Press, London and New York.
428. T. L. Hill, *J. Amer. Chem. Soc.* (1958) **80**, 2142.
429. T. L. Hill, *Proc. Nat. Acad. Sci. U.S.A.* (1967) **58**, 111.
430. D. Schneider, *Science, N.Y.* (1969) **163**, 1031.
431. K. Kurihara and L. M. Beidler, *Nature (London)* (1969) **222**, 1176.
432. J. Wyman, *Quart. Rev. Biophys.* (1968) **1**, 35.
433. J. Wyman, *J. Mol. Biol.* (1969) **39**, 523.

Chapter III

PERIPHERAL NEUROCHEMICAL TRANSMITTERS: PRELIMINARY CONSIDERATIONS

The remaining chapters of this volume are concerned primarily with the actions of the neurotransmitters, norepinephrine and acetylcholine, their analogs and antagonists, at peripheral neuroeffector sites with principal reference to the mammalian organism. A complete understanding of how these agents produce their physiological effects requires detailed analyses of their actions at the organ, cellular, subcellular and molecular levels; most of our information concerning molecular interpretations of these actions relies very heavily on observations made at the cellular and organ level.

As pointed out in the initial chapter neurotransmitters may be viewed as regulatory ligands with a primary interaction probably exerted at discrete macromolecular localizations (receptors) in the cell membrane. Thus an understanding of the molecular basis of neurotransmitter action is to be sought, initially at least, in the framework of current knowledge of macromolecular organizations and functions particularly as these relate to the cell membrane. Several aspects of these latter problems have been reviewed in Chapters I and II with the principal intention of setting the stage for a more detailed analysis of neurotransmitter action.

In considering the actions of neurotransmitters the following equation will serve as descriptive

$$A + \text{Rec.} \rightleftharpoons A\text{----Rec.} \xrightarrow{\text{n intermediate steps}} \text{Final response} \qquad \text{III-1}$$

of the total sequence of events. An initial interaction of the neurotransmitter (A) at a specific site, the receptor (Rec.), initiates the chain of events leading to the final physiological response (muscle contraction or relaxation, action potential generation etc.). Accompanying the final response are other physiological events including changes in membrane potential and ionic permeabilities and alteration of metabolic events, etc. (Fig. III-1). A major problem is that of determining the relationships existing between the various observable changes and of establishing which of them are directly involved as part of the linkage between the initial neurotransmitter-receptor interaction and the final response and which are merely epiphenomena activated through the initial receptor interaction or some subsequent event, but actually unrelated to the production of the final response. In subsequent discussion (Chapters V and VII) it will be noted for several muscle systems that it is possible to dissociate completely the contractile events from electrical changes indicating that the latter may fall into the epiphenomena category.

Because the sequence of events initiated by the neurotransmitter-receptor interaction (equation III-1) is, as yet, not completely defined and because of well-founded assumptions that these specific receptors occur at extremely low concentrations and have not, so far, been successfully characterized or isolated, knowledge of the molecular basis of this

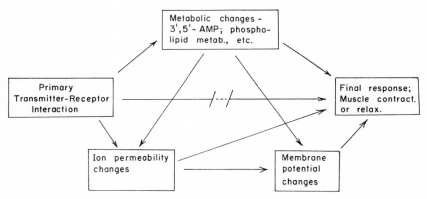

FIG. III-1. Possible interrelationships between the primary neurotransmitter-receptor interaction showing various pathways (direct and indirect) by which this interaction could activate the final physiological response (muscle contraction relaxation, glandular secretion, etc.).

primary interaction is based essentially upon observations relating to events that occur at least several steps subsequent to this primary interaction. These may be perfectly satisfactory procedures *provided* that the primary neurotransmitter-receptor interaction is determinant for the entire sequence of events leading to the production of the measured response. While this assumption seems, *a priori*, at least plausible it cannot be ignored that the initial interaction may be modified by subsequent intermediate events such that the characteristics of the final measured response relate to one or more intermediate steps. In any event it must be recognized that there are two important components of the neurotransmitter-receptor interaction—the *affinity*, determined by the strength (goodness of fit) of the mutual interaction and the *ability* of the formed complex to initiate the sequence of events. Some progress, although essentially at an empirical level has been made in separating these factors (Chapter IV, p. 267).

In the following chapters discussions will be presented of various parameters of neurotransmitter-receptor interactions including structure–activity relationships (Chapter IV), membrane potential and permeability changes (Chapter V), metabolic events (Chapter VI) and the interrelationships of neurotransmitters and Ca^{++} in excitation–contraction (relaxation) coupling (Chapter VII). Finally (Chapter VIII) a brief summary is given of recent progress towards the actual isolation and characterization of the receptors.

However, before any detailed discussion of neurotransmitter action is presented a brief and very general discussion of the peripheral nervous system, its physiological role and the sites of action of neurotransmitters and their analogs and antagonists may prove helpful.

The fundamental unit of the nervous system is the neurone, which consists essentially of a nucleated cell and a number of fibers leading from it. In general neurones are independent with functional connections occurring through close proximity of the nerve terminals: such junctions are referred to as synapses. The complexity of the vertebrate nervous system dictates that even simple nervous reflexes must involve several neurones linked together in a functional pathway. There is considerable evidence to indicate that at most synapses transmission of the nerve impulse occurs through the intermediate liberation and action of neurotransmitters.

The nervous system has two primary divisions of motor outflow: the somatic which controls reflex and volitional activities of skeletal muscle, and the autonomic, which controls smooth muscle and glands. There are several anatomical distinctions to be made between these two systems; of particular importance is the fact that autonomic nerves form peripheral, multineuronal synapses (ganglia) which are absent in the somatic nervous system. The autonomic system is further divided into two components—the thoracolumbar or sympathetic outflow and the craniosacral or parasympathetic outflow. These two divisions are distinct in many of their anatomical and physiological characteristics. The sympathetic nerves originate in the spinal cord between the eighth cervical and the third lumbar segments and they synapse in peripheral ganglia. The largest group of ganglia comprise the twenty-two pairs of vertebral ganglia: the preganglionic fibers synapse in only one ganglion which is not necessarily adjacent to the appropriate spinal segment; furthermore the post:preganglionic ratio is high so that discharge of the sympathetic system is likely to produce a diffuse and general response. In contrast the parasympathetic system is a more localized structure: the outflow from the cranial and sacral regions synapse in ganglia close to the innervated structure and the ratio of post:preganglionic innervation is unity.

The functions of the autonomic nervous system are probably best summarized as "the controlling of the internal environment" (Claude

TABLE III-1. The Effects of Sympathetic and Parasympathetic Nerve Stimulation

Effector system	Adrenergic stimulation†	Cholinergic stimulation†
Heart,		
Rate	Increased (β)	Decreased
Stroke volume	Increased (β)	Decreased
Blood vessels		
Skin	Constriction (α)	Dilatation
Skeletal muscle	Constriction (α) Dilatation (β)	Dilatation
Pulmonary	Constriction (α)	—
Abdomen	Constriction (α) Dilatation (β)	—
Lung,		
Bronchial muscle	Relaxation (β)	Contraction
Stomach,		
Motility and tone	Decrease (β)	Increase
Intestine,		
Motility and tone	Decrease (α,β)	Increase
Eye,		
Radial muscle	Contraction (mydriasis)	—
Sphincter muscle		Contraction (miosis)
Uterus	Variable (α,β)	Variable
	(very dependent on species, pregnancy and hormonal state)	
Adrenal medulla	—	Liberation of catecholamines
Liver	Glycogenolysis	—
Skin,		
Pilomotor muscles	Contraction (α)	—
Salivary glands	Thick secretion (α)	Watery secretion

† The terms "cholinergic" and "adrenergic" are often used in preference to the anatomical descriptions since, for example, some anatomically postganglionic sympathetic fibers appear to use acetylcholine as the transmitter.

Bernard, 1879) or homeostasis. The anatomical distinctions between the two divisions of the autonomic nervous system are reflected by their corresponding differences of function. The sympathetic system frequently functions as a unit particularly under conditions of acute stress: sympathetic stimulation accelerates the heart rate, increases blood pressure and volume, raises the blood sugar level, decreases intestinal mobility and, in short, prepares the animal for "fight or flight" (W. B. Cannon). However, the sympathetic system should not be regarded as being active only under traumatic conditions. The parasympathetic system is organized for localized activity and is primarily concerned with the conservation of energy. Table III-1 summarizes some of the effects of sympathetic and parasympathetic stimulation.

As far as chemical transmitters are concerned their various loci of action are shown in Fig. III-2. The actions of acetylcholine at the post-ganglionic parasympathetic neuroeffector junctions are referred to as "muscarinic" since they are mimicked by muscarine (Chapter IV, p. 325) while at the ganglia and the skeletal neuromuscular junctions the actions

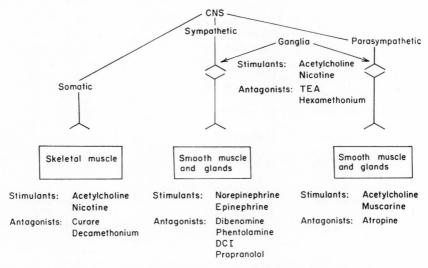

FIG. III-2. Sites of action of neurotransmitters.

are referred to as nicotinic. The neurotransmitter at most postganglionic sympathetic neuroeffector junctions is norepinephrine but it is now well established from comparisons of structure–activity data, physiological responses and the selectivity of agonist and antagonist action that there are two types of adrenergic receptor (often present in the same tissue) referred to as α- and β-receptors (Chapter IV, p. 275). Thus norepinephrine and isopropyl norepinephrine have maximum activities at α- and β-receptors respectively. It was upon essentially this type of evidence that Ahlquist introduced the α,β classification in 1948. Figure III-2 summarizes the sites of action of neurotransmitters and indicates how pharmacological distinctions may be provided through the use of selectively acting antagonists.

Chapter IV

ANALOGS AND ANTAGONISTS OF ACETYLCHOLINE AND NOREPINEPHRINE: THE RELATIONSHIPS BETWEEN CHEMICAL STRUCTURE AND BIOLOGICAL ACTIVITY

In the simplest sense, the basic assumption in the general analysis of structure–activity relationships is that the ligand molecule exhibits a degree of complementarity to its site of recognition on the macromolecular surface, and that with progressive alteration of the ligand structure appear correlatable changes in a particular biological activity; hence a "mapping", at least in general terms, of the macromolecular surface may be achieved.

In practice, the situation is rarely as simple as this. For a significant structure–activity relationship to be deduced, at whatever level of sophistication, it is necessary that certain primary requirements be met. A number of these requirements, which are not of course unique to the neurotransmitter-receptor interactions that will form the principal topic of discussion, may be summarized as follows.

The series of compounds should produce their common biological response through interaction at a common receptor system. Thus, it is now well established that many sympathomimetic amines produce their biological effects, not through interaction at the adrenergic receptor, but through the indirect mechanism of release of norepinephrine (see section on p. 217) with the latter agent producing the biological response. It is clear that this and related phenomena such as varying susceptibility to degradative enzymes (acetylcholinesterase, monoamine oxidase, etc.) or the occurrence of selective diffusion barriers can grossly perturb a structure–activity relationship.

In considering the molecular basis of the ligand–receptor interaction at least two major problems are presented. The neurotransmitters and most of their analogs are small, relatively flexible molecules, the conformations of which, *as receptor-bound species*, bear no necessary relationship to the experimentally accessible conformations in the aqueous or crystalline state (1, 2). Differences in biological activity amongst structurally related ligands may thus reflect differences in their relative abilities to attain a certain conformation rather than *intrinsic* differences in the ability of the ligands to bind at the receptor site. An interesting case that may constitute an example of this problem is cited by Greenberg (3) who argues that the relative inactivity of tryptamines (IV-2) relative to lysergic acid diethylamide (IV-1) on the Venus merceneria heart preparation may be due to the high energy barrier to C_3, C_2, C_β and C_α of the tryptamines adopting the corresponding planar configuration found in IV-1. A related problem concerns the number of modes of binding

IV-1　　　　　　　　　IV-2

available to activator ligands and the feasibility of determining whether activator and inhibitor ligands interact at the same site. The simplest assumption, of course, is that there exists but a single unique neuro-transmitter recognition site and that all the analogs and antagonists also bind to this same unique site, occupying greater or lesser areas of it according to ligand structure. However, there is actually no reason to believe that such a binding mechanism is generally operative and an increasing amount of evidence, much of it derived from enzyme–substrate–inhibitor studies, supports the concept that multiple, but overlapping, binding sites are available for substrates and that many inhibitors produce their effects through interaction at sites topo-graphically distinct from those involved in substrate binding. Some examples of these conclusions derived from several enzyme systems are discussed later in this chapter together with evidence highly suggestive of the application of similar conclusions to the interaction of neuro-transmitter analogs at their corresponding receptor sites. The importance of these conclusions to the quantitative interpretation of structure–activity relationships is quite clear; interpretations offered in terms of a common mutual complementarity between ligands and macromolecule cannot be valid if partially or totally distinct binding sites are utilized for different ligands. Furthermore, a small structural change may produce a change in binding mode: occasionally such changes may be dramatic and evidenced by, for example, changes in the chiralty of the ligand–receptor interaction; perhaps more commonly, however, the effects of such changes are more subtle as may occur in the gradual structural transition from a "polar" ligand (i.e. $CH_3COOCH_2CH_2\overset{+}{N}Me_3$) to a "non polar" ligand (i.e. $CH_3CH_2CH_2CH_2CH_2\overset{+}{N}Me_3$), where it seems likely (see section on p. 257) that a transition in binding preference for a site of reduced polarity occurs with increasing nonpolar character of the ligand.

Finally, in systems where the measure of a ligand–receptor interaction is muscle contraction, relaxation, change of membrane potential or a related process which is clearly the result of a more or less complex series of events,

$$L + Rec \underset{}{\overset{\text{Step 1}}{\rightleftharpoons}} L\text{---}Rec \xrightarrow{\text{n steps}} \text{measured physiological response} \quad (I)$$

the question must be posed as to what extent the measured response is a *direct* measure of the initial ligand–receptor interaction. This problem may be considered in the following way: the dependence of biological

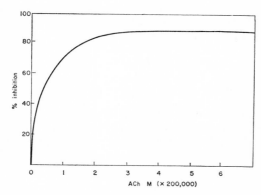

FIG. IV-1. Concentration–response curve for the action of acetylcholine on frog heart. Reproduced with permission from Clark (4).

response upon drug concentration may be expressed as a concentration–response curve (Fig. IV-1) that in many instances, as emphasized particularly by A. J. Clark (5, 6), bears a considerable resemblance to Langmuir adsorption curves. If this resemblance is more than formal and concentration–response curves actually describe the ligand saturation process at the receptor (step 1 of eqn. I is determinant for the total sequence of events initiated) then they may very simply be employed to generate quantitative data for the interaction of series of ligands with the receptor. Furthermore, deviations from hyperbolic concentration–response curves, most commonly in the direction of increased steepness of curve (6) so that $S_{0.1}/S_{0.9} < 81$ (Chapter I, see section on p. 95), could then be interpreted, although not unambiguously, according to the various treatments of cooperative ligand binding phenomena (Chapter I, see section on p. 71).

However, it is also possible to envisage that the primary ligand–receptor interaction may be determinant for the production of response but that the linkage between this interaction and the response may vary from ligand to ligand (this point is further elaborated below in the next section of this chapter). Alternatively, the concentration–response curves may also be a measure of a step (or steps) subsequent to the initial ligand–receptor interaction and which bears no necessary proportionality to this first interaction. If either of these alternatives are correct, and they cannot be eliminated by only *a priori* arguments, then quantitative information concerning the ligand–receptor interaction is not available from the concentration–response curves.

Despite these potential constraints structure–activity relationship determinations have been widely employed in attempts to define the molecular basis for neurotransmitter actions and there is now some evidence available to suggest that at least some concentration–response curves probably do represent receptor saturation curves (see section on p. 330).

QUANTITATIVE TREATMENTS OF LIGAND–RECEPTOR INTERACTIONS

From his work on the concentration–response curves of acetylcholine in the frog heart and rectus muscle preparations Clark (4, 7, 8) noted that these hyperbolic curves could be fitted rather well to the mass-action expression,

$$K[A] = \frac{r_A}{r_{max} - r_A} \tag{II}$$

an expression which also describes many adsorption phenomena (4), where $[A]$ is the acetylcholine concentration, r_A is the observed response and r_{max} is the maximum observed response of the tissue to acetylcholine. In addition, Clark (4) made the assumption that the response of the tissue to the activator ligand is proportional to the number of receptors occupied and that at maximum response all of the receptors will be occupied. Thus, equation (II) may be rewritten,

$$K[A] = \frac{r_A}{100 - r_A} \tag{III}$$

On the basis of the above assumption, and it is worth noting at this point that Clark clearly realized (9) that such assumptions might not be valid and would in any event be difficult to establish unambiguously, then the quantitative treatment of ligand–receptor interactions becomes very simple. According to Clark,

$$r_A = kY_A \tag{IV}$$

where r_A is the response produced by agonist A, and Y_A is the fraction of receptors occupied at this response level. Under saturating conditions,

$$r_A = k = r_{max} \qquad \text{(V)}$$

where r_{max} represents the maximum response and is assumed to be equal for all activator ligands (agonist) since the constant, k, applies to all agonists at one receptor. Hence,

$$Y_A = r_A / r_{max} \qquad \text{(VI)}$$

so that the ratio of observed to maximum response measures that proportion of receptors occupied by the agonist A. At half-maximum response, $Y_A = 0 \cdot 5$ and, from the mass-action expression,

$$R + A \rightleftharpoons RA,$$

$$K_A = \frac{[RA]}{[R][A]}$$

since

$$[R_{tot}] = [R] + [RA]$$
$$= [RA]\left\{1 + \frac{1}{K_A[A]}\right\}$$

and

$$Y_A = \frac{[RA]}{[R_{tot}]} = \frac{1}{\left\{1 + \dfrac{1}{K_A[A]}\right\}} \qquad \text{(VII)}$$

then

$$Y_A = 0 \cdot 5 = \frac{1}{\left\{1 + \dfrac{1}{K_A[A]}\right\}} \qquad \text{(VIII)}$$

and

$$K_A = \frac{1}{[A]_{50}} \qquad \text{(IX)}$$

thus generating the familiar finding that the affinity of the ligand may be determined directly from the agonist concentration curve producing 50 per cent of the maximum response *provided that the original assumptions are correct.*

An early recognized deficiency of the Clark treatment was that not all agonists of a given class generate the same maximum response (10–12) (Fig. IV-2: the example cited is for the alkyltrimethylammonium series but many other examples could be cited and are discussed more fully in reference 12), and hence the simple concept of agents being either agonists or antagonists was, by necessity, modified.

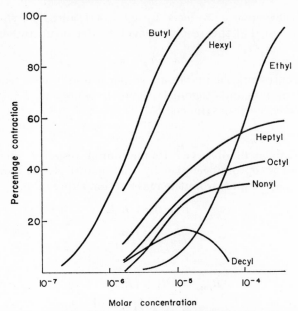

Fɪɢ. IV-2. Concentration–response curves for alkyltrimethylammonium ligands on the guinea-pig ileum. The curves all refer to one piece of ileum. Reproduced with permission from Stephenson (13).

Ariëns, in 1954 (11), introduced the concept of *intrinsic activity* whereby the effect of an agonist is presumed to depend not only upon its affinity for the receptor but also upon its ability to initiate the biological response. Thus eqn. IV may be rewritten,

$$r_A = \alpha Y_A \tag{X}$$

where α is the intrinsic activity, hence,

$$r_{max} = \alpha \tag{XI}$$

and the intrinsic activity of an agonist is equal to the maximum response that it can induce. Customarily, intrinsic activities are assigned by comparing the maximum response of agonist (B) to that produced by a standard agonist (A),

$$\frac{\alpha_B}{\alpha_A} = \frac{r_{Bmax}}{r_{Amax}} \tag{XII}$$

Since, in this treatment the fundamental assumptions made by Clark were still retained, affinity constants are still readily determinable according to eqn. IX save that $[A]_{50}$ now represents the concentration of agonist producing 50 per cent of its respective maximum response.

Stephenson (13), in 1956, preferred not to utilize the basic assumptions of Clark and developed a treatment in which he assumed that some agonists may not require 100 per cent of the available receptors to generate a maximum response and that response is not proportional to receptor occupancy. If this is correct then the possibility exists that identical responses may be produced by agonists occupying different numbers of receptors and thus comparison of response alone may obscure important differences in the agonist–receptor interaction. According to Stephenson's treatment a parameter termed the *stimulus*, S, characteristic of each agonist–receptor interaction is defined as,

$$S = eY \tag{XIII}$$

where e is termed the *efficacy* and Y, as before, is the fraction of receptors occupied to produce the response corresponding to this stimulus, it being further assumed that response is a constant function of stimulus,

$$r = fS \tag{XIV}$$

so that a given stimulus always produces the same response. The importance of the assumptions expressed in eqns. XIII and XIV is that identical responses may be produced by different agonists using different combinations of e and Y provided that they generate the same value of S. For a series of alkyltrimethylammonium ligands active at the cholinergic

TABLE IV-1. Affinities and Efficacies of Alkyltrimethylammonium Ligands (calculated by Stephenson (13))

$$\overset{+}{\text{RNMe}_3}$$

R =	Me	Et	Pr	Bu	Am	Hex	Hep	Oct	Non	Dec
Efficacy†	94	31	4·3	200	200	21	2·2	1·4	1·0	0·6
Affinity × 10^{-3}	0·24	0·63	1·6	3·8	8·5	19·0	41	63	110	190

† Guinea-pig ileum preparation.

(muscarinic) receptor Stephenson calculated (making various assumptions for details of which the original paper should be calculated) values of e and K_A (Table IV-1) from which he concluded that the peak activity observed at amyltrimethylammonium is, since the affinity constants of the ligands vary in a regular fashion, associated with the high efficacy of this ligand.‡

‡ The concept of nonequal receptor occupancy in the generation of responses had, by 1962, been explicitly recognized by Ariëns *et al.* (15, 16) who suggested that many agents classified as having equal intrinsic activities of unity actually had different intrinsic activities that were >1. Thus, conceptually, the intrinsic activity parameter had become equivalent to the efficacy parameter of Stephenson.

A variation of the Stephenson treatment was produced in 1965 by Furchgott (14) who proposed that,

$$S = \epsilon[RA] \qquad\qquad (XV)$$

where ϵ is a hybrid term termed the *intrinsic efficacy*. It is clear that

$$e = \epsilon[R]_{tot} \qquad\qquad (XVI)$$

thus introducing the further development that efficacy is dependent upon the total concentration of receptors and, therefore, that stimulus and hence response is explicitly dependent upon the absolute concentration of receptors.

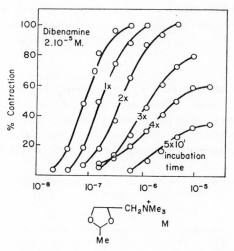

FIG. IV-3. Concentration response curves of 2-methyl-4-dimethylaminomethyl-1,3-dioxolane methiodide on the rat jejunum progressively treated with dibenamine. Note the initial parallel shift prior to declination of maximum response. Reproduced with permission from Ariëns (12).

The importance of these and other (17–21) quantitative treatments of ligand–receptor interactions is that they all attempt to provide a formal basis for obtaining such (by various experimental manipulations for details of which the original articles may be consulted) fundamental parameters as K_A for agonists from measurements of the final tissue response. As noted in the introduction of this chapter the relationship of this final event to the initial interaction for which the data is required is complex and still obscure. In any event the various treatments yield different values for such parameters as affinity, intrinsic activity and efficacy, suggesting that the various assumptions basic to each treatment must be carefully re-examined. In particular, the assumption that maximum response may be produced when only a small fraction of the total number of receptors is occupied by the activator ligand and which constitutes a basic point of departure for the Ariëns, Stephenson and Furchgott treatments seems open to serious doubt. This assumption rests essentially on one type of experimental evidence, namely that exposure of the tissue to various irreversible antagonists (Dibenamine, etc.) produces, with many agonists, an initial parallel shift of the dose–response curve prior to a reduction in the tissue response (6, 14, 16, 22, 23; Fig. IV-3). The initial parallel shift is presumed to represent irreversible inactivation of that fraction of the receptors (the receptor reserve) that is not necessary for generation of 100 per cent response, subsequent inactivation of receptors producing a loss of response. However, this interpretation is valid only to the extent that the modification of the agonist-induced response by the irreversible antagonist is attributable to specific interactions at the appropriate receptor. The general plausibility of these considerations is, however, considerably reduced by findings that such irreversible antagonists exert their pharmacological actions at a number of sites (in complete accord with knowledge of their chemical reactivity and more general concepts of antagonist–receptor interactions). These and other aspects of antagonist action will be discussed later in this chapter (see section on p. 330).

Despite these considerations it is still very useful to describe the actions of agonists in terms of the above discussed parameters: in particular, the affinity constant and intrinsic activity parameters of Ariëns are useful since, whatever their theoretical significance, they do provide a convenient summary of two important features of the relationship between tissue response and the agonist activity.

LIGANDS ACTIVE AT CHOLINERGIC AND ADRENERGIC RECEPTORS

Attention will now be turned to discussion of what has been the most widely employed approach to structure–activity relationships, namely the attempted correlation of molecular structure with the characteristics of the final physiological response (muscle contraction, relaxation, etc). Despite the comments of the previous two sections of this chapter indicating the hazards inherent in such correlations the fact remains that an extremely large quantity of very useful work has been based on this approach and has generated information of considerable interest.

AGONISTS AT THE ADRENERGIC RECEPTORS

The sympathomimetic amines—compounds generating responses more or less equivalent to those of sympathetic nerve stimulation—provide an admirable example of the necessity of establishing that

TABLE IV-2. Classification of Sympathomimetic Amines (42)

Amine	4	3	X	Y	R	Nictitating membrane	Heart rate	Blood pressure
Norepinephrine	HO	HO	HO	H	H	1	1	1
Epinephrine	HO	HO	HO	H	Me	1	1	1
Corbasil	HO	HO	HO	Me	H	1	1	—
Dihydroxyephedrine	HO	HO	HO	Me	Me	1	—	—
Dopamine	HO	HO	H	H	H	1	—	—
Epinine	HO	HO	H	H	Me	1	1	—
Isopropylnorepinephrine	HO	HO	HO	H	CH(Me)$_2$	1	1	—
Phenylephrine	H	HO	HO	H	Me	1	1	1
Synephrine	HO	H	HO	H	Me	1	1	1
Norphenylephrine	H	HO	HO	H	H	1	1-2	1
Norsynephrine	HO	H	HO	H	H	2	2	**2**
Phenylethanolamine	H	H	HO	H	H	2-3	2-3	—
Phenylpropanolamine	H	H	HO	Me	H	2	2	**2**
m-Hydroxyphenylpropanolamine	H	HO	HO	Me	H	1	2	—
p-Hydroxyphenylpropanolamine	HO	H	HO	Me	H	2	2	2
Ephedrine	H	H	HO	Me	Me	2-3	2-3	2
m-Hydroxyephedrine	H	HO	HO	Me	Me	2	2	1
p-Hydroxyephedrine	HO	H	HO	Me	Me	2	2	2
m-Hydroxytyramine	H	HO	H	H	H	2-3	2-3	2
Tyramine	HO	H	H	H	H	3	3	3
2-Phenylethylamine	H	H	H	H	H	3	3	3
Amphetamine	H	H	H	Me	H	3	3	**3**
p-Hydroxyamphetamine	HO	H	H	Me	H	—	—	**3**
N-Methylamphetamine	H	H	H	Me	Me	3	3	—

1 = direct action; 2 = mixed action; 3 = indirect actions.

agents producing a common response do so by a common mechanism. For many years interpretation of structure–activity relationships of sympathomimetic amines were frustrated in large part by the fact that a very large range of structures, in which the presence of an amino function appeared to be essentially the sole structural prerequisite, possess some degree of sympathomimetic activity (for reviews see refs 24–28). This problem has been considerably clarified over the past few years by the very thoroughly documented findings (26–55) that many sympathomimetic amines produce their pharmacological actions through the release of norepinephrine from peripheral storage sites and that the released norepinephrine, rather than the administered sympathomimetic amine, is responsible for the pharmacological actions.† Through the use of reserpine, an agent that produces depletion of adrenergic storage sites, it has been possible to provide a broad classification of sympathomimetic amines into agents that act essentially through direct interaction at the receptor, agents that act essentially through the indirect mechanism of norepinephrine release and agents that have both direct and indirect actions (Table IV-2). From this data it is clear that the basic structural requirements for direct (receptor) action among phenethylamines are the presence of the catechol group of the m-phenolic and β-hydroxyl groups. Agents lacking these features have indirect activity and the extent of the indirect activity increases with progressive molecular deviation from the structure of norepinephrine.

Thus, agonist interaction at the adrenergic receptors requires the presence of defined structural features imposed upon a basic phenethylamine pattern. Each of these structural features will now be examined.

Chirality of the Adrenergic Receptors

The absolute configurations of catecholamines (norepinephrine, epinephrine, N-isopropylnorepinephrine, N-t-butylnorepinephrine and N-methylephinephrine) have been established (56–60), the more active

IV - 3

isomers having the R (D) configuration (IV-3). The activities of some stereoisomers in α- and β-receptor preparations are listed in Table IV-3

† In this treatment it is impossible to do justice to the immense pharmacological importance of this concept and for its many ramifications. For fuller discussions the reader should consult references cited above.

9

TABLE IV-3. Activities of Norepinephrine Derivatives at α- and β-Receptors (61, 62)

$$3,4(HO)_2C_6H_3CHOHCH_2NHR$$

R	Configuration	α-Receptor (rat vas deferens)				β-Receptor (guinea-pig atrium)			
		i.a.	pD$_2$†	pA$_2$‡	D/L ratio	i.a.	pD$_2$	pA$_2$	D/L ratio
H	DL	1	5·4	—	—	1	4·0	—	20
H	D	1	5·4	—	—	—	—	—	—
H	L	1	4·8	—	4	1	4·8	—	50
Me	DL	1	5·4	—	—	1	—	—	—
Me	D	1	6·1	—	—	—	4·8	—	—
Me	L	1	5·0	—	8	—	—	—	—
Pr^i	DL	0·4	2·8	—	—	1	6·3	—	>500
Pr^i	D	1	4·0	—	—	—	—	—	—
Pr^i	L	0	—	3·4	—	1	6·9	—	>1000
CHMeCH$_2$C$_6$H$_4$OH-p	DL	0	—	5·0	—	—	—	—	—
	D	0	—	4·2	—	—	—	—	—
	L	0	—	5·3	0·1	—	—	—	—

† pD$_2$ = $-\log_{10} K_A$ (equation IX).

‡ pA$_2$ = $-\log_{10}$ concentration of antagonist to reduce effect of double agonist concentration to effect of single concentration.

from which it is apparent that the stereochemical demands of the receptor macromolecules are substantially higher at the β-receptor.
Apparently, the β-hydroxyl group is more critical for β-receptor
activation; furthermore the stereospecificity of events at the β-receptor
increases with increasing size of the N-substituent (Table IV-3) and it
has been suggested (28) that nonpolar binding of this substituent may

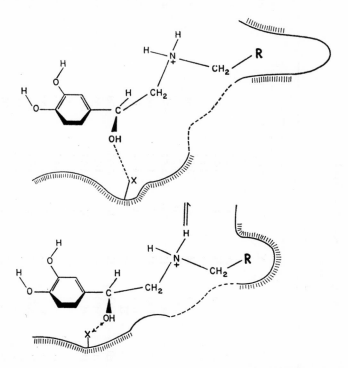

FIG. IV-4. Representation of the effect of the nonpolar groups R in β-agonists in
modifying hydrogen-bonding (X----OH) at the chiral center.

play a determinant role in the catecholamine binding conformation at
the β-receptor. Possibly the N-substituent produces a conformational
change which increases the importance of binding of the β-hydroxyl
group (Fig. IV-4); increasing bulk of the N-substituent causing progressively greater structural change and hence increasing stereoselectivity.

Nevertheless, the β-hydroxyl group may not be an indispensable
molecular function for either activity at the α- or β-receptors. This is
clearly shown in the data from Tables IV-4 and IV-5, which indicate that

TABLE IV-4. Activities of DL, D- and L-Norepinephrine Analogs in Normal and Catecholamine-Depleted Rat vas deferens (64)

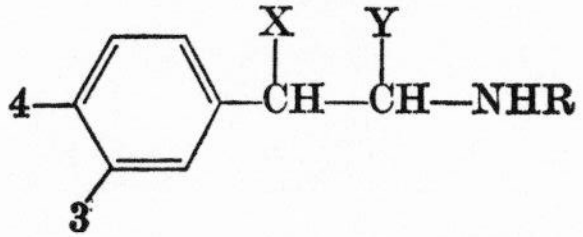

Compound	4	3	X	Y	R	Normal		Reserpinized	
						pD$_2$	Max. effect†	pD$_2$	Max. effect†
Norepinephrine D(−)	HO	HO	HO	H	H	5·23	99	4·80	100
Norepinephrine L(+)	HO	HO	HO	H	H	4·51	107	4·08	78
Desoxynorepinephrine	HO	HO	H	H	H	4·64	107	3·95	67
Epinephrine D(−)	HO	HO	HO	H	Me	5·78	84	5·39	91
Epinephrine L(+)	HO	HO	HO	H	Me	4·51	106	3·96	70
Desoxyepinephrine	HO	HO	H	H	Me	4·77	100	4·07	84
Corbasil D(−)	HO	HO	HO	Me	H	4·96	104	4·80	61
Corbasil L(+)	HO	HO	HO	Me	H	4·42	40	—‡	10
Desoxycorbasil	HO	HO	H	Me	H	4·86	89	3·94	32
Phenylephrine D(−)	H	HO	HO	H	Me	5·05	109	5·19	91
Phenylephrine L(+)	H	HO	HO	H	Me	4·16	84	—‡	7
Desoxyphenylephrine	H	HO	H	H	Me	4·71	100	—‡	6
Synephrine D(−)	HO	H	HO	H	Me	4·31	81	4·14	86
Synephrine L(+)	HO	H	HO	H	Me	4·27	45	—‡	30
Desoxysynephrine	HO	H	H	H	Me	4·61	89	—‡	12
Octopamine D(−)	HO	H	HO	H	H	4·71	102	3·62	77
Octopamine L(+)	HO	H	HO	H	H	4·36	86	—‡	12
Desoxyoctopamine	HO	H	H	H	H	4·15	97	—‡	10

† Relative to D(−)-norepinephrine.
‡ Maximal effect too low for determination of ED$_{50}$.

TABLE IV-5. Activities of L-Norepinephrine Derivatives and their Desoxy Analogs (61, 62)

$$3,4(HO)_2C_6H_3CHRCH_2NHR'$$

R	R'	Configuration	i.a.	α-Receptor pD$_2$	α-Receptor pA$_2$	α-Receptor L/Desoxy ratio	β-Receptor L/Desoxy ratio
OH	H	L	1	4·8	—	—	—
H	H		1	4·9	—	1	2–5
OH	Me	L	1	5·0	—	—	—
H	Me		1	5·0	—	1	2
OH	Pr^i	L	0	—	3·4	—	—
H	Pr^i		0	—	3·4	1	1
OH	CHMeCH$_2$C$_6$H$_4$OH-p†	L	0	—	5·3	—	—
H	CHMeCH$_2$C$_6$H$_4$OH-p		0	—	5·2	1	1–30

† The D/L ratio of this compound as an adrenergic α-antagonist is 0·1.

dopamine, deoxynorepinephrine and deoxyepinephrine have direct α- and β-adrenergic activities, albeit at a reduced level from their R-β-hydroxy analogs. Similarly, the 6,7-dihydroxytetrahydroisoquinoline (IV-4) is at least as potent as N-isopropylnorepinephrine in some β-receptor systems (63).

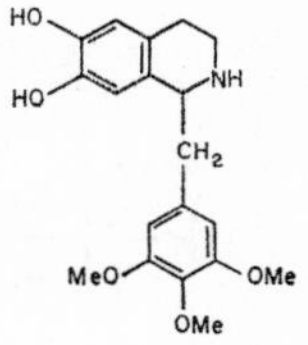

IV - 4

A stereospecific three-point binding of the catechol, β-hydroxyl and amino groups had been proposed by Easson and Stedman in 1933 (65) to account for the stereospecificity of adrenergic actions. According to this hypothesis it would be anticipated that the S-(L) isomers of catechol-amines, where β-hydroxyl binding should be absent, will have the same potency as the desoxy compounds. This has been found to be essentially true but only for those agents that interact directly at the receptors (61, 62, 64; Tables IV-4 and IV-5).

The N-substitution Pattern

In the previous chapter the activities of norepinephrine, epinephrine and N-isopropylnorepinephrine were discussed with reference to the classification of α- and β-receptors: N-isopropylnorepinephrine is most

TABLE IV-6. Effects of N-substitution in DL-Norepinephrine (68)
$3,4\text{-}(HO)_2C_6H_3CHOHCH_2NHR$

R	α-Receptors (rat vas deferens)			β-Receptors (calf trachea)	
	i.a.	pD_2	pA_2	i.a.	pD_2
H	1	5·4	—	1	6·0
CH_3	1	5·9	—	1	6·7
C_2H_5	0·9	5·2	—	1	7·2
C_3H_7	0·3	3·3	—	—	—
$C_3H_7{}^i$	0·6	3·0	—	1	7·5
C_4H_9	0	—	3·0	—	—
$C_4H_9{}^s$	0	—	3·0	—	—
$C_4H_9{}^i$	0	—	3·0	—	—
$C_4H_9{}^t$	0	—	3·0	1	7·6
$CHMeCH_2Ph$	0	—	4·4	—	—
CMe_2CH_2Ph	0	—	5·9	—	—

active at β-receptors and least active at α-receptors. The effects of N-substitution on the activities of norepinephrine at α- and β-receptors have been quantitated by a number of workers (61, 62, 66–68) and a very

TABLE IV-7. Effect of N-substitution on β-Activity of Norepinephrine Homologs
3,4-$(HO)_2C_6H_3CHOHCH_2NHR$

No.	R	Relative bronchodilator activity	Ref.
1	CH_3	40	70
2	CH_2CH_3	25	71, 72
3	$CH_2CH_2CH_3$	10	71, 72
4	$CH(CH_3)_2$	100 (standard)	—
5	$(CH_2)_3CH_3$	8	71–73
6	$CH(CH_3)CH_2CH_3$	50	73, 74
7	$C(CH_3)_3$	170	71–73
8	$(CH_2)_4CH_3$	25	71
9	Cyclopentyl	70	75
10	$(CH_2)_6CH_3$	10	76
11	$(CH_2)_8CH_3$	7	76
12	$CH_2CH_2C_6H_5$	10	72, 77
13	$CH_2CH_2C_6H_4$—OH-4	50	72
14	$CH(CH_3)CH_2C_6H_5$	100	72
15	$C(CH_3)_2CH_2C_6H_5$	100	72
16	$CH(C_2H_5)CH_2C_6H_5$	100	76
17	$C(CH_3, C_2H_5)CH_2C_6H_5$	3	72
18	$CH_2CH(CH_3)C_6H_5$	1	72
19	$CH(CH_3)CH_2$ cyclohexyl	17	76
20	$CH(CH_3)CH_2C_6H_4$—OH-4	800	72
21	$CH(CH_3)CH_2C_6H_4$—CH_3-4	50	72
22	$CH(CH_3)CH_2C_6H_4$—OCH_3-4	200	76
23	$CH(CH_3)CH_2C_6H_4O_2CH_2$-3,4	100	76
24	$C(CH_3)_2CH_2C_6H_4$—OH-4	800	72
25	$C(CH_3)_2CH_2C_6H_4$—CH_3-4	100	72
26	$(CH_2)_3C_6H_5$	50	76, 77
27	$CH(CH_3)CH_2CH_2C_6H_5$	100	72
28	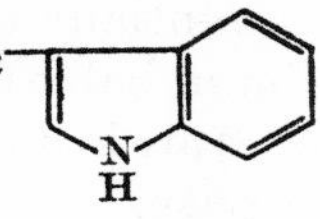	750	78

considerable quantity of data is also available concerning the activities of such compounds in other test systems also (further discussion is given in ref. 69). Thus, the data of Table IV-6 show very nicely that increasing size of N-substitution produces increased activity at β-receptors. Obviously the increasing size of the nonpolar N-substituent is of importance and the data of Table IV-7 show that the binding locus for such nonpolar groups has a defined area of at least the size of the *t*-butyl group and that whilst the introduction of further nonpolar function (e.g., 4 → 21; 7 → 15; 7 → 25 etc.) does not increase activity over *N-t*-butylnorepinephrine certain compounds appear to make contact with a polar binding area (e.g., 12 → 13, 14 → 20, 15 → 24). Thus, we may conclude tentatively that the nonpolar binding area has a limited surface in two dimensions capable of accommodating only the >CMe$_2$ structure but has greater tolerance in the third dimension and eventually permits bridging to a polar area (Fig. IV-5). However, these areas must be regarded as "extra-receptor" in the sense that they are not

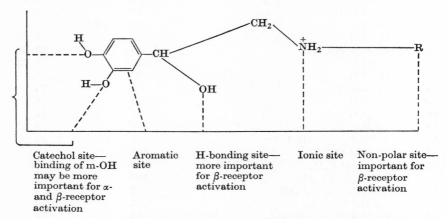

| Catechol site— binding of m-OH may be more important for α- and β-receptor activation | Aromatic site | H-bonding site— more important for β-receptor activation | Ionic site | Non-polar site— important for β-receptor activation |

FIG. IV-5. Summary of the various binding sites considered of importance in α- and β-receptor activation.

employed in the binding of the physiological transmitters, norepinephrine and epinephrine. Nevertheless, in any consideration of the transition from α- to β-mimetic activity with increasing size of the *N*-substituent a number of factors must be considered. At physiological pH norepinephrine and its *N*-alkyl homologs all exist essentially exclusively as the protonated species (68, 79); it thus appears improbable that the relatively small variations in the pK$_1$ values (Table IV-8) are in any way responsible for the dramatic variations in biological activity.

A number of workers, notably Belleau (80–83) and Bloom (84) have discussed the role of the ammonium group in both α- and β-receptor activation. Full discussion of such models is best left until further pertinent evidence concerning adrenergic events has been discussed but in principle one might expect two primary functions of the ammonium group, (a) involvement in a charge–charge interaction and (b) involvement in hydrogen bonding. The charge–charge interaction will become less effective with the increasing charge separation that will be anticipated to be caused by increased steric bulk of the N-substituent (Chapter I, p. 2) although the contribution to ionic stabilization provided by any nonpolar binding of the N-alkyl substituent will offset this to the

TABLE IV-8. pK Values of
N-Alkylnorepinephrines (68)
$3,4(HO)_2C_6H_3CHOHCH_2NHR$

R	pK_1†
H	9·18
CH_3	9·51
CH_2CH_3	9·61
$CH(CH_3)_2$	9·58
$CH_2CH_2CH_2CH_3$	9·56
$CH(CH_3)CH_2CH_3$	9·48
$CH_2CH(CH_3)_2$	9·28
$C(CH_3)_3$	9·73

† $3,4(HO)_2C_6H_3CHOHCH_2\overset{+}{N}H_2R \underset{K_1}{\rightleftharpoons}$
$3,4(HO_2C_6H_3CHOHCH_2NHR.$

extent that it occurs (Chapter I, p. 52). In contrast, hydrogen bonding will be considerably facilitated by a hydrophobic environment (Chapter I, p. 52) as would be provided by the bonding of the N-substituent of the catecholamine to a hydrophobic patch: this phenomenon has been discussed by Grunwald and his colleagues (85, 86) who have measured the rate constants for dissociation of hydrogen bonded amine–water

TABLE IV-9. Effects of Nonpolar Structure on Dissociation of Amine–Hydroxylic Solvent Hydrogen Bonds (86)

System	Temp.	$10^{-10} k_H$ sec^{-1}
NH_3—water	25°	22
CH_3NH_2—water	25°	6·2
$(PhCH_2)_2NCH_3$—water	30°	0·27
$3\text{-}MeC_6H_4NEt_2$—water	25°	0·66
$3\text{-}MeC_6H_4NEt_2$—MeOH	30°	0·043
$3\text{-}MeC_6H_4NEt_2$—Bu^{t}OH$_{aq}$	25°	0·000027

(solvent) or hydroxylic complexes as a function of nonpolar character of the amine and of the solvent;

$$\text{Amine.}ROH + \text{ROH}_{aq} \xrightarrow{k_H} \text{Amine.ROH} + ROH_{aq}$$

k_H shows considerable dependence on the nonpolar volume of both the amine and solvent (Table IV-9) and whether such data are interpreted on the basis of formation of "ordered water" around the nonpolar solute or of increased London dispersion interactions between the hydrogen bonding solvent and the nonpolar solute (Grunwald, *loc. cit.*), the magnitude of the effect makes it likely to be of considerable importance and potentially of relevance to an understanding of the interaction of the alkylamino function of catecholamines at the β-receptor.

The Catechol Substitution Pattern

It has been noted that the catechol function appears to be particularly important for activity at both α- and β-receptors. Elimination of one phenolic group generally leads to a large drop in activity (24–28); however, some evidence exists to suggest that this loss of activity is more

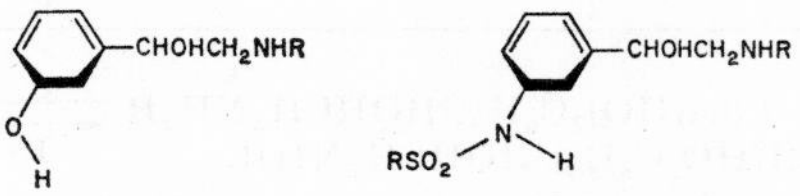

Fig. IV-6. Structural and steric analogies between sulfonamido and phenolic groups.

severe in β-receptor systems than in α-receptor systems and the catechol function may, therefore, be relatively more important for β-receptor activation (e.g., 87).

Some of the most interesting and important work on the phenolic substitution pattern has been that concerned with the incorporation of the alkyl- or arylsulfonamide substituent into the benzene ring of phenylethanolamines (88–90). The sulfonamide substituent possesses an acidic proton with a pK_a similar (0·5–1·0 pK_a units higher) to that of phenols and should also provide a close geometrical approximation to the phenolic group (Fig. IV-6). In a series of 3- and 4-(2-amino-1-hydroxyethyl)methanesulfonanilides (IV-5a,b) a remarkable dichotomy of action was observed with the 3-substituted compounds showing

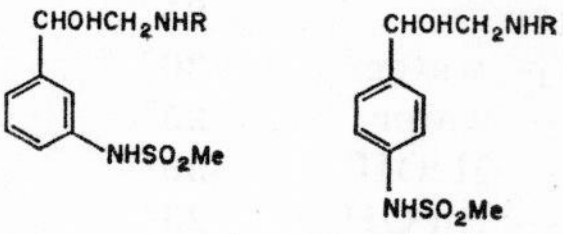

IV - 5a　　　　IV - 5b

TABLE IV-10. Adrenergic Activities of m-Alkyl(or Aryl)sulfonamidophenylethanolamines (89)

3-$RSO_2NHC_6H_4CHOHCH_2NHR'$

No.	R	R'	Adrenergic effects			
			α-Receptor		β-Receptor	
			Stimulant ED_{50} μg/ml†	Blockade ID_{50} μg/ml‡	Stimulant ED_{50} μg/ml§	Blockade $\times$ DCI¶
1	CH_3	H	320	—	60	0·07
2	$4\text{-}CH_3C_6H_4$	H	—	190	140	0·04
3	CH_3	CH_3	2·8	—	0·4	0·1
4	C_2H_5	CH_3	68	—	0·2	0·05
5	$4\text{-}CH_3C_6H_4$	CH_3	—	195	0·7	0·09
6	CH_3	C_2H_5	1500	—	0·02	0·07
7	CH_3	$CH(CH_3)_2$	—	100	0·01	1·0
8	C_4H_9	$CH(CH_3)_2$	—	97	0·7	0·1
9	$4\text{-}CH_3C_6H_4$	$CH(CH_3)_2$	—	79	0·002	1·1
10	CH_3	$CH(CH_3)CH_2OC_6H_5$	—	2·0	0·003	0·03

† Concentration required to produce contractions of the rat seminal vesicle 50 per cent as intense as that of D-epinephrine (2·0 μg/ml).

‡ Concentration required to reduce by 50 per cent the contraction of the rat seminal vesicle induced by D-norepinephrine (4·0 μg/ml); ED_{50}, phentolamine = 0·015 μg/ml.

§ Concentration required to reduce by 50 per cent the spontaneous contractions of the rat uterus; ED_{50}, isopropylnorepinephrine = 3–8×10^{-5} μg/ml.

¶ Relative β-blocking activity, DCI = 1.

essentially stimulant activity dependent upon the N-substituent at the α- and β-receptors (Table IV-10) and the 4-substituted compounds showing essentially antagonist activity at β-receptors (Table IV-11). These studies clearly indicate the importance of an acidic function in the

TABLE IV-11. Adrenergic Activities of p-Alkyl(or Aryl)sulfonamidophenyl-ethanolamines (89)

$$4\text{-RSO}_2\text{NHC}_6\text{H}_4\text{CHOHCH}_2\text{NHR}'$$

| | | | β-Receptor activity | |
No.	R	R'	Stimulation ED_{50} $\mu g/ml$[†]	Blockade $\times DCI$[‡]
1	CH_3	H	>350	0·2
2	$4\text{-}CH_3C_6H_4$	H	360	0·03
3	CH_3	CH_3	>1800	0·2
4	$4\text{-}CH_3C_6H_4$	CH_3	1·2	0·06
5	CH_3	$CH(CH_3)_2$	>900	6·0
6	$4\text{-}CH_3C_6H_4$	$CH(CH_3)_2$	>90	0·2
7	CH_3	$CH(CH_3)CH_2OC_6H_5$	195	4·0
8	CH_3	$C(CH_3)_3$	>1600	24·2

† Concentration required to reduce by 50 per cent the spontaneous contractions of the rat uterus. ED_{50}, isopropylnorepinephrine = $3\text{--}8 \times 10^{-5}$ $\mu g/ml$.

‡ Relative β-blocking activity, DCI = 1.

3-position of phenylethanolamines for stimulant activity although it is most important to note that the β-stimulants listed in Table IV-10 are very significantly less active than N-isopropylnorepinephrine. Similarly in a series of 4- or 5-(2-amino-1-hydroxyethyl)-2-hydroxyalkanesulfon-anilides (IV-6a,b), stimulant activity is again confined to those agents

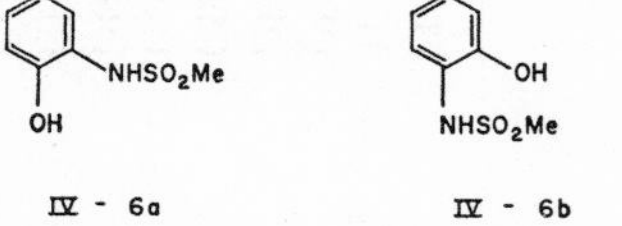

IV - 6a   IV - 6b

containing the sulfonamide substituent *meta* to the ethanolamine side chain (Table IV-12); with the *para*-substituted compounds (Nos. 11–15, Table IV-12) being essentially devoid of measured adrenergic activities. In an interpretation (90) of these findings it is suggested that binding of the more acidic benzene substituent—the alkanesulfonamide group—is determinant for the phenylethanolamine binding pattern. Thus, in the *meta*-sulfonamido series (IV-5a, IV-6a) it is assumed that this substituent

TABLE IV-12. Adrenergic Effects of Alkanesulfonamidohydroxyphenylethanolamines (90)

Structure: 4- and 3-substituted benzene ring with $CHOHCH_2NHR$

| No. | 4 | 3 | R | Relative adrenergic activity† | | | | |
| | | | | α-Receptors | | β-Receptors | | |
				Stimulant (rat seminal vesicle)	Blockade	Stimulant (rat uterus)	Stimulant (guinea-pig trachea)	Ratio T/U‡
1	HO	CH_3SO_2NH	H	7.8	—	0.003	0.005	1.7
2	HO	$C_4H_9SO_2NH$	H	0.7	—	0.0003	0.002	6.7
3	HO	CH_3SO_2NH	CH_3	12.0	—	0.001	0.03	30.0
4	HO	$C_4H_9SO_2NH$	CH_3	0.7	—	0.0001	0.003	0.8
5	HO	CH_3SO_2NH	$(CH_3)_2CH$	0.01	—	1.2	1.0	0.06
6	HO	CH_3SO_2NH	$(CH_3)_3C$	—	0.0001	0.2	1.4	7.0
7	HO	CH_3SO_2NH	$C_6H_5CH_2CH_2$	—	0.003	0.5	0.3	0.6
8	HO	CH_3SO_2NH	$3,4(CH_3O)_2C_6H_3CH_2CH_2$	—	<0.0001	0.06	0.1	1.7
9	HO	CH_3SO_2NH	$3,4(CH_3O)_2C_6H_3CH_2CH_2CH(CH_3)$	—	0.006	0.4	0.8	2.0
10	HO	CH_3SO_2NH	$3,4(CH_2O_2)C_6H_3CH_2CH_2CH(CH_3)$	—	0.04	4.0	4.0	1.0
11	CH_3SO_2NH	HO	H	inactive	—	0.00001	inactive	—
12	CH_3SO_2NH	HO	CH_3	inactive	—	inactive	inactive	—
13	CH_3SO_2NH	HO	$(CH_3)_2CH$	inactive	—	inactive	inactive	—
14	CH_3SO_2NH	HO	$C_6H_5CH_2CH_2$	inactive	—	inactive	inactive	—
15	CH_3SO_2NH	HO	$4-CH_3OC_6H_4CH_2CH_2$	inactive	—	inactive	inactive	—
			Norepinephrine	1.0	—	0.001	0.02	20.0
			Epinephrine	3.3	—	0.2	0.15	0.8
			Isopropylnorepinephrine	—	—	1.0	1.0	1.0
			Phentolamine	—	1.0	—	—	—

† Calculated as bases (Molar).
‡ Ratio of activities on trachea and uterus.

interacts with a receptor function normally responsible for binding the *m*-phenolic group of catecholamines, so ensuring "productive" inter-action of the ethanolamine side-chain with the receptor (Fig. IV-7a). In

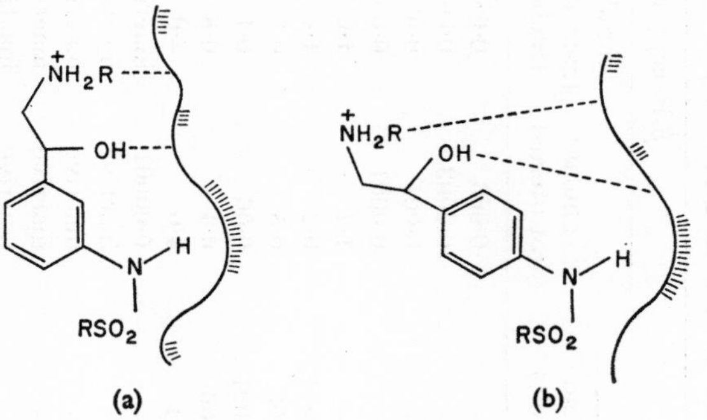

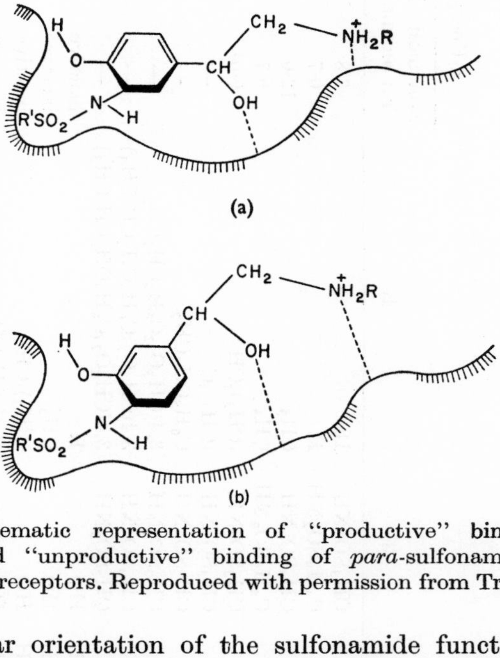

Fig. IV-7a,b. Schematic representation of "productive" binding of *meta*-sulfonamido- and "unproductive" binding of *para*-sulfonamido-agonists at adrenergic receptors. Reproduced with permission from Triggle (28).

contrast, similar orientation of the sulfonamide function of the *p*-substituted compounds (IV-5b, IV-6b) causes a "non-productive" positioning (Fig. IV-7b) of the ethanolamine side chain. Presumably, similar interpretations might be offered for the *meta*- and *para*-hydroxy-phenylethanolamines (90). However, it is clear from the very significantly lower activity of the 3-monosubstituted phenylethanolamines (Table

IV-10) relative to their 3,4-disubstituted catecholamine analogs (Table IV-12) that this proposed interaction of the 3-substituent can only be part of the interaction mechanism of the catechol nucleus. Evidence that the *meta*-sulfonamidophenylethanolamines interact at the adrenergic receptors in a manner essentially analogous to the corresponding catecholamines is provided by a comparison of the data of Tables IV-6, IV-7, IV-10, IV-11 and IV-12 which reveal that the effects of N-substitution on relative α- and β-stimulant activities are broadly similar in all three series.

The speculations offered by Larsen and co-workers (90) concerning the binding modes of catecholamine analogs are supported indirectly by several contemporary studies on ligand–enzyme interactions, including chymotrypsin (91), dihydrofolate reductase (92) amongst others and ligand–receptor interactions, including analgetic (93) and cholino-mimetic (94) agents, that indicate very strongly that a particular substituent group, polar or nonpolar, may play a determinant role in orienting the ligand at the macromolecular surface. Additionally, according to the hypothesis outlined above the sulfonamido function is able to distinguish quite selectively between those groups on the receptors that bind the *meta*- and *para*-phenolic functions of catecholamines. It is, therefore, of very considerable interest that Kappe and Armstrong (95) determined enhanced acidity (~0.5 pK$_a$ units) and reduced acidity (3–4 pK$_a$ units) for the first and second phenolic groups respectively of a catecholamine when compared to the monophenolic phenethanolamine. This data suggests that significant corresponding differences may exist between the receptor functions normally respon-sible for binding the phenolic groups of catecholamines and that the sulfanimido function can, because of its enhanced activity relative to a monophenol, distinguish these sites in a manner unavailable to the corresponding monophenolic phenethanolamines. As noted previously, however, *maximum* adrenergic activity is associated with the catechol-amines and their sulfonamide analogs rather than with the mono-substituted phenolic or sulfonamide analogs.

Larsen has offered (96) the ingenious and provocative speculation that a rationalization of the structural requirements for adrenergic α- and β-stimulant may be achieved with the assumption that a quinone methide is the required chemical species for receptor activation. Such species are readily derived from 4-hydroxybenzylalcohols and amines (97) and Larsen proposes that an initial stereoselective activation and elimination of the benzylic hydroxyl group of catecholamines occurs to generate an intermediate quinone methide (Fig. IV-8). This species is then presumed to partition between two routes—reaction with an external nucleophile (HB, Fig. IV-8) considered to represent the

β-agonist pathway and internal cyclization to an ethyleniminium ion followed by reaction with a nucleophile, HA, considered to represent the α-agonist pathway. The partitioning of the quinone methide intermediate between these two pathways is presumed dependent on the size of the

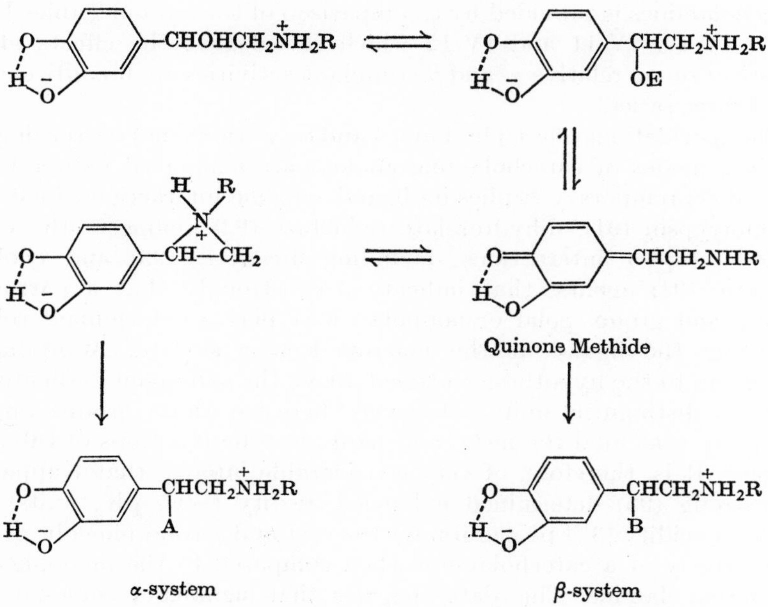

Quinone Methide

A α-system

B β-system

FIG. IV-8. Representation of various species involved in potential "chemical" interaction of catecholamines at adrenergic α- and β-receptors. After Larsen (96).

N-substituents, small substituents favoring the ethyleniminium ion pathway and hence α-agonist responses. The pathways shown in Fig. IV-8 for quinone methide formation are not available for 3-hydroxy-phenylethanolamines, a number of which, including IV-7 and IV-8 (98),

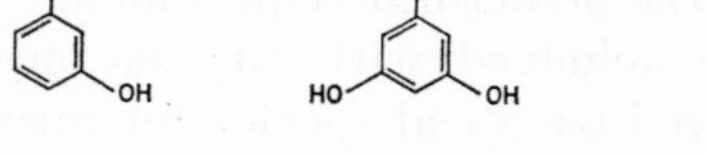

IV - 7   IV - 8

are active at α- and β-adrenergic systems respectively, although significantly less so than their catecholamine counterparts. For such systems Larsen proposes nonconjugative assisted displacement of the benzylic hydroxyl groups by the corresponding phenolate species.

Subclassification of Adrenergic Receptors

Emphasis thus far has been directed towards the concept of two classes of receptors (α and β) distinguished essentially by gross activity sequences of catecholamines and the selective actions of antagonists. However, there are an increasing number of observations (99–103) which suggest that within each of the above broad classes there may exist subclasses of receptors with species and tissue selectivity. Thus, Lands *et al.* (100) studied the activities of fifteen catecholamines on four β-receptor systems—lipolysis, cardiac acceleration, bronchodilation and vaso-depression. The activity sequences were essentially identical for

TABLE IV-13. Subclassification of β-Adrenergic Receptors According to Agonist and Antagonist Activities (101)

	Relative activities				K_B (apparent)
Tissue	ISO†	E‡	NE§	PE¶	moles/liter × 10^8
Rabbit aorta	130	65	1	0·1	3·4
Guinea-pig trachea	47	12	1	0·06	3·1 ± 0·1
Guinea-pig left atrium	3	0·5	1	<0·01	7·38 ± 0·61
Rabbit left atrium	3·5	0·5	1	—	7·45 ± 1·29
Guinea-pig duodenum	3	0·5	1	—	9·5
Rabbit duodenum	1·5	0·2	1	<0·01	49·1 ± 5·8
Rabbit stomach	2·5	1·2	1	—	56

† Isopropylnorepinephrine.
‡ Epinephrine.
§ Norepinephrine.
¶ Phenylephrine.

lipolysis–cardiac acceleration ($r = 0\cdot96$) and bronchodilation–vaso-depression ($r = 0\cdot95$) but no cross-correlations existed (i.e., cardiac acceleration–bronchodilation $r = 0\cdot31$). Furchgott (101) has determined the activities of agonists and values for the apparent dissociation constant of the antagonist 2-N-isopropylamino-1-(1-naphthyl)ethanol-(pronethalol) in a series of β-systems (Table IV-13). Both the relative activity orders of the agonists and the apparent K_B values of the antagonist suggest the existence of different β-receptor types. Similarly, it is noteworthy that 2-N-isopropylamino-1-(2,3-dimethoxyphenyl)-ethanol (IV-9, N-isopropylmethoxamine) blocks lipolysis and uterine relaxation in the rat but does not affect the β-receptors of the guinea-pig atrium (104, 105). 2-N-tert-Butylamino-1-(3-hydroxymethyl-4-hydroxy)phenylethanol (IV-10) is reported to be markedly more effective against bronchial smooth muscle than other β-receptor smooth muscle systems (106).

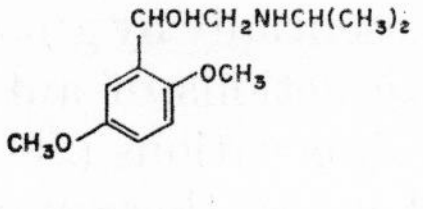

$$\text{CHOHCH}_2\text{NHCH(CH}_3)_2 \qquad \text{CHOHCH}_2\text{NHC(CH}_3)_3$$

CH₃O— ...—OCH₃   —CH₂OH / OH

IV - 9 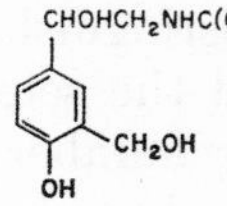   IV - 10

That receptors should vary from species to species and tissue to tissue is not surprising since the corresponding variations in enzymes and other macromolecules have been long recognized (107, 108). However, it serves to illustrate a further difficulty in the interpretation of structure–activity relationships.

AGONISTS AT THE CHOLINERGIC RECEPTORS

As was found to be the case with sympathomimetic amines a very large number of agents act as cholinomimetic agents at both the nicotinic and muscarinic receptor systems. However, unlike the sympathomimetic ligands it appears improbable that a real division into directly and indirectly acting cholinomimetic ligands exists, although some agents do release acetylcholine (109–113), a factor which may contribute to their activity. That many quaternary and tertiary ammonium salts function as cholinomimetics does not, of necessity, imply a low specificity of ligand recognition at the binding site for acetylcholine since, as will be discussed, it appears probable that there exists more than one ligand binding mode appropriate for the initiation of response.

Little point would be served by an attempt to describe all of the compounds with demonstrated activity as cholinomimetic ligands; rather, a selection will be made of those agents whose activity or molecular structure is particularly pertinent to an attempted description of the physicochemical basis of the activating or inhibitory processes at the cholinergic receptors. Several general reviews of the structure–activity relationships of cholinomimetic agents are available (12, 26, 27, 113, 116). In the following discussion various molecular modifications of the acetylcholine structure will be discussed in terms of both muscarinic and nicotinic activities.

Influence of the Ammonium Function

Quite generally the most active molecules contain the quaternary trimethylammonium structure, although some significant exceptions are known, e.g., nicotine (IV-11), arecoline (IV-12) and oxotremorine (IV-13). The role of the quaternary ammonium group has been discussed by a number of workers (114–120) and Tables IV-14–IV-18 present data for the effect of modification of quaternary group structure in several series of ligands. It has been assumed previously that the $>\overset{+}{\text{N}}\text{Me}_2$ function probably constitutes the minimal effective structure for stimulant

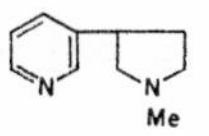

IV - 11 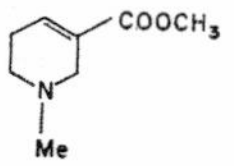   IV - 12

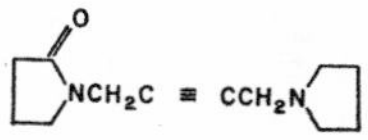

IV - 13

activity, an assumption based essentially on the data for acetylcholine where replacement of $—\overset{+}{\text{N}}\text{Me}_3$ by $—\overset{+}{\text{N}}\text{Me}_2\text{Et}$ (Table IV-14) decreases affinity slightly but does not affect intrinsic activity. Comparison of the more extensive data compiled in Table IV-18 reveals that this assumption is not generally valid and that the effects of N-methyl substitution are critically dependent upon the remaining structure of the ligand. Quite generally, the effects of incorporation of one N-ethyl group upon the

TABLE IV-14. Muscarinic and Nicotinic Activities of Ammonium Derivatives Related to Acetylcholine (114) $\text{CH}_3\text{COOCH}_2\text{CH}_2\text{R}$

	Equative molar ratios		
R	Cat bp (M)	Frog heart (M)	Frog rectus (N)
$—\overset{+}{\text{N}}\text{Me}_3$	1	1	1
$—\overset{+}{\text{N}}\text{Me}_2\text{H}$	50	40	—
$—\overset{+}{\text{N}}\text{MeH}_2$	500	1000	—
$—\overset{+}{\text{N}}\text{H}_3$	2000	20,000	—
$—\overset{+}{\text{N}}\text{Me}_2\text{Et}$	3·3	2·0	5
$—\overset{+}{\text{N}}\text{MeEt}_2$	400	2000	300
$—\overset{+}{\text{N}}\text{Et}_3$	2000	—	5000
$—\overset{+}{\text{P}}\text{Me}_3$	12	12	6
$—\overset{+}{\text{As}}\text{Me}_3$	60	80	37

TABLE IV.15. Muscarinic Activities of Quaternary Ammonium Derivatives of 1,3-Dioxolanes† (12)

No.	R	R'	$-CH_2\overset{+}{N}Me_3$			$-CH_2\overset{+}{N}Me_2Et$			$-CH_2\overset{+}{N}MeEt_2$			$-CH_2\overset{+}{N}Et_3$		
			i.a.	pD$_2$	pA$_2$	i.a.	pD$_2$	pA$_2$	i.a.	pD$_2$	pA$_2$	i.a.	pD$_2$	pA$_2$
1	H	H	1	5·3	—	1	4·9	—	0·4	3·9	—	0·1	3·5	—
2	CH_3	H	1	7·2	—	1	7·1	—	0·3	4·8	—	0	—	3·6
3	C_2H_5	H	0·9	5·3	—	0·4	5·2	—	0	—	4·6	0	—	4·2
4	C_3H_7	H	0·5	4·9	—	0	—	5·0	—	—	—	0	—	4·8
5	C_4H_9	H	0	—	4·9	—	—	—	—	—	—	—	—	—
6	C_6H_{13}	H	0	—	4·5	—	—	—	—	—	—	—	—	—
7	C_6H_5	H	0	—	4·1	0·6	4·7	4·3	—	—	—	—	—	—
8	CH_3	CH_3	1	4·3	—	0	—	4·9	0·3	4·2	—	0	—	4·2
9	C_2H_5	C_2H_5	0·5	4·6	—	0	—	6·8	—	—	—	—	—	—
10	C_3H_7	C_3H_7	0	—	6·2	0	—	7·3	0	—	6·9	0	—	6·6
11	C_4H_9	C_4H_9	0	—	6·9	—	—	—	—	—	—	—	—	—
12	C_6H_5	C_6H_5	0	—	7·1	—	—	—	—	—	—	—	—	—

† Rat jejunum preparation.

TABLE IV-16. Muscarinic Activities of Alkyltrialkylammonium salts† (12)

$$R'NR_3^+$$

R'	$-NMe_3^+$			$-NMe_2Et^+$			$-NMeEt_2^+$			$-NEt_3^+$		
	i.a.	pD_2	pA_2	i.a.	pD_2	pA_2	i.a.	pD_2	pA_2	i.a.	pD_2	pA_2
CH_3	1	3·0	—	—	—	—	—	—	—	—	—	—
C_4H_9	1	5·2	—	0·5	5·1	—	0	—	4·0	0	—	4·3
C_5H_{11}	1	5·4	—	0·4	5·2	—	0	—	4·1	0	—	4·4
C_6H_{13}	0·9	5·0	—	0	—	4·7	—	—	—	0	—	5·0
C_7H_{15}	0·1	4·6	—	0	—	5·1	—	—	—	0	—	5·5
C_8H_{17}	0	—	5·0	—	—	—	—	—	—	0	—	5·4
C_9H_{19}	0	—	5·0	—	—	—	—	—	—	0	—	5·6
$C_{10}H_{21}$	0	—	5·9	—	—	—	—	—	—	0	—	6·0
Acetylcholine	1	7·5	—	—	—	—	—	—	—	—	—	—

† Rat jejunum preparation.

TABLE IV-17. Activities of Bisquaternary Salts on Frog Rectus Abdominus Preparation (12)

Ligand	i.a.	pD_2
$Me_3\overset{+}{N}(CH_2)_{10}\overset{+}{N}Me_3$	0·7	5·4
$EtMe_2\overset{+}{N}(CH_2)_{10}\overset{+}{N}Me_2Et$	0·3	4·7
$Et_2Me\overset{+}{N}(CH_2)_{10}\overset{+}{N}MeEt_2$	0	—
$(Me_3\overset{+}{N}CH_2CH_2OOCCH_2)_2$	1	5·7
$(EtMe_2\overset{+}{N}CH_2CH_2OOCCH_2)_2$	0·9	5·0
$(Et_2Me\overset{+}{N}CH_2CH_2OOCCH_2)_2$	0	—
$(Me_3\overset{+}{N}CH_2CH_2OOCCH_2)_2CH_2$	1	6·4
$(EtMe_2\overset{+}{N}CH_2CH_2OOCCH_2)_2CH_2$	0·9	6·4
$(Et_2Me\overset{+}{N}CH_2CH_2OOCCH_2)_2CH_2$	0·4	4·3

intrinsic activity become progressively more marked as the total molecular structure becomes less polar. Thus, in acetylcholine even complete replacement of the trimethylammonium by the triethyl-ammonium group does not affect the intrinsic activity although

TABLE IV-18. Effects of *N*-Ethyl Substitution on Muscarinic Activities in Cholinergic Salts† (12)

$$R—\overset{+}{N}—R'$$

	R'							
	—Me$_3$		—Me$_2$Et		—MeEt$_2$		—Et$_3$	
R	i.a.	pD_2/pA_2	i.a.	pD_2/pA_2	i.a.	pD_2/pA_2	i.a.	pD_2/pA_2
$CH_3COOCH_2CH_2$—	1	7·0	1	6·3	1	4·2	1	4·1
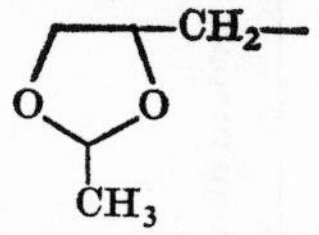 (1,3-dioxolane with —CH$_2$— and CH$_3$)	1	7·3	1	7·1	0·3	4·8	0	3·6
$CH_3CH_2OCH_2CH_2$—	1	5·8	0·8	5·3	0	4·1	0	4·0
$CH_3CH_2CH_2CH_2CH_2$—	1	5·4	0·5	5·2	0	4·1	0	4·4

† Rat jejunum preparation.

producing a large reduction in affinity; in the 2-methyl-1,3-dioxolane series only one methyl group can be substituted without reduction in intrinsic activity and in n-pentyltrimethylammonium replacement of even one methyl group leads to a reduction in intrinsic activity. These points have been explicitly emphasized by Ariëns (12). The relationship between the effects of onium group substitution and total molecular polarity of the activator structure unquestionably relates rather directly to the question of a plurality of ligand binding modes and will be re-emphasized later.

What can be said about the molecular basis of the interaction of the quaternary ammonium group with the receptor? A generally accepted assumption (119) is that an ion-pairing interaction occurs with a complementary anionic function ($-CO_2^-$, $-PO_3R_2^-$): at least two lines of evidence appear to support this assumption quite directly. The uncharged carbon isostere, 3,3-dimethylbutyl acetate (IV-14) has only 1/3000 the

$$CH_3COOCH_2CH_2C(CH_3)_3$$

IV - 14

activity of acetylcholine (119) and at least part of this extremely low activity is probably due to the ability of this agent to release acetylcholine (111). Studies of the pH dependence of the activity of such tertiary amines as oxotremorine (IV-13), arecoline (IV-12) and nicotine (IV-11) reveal (119, 121–123) that cholinomimetic activity is probably associated exclusively with the cationic species. Several attempts have been made to treat the data from experiments as described above to obtain quantitative estimates of the energy of binding of the ammonium group. Thus, Burgen (119), following an essentially identical procedure applied by Pressman et al. to hapten–antibody interactions (124, 125) and Wilson (126) and Bernhard (127) to acetylcholinesterase, determined a ΔF of -5 kcal mole^{-1} as the contribution of the ionic association to the total binding energy from a comparison of the relative activities of acetylcholine and 3,3-dimethylbutylacetate; from this figure it may be readily calculated (119, 128) that the equilibrium distance of the presumed ionic interaction is 3·3 Å which is virtually identical to that estimated from Courtauld models (119). Other estimates of the ionic contribution of binding of the quaternary nitrogen atom in systems that bear relevance to the cholinergic receptor have been obtained by comparison of acetylcholine and 3,3-dimethylbutylacetate on acetylcholinesterase (126, 127) to yield a value of $-1·2$ kcal mole^{-1}. From a study (21) of the binding of onium ions and their analogs to antibody prepared against albumin-azophenoxycholine (IV-15), comparison of choline and 3,3-dimethylbutan-1-ol and acetylcholine and 3,3-dimethylbutylacetate yielded ΔF (ionic) values of $-2·81$ and $-2·71$ kcal mole^{-1}

respectively: a second estimate was obtained from the binding of the ammonium cation, where nonpolar interactions are likely to be negligible (although hydration parameters are probably very different), of $-2 \cdot 83$ kcal mole^{-1} (129).

$$\text{Albumin} - \text{N} = \text{N} - \langle \bigcirc \rangle - \text{OCH}_2\text{CH}_2\overset{+}{\text{N}}\text{Me}_3$$

IV - 15

However, the validity of the above treatments depends essentially upon the assumption that the charged and uncharged isosteres bind to an identical site on the macromolecular system. Whilst it seems certain, in view of the negligible cholinomimetic activity of 3,3-dimethylbutyl-acetate relative to acetylcholine, that an ionic interaction is critical for activity at the cholinergic receptors, the isosterism of the trimethyl-ammonium and the tert-butyl groups cannot be used as an *a priori* argument for the assumption of equivalence of binding locus of the two groups. In fact there is an increasing amount of evidence for both the cholinergic receptor and acetylcholinesterase suggesting that this assumption is not valid. This evidence, which will be discussed in detail later (see section on p. 276), generates as its principal conclusions that acetylcholinesterase contains a binding site for positively charged ligands and a distinct, but overlapping at the esteratic function (the ammonium function is not essential here since 3,3-dimethylbutylacetate is a substrate of the enzyme), binding site for uncharged esters (Fig. IV-9a). Similarly, the cholinergic (muscarinic) receptor also contains two binding areas, one for acetylcholine and related polar ligands and another for nonpolar ammonium ligands: these areas probably overlap at an anionic site (Fig. IV-9b).†

The effects of increased size of the ammonium function upon biological activity may now be reconsidered in an attempt to interpret the apparently variable effects of N-ethyl substitution. These effects are most unlikely to be due simply to reduction in the magnitude of the ionic interaction for model measurements indicate that replacement of $-\overset{+}{\text{N}}\text{Me}_3$ by $-\overset{+}{\text{N}}\text{Et}_3$ is not likely to produce more than an $0 \cdot 8$ Å increase in the minimum interionic distance. This would correspond to an approximate energy loss of 2 kcal mole^{-1} and a fiftyfold reduction in affinity; with acetylcholine (Table IV-18) this substitution produces approximately a thousandfold loss in affinity. Thus factors other than simple ionic interactions are playing an equally important role and

---

† Such a method of organization, that of surrounding or enveloping a binding site for recognition of polar molecules by a nonpolar area, would appear to offer certain advantages in ensuring specificity of the ligand recognition process with regard both to ligand selection and correct orientation of the ligand in the polar binding site.

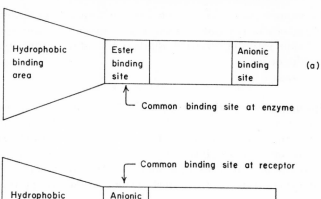

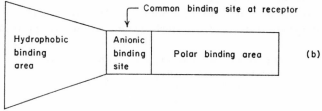

FIG. IV-9. Schematic comparison of dual binding modes at (a) acetylcholinesterase and (b) the cholinergic receptors. Both surfaces distinguish polar and nonpolar side chains orienting around a common binding site.

consideration must be given to a more detailed examination of the role of the ion-pairing mechanism.

The electrostatic ion-pairing mechanism is dependent upon ionic size and change, interionic distance and the dielectric constant (Chapter I,

TABLE IV-19. Dissociation Constants of Tetraalkylammonium Salts in Ethylene Chloride (130–132)

Salt	$K \times 10^4$		$K \times 10^4$
$\overset{+}{Me_4N}$, Pi	0·32	NO_3	—
$\overset{+}{Et_4N}$, Pi	1·59	NO_3	0·74
$\overset{+}{Pr_4N}$, Pi	1·94	NO_3	0·95
$\overset{+}{Bu_4N}$, Pi	2·26	NO_3	1·19
$\overset{+}{Am_4N}$, Pi	2·38	NO_3	1·29
$\overset{+}{Et_4N}$, Cl	0·510		
$\overset{+}{Et_4N}$, Br	0·69		
$\overset{+}{Et_4N}$, BF_4	1·05		

p. 2) and becomes progressively weaker with increasing ionic size and increasing dielectric constant. Thus for a given anionic species, the strength of the interaction with quaternary ammonium ions should decrease in the order

$$\overset{+}{R}NMe_3 > \overset{+}{R}NEt_3 > \overset{+}{R}NPr_3 > \overset{+}{R}NBu_3, \text{ etc.}$$

The comprehensive studies of Kraus, Fuoss and their co-workers (130–132) on the conductances of ammonium salts in various solvent systems lend ample confirmation. The data of Table IV-19 reveal the anticipated order of dissociation constants for a series of ammonium picrates and nitrates in ethylene chloride: the magnitude of the dissociation constant for the tetramethylammonium salt is anomalously

TABLE IV-20. Dependence of Dissociation Constant of Tetramethylammonium Picrate on Dielectric Constant (130–132)

Solvent	$K \times 10^4$	D
Nitrobenzene	400	34·8
Acetone	112	20·7
Pyridine	6·7	12·3
Ethylene Chloride	0·32	4·6

low suggesting that it is exhibiting specific ion–dipole interactions with the solvent. The dependence of dissociation constant upon anion size is also shown in Table IV-19 and the dependence upon dielectric constant is shown in Table IV-20 for tetramethylammonium picrate and in Table IV-21 for tetraisoamylammonium picrate. Thus for electrostatic ion-pairing the anticipated order of affinity listed previously is basically

TABLE IV-21. Dependence of Dissociation Constant of Tetraisoamylammonium Picrate on Dielectric Constant in Dioxane–Water Mixtures (130–132)

% H_2O	D	K
0·60	2·38	2×10^{-16}
2·35	2·90	1×10^{-12}
6·37	4·42	3×10^{-8}
14·95	8·5	1×10^{-4}
53·0	38·0	0·25

that observed for the stimulatory effects of cholinergic ligands. However, the large differences between the trimethylammonium and the differential effects of N-ethyl substitution according to the parent ligand structure (Table IV-18) remain to be accommodated. The apparently optimum fit of the trimethylammonium group is probably generated through specific Van der Waals binding of the N-methyl groups (Fig. IV-10), thus providing an anhydrous low dielectric microenvironment in which the ionic interaction will be greatly strengthened (cf., data of Table IV-21). Such specific nonpolar binding provided by the methyl groups is probably very important in supplying the driving force for desorption of highly polar ligands such as acetylcholine from an aqueous

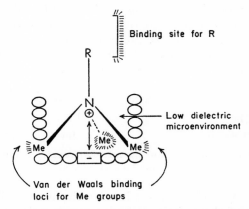

Fig. IV-10. Schematic representation of the binding of the trimethylammonium function of cholinergic activators.

environment onto an essentially polar surface. Progressive N-ethyl substitution into acetylcholine will, if the assumption of specific Van der Waals binding sites for the N-methyl groups is correct, produce an increase in the interionic distance and, more importantly, permit the intrusion of water into the ionic binding locus thus raising the dielectric of the microenvironment and causing a greater reduction in binding energy than predicted solely on the basis of the increase in interionic distance. Additionally, a dislocation of the binding of the remaining molecular structure, $CH_3COOCH_2CH_2-$, presumably also involved in rather specific binding, may also occur; this factor will also contribute to the affinity loss. Considering now the effects of similar substitution in the other ligand series listed in Table IV-18, we note the effects of N-ethyl substitution on the cholinomimetic activity become, quite generally, increasingly severe with increasing nonpolar character of the total ligand structure. That is, for the maintenance of full activity (i.a. = 1) the order of "tolerance" of N-ethyl substitution is, acetoxyethyl $>$ 1,3-dioxol-anyl $>$ ethoxyethyl $>$ pentyl (Table IV-18). Most probably this finding relates to the original suggestion by Frank (133, 134) that the tetra-alkylammonium ions should become hydrophobic structure makers as the size of the alkyl substituents increases. There is very considerable experimental evidence available derived from heat capacity (134, 135), viscosity (133, 136), partial molal volume (137–142), heats of dilution and mixing (143–145), conductance (146) and other measurements (147, 148) that the ability of these ions to modify water structure lies in the order

$$Bu_4^+N > Pr_4^+N > Et_4^+N > Me_4^+N$$

There are good indications (135, 136, 146) that a transition in properties between structure-breaking and structure-making occurs between the tetramethylammonium and tetraethylammonium ions: the smaller tetramethylammonium ion behaving like the larger alkali metal cations and anions to break down the structure of local water whilst in the

$$\text{Ionic complexes} \xrightleftharpoons{K_I} R_4^+N \xrightleftharpoons{K_N} \text{Nonpolar complexes}$$

R = Me	R > Me
Activity (agonism)	Inactivity (antagonism)

FIG. IV-11. Quaternary ammonium ligand (cholinergic) partitioning into ionic and nonpolar complexes.

larger, less polar, tetraethylammonium ion the net ordering effect on the water structure of the additional hydrocarbon residues is sufficient to overcome the structure-breaking effect.

Similarly, in a series of quaternary ammonium ions, RN^+Me_3, the transition from an ionic to a hydrophobic binding species with increasing N-ethyl substitution will be attained progressively earlier with increasing nonpolar character of the R group and thus lead to a progressively earlier reorientation of the ligand binding mode (Table IV-18). The ligand binding process may thus be represented (Fig. IV-11) as a partitioning between primarily polar complexes (active) and primarily nonpolar complexes (inactive): at a critical ratio of nonpolar:polar function partitioning of the ligand into the nonpolar complex will become significant and stimulant activity progressively weaker. A basically similar proposal has also been advanced by Smith and Williams (149) for the ligand series, RN^+Me_3. The concept of inhibitors partitioning into a hydrophobic phase has been advanced very explicitly by Canady and co-workers (Chapter I, p. 58) in their study of nonpolar inhibitors of chymotrypsin.

Finally, in this consideration of the role of the ammonium function in cholinergic activity it is most significant that with the reduction in stimulant activity produced by N-ethyl substitution appears increasing competitive *inhibitory* activity (Tables IV-15, 16 and 18). According to the above treatment, therefore, the inhibitory activity of cholinergic ligands is to be associated with the preferential formation of nonpolar complexes. Subsequent discussion will corroborate this conclusion which carries with it the implicit assumption of discrete binding loci for cholinergic stimulant and inhibitory ligands.

Influence of the Side Chain in $R\overset{+}{N}Me_3$

Acyclic Analogs. From the preceding discussion it appears, at least to a first approximation, that the requirements for the onium function are basically similar in the cholinergic receptors of skeletal muscle, smooth and cardiac muscle and ganglia.

However, when further molecular variations of cholinomimetic ligand structure are explored it is quite apparent that the structural requirements for activity in these receptor systems may diverge rather sharply. The data in Table IV-22 are for a collection of choline esters and it is apparent that the structure activity relationship is strictest at the muscarinic receptor since almost any deviation in structure from that of acetylcholine results in a reduction of activity. Quantitative data for muscarinic activities of choline esters are also presented in Table IV-23 and substantiate this point. In contrast the same molecular substitutions result in maintained or slightly increased activity in the ganglion or skeletal muscle systems. However, because these data are gathered from different sources and were obtained under differing experimental conditions, no particular significance can be necessarily attributed to *small* variations in activity. However, it is particularly interesting to compare the data for the substituted benzoyl and imidazolyl esters: in the rectus preparation, these agents have very low activity but in ganglionic preparations they are of the same order of potency as acetylcholine. However, activity of the imidazolyl ester in the ganglionic preparation can be dramatically increased by the incorporation of one or two methylene groups (Nos. 8, 9, Table IV-22). It may well be that both receptor systems have similar tolerance for large aromatic groups but exhibited at different loci relative to the onium binding site. In the benzoylcholine esters, the effects of substituents on ganglion-stimulant activity are not large but they show dependence on the Hammett substituent constant (Fig. IV-12) indicating that activity decreases with increasing electron-withdrawing capacity of the substituent.

A large number of choline ethers, aliphatic and aromatic, have also been studied (reviewed in refs 27, 115, 116, 158, 160). As ganglion stimulants the ethyl, propyl and butyl ethers are approximately equipotent with acetylcholine (151) but in muscarinic preparations (guinea-pig ileum, rat jejunum) they are less active than acetylcholine,

TABLE IV-22. Activities of Choline Esters as Cholinomimetic Agents
$$RCOOCH_2CH_2\overset{+}{N}Me_3$$

		Equiactive molar ratios (ACh = 1)					
No.	R	Frog rectus	Ref.	Ganglia†	Ref.	Rabbit intestine	Ref.
1	H	700	150	—	—	~500	150
2	CH_3	1·0	150	1	151, 156	1	150
3	CH_3CH_2	0·6	150	0·65	151, 156	33	150
4	$CH_3(CH_2)_2$	1·0	150	0·47	151, 156	400	150
5	$CH_3(CH_2)_3$	0·95	151	—	—	500	150
6	$(CH_3)_3C$	5·0	151	0·10	151, 156	inactive	152
7	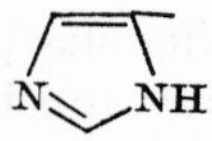	1000	154	1·2	154	negligible	154
8	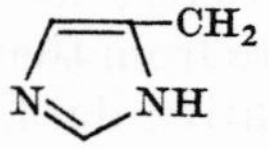	25	154	2·0	154	negligible	154
9	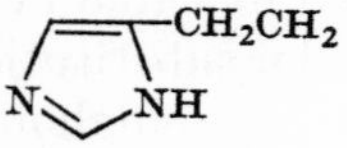	1·4	154	0·12	154	negligible	154
10	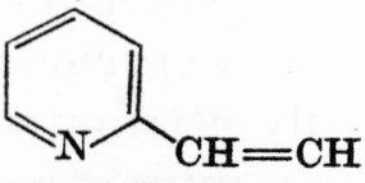	1·2	154	0·17	154	—	—
11	C_6H_5	100	155	0·88	151, 156	~1000	157
12	$3\text{-}O_2NC_6H_4$	300	155	10·0	155	inactive	153
13	$3\text{-}ClC_6H_4$	400	155	3·3	155	—	—
14	$4\text{-}ClC_6H_4$	430	155	2·2	155	—	—
15	$4\text{-}FC_6H_4$	200	155	1·7	155	—	—
16	$4\text{-}MeC_6H_4$	480	155	2·5	155	—	—
17	$4\text{-}MeOC_6H_4$	430	155	0·46	155	—	—
18	$4\text{-}MeC_6H_4$	—	—	1·7	155	—	—

† Data taken from the compilation by Barlow (158).

maximum activity being attained with the ethyl ether which is some ten times less active than acetylcholine (27, 115, 158, 161). Aromatic ethers of choline are essentially devoid of activity in muscarinic systems, but show marked activity as nicotinic stimulants. Hey (156) has studied a number of substituted phenylcholine ethers (Table IV-24) and from his

TABLE IV-23. Muscarinic Activities of
Choline Esters (159)

$$\overset{+}{RCOOCH_2CH_2NMe_3}$$

R	i.a.†	pD_2	pA_2
H	1	5·2	—
CH_3	1	7·6	—
CH_3CH_2	0·9	5·0	—
$(CH_3)_2CH$	0·4	4·1	—
$CH_3CH_2CH_2$	0·3	3·8	—
$CH_3(CH_2)_4$	0	—	4·0
$CH_3(CH_2)_{10}$	0	—	5·2

† Rat jejunum preparation.

data it is quite apparent that nicotinic activity increases with increasing electron withdrawing capacity of the substituent. It is thus quite interesting to note that the substituent effects in benzoylcholine esters and phenylcholine ethers are completely opposed. From the point of view of attempted quantitative correlations between biological activity and

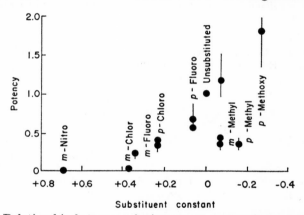

FIG. IV-12. Relationship between substituent constant and nicotinic activity in substituted benzoylcholines. Reproduced with permission from Ormerod (155).

substituent effects the phenylcholine ethers are of particular interest since they represent one of the few systems (162) in which an excellent correlation has been obtained. Fukui (163) has calculated the super-delocalizability, a measure of the ability of an atom to form a weak π bond, at the *ortho* positions of the aromatic ring (Table IV-25) and the fractional positive charge on the ether oxygen. The excellent correlation with superdelocalizability (S_o),

$$\log 1/C = 13·7\,S_o - 10·5, \qquad r = 0·994$$

TABLE IV-24. Ganglion Stimulant Activities of Substituted Phenyl-choline Ethers (156)†

$$R-\text{C}_6\text{H}_3-O(CH_2)_2\overset{+}{N}Me_3$$

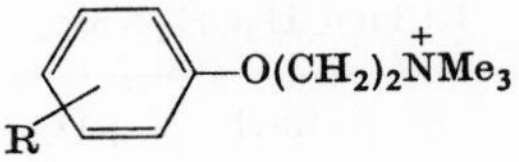

R	Equiactive molar ratio (ACh = 1) (to produce a standard rise in blood pressure)	
	Adrenal glands intact	Adrenal glands ligated
3,5-Br$_2$	0·0065	0·0045
3-Br	0·0060	0·0046
3-Cl	0·010	0·0062
H (unsubstituted)	0·022	0·012
3-Me	0·17	0·089
4-Cl	0·21	0·12
3,5-Me$_2$	0·42	0·23
4-Me	5·5	2·6

† Tying the adrenal gland alters the activity ratio relative to acetylcholine but does not significantly alter the relative sequence of activities within the ligand series.

TABLE IV-25. Nicotinic Activity, Superdelocalizability and Electronic Charge in Substituted Phenylcholine Ethers (156, 163)

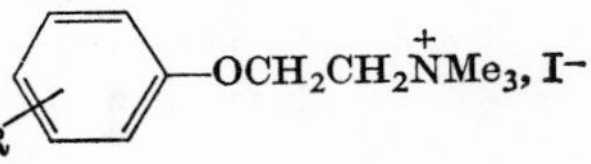

$$R-\text{C}_6\text{H}_3-OCH_2CH_2\overset{+}{N}Me_3, \text{I}^-$$

R	S_0	Positive charge on oxygen	Equiactive molar ratio† Adrenals	
			Intact	Ligated
3,5-(Br)$_2$	0·952	0·179	337	268
3-Br	0·938	0·179	370	258
3-Cl	0·931	0·180	220	192
H	0·911	0·180	100	100
3-Me	0·847	0·179	13·1	13·5
4-Cl	0·911	0·186	10·4	10·1
3,5-(Me)$_2$	0·811	0·179	5·2	5·2
4-Me	0·915	0·165	0·4	0·47

† To produce a standard bp rise (60 mm). The biological data are the same as in Table IV-24 but expressed relative to phenyl-choline ether (100).

suggests that the aromatic ring may be binding through a charge transfer mechanism (see also ref. 164).

Other modifications of acetylcholine which also reveal marked differences between the various cholinergic binding sites include the thiocholine esters. Acetylthiocholine is some five times more active as a ganglion stimulant (165), some 20–30 times less active on the rectus preparation (165) and some 300 times less active as a muscarinic agent (166). Ing, Kordik and Tudor Williams (161) have studied a series of ketones related to acetylcholine (Table IV-26): from their results it is interesting to note that these compounds are, quite generally, very significantly more active in the rectus preparation than in the ganglionic and muscarinic preparations.

TABLE IV-26. Cholinomimetic Activities of Carbonyl Analogs of Acetylcholine (161)

Ligand	Equiactive molar ratios (ACh = 1)		
	Cat bp	G.P. ileum	Frog rectus
$CH_3COCH_2CH_2CH_2\overset{+}{N}Me_3$, I^-	pressor only	80	1·1
$CH_3CH_2COCH_2CH_2\overset{+}{N}Me_3$, I^-	pressor only	670	1·3
$CH_3CH_2CH_2COCH_2\overset{+}{N}Me_3$, I^-	84, pressor after atropine	330	153
$CH_3CH_2COCH(CH_3)CH_2\overset{+}{N}Me_3$, I^-	4500, depressor after atropine	584	700
$CH_3COCH_2CH_2\overset{+}{N}Me_3$, I^-	150, pressor after atropine	167	0·7

Finally in this brief survey of acyclic trimethylammonium ligands fall the functionally simplest compounds, the alkyltrimethylammonium compounds. Their activities in a large number of cholinergic preparations have been discussed by many workers and Table IV-27 lists a representative selection of these data, although it must again be emphasized that there is a very large spread in the reported activities of these compounds. However, from this data arise two principal points of interest: activity is maximal in all three receptor systems with n-pentyltrimethylammonium and, relative to acetylcholine, there are significant differences between the activities of the members of this series in the three systems. Thus, for muscarinic receptors n-pentyltrimethylammonium is some 100 times less potent, for the receptors in the rectus some 25 times less

10

potent and for the ganglionic receptors some 6 times more potent than acetylcholine. Furthermore, in the ganglionic preparation there is comparatively little difference in the activities with variation of alkyl chain length. If these differences actually relate directly to the ligand–

TABLE IV-27. Cholinergic Activities of Alkyltrimethylammonium Ligands (151, 167–169)

$$\overset{+}{R}NMe_3$$

| R | Rat jejunum | | | Frog rectus | Dog blood pressure |
	i.a.	pD_2	pA_2	i.a.	Equiactive molar ratio
Me	1	3·0	—	1	13 000	0·5
C_2H_5	—	—	—	1	>400	2
C_3H_7	—	—	—	1	400	10
C_4H_9	1	5·2	—	1	200	0·5
C_5H_{11}	1	5·4	—	1	25	0·15
C_6H_{13}	0·9	5·0	—	0·9	35	0·2
C_7H_{15}	0·1	4·6	—	0·75	100	0·5
C_8H_{17}	0	—	5·0	0·2	>250	—
C_9H_{19}	0	—	5·0	0·1	≫250	—
Acetylcholine	1	7·5	—	1	1	1

receptor interaction then they suggest that there exists a nonpolar site of similar dimensions at the cholinergic receptors in the rat jejunum and frog rectus which is, however, of somewhat greater polarity in the muscarinic receptors. At ganglionic receptors the alkyl chain appears to make relatively little contribution to binding and it may be that interaction of the tetramethylammonium ion alone is involved.

Cyclic Analogs. There are a number of agents known which may be regarded as cyclic analogs of acetylcholine. Muscarine, the parasym

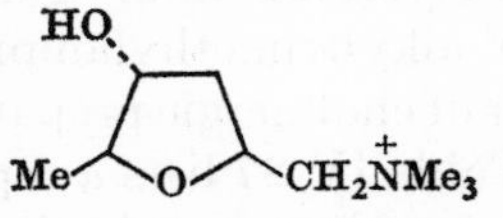

(a) Muscarine (2S, 3R, 5S)

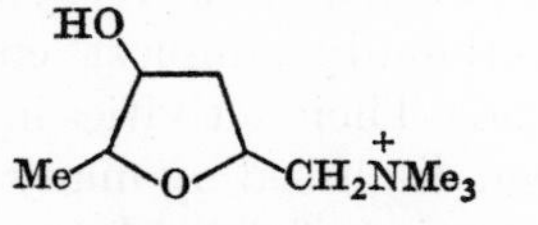

(b) *epi* Muscarine (2S, 3S, 5S)

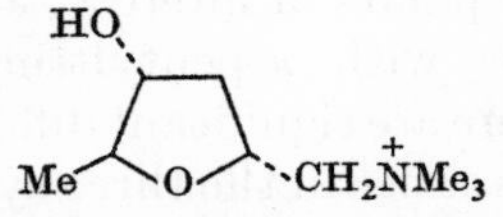

(c) *allo* Muscarine (2S, 3R, 5R)

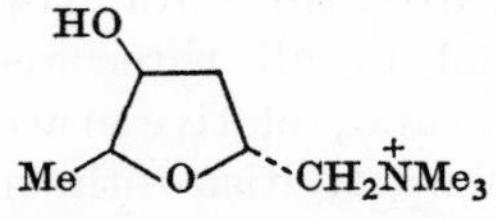

(d) *epiallo* Muscarine (2S, 3S, 5R)

IV-16

TABLE IV-28. Cholinomimetic Activities of Muscarine and Related Compounds (172, 173)

Compound	Equiactive molar ratio (ACh = 1)			
	Cat bp	Frog heart	Rabbit ileum	Frog rectus
DL-Muscarine	0·75	10	1·0	>50
L(+)-Muscarine	0·32	5	0·33	>50
D(−)-Muscarine	350	—	130	>50
DL-*epi*-Muscarine	230	≥1000	230	>200
DL-*allo*-Muscarine	130	>1000	150	>200
DL-*epiallo*-Muscarine	75	>1000	220	>100
DL-2-Desmethylmuscarine	80	>1000	—	—
DL-2-Desmethyl-*epi*-muscarine	550	≥1000	—	—
DL-2-Methylmuscarine	650	>1000	—	—
DL-4,5-Dehydromuscarine	0·76	61	—	—
DL-4,5-Dehydro-*epi*-muscarine	1·5	120	—	—

pathomimetic effects of which have been known since 1869 (170), although its structure was not elucidated until 1957 (171, 172), is representative of this class of agents. There are four pairs of enantiomers (IV-16) of which the most active and the naturally occurring compound is L(+)-muscarine (IV-16a). From the comparative data presented in Tables IV-28 and IV-29 it is evident that the activity of muscarine is highly stereospecific and actually resides almost exclusively in one isomer: the other enantiomeric pairs of isomers are only feebly active muscarinic agents. While L(+)-muscarine is not the most active muscarinic agent known† it is probably one of the most specific, being

TABLE IV-29. Affinities and Intrinsic Activities of Muscarine Isomers (174)

Compound	Rat jejunum		Frog heart		
	i.a.	pD_2	i.a.	pD_2	pA_2
DL-Muscarine	1	6·8	1	6·4	—
DL-*epiallo*-Muscarine	1	5·0	1	4·5	—
DL-*allo*-Muscarine	1	4·4	0·4	—	3·7
DL-*epi*-Muscarine	1	3·9	0·1	—	3·8
Acetylcholine	1	7·1	1	7·2	—

† It seems pertinent here to emphasize again that the comparative activities of ligands often differ quite dramatically from one tissue system to another even though, qualitatively, the receptor systems are identifiable as one class. Various factors may be involved in this, but it seems quite probable that differences in the molecular architecture of the receptor may constitute a significant contribution.

essentially devoid of nicotinic activity. From Table IV-28 it is apparent
that the 2-methyl group of muscarine plays a critical role in the control
of biological activity for its removal, as in desmethylmuscarine (IV-17)

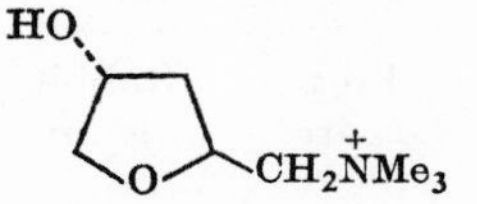

IV-17

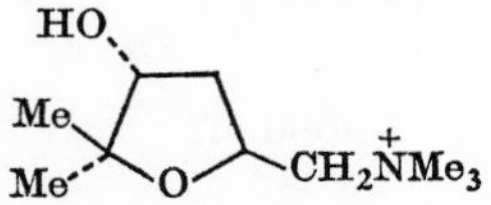

IV-18

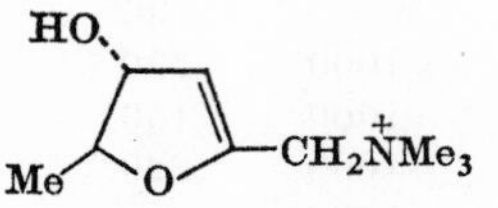

IV-19

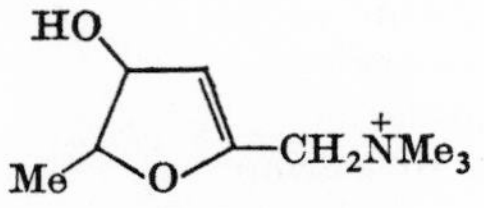

IV-20

leads to a very significant decrease in activity and the addition of a
second 2-methyl group (IV-18) leads to an even larger reduction in
activity. Similar findings are also available for the structurally related
1,3-dioxolanes that will be discussed later. In view of the large differences
in activity between (±)-muscarine and (±)-*epi*-muscarine it is noteworthy
that (±)-4,5-dehydromuscarine (IV-19) and (±)-4,5-dehydro-*epi*-mus-
carine (IV-20) are approximately equipotent to (±)-muscarine. These
findings find their counterpart in observations with the muscarones
(Table IV-30). In contrast to the high chirality exhibited by the cholinergic receptor towards the muscarine isomers the interaction between the
receptor and muscarone and related compounds is relatively nonspecific.
Thus there exist only small differences between (±)-muscarone and
(±)-*allo*-muscarone and in the ganglionic and rectus preparations
allo-muscarone appears to be more potent: the introduction of trigonal
centers, as in the dehydro-muscarines and muscarones, produces
reduction in configurational specificity. Examination of molecular

TABLE IV-30. Cholinomimetic Activities of Muscarone and Related Compounds
(172, 173, 175)

		Equiactive molar ratio (ACh = 1)			
Compound	Cat bp	Blockade of cat superior cervical ganglion	Frog heart	Rabbit ileum	Frog rectus
DL-Muscarone	0·12	0·1	4	0·13	0·5
D(−)-Muscarone	0·10	0·05	2·5	0·06	0·5
L(+)-Muscarone	0·25	—	—	0·15	2·0
DL-*allo*-Muscarone	0·25	0·075	6·1	0·28	0·2

models reveals that dehydromuscarine, dehydro-*epi*-muscarine and muscarine cannot present all potential binding groups (presumed to be the $> \overset{+}{N} <$, —OH $\searrow O \nearrow$ and —CH$_3$ functions) to an identical surface and it must, therefore, be assumed that at least some shift in the binding orientation has occurred, produced by introduction of the polarizable double bond, so that one group, probably the 3-hydroxyl group, is no longer involved in the interaction. For the muscarones there is more conclusive evidence for a change in orientation of binding for the data of Table IV-30 reveal not only a reduction in the stereospecificity of action but also an inversion so that D(—)-muscarone is the more potent isomer. Finally, it is of particular interest to note that with the transition from muscarine to muscarone appears significant nicotinic activity (Table IV-30).

A number of other cyclic analogs are known that bear considerable structural resemblance to acetylcholine and muscarine. Thus, 2-dimethylaminomethylfuran methiodide (IV-21) has quite high muscarinic

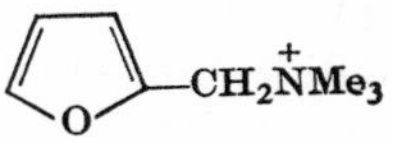

IV-21

activity (176, 177) which is substantially increased by the presence of a 5-methyl group (Table IV-31). The corresponding tetrahydrofurans are less potent by an approximately tenfold factor (Table IV-31) but it is

TABLE IV-31. Cholinomimetic Activities of Furan and Tetrahydrofuran Derivatives (176, 178)

	Equiactive molar ratio (ACh = 1)			
Compound	Cat bp	G.P. ileum	Frog heart	Frog rectus
2-Dimethylaminomethyl-furan methiodide	10–30	12	126	505
2-Methyl-5-dimethylamino-methylfuran methiodide	1–3	0·34	15	⩾1000
2-Ethyl-5-dimethylamino-methylfuran methiodide	120	35	>1000	>1000
2-Dimethylaminomethyl-tetrahydrofuran methiodide	100–300	—	—	—
2-Methyl-5-dimethylamino-methyltetrahydrofuran methiodide†	—	20	—	—

† Probably the *cis*-isomer.

TABLE IV-32. Cholinomimetic Activities of 1,3-Dioxolanes (176, 179)

Compound	Equiactive molar ratio (ACh = 1)		
	Cat bp	G.P. ileum	Frog rectus
4-Dimethylaminomethyl-1,3-dioxolane methiodide (F-2249)	60	17	21
2-Methyl-4-dimethylaminomethyl-1,3-dioxolane methiodide (F-2268)†	1·6	0·43	33
2,3-Dimethyl-4-dimethylaminomethyl-1,3-dioxolane methiodide (F-2269)	—	100	—

† cis, trans (60:40) mixture.

pertinent that the introduction of the 5-methyl group into both furan and tetrahydrofuran produces the same relative increase in activity. A further series of rather closely related compounds is the 1,3-dioxolanes (Tables IV-15, IV-32 and IV-33) where 2-methyl-4-dimethylamino-methyl-1,3-dioxolane methiodide has long been recognized as an extremely active muscarinic agent (179–182). Triggle and Belleau (183) established the relative configuration about the C_2 and C_4 centers

TABLE IV-33. Cholinomimetic Activities of 1,3-Dioxolanes and Related Compounds (183–185)

Compound	Equiactive molar ratio (ACh = 1) G.P. ileum
2-Dimethylaminomethylfuran methiodide	10
2-Methyl-5-dimethylaminomethylfuran methiodide	0·9
L-4-Dimethylaminomethyl-1,3-dioxolane methiodide	14
D-4-Dimethylaminomethyl-1,3-dioxolane methiodide	200
L-cis-2-Methyl-4-dimethylaminomethyl-1,3-dioxolane methiodide	0·2
D-cis-2-Methyl-4-dimethylaminomethyl-1,3-dioxolane methiodide	12
L-trans-2-Methyl-4-dimethylaminomethyl-1,3-dioxolane methiodide	2
D-trans-2-Methyl-4-dimethylaminomethyl-1,3-dioxolane methiodide	4
L-β-Methylacetylcholine methiodide	1
D-β-Methylacetylcholine methiodide	~1000

showing that cis-2-methyl-4-dimethylaminomethyl-1,3-dioxolane methiodide (IV-22) is some 5–10 times more potent than the $trans$-isomer. Unlike the situation with the muscarines where the relative orientation of the 2-methyl and 5-quaternary groups is of critical importance in determining activity the relative configuration of these groups in the 1,3-dioxolane does not seem critical. However, the *presence* of the

IV-22

C_2-methyl group is of great importance since its absence leads to an approximately thousandfold loss in activity (183) and the presence of a second C_2-methyl group also reduces activity (Table IV-32). To this extent the role of the C_2-methyl group appears rather similar in the 1,3-dioxolanes, furans and tetrahydrofuran (including muscarine) ligands just discussed and, in view of the general structural resemblance between these cyclic agents and acetylcholine, may be tentatively equated with the role of the similarly situated methyl group in maintaining the rather pronounced maximum of muscarinic activity of acetylcholine in the series formylcholine ≪ acetylcholine > propionylcholine. Furthermore, despite the fact that the relative lack of configurational specificity in the cis- and $trans$-2-methyl-4-dimethylaminomethyl-1,3-dioxolanes is more similar to the situation with the muscarones than the muscarines (183, 184), it is quite apparent from the almost exclusive L-chirality of interaction of the dioxolanes that binding should be considered as essentially similar (184) to that obtaining with L-(+)-muscarine.

The Chirality of the Cholinergic Receptor and the Mode of Binding of Cholinomimetic Ligands

Some passing comment has already been made of the stereospecificity of ligand interaction at the acetylcholine receptor: in this section the data will be collected and extended.

The effects of α- and β-methyl substitution into acetylcholine are of some interest since they reveal further important differences in ligand interaction at the various cholinergic junctions. The data in Table IV-34 show that DL-acetyl-α-methylcholine retains the nicotinic activity of acetylcholine but loses much of the muscarinic activity, whilst, in direct contrast, DL-acetyl-β-methylcholine retains the muscarinic activity of acetylcholine but is very significantly reduced in nicotinic activity. It is important to note, however, that the introduction of the α- or β-methyl

TABLE IV-34. Stereospecificity of Interaction of Acetyl α- and β-Methylcholines (185, 186, 188, 189)

Compound	Equipotent molar activities (ACh = 1)			
	G.P. ileum	Ratio R/S	Frog rectus	Ratio R/S
$CH_3COOCH(Me)CH_2\overset{+}{N}Me_3$ (DL)	1·6	—	180	—
$CH_3COOCH_2CH Me\overset{+}{N}Me_3$ (DL)	49	—	2	—
$S(+)CH_3COOCH(Me)CH_2\overset{+}{N}Me_3$ (L)	1·01	240	—	—
$R(-)CH_3COOCH(Me)CH_2\overset{+}{N}Me_3$ (D)	240	—	—	—
$S(-)CH_3COOCH_2CH(Me)\overset{+}{N}Me_3$ (L)	232	0·13	—	0·60
$R(+)CH_3COOCH_2CH(Me)\overset{+}{N}Me_3$ (D)	28	—	—	—
	Rat jejunum			
	i.a.	pD_2		
$S(+)CH_3COOCH(Me)CH_2\overset{+}{N}Me_3$ (L)	1	6·9		
$R(-)CH_3COOCH(Me)CH_2\overset{+}{N}Me_3$ (D)	1	4·4		

group does not produce any significant increase in activity relative to acetylcholine. Thus in any consideration of the stereospecificity of action of these ligands (Table IV-34) the role of the methyl substituents is probably to be regarded in the negative sense that they permit, in one enantiomer, an effective interaction but prevent, in the other enantiomer, this interaction. It should be noted that the different activities of the acetyl α- and β-methylcholines seems quite unrelated to their ability to act as substrates or inhibitors of acetylcholinesterase (Table IV-35).

TABLE IV-35. Rates of Hydrolysis of Acetyl α- and β-Methylcholines by Acetylcholinesterase (186, 190)

Compound	[S]optimum × 10^3 M	Rate of hydrolyses (ACh = 1)
Acetylcholine	4·9	100
$S(+)CH_3COOCH(Me)CH_2\overset{+}{N}Me_3$	10·0	54
$R(-)CH_3COOCH(Me)CH_2\overset{+}{N}Me_3$	—	weak inhibition
$S(-)CH_3COOCH_2CH(Me)\overset{+}{N}Me_3$	6·7	97
$R(+)CH_3COOCH_2CH(Me)\overset{+}{N}Me_3$	6·7	78

TABLE IV-36. Stereospecificity of Muscarinic Activities

Ligand (active isomer)	Equipotent molar ratio(−/+)
S(+)-Acetyl-β-methylcholine†	240§
2S.3R.5S-(+)-Muscarine‡	350
2S.4R-(+)cis-2-Methyl-4-dimethylamino-methyl-1,3-dioxolane methiodide†	100¶

† Guinea-pig ileum (185, 186).
‡ Rabbit ileum (191).
§ A ratio of 400 is observed for rat jejunum (189, 190).
¶ A ratio of 150 is observed for rat jejunum (192).

From the data of Table IV-36 it will be noted that the activities and stereospecificities of acetyl-β-methylcholine, muscarine and cis-2-methyl-4-dimethylaminomethyl-1,3-dioxolane methiodide are basically very similar. The chiral equivalence of the asymmetric centers in the active isomers of the cis-dioxolane and acetyl-β-methylcholine with the corresponding centers in 2S, 3R, 5S-muscarine, strongly suggest equivalent binding environments for the asymmetric centers. Thus muscarine and the cis-dioxolane probably have an almost identical binding mode (Fig. IV-13). Although not directly inferrable from the

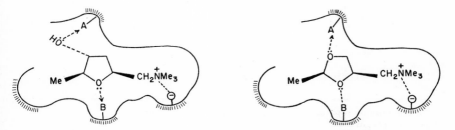

FIG. IV-13. Schematic representation of analogous binding mechanisms of muscarine (left) and the dioxolane (right).

chirality data acetyl-β-methylcholine can also fit the binding pattern represented in Fig. IV-13 so that the methyl group becomes equivalent to the 2-methyl group of the cis-dioxolane and muscarine. Examination of models shows that in this conformation the carboxyl, ether and hydroxyl functions of S-acetyl-β-methylcholine, 2S:4R-cis-dioxolane and 2S:3R:5S-muscarine can all bind to a symmetrically disposed hydrogen-bonding group. Support for this proposal is found in the data of Table IV-37 which reveals that the effects of methyl substitution into the presumed equivalent positions of acetylcholine, muscarine and the

10*

cis-dioxolane are remarkably similar, suggesting an identical and highly specific binding locus for this methyl group (the differences are not, however, as marked with the furan derivative see p. 255).

The introduction of the α-methyl group into acetylcholine produces a decrease in muscarinic activity and, as in the previously cited comparison of muscarine and muscarone, a loss and inversion of optical specificity (Table IV-34). This information suggests quite clearly that an alternative

TABLE IV-37. Effects of Methyl Substitution on the Muscarinic Activities of Acetylcholine and Related Ligands

Ligand	R = H		R = Me		R = Et	
	i.a.	pD$_2$	i.a.	pD$_2$	i.a.	pD$_2$
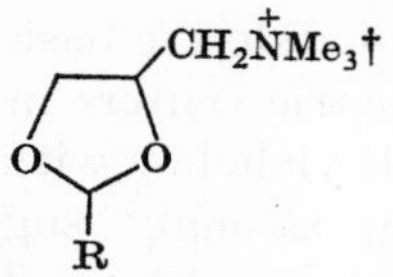 ![dioxolane] CH$_2$$\overset{+}{N}Me_3$†	1	5·3	1	7·2	0·9	5·3
RCOOCH$_2$CH$_2$$\overset{+}{N}Me_3$†	1	5·2	1	7·6	0·9	5·0

HO, tetrahydrofuran R′ —CH$_2$$\overset{+}{N}Me_3$‡ (DL)	Equipotent molar activities (ACh = 1)		
	R = H	R = Me	R = Et
	125	1	—
R— furan —CH$_2$$\overset{+}{N}Me_3$§	12	0·34	35

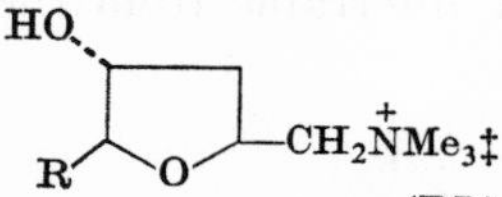

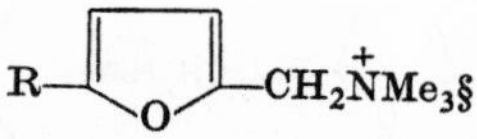

† Rat jejunum preparation (159, 193, 194).
‡ Cat bp preparation (172).
§ G.P. ileum preparation (176).

mode of binding to that represented in Fig. IV-13 has become available for muscarone and acetyl-α-methylcholine (184). The simplest rationalization of this phenomenon is that the alternative binding mode is that shown in Fig. IV-14 (shown relative to muscarine) whereby a number of common binding sites are still shared (α-methyl, ring oxygen and $\overset{+}{N}$Me$_3$). The almost complete lack of stereospecificity shown by muscarone suggests that it can probably adopt, with approximately equal ease, either this latter conformation or that proposed for muscarine (Fig. IV-13): acetyl-α-methylcholine, which shows an eightfold activity difference between the isomers would, according to this hypothesis, favour binding conformation B (Fig. IV-14) by approximately 1 kcal. In this connection it is interesting to note that acetyl-α-methylcholine shows no apparent stereospecificity in its nicotinic actions (Table IV-34).

In a more general consideration of cholinomimetic ligand binding it has been noted that quite diverse structures, which in general possess the common structural feature $\overset{+}{-}NMe_3$ (in the most active compounds), constitute active species. In fact, there is in such compounds an essential continuum of molecular variation in $R\overset{+}{-}NMe_3$ such that R varies from the nonpolar (alkyl, alkaryl) to the highly polar ($CH_3COOCH_2CH_2$) and the major question to be asked is to what extent such structurally diverse ligands may be anticipated to possess common characteristics of binding. Whilst it does not seem possible at the present time to define in any

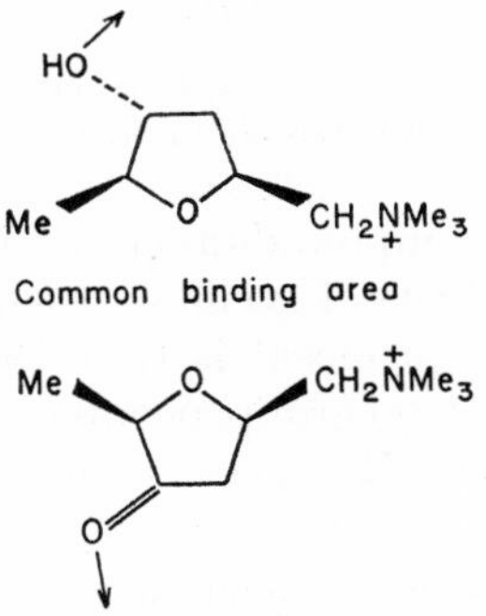

FIG. IV-14. Schematic representation of the opposing stereoselectivity of L-muscarine (top) and D-muscarone (bottom) showing how the methyl, ring oxygen and quaternary ammonium groups in the two compounds can occupy identical sites (common binding area).

rigorous sense the mode of binding of any one ligand or class of ligands, general considerations, derived in particular from the study of enzyme–substrate and enzyme–inhibitor relationships, do indicate quite clearly the basic improbability that there exists a single unique binding mode for all cholinomimetic ligands active at a single receptor system. It seems more probable that in structures of the general class $R\overset{+}{-}NMe_3$ there will exist at least two binding modes, sharing a common onium binding locus, available for polar and nonpolar R functions. Such pluralities of substrate and inhibitor binding modes have been proposed for a number of enzyme systems including carboxypeptidase (195), trypsin (196) dihydrofolate reductase (197), lysozyme (198), etc. Several lines of experimental evidence lend considerable support to this concept of cholinomimetic ligand binding.

Early studies (169, 199) of the structural requirements for muscarinic activity suggested the importance of the "5-atom" rule whereby maximum stimulant activity is associated with an effective 5-carbon chain length attached to the quaternary nitrogen function. This rule

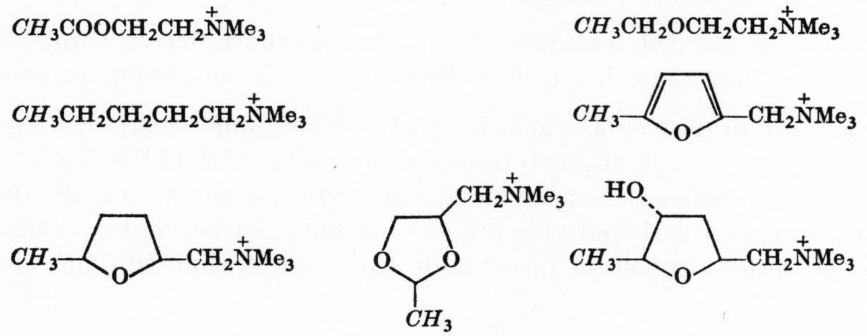

$$CH_3COOCH_2CH_2\overset{+}{N}Me_3 \qquad\qquad CH_3CH_2OCH_2CH_2\overset{+}{N}Me_3$$

$$CH_3CH_2CH_2CH_2CH_2\overset{+}{N}Me_3$$

FIG. IV-15. Muscarinic ligands which approximate to the "5-atom" rule of Alles and Knoefel and Ing.

certainly applies to such compounds as shown in Fig. IV-15 (after making some allowance for the effects of cyclic structure on chain length) and the clear implication of this proposal is that the five atom chain, which always terminates in a methyl group, occupies a common complementary structure on the receptor. However, a more detailed examination of

TABLE IV-38. Contributions of Terminal Methyl Group to Binding of Cholinomimetic Ligands (200)

Ligand	R = CH$_3$ $\Delta F°$ kcal mole^{-1}	R = H $\Delta F°$ kcal mole^{-1}	$\Delta\Delta F°$
RCOOCH$_2$CH$_2$$\overset{+}{N}Me_3$	10·0–10·8	7·4	2·6–3·4
R—⟨dioxolane⟩—CH$_2$$\overset{+}{N}Me_3$	10·4	7·5	2·9
R—⟨furan⟩—CH$_2$$\overset{+}{N}Me_3$	10·2	8·4–8·7	1·5–1·8
RCH$_2$CH$_2$OCH$_2$CH$_2$$\overset{+}{N}Me_3$	9·7	7·5	1·2
⟨pyridine⟩	8·8	7·7	1·1
RCH$_2$CH$_2$CH$_2$CH$_2$$\overset{+}{N}Me_3$	7·7	7·4	0·3

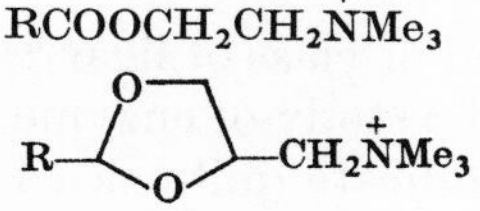

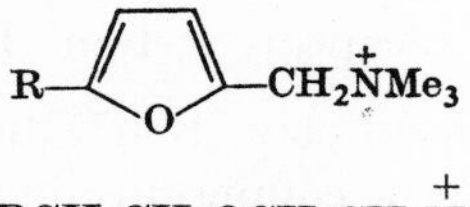

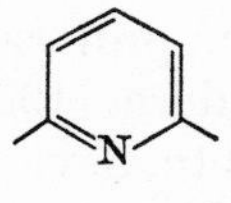

these and related compounds reveals a fundamental inconsistency: the data of Table IV-38 show that the differences in activity (expressed as $\Delta F°$ calculated from $\Delta F° = -RT\ln K$)† in a series of pairs of ligands differing only in the presence or absence of a terminal methyl group become less pronounced with decreasing polar character of the ligand structure. If the terminal methyl group in these compounds, which is in each case approximately equidistant from the $\overset{+}{-}NMe_3$ group were occupying a common site then the increment in activity might be expected to be essentially constant. That this is clearly not so is at least in accord with the hypothesis that a transition in binding environment of the R substituent is occurring in the progression from polar to non-polar character. Whether this indicates a continuum of binding sites of varying polarity surrounding a common anionic site (Fig. IV-16a) or a duality of binding sites (Fig. IV-16b) in which progressive alteration in

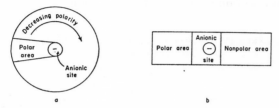

a   b

FIG. IV-16. Schematic representations of ligand binding areas at the cholinergic receptor. In (a) there exists an essential continuum of binding sites for the side chain whilst in (b) there exists only two defined binding areas for the side chains.

ligand polar character causes a progressive reduction in the free energy difference ($\Delta\Delta F°$) of ligand recognition at the two sites cannot be determined from this data. A further point of some interest that arises from the data of Table IV-38 concerns the magnitude of the binding increments ($\Delta\Delta F°$) for the methyl groups which, for the first two ligands, are significantly greater than the maximum contribution of Van der Waals and hydrophobic interactions of ~1400 cal (Chapter I, see section p. 25). This may indicate that the binding of these methyl groups produces stabilization of other binding forces perhaps by a water displacement process facilitating hydrogen bond formation by the oxygen functions in acetylcholine and the 1,3-dioxolane. A number of other lines of evidence also suggest the occurrence of alternative binding modes for cholinomimetic ligands. Schueler *et al.* (201, 202) found the "reversed ester" analog (IV-23) of acetylcholine to be approximately

† The validity of these calculations depend, of course, upon the correctness of the assumption that affinity constants can be calculated directly from dose–response curves (p. 212). Evidence to support the assumption will be presented later in this chapter.

equiactive with acetylcholine as a muscarinic agent; however, introduction of a β-methyl group to give IV-24 reduced activity by a factor of 10,000, whereas, the same substitution into acetylcholine leaves muscarinic activity unchanged (Table IV-34). Apparently, acetylcholine and its reversed analog do not bind in identical environments. More

$$CH_3OOCCH_2CH_2\overset{+}{N}Me_3 \qquad\qquad CH_3OOCCH(Me)CH_2\overset{+}{N}Me_3$$

IV-23   IV-24

recently it has been shown that the R and S isomers of 2-methylbutyl- and 2-methylamyltrimethylammonium do not differ significantly in their activity (Table IV-39) and that an actual inversion of chirality of interaction has occurred with the 2-methylamyltrimethylammonium ligand. These results also suggest that acetylcholine and the alkyltrimethylammonium ligands bind in different environments. Other lines of evidence that also lend strong support to this conclusion are discussed elsewhere in this volume (Chapter V, see section p. 444).

TABLE IV-39. Stereoselectivity of Interaction of
Muscarinic Ligands

Ligand	Activity ratio[†] L/D
$CH_3COOCH(Me)CH_2\overset{+}{N}Me_3$	400
$CH_3CH_2CH(Me)CH_2\overset{+}{N}Me_3$	10
$CH_3CH_2CH_2CH(Me)CH_2\overset{+}{N}Me_3$	0·05

[†] Rat jejunum preparation (unpublished data of
J. F. Moran and D. J. Triggle).

As indicated previously, the concept of multiple ligand binding modes centered around a common functional or catalytic center has received general support from both enzyme and receptor systems. For carboxypeptidase, which hydrolyses both dipeptide and ester substrates Vallee and his co-workers have proposed (195) a model that accommodates a great deal of the apparently contradictory evidence in this field: in their model, nonidentical, but overlapping, binding sites are presumed to exist for the peptide and ester substrates and are shown schematically in Fig. IV-17. Such an arrangement of binding sites accounts for many observations, e.g., that ester substrates inhibit peptidase activity and *vice versa* and that esterolytic activity can be inhibited without affecting peptidase activity and *vice versa*. Similarly, trypsin has long been known

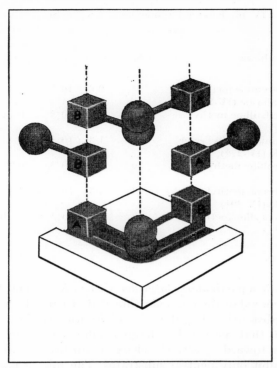

Fig. IV-17. Model of carboxypeptidase showing dual substrate binding sites which consist at a common catalytic site (center) and nonoverlapping binding sites for the side chains. The lowest portion of the figure shows ester (A) and peptide (B) binding modes (the balls represent the site of enzyme attack) and the upper figures two of many possible ways in which substrate interactions could occur to produce inhibition. Reproduced with permission from Vallee *et al.* (195).

(203, 204) to exhibit high specificity towards esters derived from L-lysine and L-arginine: however, neutral substrates (Fig. IV-18) are also hydrolysed (Chapter I, see section p. 62) but the absence of the positive

$$\underset{H_2N\overset{\overset{\displaystyle X}{\|}}{C}(CH_2)_3CH}{\overset{\diagup NHR}{\diagdown COOMe}}$$

IV-25 R = C_6H_5CO; X = $\overset{+}{N}H_2$

IV-27 R = $4\text{-}MeC_6H_4SO_2$; X = $\overset{+}{N}H_2$

IV-26 R = C_6H_5CO; X = O

IV-28 R = $4\text{-}MeC_6H_4SO_2$; X = O

$$\underset{X(CH_2)_4CH}{\overset{\diagup NHR}{\diagdown COOMe}}$$

IV-29 R = C_6H_5CO; X = $\overset{+}{N}H_3$

IV-30 R = C_6H_5CO; X = CH_3

Fig. IV-18. Positively charged and neutral substrates of trypsin.

TABLE IV-40. Kinetic Parameters of Trypsin Substrates (196)

Substrate	Charge	K_o M	k_o sec^{-1}	k_o/K_o (M^{-1} sec^{-1})
N^α-Benzoyl-L-arginine methyl ester hydrochloride (IV-25[†])	+	9.6×10^{-6}	9.3	9.7×10^5
N^α-Benzoyl-L-citrulline methyl ester (IV-26[†])	0	4.1×10^{-2}	0.14	3.5
N^α-Tosyl-L-arginine methyl ester hydrochloride (IV-27[†])	+	1.3×10^{-5}	60	4.8×10^6
N^α-Tosyl-L-citrulline methyl ester (IV-28[†])	0	9.1×10^{-2}	0.39	4.3
N^α-Benzoyl-L-lysine methyl ester hydrochloride (IV-29[†])	+	5.5×10^{-5}	1.8	3.3×10^4
N-Benzoyl-L-heptyline methyl ester (IV-30[†])	0	1.0×10^{-4}	9.4×10^{-3}	9.0

[†] See Fig. IV-18.

charge results in a particularly large decrease in K_o (>1000, Table IV-40) suggesting removal of the nonpolar side chain to an alternative binding site. This is substantiated by data from inhibition studies (Table IV-41) which reveal that positively charged inhibitors show competitive behavior only towards positively charged substrates and that neutral inhibitors inhibit only neutral substrates. The role of nonpolar interactions as a determinant for substrate binding has also been discussed in a previous section of this volume (Chapter 1, see section, p. 52).

Finally, in this brief discussion of enzymes with multiple-binding possibilities may be mentioned acetylcholinesterase, a system of obvious relevance to any discussion of cholinomimetic ligands even if, as in the

TABLE IV-41. Effect of Inhibitors on Substrate Hydrolysis by Trypsin (196)

Modifier	Charge	Substrates (K_I) Benzoylarginine methyl ester (+)	Benzoylcitrulline methyl ester (0)
Phenylguanidinium nitrate	+	7.2×10^{-5} M competitive	2.0×10^{-4} M noncompetitive
Ethylammonium chloride	+	6.2×10^{-2} M competitive	6.6×10^{-2} M noncompetitive
Phenol	0	12×10^{-2} M noncompetitive	5.4×10^{-2} M competitive
Phenyl urea	0	No effect at 10^{-1} M	1×10^{-1} M competitive

present context, no consideration is given to possible interrelationships of esterase and receptor function (Chapter VI). In a previous chapter (Chapter I, see section, p. 62) some mechanistic aspects of acetylcholinesterase were discussed from which it seems probable that the quaternary ammonium structure of acetylcholine and related substrates is playing the role of an internal regulatory group thereby facilitating the ester hydrolysis. However, acetylcholinesterase also hydrolyses neutral esters including aliphatic esters, aryl acetates, indophenol acetate, etc., which clearly cannot be assumed to occupy the complete binding site utilized by acetylcholine. Nevertheless, the same esteratic site is apparently occupied by all esters since their hydrolyses are facilitated by

$$C_6H_5CH\!\!-\!\!-\!\!CH_2 \qquad\qquad C_6H_5CH\!\!-\!\!-\!\!CH_2$$
$$\underset{\overset{+}{N}Me_2}{} \qquad\qquad \underset{\overset{+}{N}MeCH_2CH_2Cl}{}$$

IV-31 IV-32

the addition of quaternary ammonium functions: first demonstrated by Wilson *et al.* (Chapter I, see section, p. 62) for the alkanesulfonyl fluoride interaction at the enzyme esteratic site. Similarly, Purdie and McIvor (205, 206) O'Brien (207) and Belleau (208) have shown that irreversible occupation of (presumably) the anionic site by IV-31 and IV-32 potentiates the hydrolysis of neutral substrates whilst inhibiting the hydrolysis of positively charged substrates. Thus, the substrate

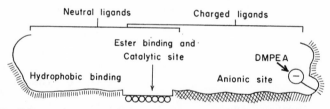

FIG. IV-19. Schematic representation depicting how acetylcholinesterase might bind, at partially overlapping sites, neutral and positively charged substrates.

binding site of acetylcholinesterase recognizes at least two classes of ligands and may be schematically represented as in Fig. IV-19.

The detailed studies by Purdie (206) on acetylcholinesterase inhibited irreversibly to acetylcholine by IV-31 (DMPEA) reveal several points of great interest concerning ligand binding to this enzyme system. The DMPEA enzyme is resistant to inactivation by Amiton (IV-33) whereas Sarin (IV-34), Tepp (IV-35) and related "neutral" organophosphate inhibitors are still potent inhibitors. Similar conclusions have been reached by O'Brien (207) using the enzyme inhibited by an essentially similar agent IV-32 and his data (Table IV-42) clearly reveal the very large variations in ability of organophosphates to react with the inhibited enzyme. Thus it is quite apparent that two binding modes exist among these inhibitors, one available for positively charged and one available for neutral substrates. Similar behavior is also found with substrates of acetylcholinesterase and from the quantitative data of

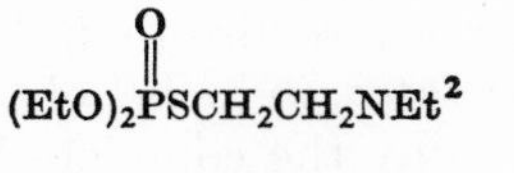

$$(EtO)_2\overset{O}{\overset{\|}{P}}SCH_2CH_2NEt^2$$

IV-33

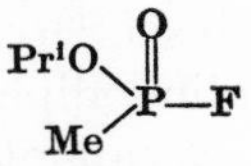

$$\underset{Me}{\overset{Pr^iO}{\diagdown}}\overset{O}{\overset{\|}{P}}\text{---}F$$

IV-34

$$(C_2H_5O)_2\overset{O}{\overset{\|}{P}}O\overset{O}{\overset{\|}{P}}(OC_2H_5)_2$$

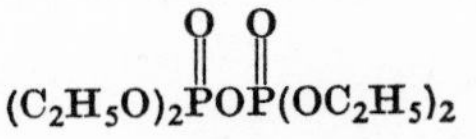

IV-35

Table IV-43 it is quite apparent that DMPEA treatment modifies to quite different extents the kinetic parameters of substrate binding and catalysis.

The studies of Bracha and O'Brien (209, 210) on the structure–activity relationships of organophosphate inhibitors of acetylcholinesterase related to O,O-diethyl-5-(2-diethylaminoethyl)-phosphorothiolate

TABLE IV-42. Effect of N-2-Chloroethyl-N-methyl-2-Chloro-2-phenylethylamine on the Susceptibility of Acetylcholinesterase to Inhibition by Organophosphates (207)

	Bimolecular rate constant, k_1, min^{-1} mole^{-1} 1 × 10^{-3}		
Organophosphate	Control	Enzyme alkylated at 0·1 mM	Control/ alkylated ratio
Paraoxon (diethyl-p-nitrophenyl phosphate)	734	78·0	9
Malaoxon (S-1,2-bis(ethoxycarboxyl)ethyl-O,O-dimethylphosphorothiolate)	138	5·0	27
Amiton (S-(diethylaminoethyl)-O,O-diethyl-phosphorothiolate)	114	0·125	913
PB72 (S-5,5-dimethylhexyl-O,O-diethyl-phosphorothiolate)	228	6·9	33

(Amiton) and the quaternary analogs lends further support to this multibinding hypothesis. The high inhibitory activity of Amiton is assumed to relate to its structural resemblance to acetylcholine, the high affinity compensating for the relatively poor phosphorylating ability.

However, uncharged carbon isosteres of Amiton show similarly high activity suggesting that in these analogs hydrophobic binding only is of importance. In a series of diethyl-n-alkyl phosphates (IV-36, R = alkyl) and diethyl-n-alkyl-phosphorothiolates (IV-37, R = alkyl) inhibitory activity was found to increase with length of the carbon chain and to

TABLE IV-43. Kinetic Constants of Ester Hydrolysis by Acetylcholinesterase Modified by N,N-Dimethyl-2-chloro-2-phenylethylamine (206)

Substrate	K_m (approx.) mM		Relative k_{cat}	
	Control	Alkylated	Control	Alkylated
Ethyl acetate	500	156	very low	0·10
n-Propyl acetate	200	18·5	0·10	0·10
n-Butyl acetate	38	11·5	0·09	0·09
3,3-Dimethylbutyl acetate	4·0	4·4	0·55	0·07
Acetylcholine	0·19	no reaction	1·00	no reaction
Phenyl acetate	1·6	3·3	0·92	0·12

plateau at the C_6 level (Fig. IV-20) yielding a value of $\Delta F = -600$–800 cal mole^{-1} in excellent agreement with accepted values for the hydrophobic contributions of methylene groups (Chapter I, see section, p. 25).

Finally, Belleau (208) has demonstrated that of a large series of cholinomimetic ligands containing the —$\overset{+}{\text{N}}\text{Me}_3$ group (including esters, dioxolanes and alkylammonium compounds) *only* acetylcholine and butyrylcholine protect acetylcholinesterase from inactivation by methanesulfonyl fluoride: the other ligands, all of which are known to be

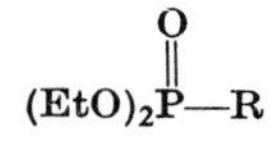

$$(EtO)_2\overset{\overset{O}{\|}}{P}\text{—R}$$
IV-36

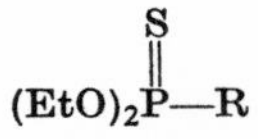

$$(EtO)_2\overset{\overset{S}{\|}}{P}\text{—R}$$
IV-37

competitive inhibitors of acetylcholinesterase, must therefore adopt a binding orientation that is at least partially distinct from that adopted by acetylcholine and butyrylcholine.

The most important features of these several studies with acetylcholinesterase are that a broad classification of substrates and inhibitors into cationic and neutral species is possible which, in all probability, reflects also a similar classification of binding sites. A second point of equal importance, to which attention will also be directed elsewhere (p. 339) is that within a given ligand class susceptibility to hydrolysis is differentially affected by the same inhibition procedure: in more general terms, the same chemical modification at the same macromolecular site(s) will modify subsequent ligand interaction, the nature and magnitude of such modification being dependent upon the particular ligand structure. As a final comment on the concept of multiple binding

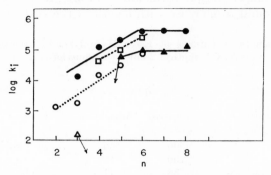

Fig. IV-20. The relationship between anticholinesterase activity (K_i) and the number of carbon atoms in the longest chain: ●, O,O-diethyl-S-(ω-3-pentylalkyl)-phosphorothiolates; ▲, diethyl-ω-(3-pentylalkyl)phosphates; □, O,O-diethyl-S-(ω-t-butylalkyl)phosphorothiolates; ○, diethyl-(ω-t-butylalkyl)phosphates. Reproduced with permission from Bracha and O'Brien (210).

modes of ligands at receptor sites it should be noted that Portoghese (211) explicitly advanced this concept to accommodate narcotic analgesic interactions. In his model the analgesics were assumed to bind to a

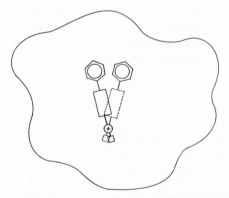

Fig. IV-21. Representation of various analgesic binding modes centered around a common anionic site. Reproduced with permission from Portoghese (211).

common anionic site which serves as an anchoring site around which various binding modes are possible (Fig. IV-21). A basic argument for this model was that in a series of analgesics (IV-38–IV-41) identical binding would indicate that the effects of N—R modification should produce, according to the simplest considerations, parallel changes in activity. Of the series studied parallel changes in activity with N-substitution were observed with the ligands represented by IV-38 and IV-39–IV-41 respectively, but these were not identical. Thus the data suggest at least two binding modes for narcotic analgesic structures. The conclusions drawn by Portoghese for analgesic interaction are thus essentially similar to those discussed earlier for the effect of N-alkyl-substitution on cholinomimetic activity and lend further support to the concept of structure-dependent multiple binding modes for ligands.

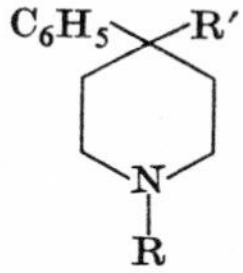

R′ = CO₂Et, OCOEt, OCOMe
R = alkyl, alkaryl

IV-38

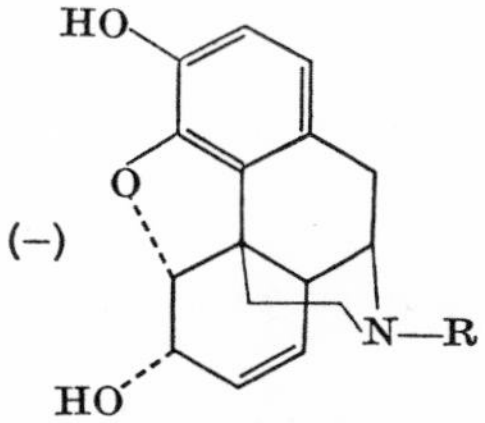

R = alkyl, alkaryl

IV-39

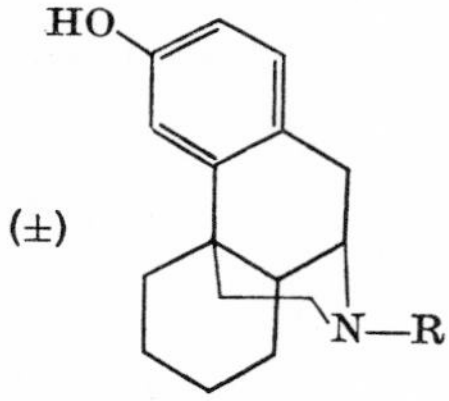

R = alkyl, alkaryl
IV-40

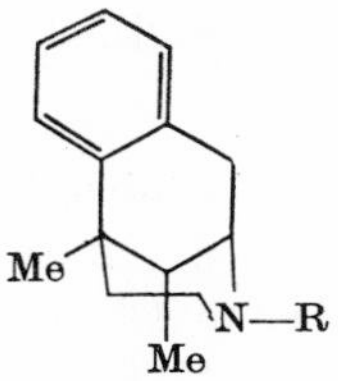

R = alkyl, alkaryl
IV-41

Turning from the general problem of defining the possible multiplicity of binding sites for cholinomimetic ligands at the cholinergic receptor to the more specific problem of the conformation of receptor-bound ligand it seems clear from the preceding discussion that a single conformation of bound ligand is most unlikely. However, it may be anticipated that the "active" conformations adopted by ligands of similar structure and activity may well be essentially similar. This conclusion is well supported by the chirality data for muscarine, acetyl-β-methylcholine, cis-2-methyl-4-trimethylammoniummethyl-1,3-dioxolane and, by extension, for acetylcholine; as noted, however, muscarone adopts a binding site (but not necessarily a binding conformation) that is at least partially distinct from the above ligands. Furthermore, the molecular constraints imposed by the ring structure of muscarine and the dioxolane serve as a partial characterization of the conformation of the non-rigid analogs, acetylcholine and acetyl-β-methylcholine.

A number of attempts have been made to further define the conformation of receptor-bound ligands: none of the methods employed is free from objection.

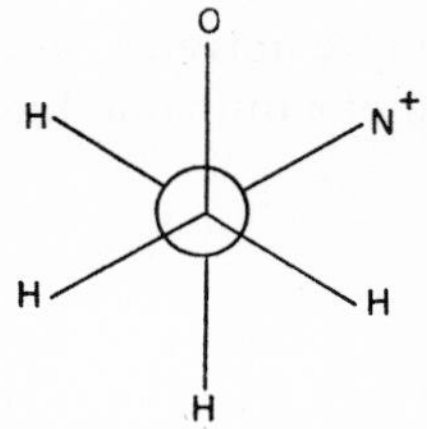

FIG. IV-22. Gauche conformation of O—C—C—N$^+$ function.

X-ray crystallography has been employed by several workers (212, 213) to elucidate the structures of the cholinomimetic ligands in the crystalline state. Amongst the molecules thus studied are acetylcholine (214), L(+)-acetyl-β-methylcholine (215), L(+)-muscarine (216), D(−)-acetyl-α-methylcholine (217), α-lactoylcholine (218), acetylthiolcholine,

TABLE IV-44. Torsion Angles of Some Cholinomimetic Ligands (214–221)

Cholinomimetic Ligand	O—C—C—$\overset{+}{\text{N}}$	C—O—C—C
L-Acetyl-β-methylcholine iodide	+85	−147
L-cis-2-Methyl-4-dimethylaminomethyl-1,3-dioxolane methiodide†	+68	+100
L-Lactoylcholine iodide	+85	+157
L-Muscarine iodide†	+73	+144
Acetylcholine bromide	+77	+79
D-Acetyl-α-methylcholine iodide	+90 (A)	+170
	−148 (B)	+176
Acetylthiolcholine (S—C—C—$\overset{+}{\text{N}}$)	+171°	+150
Acetylselenolcholine (Se—C—C—$\overset{+}{\text{N}}$)	+175°	+155

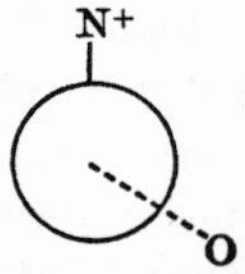

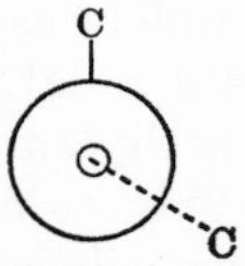

† For cyclic molecules this torsion angle refers to the atoms corresponding to those in acetylcholine.

acetyl selenolcholine (219, 220) and *cis*-2-(S)-methyl-4-(R)dimethyl-aminomethyl-1,3-dioxolane methiodide (221). For a large number of structures containing the O—C—C—$\overset{+}{N}$ function a *gauche* (synclinal) conformation (Fig. IV-22) has been established, it being presumed that an electrostatic stabilization occurs in $\overset{+}{N}$----O and which has been associated with the occurrence of cholinomimetic activity (218, 222); Table IV-44). However, a number of exceptions to this generalization are known: thus, choline exists in a gauche conformation yet is inactive and acetylthiolcholine and acetylselenolcholine exist in the *trans*-conformations with acetylthiolcholine being active and acetylselenol-choline relatively inactive as depolarizing agents in the electric eel electroplax preparation (223, 224). As noted previously, acetylthiocholine is inactive as a muscarinic agent. It is thus quite apparent that differences in electron distribution and polarizability caused by the sulfur or selenium substitution are factors that are probably of greater importance

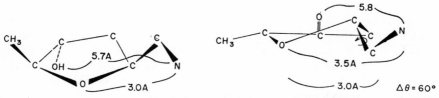

FIG. IV-23. Calculated conformations of L-muscarine (left) and D-muscarone (right). Reproduced with permission from Kier (226).

than the conformation in the solid state. In any case the relevance of the application of structural data obtained for the crystal lattice to considerations of the conformations of receptor bound ligand may be seriously questioned: there can be, by virtue of the undoubtedly low rotational barriers existing in such compounds (225–227), no *necessary* relationship between the ligand conformations in the two physical states and it may well be that the conformation adopted at the receptor is thermodynamically unstable relative to that in the solid state (1, 2). The same criticisms may also be directed against extrapolations of con-formational data obtained for acetylcholine in aqueous solution by PMR methods (228, 229). Similarly, the relevance of theoretical (extended Hückel) calculations of the conformations of acetylcholine, L-muscarine and D-muscarone (226, 230) which refer essentially to these molecules in vacuum is also open to discussion. This has been explicitly recognized by Kier (226, 230, 231); however, it is interesting to note that the Hückel calculations generate conformations for these ligands that are in good agreement with the X-ray data (Fig. IV-23) suggesting the basic soundness of the approach and offering the exciting possibility that it may be possible to extend such calculations to include interactions between the ligand, water, and functional groups of potential relevance to receptor systems (231).

An alternative experimental approach is through the synthesis of structurally rigid analogs of acetylcholine in which the possibilities of conformational variation are eliminated or greatly reduced. Whilst it is a simple matter to find rigid skeletons into which may be incorporated the appropriate functional groups for potential cholinomimetic activity, it is obviously important that the production of conformational restriction be unaccompanied by significant additional molecular

IV-42a   IV-42b

structure relative to the parent ligand (232, 233) to avoid the appearance of antagonistic properties. An additional limitation to this approach is that the molecular changes necessary to produce the conformationally restricted analog may serve to alter the mode of binding to the receptor. Thus, for both of these reasons it appears important that the conformationally restricted analog deviate as little as possible from the structure of acetylcholine or an analogous ligand.

Few compounds synthesized fulfill these requirements (233–235). Amongst the most interesting are the *cis*- and *trans*-2-acetoxycyclopropyltrimethylammoniums (IV-42a, IV-42b) which may be regarded as a hybrid analog of acetyl-α- and acetyl-β-methylcholine (236, 237). The reported activities (Table IV-45) clearly indicate that the *trans*-isomer is primarily muscarinic in its actions and hence to be regarded more as an

TABLE IV-45. Cholinomimetic Activities of *cis*-and *trans*-2-Acetoxycyclopropyltrimethylammonium (ACTM) (237)

Compound	Equipotent molar activities (ACh = 1)	
	G.P. ileum	Frog rectus
Acetylcholine	1	1
(+)-*trans*-ACTM	1·13	0·013
(−)-*trans*-ACTM	0·0022	0·0028
(±)-*cis*-ACTM	0·00010	0·0042

analog of acetyl-β-methyl choline. (However, inspection of Dreiding models reveals clearly that the 3-CH$_2$ of the cyclopropane *cannot* achieve full geometric equivalence with the β-CH$_3$ of acetyl-β-methyl-choline or the corresponding group in muscarine or the 1,3-dioxolane.)

TABLE IV-46. Cholinomimetic Activities of 1,3-Dioxolanes (2, 232, 238)

Dioxolane	Equipotent molar activity (ACh = 1) Rat jejunum	Distances[†] Å	
		$\overset{+}{Me_3N} \to O_1$	$\overset{+}{Me_3N} \to O_2$
Acetylcholine			
CH$_2\overset{+}{N}$Me$_3$	1	—	—
(dioxolane, Me)	1	3·6	4·6‡
CH$_2$ / +NMe$_2$ / (CH$_2$)$_n$ $n = 1$	inactive	2·5 / 2·8	3·3§ / 2·8¶
IV-42c (n = 1); IV-42d (n = 2) $n = 2$	80	2·5 / 2·85	3·9‖ / 3·5††
Me~~ / +NMe$_2$	*endo* 2400 / *exo-* 240	3·2–3·5	
+NMe$_2$ (dioxolane, Me) IV-42e	9·9 (i.a., 1·0)	3·4	4·5
Me / CH$_2\overset{+}{N}$Me$_3$ (dioxolane, Me) IV-42f	308 (*cis, trans*) (i.a., 0·56)		

† Measured from Dreiding models.

‡ Measured for conformation in which $\overset{+}{N}$ is at maximum distance from O$_1$ and O$_3$.

§ Morpholine ring in boat conformation.

¶ Morpholine ring in chair conformation.

‖ 1,4-Oxaazacycloheptane ring in "boat" conformation.

†† 1,4-Oxaazacycloheptaine ring in "chair" conformation.

The data of Table IV-45 reveal that muscarinic activity is confined to the *trans*-isomers and that there is a marked stereospecificity of interaction with the (+)-isomer being equipotent with acetylcholine; this stereospecificity is actually greater than that observed with acetyl-β-methylcholine, muscarine, etc. Thus it may well be that *trans*-2-acetoxycyclopropyltrimethylammonium serves to define the geometry of —$\overset{+}{N}Me_3$ and >O (torsion angle approximately 180° and separated by 3·8 Å) and a relative area for binding of the acetyl group in the bound conformation of acetylcholine.

A series of compounds structurally related to the highly active *cis*-2-methyl-4-dimethylaminomethyl-1,3-dioxolane methiodide (IV-22) has also been studied (Table IV-46). From this data it appears probable that the active conformation of IV-22 is that in which the quaternary head is maximally extended from O_1 and O_3 of the dioxolane ring. In particular the inactivity of IV-42c and IV-42d (Table IV-46) should be noted: the *spiro*-azetidinium analog (IV-42e, Table IV-46) is some tenfold less active than IV-22, but if allowance is made for the possibly detrimental effect of 4,4-substitution in the *spiro* analog, through comparison with IV-42f (Table IV-46), then the extended conformation thus represented is probably a close approximation to the active conformation adopted by IV-22.

A Molecular Basis for Cholinomimetic Ligand Interaction

In the preceding treatment of cholinomimetic ligand interactions discussion has been essentially qualitative, a treatment which is probably quite appropriate to the information currently available. However, this discussion is certainly suggestive that a number of binding modes may be available for cholinomimetic ligands and it would be clearly desirable to have available more quantitative descriptions of the ligand–receptor interactions.

Quite recently the studies by Belleau and his co-workers (239–242) of the thermodynamics of ligand binding to acetylcholinesterase have provided a framework of a quantitative model according to which the interactions of these same ligands with the cholinergic receptor may be interpreted. It should be emphasized immediately that such treatments imply no necessary functional connection between acetylcholinesterase and the cholinergic receptor (this question is dealt with in greater detail in Chapter VI), but are based essentially on the less dramatic conclusion that the ligand binding mechanisms operative in the two systems may be very similar.

As noted by Belleau, the alkyltrimethylammonium series is peculiarly appropriate for such studies since it represents a well-defined structure–activity relationship in which the sole molecular variation is the progressive addition of methylene groups. The data of Table IV-47 for the inhibition of acetylcholinesterase by these ligands reveals a relatively constant free energy of binding which is thus uninformative as

TABLE IV-47. Thermodynamic Parameters for Binding of Alkyltrimethylammonium ligands to Acetylcholinesterase at $25°$ C (241)

$$C_nH_{2n+1}\overset{+}{N}Me_3$$

n	ΔF kcal mole^{-1}	ΔH kcal mole^{-1}	ΔS† e.u.
1	−3·59	−6·60	−10·1
2	−3·81	−6·45	−8·9
3	−3·92	−6·32	−8·1
4	−4·20	−5·22	−3·4
5	−3·76	−5·40	−5·5
6	−3·92	−4·55	−2·1
7	−4·08	−4·49	−1·4
8	−4·34	−4·40	−0·2
9	−4·53	−4·40	+0·44
10	−4·97	−4·26	+2·4

† $\Delta S_u = \Delta S + 7·98$ (cratic term; Chapter I, see Section, p. 16).

to the nature of the interaction; however, the enthalpy and, in particular, the entropy changes do show marked and fairly regular changes with increasing alkyl chain length. Furthermore, if the *assumption* is made that the contributions by the alkyl and tetramethylammonium functions to the free energy of interaction are independent and additive,

$$\Delta H_{tot} = \delta\Delta H_{Me_4\overset{+}{N}} + \delta\Delta H_{alkyl} \qquad (XVII)$$

$$\Delta S_{tot} = \delta\Delta S_{Me_4\overset{+}{N}} + \delta\Delta S_{alkyl} \qquad (XVIII)$$

then it is possible to isolate these individual values (Table IV-48). From this data it is clear that the contribution to interaction made by the alkyl chain is endothermic and entropy-driven, features characteristic (Chapter I, see section, p. 16) of processes involving the reorientation of water. Furthermore, the variations in $\delta\Delta H$ and $\delta\Delta S$ reveal themselves as two isoequilibrium relationships (Fig. IV-24), one for C_2–C_5 and the other for C_6–C_{10} with markedly different slopes of $\beta = 288°$ K and $60°$ K respectively. From the previous discussion of such isoequilibrium relationships (Chapter I, see section, p. 35), it is possible that this

TABLE IV-48. Contributions to Enthalpies and Entropies of Interaction of the Alkyl Residues of Alkyltrimethylammonium Ligands at 25° C (241)

n	$\delta\Delta H$ cal mole^{-1}	$\delta\Delta H/CH_2$ cal mole^{-1}	$\delta\Delta S$ e.u.	$\delta\Delta S/CH_2$ e.u.
2	150		1·2	
		130		0·8
3	280		2·0	
		1100		4·7
4	1380		6·7	
		−180		−2·1
5	1200		4·6	
		850		3·1
6	2050		7·7	
		50		1·0
7	2100		8·7	
		100		1·2
8	2200		9·9	
		0		0·6
9	2200		10·5	
		140		2·0
10	2340		12·5	

bifunctional isoequilibrium relationship indicates that two different types of water reorganization are being promoted in the interaction of the alkyl chains of these ligands with acetylcholinesterase. An isokinetic temperature of $\beta = 288°\,K$ lies in the range commonly observed for a

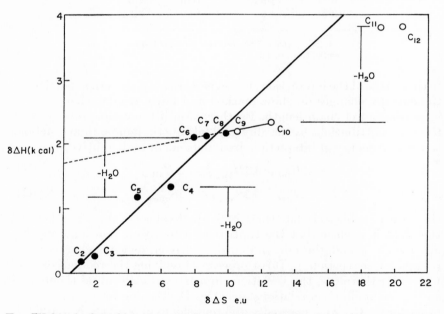

FIG. IV-24. A plot of increments of binding enthalpies and entropies of alkyltrimethylammonium ligands to bovine erythrocyte acetylcholinesterase. Reproduced with permission from Belleau (241).

variety of processes involving reorganization of protein structure and a temperature of $\beta = 60°$ K is basically similar to the values found for the transfer of hydrocarbon from water to a nonpolar solvent (Chapter I, see section, p. 16). From the standpoint of the relationship of ligand interaction at acetylcholinesterase and the cholinergic receptor, it is particularly intriguing, as noted by Belleau (241), that this transition in interaction mechanisms also marks a transition from stimulant to inhibitory activity at the cholinergic receptor (Table IV-16). Thus the determinant for stimulant or inhibitory activity in this ligand series may be, in addition to the interaction of the $-\overset{+}{\text{N}}\text{Me}_3$ function, the type of water reorganization produced at the macromolecular surface. Although it is not possible to define with real certainty these patterns of water reorganization, it seems clear that they are different and that the process associated with $\beta = 288°$ K may involve water reorganization similar in kind, if not extent, to that involved in protein denaturation whilst the process associated with $\beta = 60°$ K may simply reflect the loss of water associated with insertion of a hydrocarbon function into a nonpolar area in the macromolecular system. Such differences in interaction could well provide the basis for the difference between activator and antagonist ligands and are in agreement with Belleau's earlier speculations (239) of ligand–receptor interactions in terms of "specific" and "nonspecific" macromolecular perturbations.

Differences in binding mechanisms are further revealed by a more detailed examination of the $\delta \Delta H$ and $\delta \Delta S$ contributions (Table IV-48, Fig. IV-24). These reveal that at $\delta \Delta S = 0$ the enthalpy contribution to interaction in the C_2–C_5 series is practically zero indicating that the interaction is almost exclusively entropy driven: furthermore, in this series the relative contributions to $\delta \Delta H$ and $\delta \Delta S$ are not uniform. In the C_6–C_{10} series interaction is characterized by very minor changes in $\delta \Delta H$ accompanied by regular increases in $\delta \Delta S$. According to Belleau (241) the negligible differences observed in the series $\text{Me}_4\overset{+}{\text{N}} \rightarrow \text{Pr}^n\overset{+}{\text{N}}\text{Me}_3$ indicates that interaction is determined primarily by the quaternary ammonium function. However, the transition from $\text{Pr}^n\overset{+}{\text{N}}\text{Me}_3 \rightarrow \text{Bu}^n\overset{+}{\text{N}}\text{Me}_3$ which is characterized by $\delta \Delta H$ and $\delta \Delta S$ values of 1400 cal mole^{-1} and 5 e.u. respectively suggests the appearance of a new interaction associated with the introduction of the terminal methyl group: this might be interpreted as the melting of one mole of ice ($\Delta S = 5$ e.u., $\Delta H = 1400$ cal mole^{-1}) but as noted previously (Chapter I, see section, p. 16) it is more probable that these thermodynamic values reflect the reorganization of several moles of water less structured than ice. However, it is particularly intriguing that the transition from $\text{Pr}^n\overset{+}{\text{N}}\text{Me}_3$ to $\text{Bu}^n\overset{+}{\text{N}}\text{Me}_3$ represents a marked increase in cholinomimetic activity in the alkylammonium series (Table IV-16) so that a particularly important role is assigned to this methyl group both in promoting water reorganization at acetylcholinesterase and stimulant activity at the cholinergic receptor.

The interaction of the C_6–C_{10} series is characterized by negligible (75 cal/CH_2 group) changes in $\delta\Delta H$ and $\delta\Delta S$ values of some 1·3 e.u./CH_2 group, thus indicating that this portion of the alkyl chain is interacting with a nonpolar area on the enzyme through a typical hydrophobic mechanism (Chapter I, see section, p. 16). As previously noted this

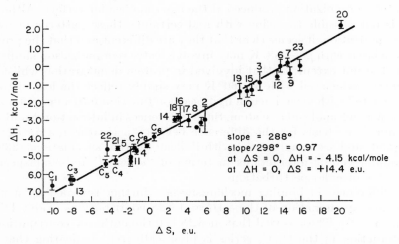

FIG. IV-25. Isoequilibrium plot for binding of the compounds listed in Table IV-49 to bovine erythrocyte acetylcholinesterase. Reproduced with permission of the National Research Council of Canada and the authors from Belleau and Lavoie, *Can. J. Biochem.* **46**, 1403 (1968).

switch in interaction mechanisms at the level of acetylcholinesterase finds its counterpart in the transition from activator to inhibitor ligands at the cholinergic receptor and accords with the general conclusion previously drawn (p. 246) that the polar:nonpolar molecular ratio in the ligand is a principal determinant of cholinomimetic activity.

An isoequilibrium relationship is also observed (242) with a series of functional trimethylammonium ligands (Fig. IV-25; Table IV-49) and, similarly to the C_2–C_6–$\overset{+}{N}Me_3$ series, β is found to be 288° K, again implicating the probable role of these ligands in the production of conformational change through the reorganization of water structure. However, unlike the alkyltrimethylammonium series the ΔH–ΔS couple

TABLE IV-49. Thermodynamic Parameters for Quaternary Ligand Interaction with Acetylcholinesterase at 25° C (242)

No.	Ligand	ΔF kcal mole^{-1}	ΔH kcal mole^{-1}	ΔS† e.u.
1	cycloButyl-$\overset{+}{N}$Me$_3$	−4·75	−3·1	+5·6
2	cycloPentyl-$\overset{+}{N}$Me$_3$	−4·79	−3·0	+5·9
3	cycloHexyl-$\overset{+}{N}$Me$_3$	−4·34	−0·85	+11·7
4	cycloHeptyl-$\overset{+}{N}$Me$_3$	−4·29	−4·65	−1·3
5	cycloOctyl-$\overset{+}{N}$Me$_3$	−4·44	−5·0	−1·9
6	2-Furyl-$\overset{+}{N}$Me$_3$	−4·80	−0·35	+14·9
7	5-Me-2-furyl-$\overset{+}{N}$Me$_3$	−4·46	−1·4	+10·4
8	L-1,3-Dioxolane-4-CH$_2\overset{+}{N}$Me$_3$	−3·98	−6·4	−8·1
9	D-1,3-Dioxolane-4-CH$_2\overset{+}{N}$Me$_3$	−3·78	−2·95	+2·7
10	L-cis-2-Me-1,3-dioxolane-4-CH$_2\overset{+}{N}$Me$_3$	−4·52	−1·3	+10·8
11	D-cis-2-Me-1,3-dioxolane-4-CH$_2\overset{+}{N}$Me$_3$	−3·85	−2·85	+3·4
12	L-trans-2-Me-1,3-dioxolane-4-CH$_2\overset{+}{N}$Me$_3$	−3·73	−2·75	+3·3
13	D-trans-2-Me-1,3-dioxolane-4-CH$_2\overset{+}{N}$Me$_3$	−3·76	−2·84	+3·1
14	L-Acetyl-β-Me-choline	−3·82	+2·2	+20·2
15	D-Acetyl-β-Me-choline	−3·58	−4·56	−3·29
16	2-Thienyl-$\overset{+}{N}$Me$_3$	−4·69	−5·25	−1·9

† $\Delta S_u = \Delta S + 7\cdot98$ (cratic term; Chapter I, see section, p. 16).

TABLE IV-50. Effects of Substituent and Chiral Changes on Thermodynamic Parameters of Quaternary Ligand Binding Interaction with Acetylcholinesterase (242)

Entry no.	Ligand pair (from Table IV-49)	Effect	$\delta\Delta H$ cal mole^{-1}	$\delta\Delta S$ e.u.
1	8–9	Config. inversion	+3400	+10·8
2	14–15	Config. inversion	+6500	+23·5
3	8–10	Addition of cis-Me (L)	+5100	+18·9
4	8–12	Addition of trans-Me (L)	+3400	+11·2
5	9–11	Addition of cis-Me (D)	+100	+0·7
6	9–13	Addition of trans-Me (D)	+100	+0·4
7	6–16	Replacement of >0 by >S	−4900	−16·8

in this ligand series is markedly sensitive to substituent and chiral changes that would be anticipated to produce only small effects in the absence of specific interactions with the protein surface. A number of such effects are listed in Table IV-50. Thus inversion of configuration in the dioxolane (No. 1) or acetyl-β-methylcholine series (No. 2) has large positive effects on both $\delta \Delta H$ and $\delta \Delta S$; addition of a *cis*- or *trans*-2 methyl group to the L-dioxolane series (Nos. 3 and 4) has similar effects on $\delta \Delta H$ and $\delta \Delta S$ whereas, in marked contrast the same substitutions in the D-dioxolane series (Nos. 5 and 6) has only small effects. Finally, replacement of oxygen by sulfur (No. 7) has very prominent and negative effects on $\delta \Delta H$ and $\delta \Delta S$.

It is, of course, of more than passing interest that these selected examples are also those in which the cholinomimetic activities of the ligands are also markedly sensitive to substituent or chiral character. As previously discussed (see section, p. 257) the L-isomers of the dioxolanes and acetyl-β-methylcholine are the most potent and the addition of a *cis*- or *trans*-2-methyl group to the L-dioxolanes also produces a marked increase in activity. It will be noted from Table IV-50 that these substituent changes are endergonic entropy driven processes indicating that these specified molecular variations produce particularly *specific* reorganizations of the water structure associated with the macromolecular system. In contrast comparison of the furan and thiophene ligands indicates that the sulfur substitution is exergonic but accompanied by an unfavorable entropy change suggesting that any perturbation of water structure achieved by the furan is not paralleled in the sulfur isostere. Again it is of interest that this substitution pattern is known to produce marked loss of (muscarinic) cholinomimetic potency but has lesser effect on nictonic activities. Certainly, oxygen–sulfur substitution is known to produce equally dramatic variations in other systems as, for example, in subtilisin and thiol-subtilisin (serine-OH $\rightarrow$ serine-SH) where the latter enzyme is completely inert towards natural substrates (243).

Finally, the isoequilibrium relationship suggests the nature of the quaternary ammonium group binding; from the isoequilibrium plot (Fig. IV-25) at $\Delta S = 0$, $\Delta H = -4 \cdot 15$ kcal mole^{-1} which represents, therefore, the enthalpic contribution of interaction of these ligands *in the absence of solvent interactions*. Since for tetramethylammonium $\Delta H = -6 \cdot 6$ kcal mole^{-1} and $\Delta S = -10 \cdot 1$ e.u. (Table IV-47) it follows that the differences, $\Delta H = -2 \cdot 5$ kcal mole^{-1} and $\Delta S = -10 \cdot 1$ e.u., must represent the reorientation of a water-sheath around the ammonium ion subsequent to its ionic binding interaction (242). Previous qualitative considerations from structure–activity data (p. 245) here also suggested the importance of nonpolar contributions to such ionic interactions.

STRUCTURE–ACTIVITY RELATIONSHIPS OF ANTAGONIST LIGANDS

From the molecular standpoint the fundamental rationale for the study of structure–activity data of antagonist ligands is the elucidation of the macromolecular structure and function of the sites at which these ligands interact. As with activator ligands it is, therefore, particularly important that attention be directed to sites at which the antagonist may bind and affect biological activity: this is important in both the relative sense of interactions within a given antagonist series and in the absolute sense of the relationship between activator and antagonist ligand binding sites. In a discussion of the various types of antagonism it is possible to establish, exactly as in the case of enzyme–substrate and enzyme–inhibitor interactions, formal mathematical representations of the various antagonisms which, quite generally, individually permit expression by more than one physical model.

A large body of agonist–antagonist interaction data can be said to describe a competitive interaction between the two ligands for the agonist binding site. This was specifically noted by Gaddum (244–247) and, using the notation of the section on Quantitative Treatments (p. 212), this type of antagonism may be described by eqn. XVIV for the fraction of receptors occupied by agonist (Y_A) in the presence of antagonist concentration $[B]$ with affinity constant K_B

$$Y_A = \frac{[RA]}{[R_{tot}]} = \frac{1}{1 + \dfrac{1}{K_A[A]} + \dfrac{K_B[B]}{K_A[A]}} \qquad \text{(XVIV)}$$

so that the fraction of receptors occupied by A and hence the apparent affinity of A is reduced by the factor $K_B[B]/K_A[A]$. In the simplest situation where only ligand A possesses agonist activity eqn. XVIV generates a simple set of parallel curves (Fig. IV-26) which show the characteristic features of competitive antagonism—the apparent reduction in affinity for A and the maintained ability of A to generate, at higher concentrations, the same intrinsic maximum response in the absence and presence of B.

To assign comparable quantitative parameters to competitively antagonistic ligands Clark and Raventos (248) suggested the use of a null method in which the concentration of antagonist required to alter by a given extent the amount of agonist to produce equal response is determined: if response is determined by Y_A then this proposal presumes, since equal responses are being compared, that the fraction of receptors occupied by the agonist in the presence and absence of the antagonist

11

remains constant. This concept forms the basis of the pA_x scale introduced by Schild (249, 250) to quantitatively define competitive antagonism: pA_x is defined as the negative logarithm of the molar concentration

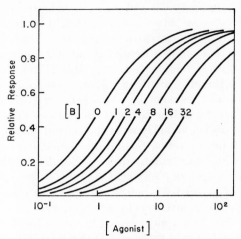

FIG. IV-26. Theoretical concentration–response curves of agonist A in the presence of the competitive antagonist B at varying concentrations indicated ($K_A = K_B = 1$). Reproduced with permission from Ariëns (12).

of an antagonist that will reduce the effect of a multiple concentration (x) of an agonist to that of a unit concentration,

$$pA_x = -\log_{10}[B]_x \qquad \textbf{(XX)}$$

$$= \log_{10} K_B - \log_{10}(x - 1) \qquad \textbf{(XXI)}$$

so that when x = 2,

$$pA_x = \log_{10}K_B \qquad \textbf{(XXII)}$$

and a plot of $\log_{10}(x - 1)$ against pA_x should yield a straight line with intercept equal to $\log_{10} K_B$ provided that the reaction is bimolecular. The dose ratio (DR) which is defined as the concentration by which the agonist, in the presence of antagonist, needs to be increased to generate the standard response (252) is directly related: if it is assumed that the fraction of receptors occupied by antagonist, B, is Y_B then that proportion available for agonists is $1 - Y_B$ and if the effect of the agonist is proportional both to its concentration and to $1 - Y_B$ then the standard response can be generated, in the presence of B, by increasing the agonist concentration by $1/(1 - Y_B)$. Thus,

$$DR = \frac{1}{(1 - Y_B)} \qquad \textbf{(XXIII)}$$

Clearly when $DR = 2$, that concentration of antagonist has occupied 50 per cent of the receptors and is equal to pA_2.

A second major class of antagonist interactions may be described as noncompetitive implying that competition between the agonist and antagonist does not exist, that, in the simplest sense, there are separate recognition sites for the agonist and antagonist ligands and that inter-action of the antagonist hinders or prevents effective interaction of the agonist ligand at its recognition site. Ariëns has produced a detailed treatment of this type of interaction mechanism in which the concen-tration of antagonist–receptor complex is given by

$$[R_B B] = \frac{[R_{tot}]}{1 + \dfrac{1}{K_B[B]}} \tag{XXIV}$$

and with the assumption that the change in r_A as a result of the for-mation of $R_B B$ is proportional to the concentration of the latter species, then

$$r_{AB} = r_A \left(1 + \frac{[R_{tot}]\beta}{1 + \dfrac{1}{K_B[B]}} \right) \tag{XXV}$$

where β is a coefficient, analogous to intrinsic activity, describing the modulating effect of $R_B B$ formation upon the "apparent" intrinsic activity of A. Some representative concentration–response curves plotted from eqn. XXV are presented in Fig. IV-27. It must be recog-nized, however, that the description of noncompetitive antagonism in receptor systems is apt to be substantially more complex than for enzyme systems for according to eqn. I (p. 211) the initial agonist–receptor interaction sets into operation a sequence of linked events: interference by the antagonist of steps subsequent to the primary interaction will also generate noncompetitive systems and, furthermore, the assumptions made in the deduction of eqn. XXIV, that the change in r_A is proportional to $R_B[B]$ may not be true for all antagonist species or the proportionality factor may vary between antagonists even when interaction occurs at a common site.

It is to be emphasized also that the concept of competitive interaction between agonist and antagonist does not necessarily imply physical competition for the same binding site. Monod et al. (253) have indicated very specifically in their discussion of allosteric proteins (Chapter I, see section, p. 82) that

... an allosteric effector, since it binds at a site altogether distinct from the active site and since it does not participate at any stage in the reaction activated by the protein, need not bear any particular chemical or metabolic relation of any sort with the substrate itself.

This is a point of considerable importance for it will become quite apparent that many antagonists of acetylcholine and norepinephrine have, at best, a distant structural relationship to the agonist ligands. That such "peripheral" antagonist binding sites may be relatively common is not surprising given the principles of macromolecular organization outlined previously (Chapter I, p. 1) in which only a small fraction of the protein residues are directly involved in the active site binding pattern. Accordingly significant areas of the remaining

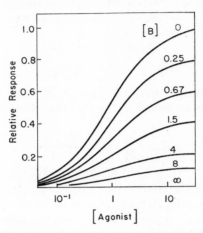

FIG. IV-27. Theoretical concentration–response curves of agonist A in the presence of the noncompetitive antagonist B at varying concentrations indicated. Reproduced with permission from Ariëns (12).

protein may be available for binding of other ligands whose interaction is likely to perturb the delicate pattern of intermolecular interactions serving to maintain the native functionality of the macromolecular system. This is likely to be of particular importance for receptor sites which constitute part of the cell membrane.

ANTAGONISTS TO ADRENERGIC RECEPTOR-MEDIATED RESPONSES

Substantial effort has been expended in the search for antagonists to the responses initiated at both the α- and β-adrenergic receptors (254–258). However, from the standpoint of structure–activity analyses, many of the compounds investigated have not been of great utility, primarily because their sites and mechanisms of action remain to be elucidated and because in many cases a very limited number of compounds have been investigated.

It is interesting to note that a rather diverse collection of molecular structures serves as antagonists of α-receptor mediated responses

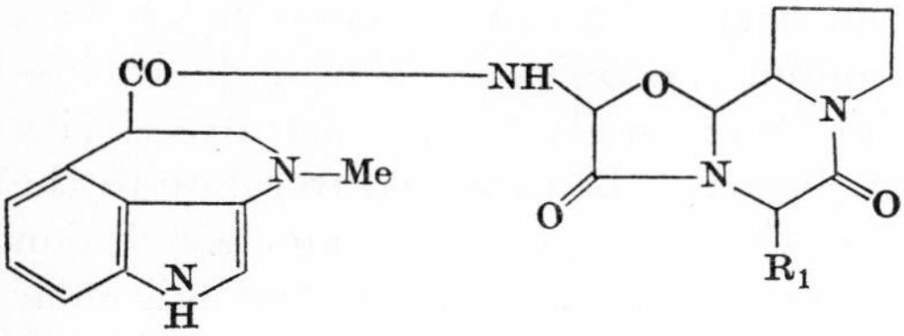

IV-43   (259, 260)

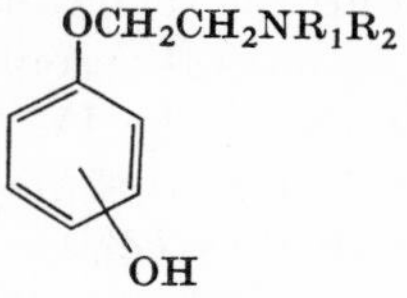

IV-44   (261, 262)

$R_1 = H, Me, R_2 = H, Me$

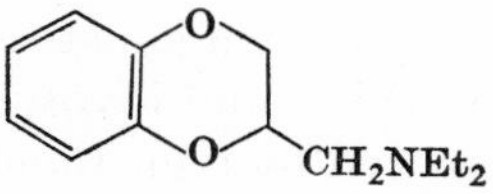

IV-45   (262, 263)

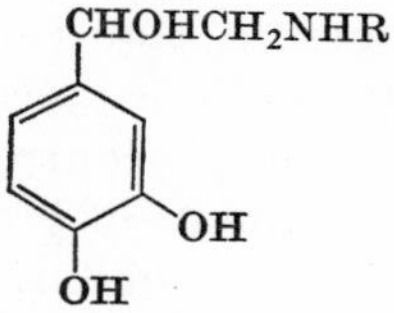

IV-46

(PhCH$_2$)$_2$NCH$_2$CH$_2$Cl

IV-47   (264)

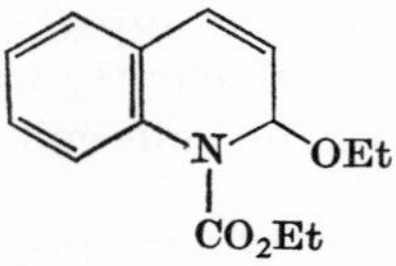

IV-48   (265)

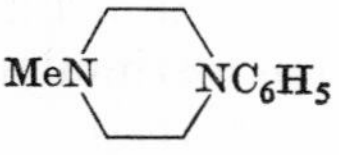

IV-49   (266)

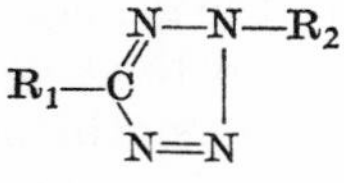

IV-50   (R$_1$, R$_2$ = alkyl, aryl, 267)

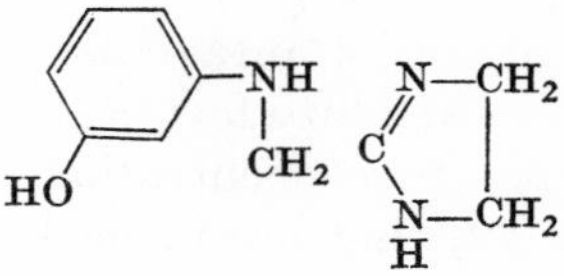

IV-51   (268)

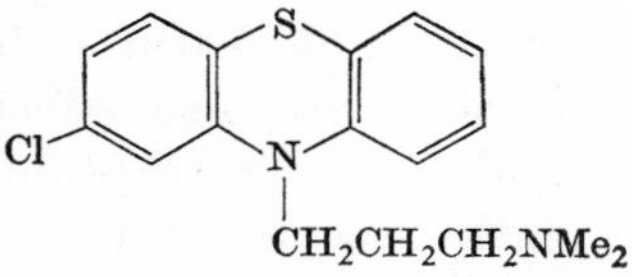

IV-52   (269)

FIG. IV-28. Structural formulae of some adrenergic α-receptor antagonists.

(Fig. IV-28) whilst antagonists of β-receptor mediated responses are (to date) a relatively select group of agents bearing a generally obvious structural resemblance to the potent β-agonist, N-isopropylnorepinephrine (Fig. IV-49). For the latter agents analyses of structure–activity relationships may, with some justification, be expected to relate to the site of catecholamine interaction at the β-receptor. The same conclusion cannot be drawn for the majority of α-antagonists where the molecular resemblance to norepinephrine is minimal; for these agents it is highly probable that their structure–activity relationships refer to sites other than the agonist binding site but at which modulation of some stage or stages in the sequence of events initiated by the agonist–receptor interaction can occur. As discussed previously this could involve direct or allosteric control of any of the steps represented by eqn. I and hence the number of potential sites of interaction is rather large. For such agents the analysis of structure–activity relationships is not likely to be particularly helpful unless some evidence concerning their sites of interaction is available. For these reasons the subsequent discussion of adrenergic antagonists will be directed towards those agents which have been sufficiently well investigated to permit at least some deductions to be made concerning their site of action.

Adrenergic α-Receptor Antagonists

A partial listing of the molecular structures reported effective in antagonizing α-receptor mediated responses is presented in Fig. IV-28. Among the structures listed, the transition from α-stimulant to α-antagonistic activities in catecholamines with progressive bulk of N-substitution (IV-46) has been discussed previously (p. 224): it seems quite probable that these compounds act by competition for the agonist binding site proper. However, it is highly relevant to the general understanding of antagonist interactions that such antagonists as catecholamines, benzodioxans and promethazine and related phenothiazines all generate concentration–response curves against norepinephrine (Fig. IV-29) that are typical of competitive interaction (270) although it is obviously improbable that they all interact at a common binding site with norepinephrine. Indeed, one of the most remarkable features about antagonists such as chlorpromazine is that they are also effective antagonists against acetylcholine, histamine and 5-hydroxytryptamine, suggesting quite strongly that they bind to "extra-receptor" areas (270) that may be structurally similar for a number of receptors.

Undoubtedly, the best investigated class of antagonists are the 2-halogenoethylamines (e.g., Dibenamine, IV-47; see Fig. IV-28): because of their importance as pharmacological tools in receptor classification, ligand–receptor quantitation, etc., they will form a

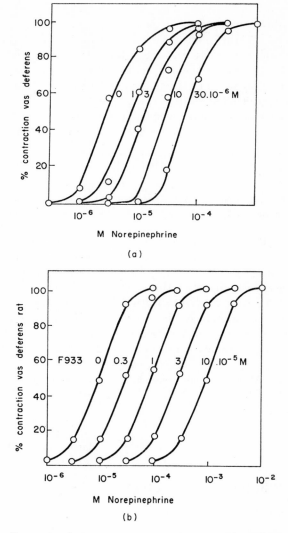

FIG. IV-29. A. Concentration–response curves for norepinephrine in the presence of increasing concentrations (as indicated) of phenothiazine (N-substituent is $\overset{+}{C}H_2CH(Me)CH_2NMe_2Et$). B. In the presence of 2-piperidinomethyl-1,4-benzo-dioxan. Reproduced with permission from Ariëns (12).

principal focus of discussion in this section. The remaining structures (IV-43–IV-46 and IV-48–IV-52; see Fig. IV-28) will not receive any significant attention.

The 2-Halogenoethylamines. The α-antagonistic properties of N,N-dibenzyl-2-chloroethylamine (Dibenamine) were first reported by Nickerson (264, 271) who emphasized the characteristic slow onset and prolonged duration of action and suggested, by analogy with the nitrogen mustards (272–274), that the etyleniminium ion derived from Dibenamine should be regarded as the pharmacologically active species acting to alkylate a constituent group of the α-receptor (Fig. IV-30). That these conclusions are essentially correct has been demonstrated by a number of workers (for reviews see references 255, 256, 275–278) who have

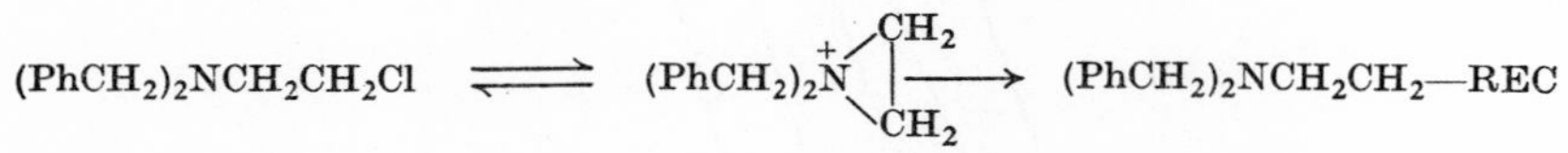

$$(PhCH_2)_2NCH_2CH_2Cl \rightleftharpoons (PhCH_2)_2\overset{+}{N}\underset{CH_2}{\overset{CH_2}{|}} \longrightarrow (PhCH_2)_2NCH_2CH_2—REC$$

Fig. IV-30. The reaction of N,N-dibenzyl-2-chloroethylamine, through the intermediate etyleniminium ion, to give an alkylated receptor.

demonstrated that only those compounds that can generate the etyleniminium ion produce the characteristic antagonism produced by Dibenamine: the structural requirements for etyleniminium ion formation are essentially that there be a relatively easily displaceable group (Cl, Br, I, mesyl, tosyl, etc.) situated *beta* to an appropriately basic amino function, nondisplaceable groups (β-OH, —OC_2H_5; CN etc.) or greatly reduced basicity of the amino function (N-benzyl-N-2-chloroethylaniline) lead to inactive compounds (275, 279, 280). However, the

TABLE IV-51. Antinorepinephrine Activities of N-(o-, m- or p-) Chlorobenzyl-N-ethyl-2-chloroethylamines and the Derived Etyleniminium Ions (286)

Compound	ED_{50} Rat bp preparation g moles/kg $\times 10^6$
2-$ClC_6H_4CH_2N(C_2H_5)CH_2CH_2Cl$	23·9
E^+ ion	0·66
3-$ClC_6H_4CH_2N(C_2H_5)CH_2CH_2Cl$	4·9
E^+ ion	0·85
4-$ClC_6H_4CH_2N(C_2H_5)CH_2CH_2Cl$	36·6
E^+ ion	1·22

converse of this argument, that all etyleniminium ions are active, is not true and thus etyleniminium ion formation is a necessary, but not a sufficient prerequisite, for irreversible α-antagonism. Sodium thiosulfate, known to react rapidly with etyleniminium ions (281, 282), prevents the establishment of irreversible antagonism, but does not reverse an established blockade (283–285). Impressive evidence that the ethyleniminium ion derived from the 2-halogenoethylamines is the pharmacologically active species has been obtained by Graham (286), who has been able to demonstrate a quantitative relationship between the anti-norepinephrine and anti-epinephrine activities of 2-halogeno-ethylamines in terms of the concentration of the derived ethyleni-minium ion (Figs IV-31, IV-32). Graham has also demonstrated that the

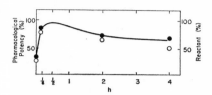

FIG. IV-31. The relationship between ethyleniminium ion concentrations and anti-norepinephrine (○) and anti-epinephrine (●) activities of *N*-*p*-chlorobenzyl-*N*-ethyl-2-chloroethylamine. Reproduced with permission from Graham (286).

ethyleniminium ions, isolated as the picrylsulfonates (287, 288) from the *N*-(*o*-, *m*- or *p*-) chlorobenzyl-2-chloroethylamines, are more potent than the parent 2-halogenoethylamines (Table IV-51). There have been many demonstrations (277) that the hydrolysis products (alcohols, piper-azinium and other quaternary salts) are inactive.

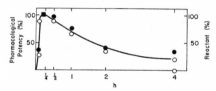

FIG. IV-32. The relationship between ethyleniminium ion centrations and anti-norepinephrine (○) and anti-epinephrine (●) activities of *N*-ethyl-*N*-(9-fluorenyl) 2-chloroethylamine. Reproduced with permission from Graham (286).

Since the discovery of Dibenamine a very large number of more or less structurally related agents have been investigated. However, from the point of view of elucidating a molecularly significant structure–activity relationship a number of difficulties are encountered. Much of the pharmacological data refers to different tissues and species and hence it is often impossible to cross-correlate data save for a few widely used compounds. From Graham's data and from the nonreactive com-pounds cited (p. 290), which do not exhibit any significant α-antagonism even of the competitive kind, it seems clear that the initial interaction of the 2-halogenoethylamine at its binding site(s) is as the ethyleniminium

11*

ion rather than as the parent compound. Thus, in comparing activities it is essential that attention be given to relative rates of cyclization to and hydrolysis of ethyleniminium ions.

This problem has been fairly extensively studied (280, 285, 286–290): as anticipated, the ease of displacement of halide ion from a 2-halogeno-ethylamine lies in the order $I > Br > Cl \gg F$, although the final extent of

TABLE IV-52. Adrenergic Blocking Activity of 2-Halogenoethylamines (255)
$ARCH_2N(C_2H_5)CH_2CH_2X$

			Activities in rat bp preparation	
Ar	X	Max. X⁻ liberated	Anti-epinephrine ED_{50} g moles $\times 10^6$	Anti-norepinephrine ED_{50} g moles $\times 10^6$
4-ClC_6H_4	Cl	71	36·6	39·6
4-ClC_6H_4	Br	98	3·5	5·3
4-ClC_6H_4	I	95	4·1	4·9
3-ClC_6H_4	Cl	61	49·0	6·0
3-ClC_6H_4	Br	95	2·1	2·2
3-ClC_6H_4	I	90	1·6	1·4
2-ClC_6H_4	Cl	70	23·9	22·1
2-ClC_6H_4	Br	98	2·1	2·6
2-ClC_6H_4	I	93 (500 min)	1·5	2·1
9-Fluorenyl	Cl	56	0·32	0·45
9-Fluorenyl	Br	100	0·06	0·10
9-Fluorenyl	I	88	0·03	0·04
1-$C_{10}H_7$	Cl	87	0·60	—
1-$C_{10}H_7$	Br	100	0·62	—
1-$C_{10}H_7$	I	100	0·12	—
2-$C_{10}H_7$	Cl	77	31·3	—
2-$C_{10}H_7$	Br	100	14·2	—
2-$C_{10}H_7$	I	99	9·6	—
$PhCHXCH_2N(CH_2Ph)_2$	Cl	96	2·4	1·1
	Br	79	1·53	1·74
	I	34 (360 min)	0·34	0·22

release may show a partial of this order, and this generally reflects the order of pharmacological activity (Table IV-52). However, there is obviously no correlation of cyclization rates and pharmacological activity from one series of compounds to another.

The production of irreversible antagonism by the derived ethyleni-minium ion is dependent upon two factors: the affinity (k_1/k_2) of the ion for the binding site and the rate of alkylation (k_3) by the bound ion

(Fig. IV-33). Thus, both K_I (k_1/k_2) and k_3 are to be considered as controlling the structure–activity relationship of 2-halogenoethyl-amines. Kinetic techniques, developed by Kitz and Wilson (291) and Main (292, 293) for the irreversible inactivation of acetylcholinesterase

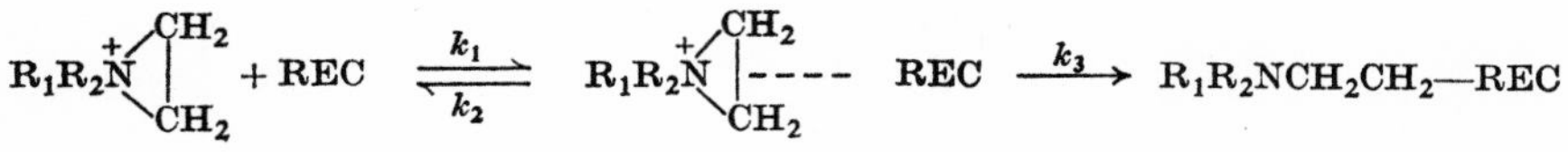

$$\begin{array}{c}
\underset{CH_2}{\overset{CH_2}{R_1R_2\overset{+}{N}}} + REC \underset{k_2}{\overset{k_1}{\rightleftharpoons}} \underset{CH_2}{\overset{CH_2}{R_1R_2\overset{+}{N}}} ---- REC \overset{k_3}{\longrightarrow} R_1R_2NCH_2CH_2\text{—}REC
\end{array}$$

FIG. IV-33. Receptor alkylation by an ethyleniminium ion.

and applied to a number of similar processes (293a,b–294) are available to obtain separate values of K_I and k_3 for irreversible antagonists. The velocity of irreversible inactivation within the macromolecule–antagonist complex is given by,

$$V = k_3[R\text{---}I] \tag{XXVI}$$

and from eqn. XXIV

$$r = \frac{k_3[R_{tot}]}{K_I/[I] + 1} \tag{XXVII}$$

and since

$$k_{obs} = \frac{V}{[R_{tot}]} \tag{XXVIII}$$

where k_{obs} is the observed first-order rate constant of inactivation then,

$$k_{obs} = \frac{k_3}{K_I/[I] + 1} = \frac{k_3[I]}{K_I + [I]} \tag{XXIX}$$

and

$$\frac{1}{k_{obs}} = \frac{K_I}{k_3} \cdot \frac{1}{[I]} + \frac{1}{k_3} \tag{XXX}$$

so that a plot of $1/k_{obs}$ versus $1/[I]$ should generate a straight line of slope K_I/k_3 and intercept $1/k_3$.

The importance of determining k_3 and K_I for irreversibly acting agents is well demonstrated by the data of Schaeffer (294, 295) for the inactivation of adenosine deaminase by IV-53–IV-55 (Table IV-53): if comparisons of "inhibitory activity" had been made at only one inhibitor concentration (0·1 mM) then the order of effectiveness would be $55 > 54 > 53$ but at 0·03 mM the order of effectiveness would be $55 > 53 > 54$. This is simply because k_{obs} is a function of both K_I and k_3 so that unless K_I happens to be equal for a series of compounds it is unjustifiable and misleading to simply utilize the observed inactivation rates as a measure of inhibitory activity.

To date this procedure has not been applied to antagonists of receptors and a number of complicating factors appear to obviate its immediate applicability. As noted previously (p. 212) the relationship between receptor occupancy and response is presumed by many workers

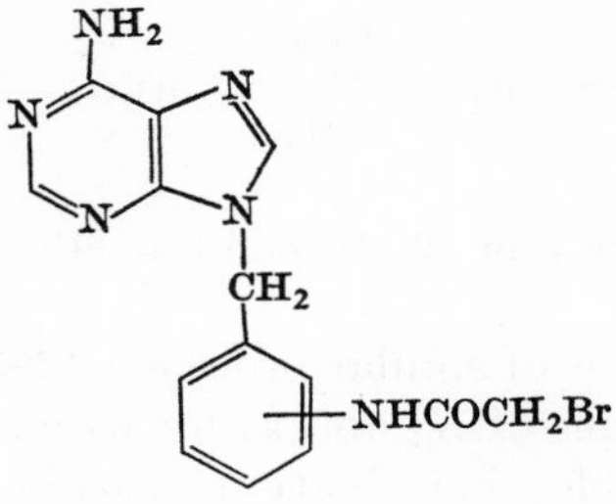

IV-53 *p*-isomer
IV-54 *o*-isomer
IV-55 *m*-isomer

to be complex so that the kinetics of loss of response may not be directly relatable to the kinetics of receptor alkylation. More serious, however, are the findings that these irreversible α-receptor antagonists can

TABLE IV-53. Kinetic Constants for Reversible and Irreversible Inhibition of Adenosine Deaminase (294, 295)

Compound	$k_3 \times 10^2$[†] min^{-1}	$K_I \times 10^5$ M
IV-53	1·1	1·4
IV-54	7·7	43
IV-55	28	72

† The use of 4-(*p*-nitrobenzyl)pyridine as the nucleophilic reagent reveals that all three compounds have similar reactivities (294, 295). Thus the differences found in the enzyme system are presumably due to different orientations in the complex.

eliminate the agonist-induced response by interaction at more than one site: thus the kinetics of inactivation will be a complex reflection of the several K_I and k_3 constants involved in the interactions.

Thus much of the discussion of the 2-halogenoethylamines as α-receptor antagonists has to be on a qualitative basis although this does not mean that useful information has not been obtained.

Structure–Activity Relationships of 2-Halogenoethylamines. Little purpose
would be served here by attempting either to list all of the 2-halogeno-
ethylamines synthesized and examined as α-antagonists or to discuss all

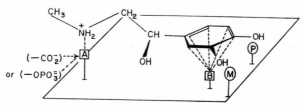

FIG. IV-34. Presumed interaction of epinephrine at the adrenergic α-receptor
according to Belleau (296).

of the attempts to define structure–activity relationships. Rather,
attention will be focused on the more important developments in the
field.

A comprehensive rationalization of the action of these agents was first
advanced by Belleau in 1958 (296) in a treatment containing the basic

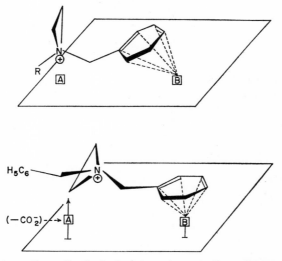

FIG. IV-35. Interaction of ethyleniminium ion at the adrenergic α-receptor
showing the rearrangement of the initially formed complex to the transition state
for alkylation. Reproduced with permission from Belleau (296).

assumption that interaction occurs at the norepinephrine binding site of
the α-receptor. (This basic assumption will be examined in detail in a
subsequent section.) According to Belleau's treatment the interaction

of norepinephrine at the α-receptor is as represented in Fig. IV-34: attachment of the ethyleniminium ion is presumed to occur initially through the interaction shown in Fig. IV-35a, a binding configuration presumed to rearrange slowly to the complex shown in Fig. IV-35b, best

TABLE IV-54. Structure, Predicted and Observed Activities of Dibenamine Analogs (296)

$$ArCH_2N(C_2H_5)CH_2CH_2Cl$$

	Substituent character	Steric compatibility	Predicted activity	Observed activity
Ar = 2-$CH_3C_6H_4$	+I	+	act.	act.
2-$CH_3OC_6H_4$	+E, −I	+	act.	act.
4-$CH_3OC_6H_4$	+E, −I	+	act.	inact.
3-$CF_3C_6H_4$	−I	+	act.	act.
3-ClC_6H_4	−I, +E	+	act.	act.
4-$C_2H_5C_6H_4$	+I	−	inact.	inact.
4-ClC_6H_4	−I, +E	?	inact.	slight act.
3,4-$(CH_3O)_2C_6H_3$	+E, +E	+	slight act.	slight act.
3,4-$(CH_2O)_2C_6H_3$	+E, +E	+	act.	slight act.
	$(ArCH_2)N(CH_2Ph)CH_2CH_2Cl$			
Ar = 2-$CH_3OC_6H_4$	+E	+	act.	act.
3-$CF_3C_6H_4$	−I	+	act.	slight act.
3-IC_6H_4	−I, +E	−	act.	act.
4-$CH_3C_6H_4$	+I	+	act.	act.
4-$CH_3OC_6H_4$	+E, −I	+	act.	act.
3,4-$(CH_3O)_2C_6H_3$	+E, +E	+	act.	act.
3,4-$(CH_2O)_2C_6H_3$	+E, +E	+	act.	slight act.
	$(ArCH_2)_2NCH_2CH_2Cl$			
Ar = 2-$CH_3C_6H_4$	+I	+	act.	act.
3-$CH_3C_6H_4$	+I	+	act.	act.
3-$CF_3C_6H_4$	−I	+	act.	slight act.
3-ClC_6H_4	−I, +E	+	act.	slight act.
4-$CH_3C_6H_4$	+I	+	act.	act.
4-$C_2H_5C_6H_4$	+I	−	inact.	inact.
4-$CH_3OC_6H_4$	+E, −I	+	act.	act.
2,4-$Cl_2C_6H_3$	−I, −I, +E	?	inact.	inact.
3,4-$Cl_2C_6H_3$	−I, −I, +E	?	inact.	inact.

represented as the transition state for the alkylation process and which satisfies those geometrical requirements (the phenylethylamine pattern of Fig. IV-34) presumed to be important for effective agonist interaction. According to this proposal the effects of substituents in the aromatic ring of the antagonists should, apart from any chelation or other chemical reaction that the catechol nucleus might undergo (see section, p. 228), approximate the phenolic groups in steric and electronic characteristics. Belleau argued that steric interactions should be progressively less important in the *para-*, *meta-* and *ortho-*positions and, furthermore, that

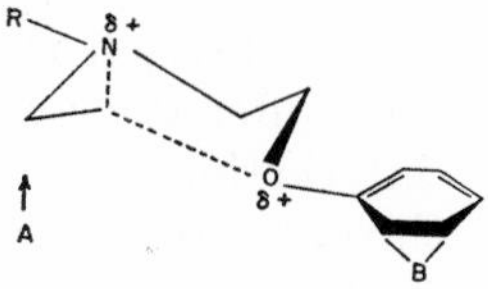

FIG. IV-36. The stabilization of the ethyleniminium ion from phenoxybenzamine to preserve the phenylethylamine pattern.

Dibenamine analogs carrying substituents in only one phenyl ring will be capable of interacting with site B through either ring and hence avoid unfavorable substituent interactions. From these arguments a number

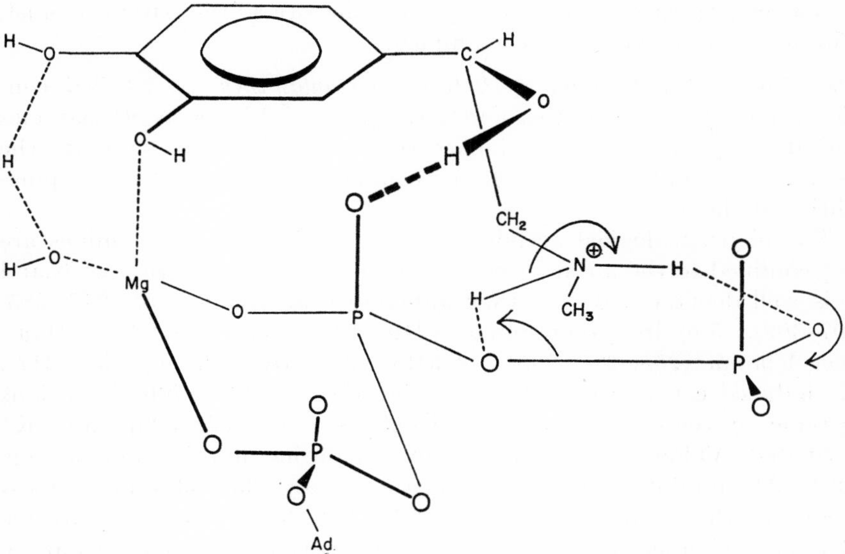

FIG. IV-37. The process of α-agonism according to Bloom and Goldman (299) in which epinephrine catalyses the hydrolysis of ATP on a phosphorolytic enzyme surface (not shown).

of fairly satisfying qualitative correlations of structure and activity were obtained (Table IV-54). The increased activity of Dibenamine analogs with polynuclear or heteronuclear aromatic residues was rationalized on the basis that interaction with site B increased with electron density. The high activity of N-alkyl(or alkaryl)-N-2-phenoxy-ethyl-2-halogenoethylamines (phenoxybenzamine analogs) which appear not to fit the phenylethylamine pattern are accommodated on the basis of the transition state shown in Fig. IV-36 where the phenyl-ethylamine pattern is maintained through a $\overset{\delta+}{C}$---O interaction (297, 298). Bloom and Goldman (299) have offered a rather different concept of the norepinephrine–α-receptor interaction in which it is assumed that the catecholamine promotes, through hydrogen-bonding and ion-pairing functions (300–302), the hydrolysis of ATP (by a "metaphosphate" type mechanism) bound as a Mg^{++} complex to an ATPase (Fig. IV-37). Since monoesters are much more susceptible to attack by external nucleophiles than diesters (303–306) it was argued that the 2-halogenoethyl-amines functioned through alkylation of the terminal phosphate of ATP thus converting it to a stabilized diester analog. Despite the fundamental differences between the original treatment of Belleau and that of Bloom and Goldman both involve the fundamental assumption that the 2-halogenoethylamines interact at the same site as the parent agonist. This assumption will now be examined.

The Site(s) of Interaction of 2-Halogenoethylamines. A detailed consideration of the activities and structures of 2-halogenoethylamines reveals surprisingly little evidence that unambiguously supports the assumption that these agents share a common binding site with norepinephrine at the α-receptor.

The pharmacological activities of many 2-halogenoethylamines are not confined to the antagonism of adrenergic α-receptor responses and it is well documented that they antagonize histamine (255, 277, 285, 307–309), 5-hydroxytryptamine (246, 255, 277, 285, 310, 311a), acetylcholine (255, 277, 285, 312–316), vasoactive polypeptides (317), K^+-induced contractures of smooth muscle (318–321), inhibit various enzyme systems including acetylcholinesterase (322–325), Na^+–K^+ activated ATPase (326) inhibit norepinephrine uptake and storage (327–334), inhibit base-transport in the kidney (335–337) and possess local anesthetic properties (255, 285, 312, 322, 338). The diverse character of processes affected by these agents would appear to argue quite strongly against their interacting specifically with each ligand binding site: interaction at a site common to all of these processes is possible but unlikely since a universal structure–activity relationship is not observed. Thus it is likely that at least a part of the biological activity of these agents is best attributed to a relatively nonspecific binding at a variety of macromolecular sites producing antagonism by nonspecific allosteric interactions (253). The relative contribution of any particular interaction to antagonism of a particular ligand-induced

TABLE IV-55. Agonist Protection Against Irreversible Inactivation (311, 312)

Agonist	g/ml	Antagonist	g/ml	Tissue	% Remaining sensitivity
Norepinephrine	0	Dibenamine	10^{-6}	Rabbit aortic strip	~0
Norepinephrine	3×10^{-5}	Dibenamine	10^{-6}	Rabbit aortic strip	7–30
Epinephrine	0	Dibenamine	3×10^{-6}	Rabbit aortic strip	0
Epinephrine	10^{-4}	Dibenamine	3×10^{-6}	Rabbit aortic strip	3–114
Isopropylnorepinephrine	0	Dibenamine	10^{-6}	Rabbit aortic strip	0
Isopropylnorepinephrine	10^{-4}	Dibenamine	10^{-6}	Rabbit aortic strip	10
Histamine	0	Dibenamine	3×10^{-6}	Rabbit aortic strip	~0
Histamine	10^{-4}	Dibenamine	3×10^{-6}	Rabbit aortic strip	2–100
Acetylcholine	0	Dibenamine	10^{-5}	Rabbit aortic strip	~0
Acetylcholine	10^{-3}	Dibenamine	10^{-5}	Rabbit aortic strip	6–33
5-Hydroxytryptamine	0	Dibenamine	10^{-6}	Rabbit aortic strip	~0
5-Hydroxytryptamine	10^{-4}	Dibenamine	10^{-6}	Rabbit aortic strip	1–10
Epinephrine	0	Phenoxybenzamine	5×10^{-8}	Cat spleen	~0
Epinephrine	10^{-4}	Phenoxybenzamine	5×10^{-8}	Cat spleen	30–81 (45)
5-Hydroxytryptamine	0	Phenoxybenzamine	5×10^{-8}	Cat spleen	~0
5-Hydroxytryptamine	5×10^{-3}	Phenoxybenzamine	5×10^{-8}	Cat spleen	12–81 (30)
Acetylcholine	0	Phenoxybenzamine	5×10^{-8}	Cat slpeen	~0
Acetylcholine	10^{-4}	Phenoxybenzamine	5×10^{-8}	Cat spleen	50–85 (65)
Histamine	0	Phenoxybenzamine	5×10^{-8}	Cat spleen	~0
Histamine	10^{-4}	Phenoxybenzamine	5×10^{-8}	Cat spleen	21–100 (50)

response would be anticipated to depend upon the ligand in question.

Much of the evidence normally cited to support the concept of a common interaction site is based very largely on protection experiments in which it is found that the agonist offers protection against inactivation by the antagonist (Table IV-55) and that cross-protection (i.e., protection by norepinephrine or histamine against inactivation of the response to acetylcholine does not occur (Table IV-56): many other examples of protection will be found scattered throughout pharmacological literature. The interpretation of such experiments is, however,

TABLE IV-56. Cross-protection by Agonists Against Irreversible Interaction (311)

	Residual response to agonist (% control)†						
	E		5-HT		ACh		Hist	
Protecting agent	U†	P†	U	P	U	P	U	P
E (10^{-4} g/ml)	1	45	~0	78	—	—	—	—
5-HT (5×10^{-3} g/ml)	1	23	~0	30	~0	~0	~0	~0
ACh (10^{-4} g/ml)	2	1	~0	~0	5	65	0	0
Hist (10^{-4} g/ml)	1	2	0	0	0	2	0	50

† Cat spleen preparation; U, unprotected; P, protected. E, epinephrine; 5-HT, 5-hydroxytryptamine; ACh, acetylcholine; Hist, histamine.

ambiguous as was explicitly recognized by Waud in 1962 (339, 340). The degree of protection observed is often low and usually extremely variable: furthermore, the concentrations of protecting agent (agonist) employed are understandably very high since the competition is between a reversible and an irreversible reaction. However, at such high concentrations it is not possible to assume that the agonist interaction is confined solely to the receptor and hence protection against the antagonist must be occurring at many additional sites. Thus protection of the response may well occur from protection of both receptor and nonreceptor sites. Reversible α-receptor antagonists such as phentolamine (IV-51; see Fig. IV-28) afford better and more consistent protection against inactivation by the irreversible antagonists (341, 342): Patil et al. (342) found that phentolamine (3×10^{-7} M) afforded almost complete protection against loss of the α-receptor response in the rat vas deferens from Dibenamine (10^{-6} M, 10 min). However, the pharmacological protection offered in such experiments represents but a small fraction of the total alkylation of the tissue (Table IV-57; also 343, 344).

Furthermore, since it is not established whether phentolamine acts at the norepinephrine recognition site of the α-receptor the fact that it affords pharmacological protection against the irreversible antagonists does not determine the site of action of the latter agents. The cross-protection experiments described previously are similarly ambiguous for it must be recognized that the receptor sites for neurotransmitter molecules are, of

TABLE IV-57. ^{3}H-Phenoxybenzamine† Labelling of Protected and Unprotected Rat Seminal Vesicle (341)

Protecting agent	Tissue radioactivity dpm/g ±SE
None	13,659 ± 599
Phentolamine (1 μg/ml)‡	11,496 ± 525
Norepinephrine (100 μg/ml)§	11,687 ± 1964

† 0·1 μg/ml/10 min.
‡ Almost complete pharmacological protection.
§ $\simeq$ 20% pharmacological protection offered relative to control.

necessity, highly specific in their recognition capabilities so that cross-interaction of different ligands at these sites is unlikely to occur even in elevated concentrations. It is also to be anticipated that nonreceptor sites occupied at higher concentrations of agonists will also be discriminatory in their binding capabilities so that the absence of cross-protection by, for example, norepinephrine, of acetylcholine-induced responses is scarcely surprising and is not uniquely interpretable in terms of specific antagonist binding at receptor sites. It is also of interest that several studies (343, 344) of the uptake of labelled 2-halogenoethyl-amines into tissues shows no detectable break (Fig. IV-38) at the concentrations which are effective in antagonizing the response.

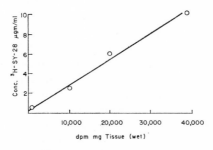

FIG. IV-38. The uptake of ^{3}H-SY-28 into rabbit vas deferens as a function of concentration.

The general absence (but see section on p. 308) of any gross structural relationship between the 2-halogenoethylamines and the various agonists which they antagonize has already received a general comment. A more detailed view strengthens further the previous suggestions: in considering the actions of quaternary ethyleniminium ions it is most unlikely that they bind at the site occupied by the primary or secondary ammonium function of norepinephrine or epinephrine for it is well established that increased N-substitution markedly decreases α-stimulant activity (p. 224) and the quaternary analog of norepinephrine $(3,4(HO)_2C_6H_3CHOH\ CH_2\overset{+}{N}Me_3)$ is devoid of activity (68). Quite

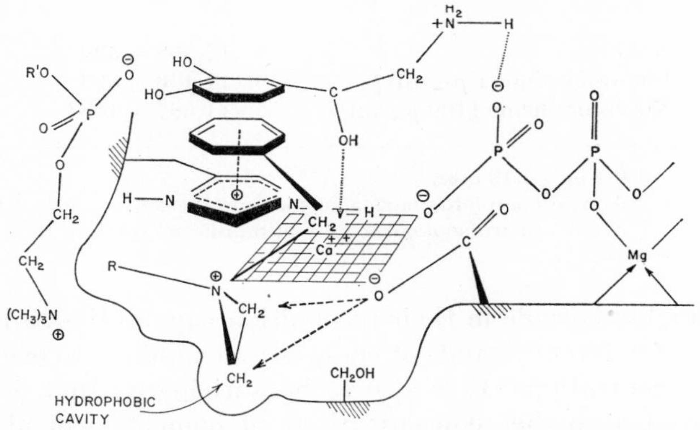

FIG. IV-39. A composite picture of adrenergic α-agonism and antagonism after Belleau (83). A key feature of this model is that binding of the cationic groups of norepinephrine and the ethyleniminium ions occurs at different sites. A prominent feature of this model is the central role of Ca^{++} which is presumed to be displaced during the interaction of norepinephrine.

generally, the forces operative in the binding of such large quaternary ions as the N,N-dibenzylethyleniminium ion, which are to be recognized as hydrophobic ions (Chapter I, p. 48), will be fundamentally different from those operative in binding of primary ammonium groups where hydrogen binding and specific hydration by water molecules will represent a major contribution to the interaction energy. Thus the binding site for ethyleniminium ions will be anticipated to be characteristically less polar than that for ammonium ions. Essentially this reasoning led Belleau to propose (83) a model for the norepinephrine α-receptor which includes as an integral feature a binding site for the ethyleniminium ions which is topographically partially distinct from the catecholamine binding site. This binding site was presumed to be that normally occupied by a choline residue of a phospholipid (Fig. IV-39), although it is not entirely clear whether the trimethylammonium group is a structure-making ion (Chapter I, p. 48), and relates rather directly to the role of Ca^{++} in adrenergically mediated processes and is more profitably discussed in Chapter VII.

Quite similar reasoning to that outlined above suggests also that the binding sites for the primary amino function of histamine and 5-hydroxy-tryptamine are unlikely to be those alkylated by the irreversible antagonists. In contrast, of course, a binding site for a quaternary ammonium function is an integral feature of the cholinergic receptor and thus, from this consideration alone, some structural analogy exists between the cholinergic agonists and certain ethyleniminium ions.

Duration of Action of 2-Halogenoethylamines. A characteristic feature of the action of Dibenamine and related compounds is their prolonged duration of action which is consistent with their proposed mode of action via alkylation of a nucleophilic site whether at the receptor itself or at some peripheral but linked site. More detailed examination reveals, however, that the irreversible blockade is actually more or less slowly reversed with time. Furchgott observed (312) that following complete blockade of aortic strips to epinephrine by Dibenamine some 12–30 per

TABLE IV-58. Cyclization Rates and Times of Onset and Duration of Action of 2-Halogenoethylamines

Compound	Rate of cyclization	Onset time (min)	Duration (approx.)
$(PhCH_2)_2NCH_2CH_2Cl$	Extremely slow	~30	~24–72 h
$PhOCH_2CH(Me)N(CH_2Ph)CH_2CH_2Cl$	Slow	~10	~24–48 h
$PhCHClCH_2N(Me)CH_2Ph$	Fast	~5	~24 h
$PhCHClCH_2NMe_2$	Very fast	~1	1–2 h

cent of the original response returned in 18 h: Nickerson has made (345) similar observations with phenoxybenzamine. A general correlation appears to exist between the relative ease of formation of ethyleni-minium ion, the time for onset and the duration of action of irreversible antagonism (Table IV-58) suggesting (255, 296, 316, 346) that the same molecular features may control both the formation of the ethyleni-minium ion and the stability of the alkylated complex. This is qualita-tively consistent with the proposal that the site(s) alkylated may be carboxylate or phosphate anionic groups, *whether or not these represent the anionic sites proposed as binding groups for the ammonium functions of the α-receptor*, since the esters so formed will be anticipated to hydrolyse spontaneously through intramolecular pathways (Fig. IV-40). There is particularly abundant evidence for the existence of intramolecular facilitation by amino groups of the hydrolysis of carboxylic acid esters

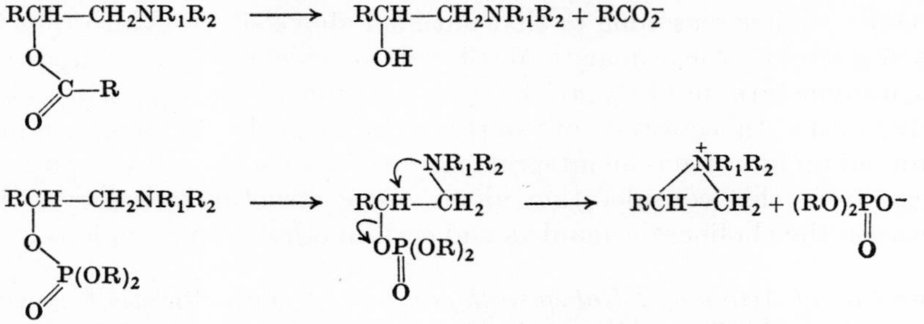

FIG. IV-40. Intramolecular hydrolyses of β-dialkylamino carboxyl and phosphate esters that may represent mechanisms for recovery of response from irreversible α-receptor blockade.

(346, 346a, 347) for which several mechanisms may be written (347; Fig. IV-41);

(a) intramolecular nucleophilic participation;
(b) intramolecular general-base catalysis;
(c) intramolecular acid-base catalysis and;
(d) electrostatic facilitation.

The latter mechanism is the only one available for quaternary amines. Table IV-59 presents some data for the effects of β-dialkylamino

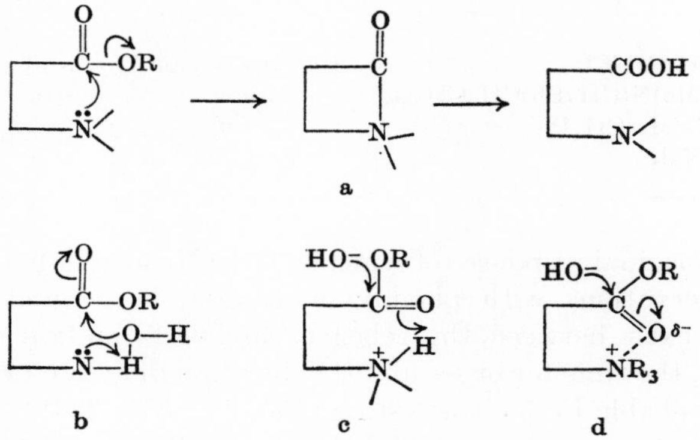

FIG. IV-41. Neighboring amino group participation [in ester hydrolysis: a, nucleophilic attack; b, general base catalysis; c, general acid-specific base catalysis; d, electrostatic assistance.

substitution on the alkaline hydrolysis of ethyl acetate from which it is apparent that the reaction rate is relatively insensitive to the size of the amino group: thus, the very marked differences in duration of action of the irreversible α-antagonists are not likely to represent the operation of intramolecular general base on acid-base catalysed hydrolysis of N-substituted-β-amino esters.

TABLE IV-59. Rate Constants for Base-catalysed Hydrolysis of Dialkylamino Acetates (348)

Compound	$\log k_1$† liter mole^{-1} sec^{-1}	$\log k_2$‡ liter mole^{-1} sec^{-1}
$CH_3COOCH_2CH_3$	−1·0	—
$CH_3COOCH_2CH_2NMe_2$	−1·0	1·63
$CH_3COOCH_2CH_2NEt_2$	—	1·56
$CH_3COOCH_2CH_2NPr^i_2$	—	1·47

† OH⁻ plus unprotonated base.
‡ OH⁻ plus protonated base.

The rate of recovery of response following agents of the N,N-dialkyl-2-bromo-2-arylethylamine class have been studied in several tissues and have been shown to follow first order kinetics (316, 346, 349–351), that for N,N-dimethyl-2-bromo-2-phenylethylamine (Fig. IV-42) being very

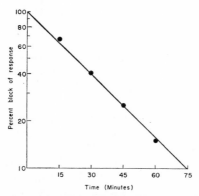

FIG. IV-42. Recovery of response of norepinephrine to blockade by N,N-dimethyl-2-bromo-2-phenylethylamine.

similar in rate to the neutral hydrolysis of the acetate ester of N,N-dimethyl-2-hydroxy-2-phenylethylamine (352). Furthermore, no recovery of response is observed from antagonism produced by N-methyl-2-bromo-2-phenylethylamine and in this case (Fig. IV-43) the possibility of $O \rightarrow N$ migration to give a stable amide derivative exists (346, 347, 353).

Attention must also be directed to a possible mechanism, apparently not previously considered, to account for the recovery of α-receptor function. In this mechanism a neighboring imidazoyl function may

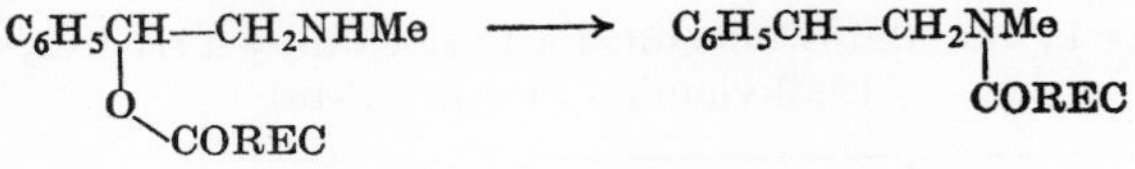

$$C_6H_5CH\text{---}CH_2NHMe \longrightarrow C_6H_5CH\text{---}CH_2NMe$$

FIG. IV-43.

function as the group facilitating ester hydrolysis (Fig. IV-44). Intramolecular catalysis by imidazole groups is rather well documented (346, 347) and of particular interest is the accelerated hydrolysis of esters of 4-(2^1-hydroxyethylimidazole (Fig. IV-45; 354).

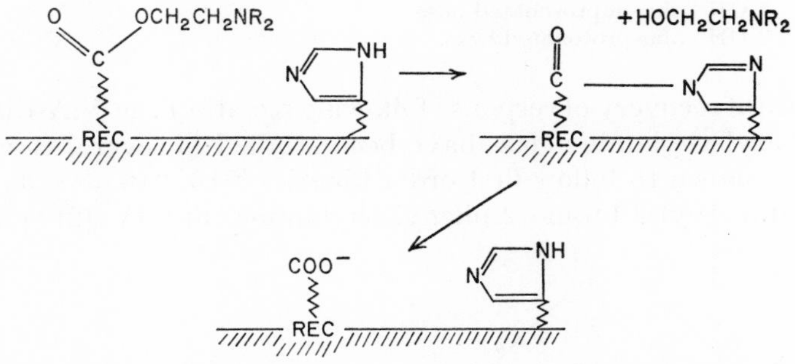

FIG. IV-44. A possible role of neighboring imidazole functions in promoting hydrolysis of esters presumed to be formed by alkylation of the adrenergic α-receptor.

Less data is available for amino-group participation in phosphate ester hydrolysis: however, β-aminophosphate triesters appear to be unstable species. Thus Brown and Osborne (355) have described the spontaneous breakdown of the diethyl, diphenyl and dibenzyl phosphate O-esters of 2-aminoethanol to give ethylenimine and the phosphate ester according to the reaction shown in Fig. IV-46: similarly, dimethyl uridine 3'-phosphate undergoes spontaneous hydrolysis (356). Fukuto

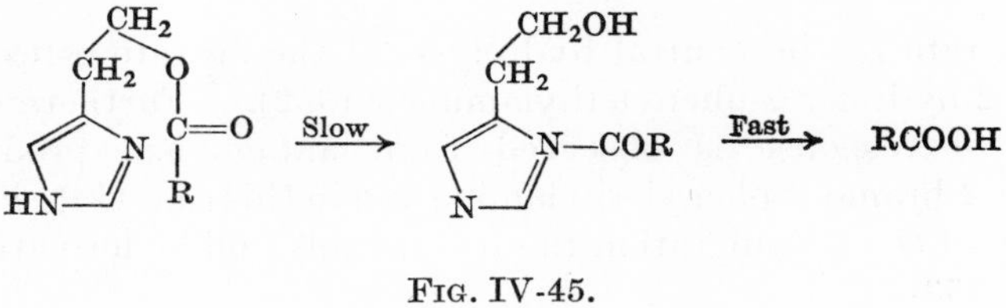

FIG. IV-45.

and Stafford have shown (357) that O,O-diethyl-O-2-diethylaminoethyl phosphorothionate (IV-56; see Fig. IV-47) rearranges to IV-57 (see Fig. IV-47) through the intermediacy of an imminium ion (Fig. IV-47)

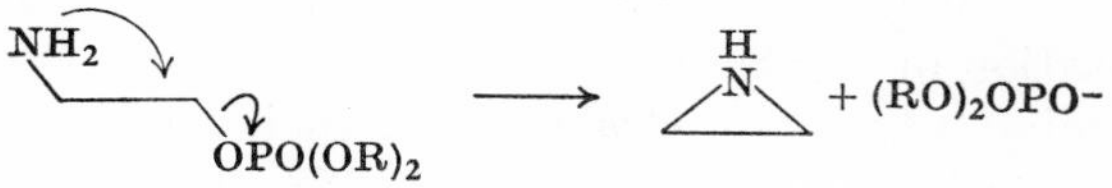

FIG. IV-46.

and Baer and Maurukas (358) have observed that methylation of certain cephalins (IV-58, R = 2-aminoethyl or O-seryl) leads to the corresponding diacylglycerol-1-(dimethyl)phosphate (IV-59) presumably because the first formed triester is unstable and eliminates R as an ethylenimine (359).

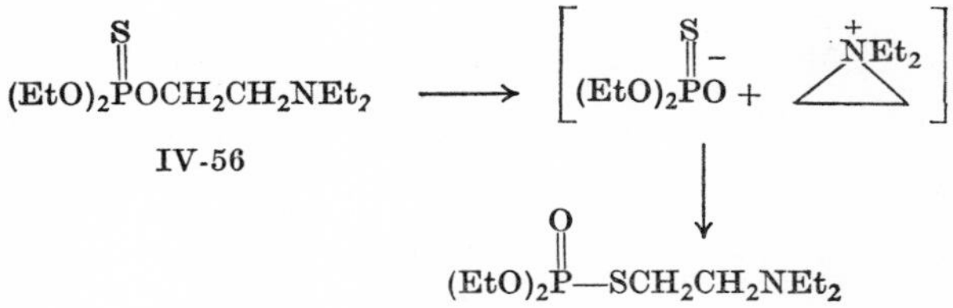

IV-56

IV-57

FIG. IV-47.

The precise significance of the facilitated reactions described above to the process of recovery of α-adrenergic response following alkylation remains to be determined and in any event is complicated by at least two factors. These agents have been demonstrated to have at least two sites, characterized by different selectivities and kinetics, at which interaction

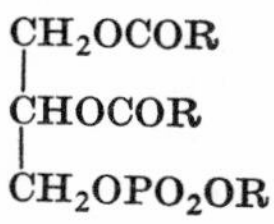

IV-58

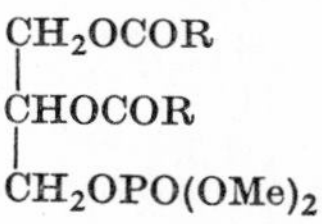

IV-59

with the antagonist can lead to the elimination of the α-response (p. 336) and, in any event, the interpretation of the rates of recovery of response in molecular terms rests very heavily on assumptions made concerning the receptor occupation and pharmacological response (p. 212). The latter assumptions will be re-examined in detail later (p. 330) following discussion of the antagonist properties of the N,N-dialkyl-2-bromo-2-arylethylamines which form a group of compounds which are in many ways uniquely different from the better known Dibenamine class of structures.

The N,N-Dialkyl-2-halogeno-2-arylethylamines. Following the original reports by Hunt (360) and Ferguson (361, 362) of the immediate onset and short duration of blockade produced by *N,N*-dimethyl-2-chloro-2-phenylethylamine, Chapman, Graham and their respective co-workers prepared (363, 364) and examined (256, 288, 309) a large series of related compounds which are listed in Tables IV-60 and IV-61. These

TABLE IV-60. α-Antagonistic Activities of *N,N*-Dimethyl-2-bromo-2-arylethyl-amines (285, 309)
ArCHBrCH₂NMe₂,HBr

No.	Ar	ED_{50}, moles $\times 10^9$/kg rat bp preparation†		$\sum\sigma$	$\sum\pi$
		Epinephrine	Norepinephrine		
1	C_6H_5	35·0	56·0	0·0	0·0
2	$4\text{-}FC_6H_4$	7·0	7·4	0·06	0·15
3	$4\text{-}ClC_6H_4$	2·10	2·10	0·23	0·70
4	$4\text{-}BrC_6H_4$	1·30	1·30	0·23	1·02
5	$4\text{-}IC_6H_4$	0·56	0·51	0·28	1·26
6	$3\text{-}FC_6H_4$	30·0	32·0	0·34	0·13
7	$3\text{-}ClC_6H_4$	7·0	7·10	0·37	0·76
8	$3\text{-}BrC_6H_4$	5·0	5·0	0·39	0·94
9	$3\text{-}IC_6H_4$	4·0	4·0	0·35	1·15
10	$3,4\text{-}(F)_2C_6H_3$	—	7·51	—	—
11	$3,4\text{-}(Cl)_2C_6H_3$	2·80	2·80	0·60	1·46
12	$3,4(Br)_2C_6H_3$	0·45	0·50	0·62	1·96
13	$4\text{-}F,3\text{-}Cl\text{-}C_6H_3$	6·40	6·40	0·43	0·91
14	$4\text{-}F,3\text{-}BrC_6H_3$	2·70	2·70	0·45	1·09
15	$4\text{-}F,3\text{-}MeC_6H_3$	1·50	1·50	−0·01	0·66
16	$4\text{-}Cl\text{-}3\text{-}BrC_6H_3$	1·20	1·20	0·62	1·64
17	$4\text{-}Cl,3\text{-}MeC_6H_3$	1·10	1·10	0·16	1·21
18	$4\text{-}Br,3\text{-}ClC_6H_3$	1·00	1·00	0·60	1·78
19	$4\text{-}Br,3\text{-}MeC_6H_3$	0·60	0·60	0·17	1·53
20	$4\text{-}C_6H_5C_6H_4$	30·0	30·0	0·01	1·89
21	$3\text{-}MeC_6H_4$	3·50	3·00	−0·07	0·51
22	$4\text{-}MeC_6H_4$	0·50	0·53	−0·17	0·52
23	$3,4\text{-}Me_2C_6H_3$	0·50	0·50	0·24	1·03
24	$1\text{-}C_{10}H_7$	20·0	20·0	—	—
25	$2\text{-}C_{10}H_7$	20·0	60·0	—	—
26	$C_6H_5CH(NMe_2)CH_2Br$	40·0	50·0	—	—
27	$C_6H_5CHOHCH_2NMe_2$	>1000	>1000	—	—
28	$3,4Br_2C_6H_3CHOHCH_2NMe_2$	>1000	>1000	—	—

† Antagonism to the pressor effect of norepinephrine and epinephrine (1 μg/kg) in the spinal rat.

data reveal that a number of these compounds are extraordinarily active (in the rat bp preparation), maximum activity being found with 12, 22 and 23 of Table IV-60 and that increasing bulk of N-substitution produces marked decreases in activity (Table IV-61).

TABLE IV-61. α-Antagonistic Activities of N,N-Dialkyl-2-bromo-2-phenylethlamines (285)

$$C_6H_5CHBrCH_2NR_2$$

NR$_2$	ED$_{50}$, moles $\times$ 10^9/kg rat bp preparation†		$\sum\sigma$	$\sum\pi$
	Epinephrine	Norepinephrine		
—NMe$_2$	35·0	56·0	0·00	1·00
—NEt$_2$	5000	1800	−0·20	2·00
—NPr$_2$	1000	1300	−0·23	3·00
—NPr$^i_2$	30,000	22,000	−0·38	2·60
—NBu$_2$	4400	4500	−0·26	4·00
—NMeEt	2800	3000	−0·10	1·50
—piperidino	15,000	14,000	—	—
—morpholino	4000	4500	—	—
—NHMe	600	500	0·49	0·50
—NHEt	100,000	80,000	0·39	1·00
—NHPr	250,000	250,000	0·37	1·50
—NHBu	200,000	200,000	0·36	2·00
—NHCH$_2$Ph		2800	0·71	2·63
—N(CH$_2$Ph)$_2$	2400	1700	0·43	5·26
—N(Me)CH$_2$Ph	220	390	0·22	3·13

† Antagonism to the pressor effect of norepinephrine and epinephrine (1 μg/kg) in the spinal rat.

Detailed kinetic studies (363) revealed that cyclization is extremely rapid so that in neutral solution ethyleniminium ion formation is almost instantaneous, and that solvolysis proceeds through the intermediacy of a carbonium intermediate (Fig. IV-48). Graham (*loc. cit.*) demonstrated that the amino-alcohols corresponding to the 2-halogenoethylamines are inactive, that the picrylsulfonates of several of the

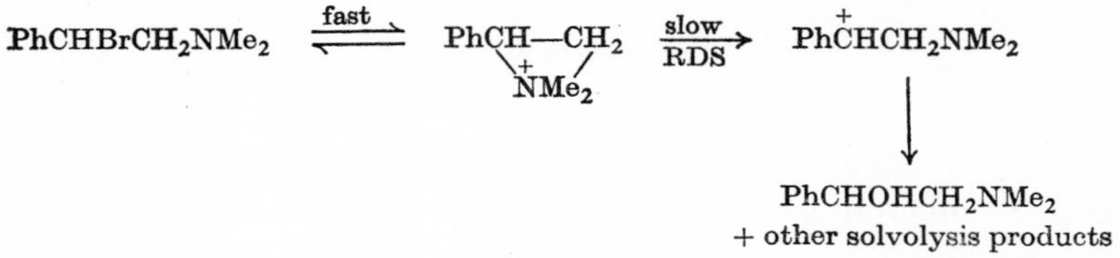

$$\text{PhCHBrCH}_2\text{NMe}_2 \underset{\longleftarrow}{\overset{\text{fast}}{\longrightarrow}} \underset{\overset{+}{\text{NMe}_2}}{\text{PhCH—CH}_2} \overset{\text{slow}}{\underset{\text{RDS}}{\longrightarrow}} \text{PhĊHCH}_2\text{NMe}_2$$

$$\downarrow$$

$$\text{PhCHOHCH}_2\text{NMe}_2$$
+ other solvolysis products

FIG. IV-48. The solvolysis of N,N-dimethyl-2-bromo-2-phenylethylamine.

derived ethyleniminium ions are active and that there is a direct proportionality between the concentration of the ethyleniminium ions in solution and the norepinephrine antagonistic activity. Furthermore, the isomeric compounds (Table IV-60, Nos. 1 and 26) which cyclize to the same ethyleniminium ion are found to be equiactive.

From their kinetic studies Chapman and Triggle suggested that the carbonium ion was the actual alkylating species although in view of its transient existence it must be presumed to act as such only if derived from the ethyleniminium ion in the bound state. This possibility was strengthened by the finding that the enantioners of N,N-dimethyl-2-chloro-2-phenylethylamine are equiactive as antagonists (365).

TABLE IV-62. Electronic and Kinetic Parameters and α-Antagonistic Activity in N,N-dimethyl-2-arylaziri-dinium Ions (309, 363)

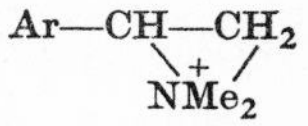

$$\text{Ar—CH—CH}_2$$
$$\underset{\text{NMe}_2}{\overset{+}{\diagdown \diagup}}$$

Ar	σ	$10^3 k_1$ min^{-1}	ED$_{50}$ (NE) moles $\times 10^9$/kg rat bp preparation
C_6H_5	0·00	14·5	56·0
4-FC$_6$H$_4$	0·06	17·7	7·4
4-BrC$_6$H$_4$	0·23	13·8	1·30
4-MeC$_6$H$_4$	−0·17	30·6	0·53

It is clear that of all the irreversible α-antagonists discussed so far those of the N,N-dimethyl-2-halogeno-2-arylethylamine class bear the greatest structural resemblance to norepinephrine. The effects of aryl substituents in this series of compounds is quite marked yet there is no obvious correlation between the σ values of the substituents, their effect on ethyleniminium stability and their biological activity (Table IV-62). However, Hansch and Lien (366) have demonstrated a correlation between the biological activity and the hydrophobic character of the substituent as measured by π (Table IV-60). Equation XXXI reveals that the σ value

$$\log \frac{1}{C} = -0·034\sigma + 8·704 \qquad (n = 22, r = 0·022, s = 0·583) \quad \textbf{(XXXI)}$$

is of little significance in determining the effect of substituents and eqn. XXXII reveals π to be of dominant importance,

$$\log \frac{1}{C} = 0·770\pi + 7·931 \qquad (n = 22, r = 0·724, s = 0·402) \quad \textbf{(XXXII)}$$

and that π and σ together,

$$\log\frac{1}{C} = 1 \cdot 221\pi + 1 \cdot 587\sigma + 7 \cdot 888 \qquad (n = 22, r = 0 \cdot 918, s = 0 \cdot 238)$$

(XXXIII)

give a rather better correlation than π alone. The most noteworthy feature of eqns. XXXII and XXXIII is their close similarity to the eqns. XXXV and XXXVI describing the effects of aryl substituents on the β-adrenergic antagonism exhibited by the N-isopropyl-2-aryl-2-hydroxyethylamines (p. 315). Thus the aryl binding sites for these two sets of substituents may be very similar or identical, a conclusion strengthened by the finding that in both series of compounds 4-phenyl substitution is unfavorable to activity despite its favorable $\sum\pi$ index. Furthermore, it has been found that the effects of methanesulfonamido substitution in N,N-dimethyl-2-chloro-2-phenylethylamine (IV-60, 61)

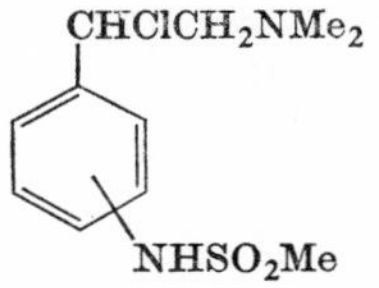

CHClCH$_2$NMe$_2$

NHSO$_2$Me

IV-60 (meta)
IV-61 (para)

parallel the effects of the same substituent on the α-agonist activity of phenylethanolamines with only the meta compound (IV-60) being active as an irreversible α-blocker (316). These lines of evidence provide some

TABLE IV-63. Local Anesthetic Activities of some 2-Halo-genoethylamines and their Corresponding Alcohols (288)

Compound	Anesthetic potency†
Procaine	1·0
$(PhCH_2)_2NCH_2CH_2Cl$	0·5
$(PhCH_2)_2NCH_2CH_2OH$	0·0
$1\text{-}C_{10}H_7CH_2N(Et)CH_2CH_2Br$	0·75
$1\text{-}C_{10}H_7CH_2N(Et)CH_2CH_2OH$	0·0
$C_6H_5CHBrCH_2NMe_2$	1·16
$C_6H_5CHOHCH_2NMe_2$	100·0
$C_6H_5CHBrCH_2NEt_2$	7·2
$C_6H_5CHBrCH_2NBu_2$	0·21
$C_6H_5CHBrCH_2NHPr$	95

† Determined by the method of Bülbring and Wajda (367).

indication that alkylating agents of the N,N-dimethyl-2-halogeno-2-arylethylamine class may well interact at the norepinephrine recognition site of the α-receptor. This is in marked contrast to the Dibenamine class of agents where evidence for this assumption is far less convincing.

However, agents of this class do have effects at other receptor sites although to a noticeably less marked degree than the Dibenamine-type agents. In general, the agents listed in Tables IV-60 and IV-61 do not exhibit marked activity at cholinergic junctions and whilst they possess antihistamine activity this is not apparently of the irreversible type (309) and is, in fact, probably due to the derived products of hydrolysis, the N,N-dimethyl-2-hydroxy-2-arylethylamines. Local anesthetic activity is prominent in this series of compounds but appears to be principally due to the amino alcohol hydrolysis products (Table IV-63).

Reversible Antagonist at Adrenergic β-Receptors

Following the discovery (368, 369) of the β-antagonism exhibited by the 3,4-dichloro analog (IV-62; see Fig. IV-49) of isopropylnorepinephrine a very considerable number of related agents have been synthesized and studied (IV-62–IV-68 are representative examples; see

CHOHCH$_2$NHCHMeCH$_2$Ph

α   β

αR, βR and αR, βS active

(379)   IV-66

Fig. IV-49) and a selection of such structure–activity data is presented in Tables IV-64–IV-70. It is quite evident, in marked contrast to the adrenergic α-antagonists previously discussed, that the β-antagonists maintain a very considerable structural resemblance to the corresponding agonist, isopropylnorepinephrine. It will be observed from this data that the effects of N-substitution on β-antagonism generally parallel the effects of the same substituents on β-agonism in the catecholamine and sulfonamidophenylethanolamine series (p. 224). This is certainly suggestive that a common binding site is involved for both agonist and antagonists at least as far as the alkanolamine side chain is concerned, a conclusion strengthened by the stereoselectivity of β-antagonism (Fig. IV-49) which, for those agents whose absolute configuration has been established reveals the more active isomers to have the R-configuration. Several general reviews of the structure–activity relationships of β-adrenergic antagonists are available (257, 385, 386) which treat the preceding discussion in rather more detail.

In consideration of the structural requirements of the aryl residue of β-antagonists the data of Table IV-67 reveal in a qualitative sense, the

TABLE IV-64. Adrenergic β-Blocking Activities of N-Substituted-2-amino-1-(2-naphthyl) ethanols (379)

CHOHCH$_2$NRR$_1$

No.	R	R$_1$	Infusion rate μg/kg/min†	% Change in heart rate	% Inhib. tachycardia
1	H	H	400	+7	55
2	H	CH$_3$	400	−10	57
3	H	CH$_2$CH$_3$	100	−9	4
4	H	CH$_2$CH$_2$CH$_3$	400	−24	45
5	H	CH(CH$_3$)$_2$	50	−15	45
6	H	(CH$_2$)$_3$CH$_3$	100	−16	29
7	H	CH(CH$_3$)CH$_2$CH$_3$	50	−12	61
8	H	C(CH$_3$)$_3$	50	0	84
9	H	(CH$_2$)$_4$CH$_3$	200	−7	46
10	H	Cyclopentyl	100	−10	44
11	H	Cyclohexyl	400	−12	60
12	H	Cyclopropyl	100	−11	54
13	CH$_3$	CH$_3$	200	−11	0
14	CH$_3$	CH(CH$_3$)$_2$	1000	−16	69
15	CH(CH$_3$)$_2$	CH(CH$_3$)$_2$	400	−21	45
16	H	CH$_2$C$_6$H$_5$	800	−7	7
17	H	CH$_2$CH$_2$C$_6$H$_5$	800	−21	52
18	H	(CH$_2$)$_3$C$_6$H$_5$	100	+9	51
19	H	CH(CH$_3$)CH$_2$C$_6$H$_5$	50	−4	34
20	H	CH(CH$_3$)CH$_2$CH$_2$C$_6$H$_5$	25	−6	65
21	H	C(CH$_3$)$_2$CH$_2$C$_6$H$_5$	100	0	59
22	H	CH(CH$_3$)CH$_2$OC$_6$H$_5$	100	+8	53
23	H	(CH$_2$)$_2$C$_6$H$_3$(OCH$_3$)$_2$-3,4	100	+4	56
24	H	CH(CH$_3$)CH$_2$C$_6$H$_4$OCH$_3$-4	200	0	43
25	H	CH(CH$_3$)CH$_2$C$_6$H$_4$OH-4	100	0	56
26	H	CH(CH$_3$)(CH$_2$)$_2$C$_6$H$_4$OCH$_3$-4	50	−5	62
27	H	CH$_2$C$_6$H$_3$O$_2$CH$_2$-3,4	20 mg/kg (intraduod.)	0	18

† Tachycardia was induced by isopropylnorepinephrine in cats and the compound introduced i.v. continuously for 20 min. Isopropylnorepinephrine was then readministered and the activity of the compounds is expressed as the percentage inhibition of the control tachycardia.

limited dimensions of the presumed aryl binding site: a steady decrease in activity in a series of pronethalol analogs is observed as the aryl residue varies from naphthyl to fluorenyl. Since these changes are not very large the progressive loss of activity is indicative that the binding site is of quite restricted dimensions. In the phenylethanolamines of Table IV-68 β-antagonistic activity reaches a maximum at the 4-methyl, 3,4-dimethyl and dichloro analogs and decreases very sharply with the 3,4-diethyl series. In the phenoxypropanol series (Table IV-69) an

TABLE IV-65. Adrenergic β-Blocking Activities of N-Substituted-1-amino-3-(1-naphthoxy)-2-propanols (380)

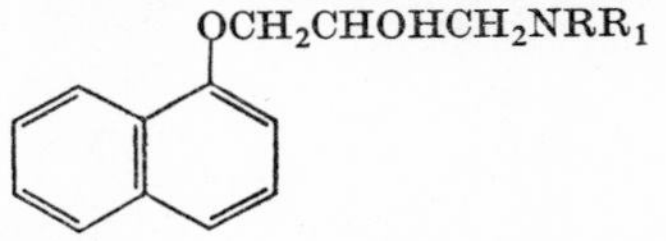

$$OCH_2CHOHCH_2NRR_1$$

No.	R	R_1	Infusion rate $\mu g/kg/min$	% Inhib. tachycardia
1	H	H	100	53
2	H	CH_3	20	17
3	H	CH_2CH_3	20	83
4	H	$CH_2CH_2CH_3$	20	57
5	H	$CH(CH_3)_2$	2·5	57
6	H	$CH_2CH_2CH_2CH_3$	50	56
7	H	$C(CH_3)_3$	2·5	65
8	H	$CH_2C_6H_5$	5	0
9	H	$(CH_2)_2C_6H_5$	10	50
10	H	$CH(CH_3)CH_2C_6H_5$	20	53
11	H	$CH_2C_6H_4OCH_3$-4	20	35
12	CH_3	CH_3	20	25
13	$CH(CH_3)_2$	$CH(CH_3)_2$	10	0
14	H	$CH(CH_3)_2$ (2-naphthoxy isomer)	50	50

essentially similar structure–activity relationship is observed with very definite indications that substitution of halogen, alkyl or alkoxy groups into the 2-position of the benzene ring produces optimum activity and that the 3- and 4- positions are progressively more sensitive to the steric bulk of substitution. This may be a reflection of the intuitive anticipation (296) that steric interactions of substituents at the catechol binding site of the adrenergic receptor should be in the order $o < m < p$.

Pratesi and his co-workers (388–392) have provided a quantitative analysis of the β-adrenergic activities of a series of substituted N-isopropyl-2-phenyl-2-hydroxyethylamines (Table IV-71) together with an analysis of the nonspecific spasmolytic activities of these compounds. This latter activity is described by the regression equation (Fig. IV-50)

$$pD_2' = 0.766\pi + 2.670 \qquad (SD = \pm 5 \text{ per cent}) \qquad \textbf{(XXXIV)}$$

showing that, within the series of compounds listed, activity is solely dependent upon π, the measure of hydrophobic activity.

TABLE IV-66. Adrenergic β-Blocking Activities of Sulfonamidophenylethanol-amines (89)

No.	R	R_1	R_2	β-Blocking effect ($\times$DCI)†
			3-$RSO_2NHC_6H_4CHOHCHR_1NHR_2$	
1	CH_3	H	H	0·07
2	CH_3	H	CH_3	0·1
3	CH_3	H	CH_2CH_3	0·1
4	CH_3	H	$CH(CH_3)_2$	1·0
5	CH_3	H	$CH(CH_3)CH_2OC_6H_5$	0·03
6	CH_3	CH_3	CH_3	0·1
7	4-$CH_3C_6H_4$	H	H	0·04
8	4-$CH_3C_6H_4$	H	CH_3	0·09
9	4-$CH_3C_6H_4$	H	$CH(CH_3)_2$	1·1
			4-$RSO_2NHC_6H_4CHOHCHR_1NHR_2$	
10	CH_3	H	H	0·2
11	CH_3	H	CH_3	0·2
12	CH_3	H	$CH(CH_3)_2$	6·0
13	CH_3	H	$CH_2C_6H_5$	0·01
14	CH_3	H	$CH(CH_3)CH_2OC_6H_5$	4·0
15	4-$CH_3C_6H_4$	H	H	0·03
16	4-$CH_3C_6H_4$	H	CH_3	0·06
17	4-$CH_3C_6H_4$	H	$CH(CH_3)_2$	0·2
18	CH_3	CH_3	CH_3	2·4
19	CH_3	CH_3	CH_3	0·001
20	CH_3	CH_3	$CH(CH_3)_2$	1·3
21	CH_3	C_2H_5	$CH(CH_3)_2$	0·4

† Relative β-blocking activity relative to DCI (=1) to inhibit by 50 per cent the relaxant action of isoprotorenol (0·01 μg/ml) on the guinea-pig tracheal spiral.

It is particularly interesting that the β-antagonistic activities of those compounds from Table IV-71 whose aryl substituents have approximately equal steric identity are also correlated quite satisfactorily by an equation involving a π-term only,

$$pA_2 = 0.671\pi + 5.554 \qquad (SD = \pm 3.7 \text{ per cent}) \qquad \textbf{(XXXV)}$$

TABLE IV-67. Adrenergic β-Blocking Activities of N-Isopropyl-2-aryl-2-hydroxy-
ethylamines (381)

$$ArCHOHCH_2NHCH(CH_3)_2$$

No.	Ar	Infusion rate $\mu g/kg/min$	% Change heart rate	% Inhib. tachycardia
1		50	+12	76
2		50	−15	45
3		50	+2	72
4		50	−6	45
5		50	+2	73
6		200	−14	20
7		200	−28	48
8		200	−7	45
9		400	0	48
10		400	0	32
11		200	−14	60

† Increased heart rate characteristic of all 1-naphthyl derivatives irrespective of
N-substitution.

and with somewhat better precision by an inclusion of the pK_a term (Fig. IV-51).

$$pA_2 = 0.662\pi - 1.528\, pK_a + 19.858 \qquad (SD = \pm 2 \text{ per cent}) \qquad (XXXVI)$$

Examination of the pK_a values reveal only a very small variation so that this must correspond to the contribution of a very small substituent term σ in eqn. XXXIII (p. 311). Examination of Table IV-71 reveals that a number of compounds (not included in the deduction of eqn. XXXVI)

TABLE IV-68. Adrenergic β-Blocking Activities of Substituted Phenylethanolamines (382)

R—⟨C₆H₃⟩—CHOHCHR₂NHR₃
R₁

No.	R	R_1	R_2	R_3	β-Receptor blocking activity (DCI = 1)	Antiarrhythmic activity
1	Cl	Cl	H	Pr^i	1·0	—
2	Cl	Cl	CH_3	Pr^i	0·08	2
3	Cl	Cl	C_2H_5	Pr^i	0·15	2
4	CH_3	H	H	Pr^i	1·2	0·5
5	CH_3	H	CH_3	Pr^i	0·2	1
6	CH_3	CH_3	H	Pr^i	1·2	0·1
7	CH_3	CH_3	CH_3	Pr^i	0·2	0·5
8	C_2H_5	H	H	Pr^i	0·15	—
9	C_2H_5	H	CH_3	Pr^i	0·2	2·5
10	C_2H_5	C_2H_5	H	Pr^i	0·08	1
11	$CH(CH_3)_2$	H	H	Pr^i	0·2	0·5
12	Cl	CH_3	H	Pr^i	1·0	—
13	CH_3	Cl	H	Pr^i	1·0	—

deviate very markedly from the theoretical slope. In particular the deviations of compounds 29–31 and 33 confirm the limited dimensions of the nonpolar binding site since the $\sum\pi$ values should correspond to higher pA_2 values than experimentally found. In contrast the deviations of compounds 10, 13 and 18 (Table IV-71) indicate the role of specific polar interactions in determining affinity since these compounds are significantly more active than their $\sum\pi$ values would indicate. Thus the binding of the aryl residue of the arylethanolamines is not equivalent to a simple partitioning into a nonpolar binding area, but rather to partitioning into a nonpolar area of critical dimensions in which highly specific polar interactions are possible. The critical dimensions of the nonpolar binding area are reflected in the anomalously high activities of pronethalol (No. 32) and propranolol (No. 34) and in the comparison of pronethalol with its 5,6,7,8-tetrahydro analog (No. 33) where relatively small changes in the shape of the aromatic ring system are accompanied, despite the increased $\sum\pi$ of 33, by decreased β-antagonistic activity.

TABLE IV-69. Adrenergic β-Blocking Activities of 1-Amino-3-(substituted phenoxy)-2-propanols (383)

$$RC_6H_4OCH_2CHOHCH_2NR_1R_2$$

No.	R	R_1	R_2	Dose μg/kg/min	% Inhib. tachycardia
1	3-CH$_3$	H	CH$_2$CH$_2$CH$_3$	40	53
2	3-CH$_3$	H	CH(CH$_3$)$_2$	10	80
3	3-CH$_3$	H	C(CH$_3$)$_3$	5	55
4	4-CH$_3$	H	CH(CH$_3$)$_2$	2·5	74
5	2-C$_2$H$_5$	H	CH$_2$CH$_2$CH$_3$	10	63
6	2-C$_2$H$_5$	H	CH(CH$_3$)$_2$	2·5	74
7	2-C$_2$H$_5$	H	C(CH$_3$)$_3$	2·5	82
8	2-C$_2$H$_5$	H	CH(CH$_3$)CH$_2$OC$_6$H$_5$	10	71
9	2-C$_2$H$_5$	H	CH(CH$_3$)CH$_2$C$_6$H$_4$—OCH$_3$-4	20	47
10	3-OCH$_3$	H	CH$_2$CH$_2$CH$_3$	10	50
11	3-OCH$_3$	H	CH(CH$_3$)$_2$	2·5	55
12	3-OCH$_3$	H	C(CH$_3$)$_3$	2·5	72
13	2-OC$_2$H$_5$	H	CH$_2$CH$_2$CH$_3$	10	60
14	2-OC$_2$H$_5$	H	CH(CH$_3$)$_2$	2	83
15	2-OC$_2$H$_5$	H	C(CH$_3$)$_3$	2·5	72
16	4-CH(CH$_3$)$_2$	H	CH(CH$_3$)$_2$	20	43
17	2-Cl	H	CH(CH$_3$)$_2$	2·5	99
18	3-Cl	H	CH(CH$_3$)$_2$	5	82
19	4-Cl	H	CH(CH$_3$)$_2$	20	46
20	2-CF$_3$	H	CH(CH$_3$)$_2$	5	64
21	3-CH$_3$	H	CH(CH$_3$)$_2$	20	86
22	2-OC$_6$H$_5$	H	CH(CH$_3$)$_2$	2·5	80
23	3-OC$_6$H$_5$	H	CH(CH$_3$)$_2$	10	64
24	2,3-Me$_2$	H	CH(CH$_3$)$_2$	10	60
25	2,4-Me$_2$	H	CH(CH$_3$)$_2$	10	50
26	2,5-Me$_2$	H	CH(CH$_3$)$_2$	10	41
27	3,5-Me$_2$	H	CH(CH$_3$)$_2$	5	61
28	3,4-Me$_2$	H	CH(CH$_3$)$_2$	5	50
29	3,5-OMe$_2$	H	CH(CH$_3$)$_2$	40	50
30	2,3-OMe$_2$	H	CH(CH$_3$)$_2$	10	65

Finally, the large difference in activity of the 1- and 2-naphthyl isomers of pronethalol serves as a further indication of the rigid steric requirements of this nonpolar binding surface.

Of great interest is a comparison of the structural requirements of aromatic substitution in the β-antagonistic phenylethanolamines of

Table IV-71 with the irreversible α-antagonistic N,N-dimethyl-2-bromo-2-arylethylamines discussed previously (Table IV-60). Comparison of the two sets of data reveals that the determinant contribution to the activities of both series of compounds is made by the $\sum\pi$ values so that activity is enhanced in both series of compounds by the same substituents (compare eqns. XXXIII and XXXVI). Since an effective argument can be raised that β-antagonists of Fig. IV-49 bind to the β-receptor site proper the above comparison suggests that the irreversible α-antagonists of the N,N-dimethyl-2-bromo-2-arylethylamine class also

TABLE IV-70. Adrenergic β-Blocking Activities of Side Chain Substituted Derivatives of Pronethalol and Propranolol (384)

$$2\text{-}C_{10}H_7CHOHCHRNHR_1$$

No.	R	R_1	Infusion rate μg/kg/min	% Change heart rate	% Inhib. tachycardia
1	H	H	400	+7	55
2	CH_3	H (erythro)	200	−12	71
3	H	CH_3	400	−10	57
4	CH_3	CH_3 (erythro)	100	+1	33
5	H	$CH(CH_3)_2$	50	−15	45
6	CH_3	$CH(CH_3)_2$ (erythro)	100	−3	30
7	CH_3	$CH(CH_3)_2$ (threo)	100	−2	10
8	CH_3	$C(CH_3)_3$ (threo)	100	+2	8
		$1\text{-}C_{10}H_7OCH_2CHOHCHRNHR_1$			
9	H	$CH(CH_3)_2$	2·5	—	57
10	CH_3	$CH(CH_3)_2$	50	−34	69

bind at the receptor proper. That substituents should be similarly effective in promoting interaction of two antagonist series at both the α- and β-adrenergic receptors is in agreement with the conclusion drawn previously from structure–activity data of adrenergic agonists (p. 228) that the binding site for the catechol nucleus (or its equivalent is identical or closely similar at both α- and β-adrenergic receptors.

Despite the above generalizations concerning the structure–activity relationships of β-antagonists it must be emphasized that a number of extremely important exceptions exist. Most notable is the methoxamine series of compounds (IV-69; see Fig. IV-49): isopropylmethoxamine and tert-butylmethoxamine antagonize (393–395) the metabolic responses mediated through β-adrenergic receptors (Chapter VI, see section, p. 476) and are very significantly less active at other β-receptor systems, notably cardiac preparations (378, 393–399): however, isopropyl-methoxamine antagonizes the rat uterine inhibitory response to

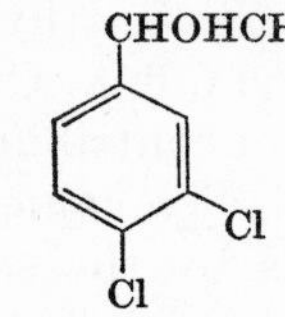

CHOHCH₂NHPrⁱ

DCI   (368, 369)
(−)/(+) = 40–60   (370)

IV-62

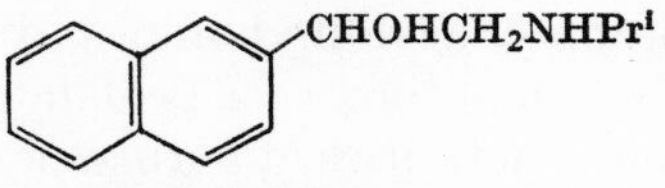

CHOHCH₂NHPrⁱ

Pronethalolol (371)
(−)/(+) = 60–100   (372)

IV-63

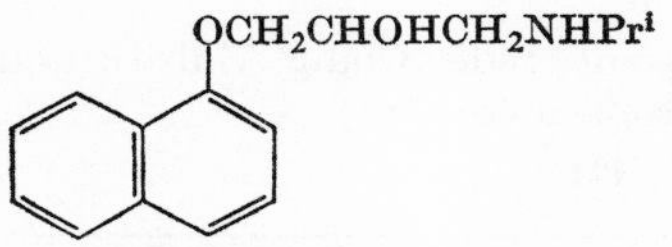

OCH₂CHOHCH₂NHPrⁱ

Propranolol (373)
R(−)/S(+) = 60–100   (372)

IV-64

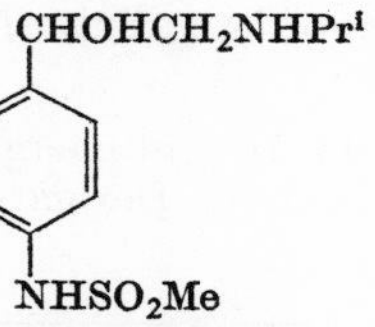

CHOHCH₂NHPrⁱ

NHSO₂Me
MJ. 1999 (88)
(−)/(+) = 20–30   (374)

IV-65

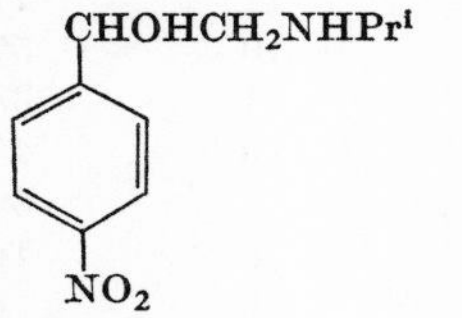

CHOHCH₂NHPrⁱ

NO₂
INPEA   (375)
R(−) active/S(+) inactive   (376)

IV-67

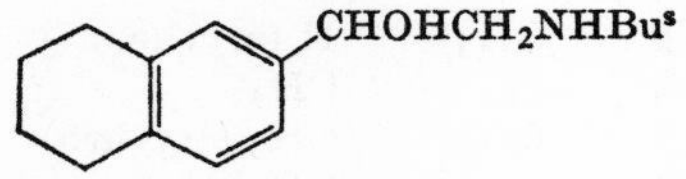

CHOHCH₂NHBuˢ

(377)

IV-68

CHOHCH(Me)NHR
OMe

MeO

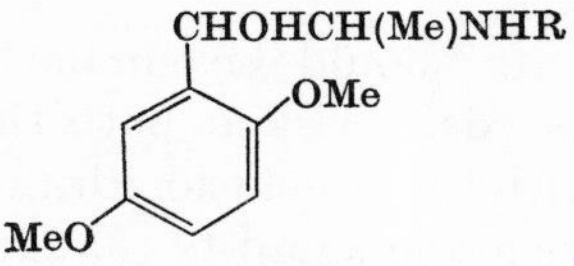

(a) R = H, Methoxamine (378)
(b) R = Prⁱ, isopropylmethoxamine
(c) R = Buᵗ tert-butoxamine

IV-69

FIG. IV-49. Structural formulae of some adrenergic β-receptor antagonists together with isomer potency ratios.

catecholamines (395) and the isopropylnorepinephrine-induced relaxation of tracheal chain (400), whilst tert-butylmethoxamine antagonizes some vasodilator responses (396, 398). The 2,4-dimethyl (IV-70) analog

TABLE IV-71. Biological Activities and Physicochemical Parameters of N-Isopropyl-2-(3,4-Disubstituted)phenylethylamines (392)

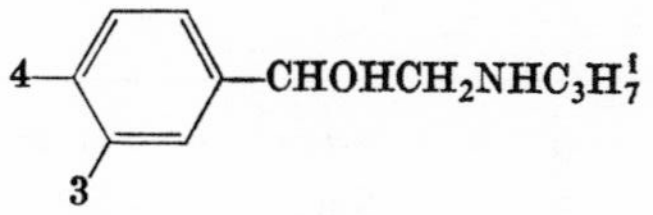

$$CHOHCH_2NHC_3H_7^i$$

(benzene ring, positions 4 and 3 substituted)

No.		4	3	β-Receptor activity						Nonspecific spasmolytic activity Intestine (rat) pD_2'	$\Sigma\pi$	pK_a†
				Atria (guinea-pig)			Trachea (calf)					
				i.a.	pD_2	pA_2	i.a.	pD_2	pA_2			
1	D(−)	OH	OH	high	8·4	—	1	7·6	—	—	−1·05	9·58
2	DL	OH	H	high	6·1	—	—	—	—	—	−0·52	9·26
3	DL	H	OH	high	6·1	—	—	—	—	—	−0·53	9·54
4	DL	OCH₃	OCH₃	high	6·2	—	1	5·7	—	<3	−0·46	9·58
5	DL	OCH₃	OH	high	6·4	—	1	5·8	—	<3	−0·57	9·58
6	DL	SO₂NH₂	H	none	—	4·5	—	—	—	<3	−1·82	9·26
7	DL	SO₂CH₃	H	none	—	5·1	0	—	5·1	<3	−0·88	9·25
8	DL	NH₂	H	high	5·4	—	1	4·9	—	<3	−1·23	9·74
9	DL	NHCOCH₃	H	none	—	4·7	—	—	—	<3	−0·84	9·50
10	DL	NHSO₂CH₃	H	none	—	6·6	0	—	6·8	<3	−1·5	9·98
11	DL	H	CN	low	5·3	5·3	1	5·8	—	<3	−0·35	9·33
12	DL	CN	H	none	—	5·5	0	—	5·6	3·1	−0·44	9·28
13	DL	COOCH₃	H	none	—	5·7	0	—	6·6	3·0	−0·01	9·43
14	DL	H	H	high	5·2	—	0·9	5·4	—	3·0	0·00	9·50
15	DL	OCH₃	H	none	—	5·2	—	—	—	<3	−0·004	9·26
16	DL	OCH₃	OCH₃	none	—	5·1	0	—	5·4	2·5	0·02	9·58
17	DL	H	OCH₃	none	—	5·4	—	—	—	<3	0·06	9·54

[continued on p. 322]

TABLE IV·71—continued

No.		4	3	β-Receptor activity						Nonspecific spasmolytic activity Intestine (rat) pD₂′	Σπ	pKₐ†
				Atria (guinea-pig)			Trachea (calf)					
				i.a.	pD₂	pA₂	i.a.	pD₂	pA₂			
18	DL	NO_2	H	none	—	6·2	0	—	6·4	3·0	0·16	9·27
19	DL	F	F	low	—	5·6	0·7	4·5	5·5	2·8	0·21	9·36
20	DL	CH_3	H	low	—	5·9	0·7	5·3	—	3·0	0·49	9·35
21	DL	H	CH_3	low	—	5·7	0·9	5·4	—	3·0	0·53	9·45
22	DL	SCH_3	H	none	—	6·2	0	—	6·9	3·0	0·62	9·06
23	DL	CH_3	CH_3	low	—	6·3	0·3	—	5·7	3·1	1·02	9·38
24	DL	CF_3	H	none	—	6·2	0	—	6·1	3·6	1·09	9·34
25	DL	Cl	Cl	low	—	6·7	0·7	5·5	6·5	3·3	1·58	9·27
26	DL	Br	Br	none	—	6·1	0·8	4·2	5·4	4·1	1·91	9·29
27	DL	I	I	none	—	6·2	0·7	5·0	5·9	4·6	2·50	—
28	DL	C_6H_5	H	none	—	5·1	1	4·2	5·1	4·0	1·89	9·49
29	DL	H	C_6H_5	none	—	5·1	1	4·3	4·5	4·4	1·89	9·20
30	DL	H	C_6H_{11}	none	—	5·0	1	4·1	4·6	4·7	2·51	9·06
31	DL	OC_4H_9	OC_4H_9	none	—	5·2	0	—	4·9	4·9	2·56	9·58
32	DL	$CH{=}CH{-}CH{=}CH$		none	—	7·0	0	—	7·2	3·7	1·24	9·51
33	DL	$CH_2CH_2CH_2CH_2$		none	—	6·3	0	—	6·4	3·7	1·39	9·26
34	DL	Propranolol		none	—	7·4	0	—	7·9	4·2	1·24	9·50

† pK_a $\overset{+}{R}NH_3 \rightleftharpoons RNH_2 + H^+$.

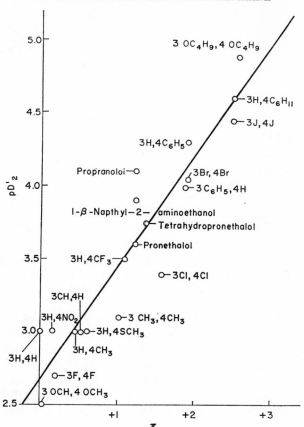

FIG. IV-50. Dependence of pD_2' (rat intestine and vas deferens upon π for a series of β-antagonists (Table IV-71). Reproduced with permission from Pratesi, Grana and Villa (392).

of isopropylmethoxamine appears to have similarly selective β-antagonistic properties (397) as does 1-(4-methylphenyl)-2-isopropylamino-propanol (401; IV-71).

Whilst a number of explanations may be offered to accommodate such selective behavior the most plausible would appear to be that within the

CHOHCHMeNHPr^i CHOHCHMeNHPr^i

IV-70   IV-71

12*

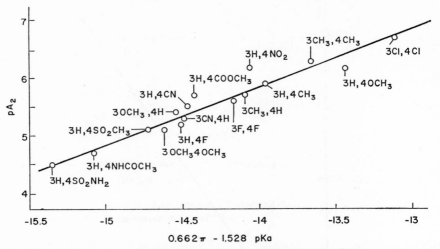

FIG. IV-51. Dependence of pA_2 values (guinea-pig atria) upon $0662\pi - 1.528$ pK_a for a series of β-antagonists (Table IV-71). Reproduced with permission from Pratesi, Grana and Villa (392).

general β-adrenergic receptor classification there exist a number of subdivisions (394–396, 402) that may be delineated by the use of appropriate stimulant or antagonist ligands (see section, p. 235). It may be important that the agents described above having this high degree of selective β-antagonism possess an α-methyl group as a common structural feature. Furthermore, 1-(3,4-dichlorophenyl)-2-isopropyl-aminopropanol (IV-72; α-methyl DCI) also possesses, but to a lesser

IV-72

IV-73

extent, selective β-antagonistic properties since it is equiactive with DCI in the inhibition of adrenergically-induced vasodilatation but is only one-fifteenth as active as DCI on cardiac tissue (398, 403, 404). According to this hypothesis only certain β-receptors are capable of binding agents containing the α-methyl group and only at these sites will antagonism be exhibited. A number of other examples of selective β-antagonism have also been described: 4-(2-hydroxy-3-isopropylaminopropoxy)acetanil-ide (IV-73) is slightly less active than propranolol in depressing myocardial function and free fatty acid elevation in the plasma but is some 150–370 times less active in antagonizing tracheal relaxation and peripheral vasodilation (405, 406). Similarly, in a comparison of IV-71, IV-73 and IV-74, Levy and Wilkenfeld (407) found that IV-74 blocked the positive

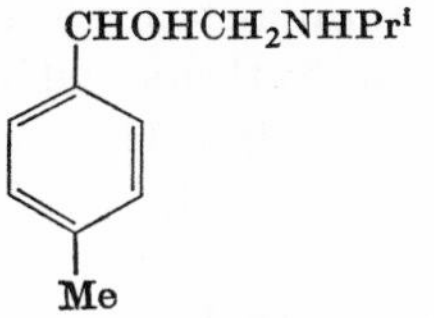

CHOHCH$_2$NHPr^i

Me

IV-74

chronotropic, vasodepressor and intestinal inhibitory responses to isopropylnorepinephrine in the dog, IV-73 blocked only the chronotropic and inhibitory responses whilst IV-71 blocked only the vasodepressor responses.

Further evidence for differences amongst β-receptors comes from the work of Bristow *et al.* (408) who have determined K_B values for four

TABLE IV-72. Apparent K_B Values for β-Antagonists in Rabbit Tissues (408)

| | Apparent K_B (mean $\pm$ SE) | | | |
	IV-64 M $\times$ 10^9	IV-73 M $\times$ 10^7	IV-75 M $\times$ 10^7	IV-76 M $\times$ 10^7
Atrium	$1\cdot35 \pm 0\cdot24$	$1\cdot67 \pm 0\cdot17$	$5\cdot88 \pm 0\cdot49$	$4\cdot38 \pm 1\cdot19$
Aorta	$1\cdot09 \pm 0\cdot19$	1100 ± 100	$2\cdot26 \pm 0\cdot36$	no activity
Stomach	180 ± 51	no activity	†	no activity
Trachea	†	$26\cdot4 \pm 6\cdot0$	†	no activity

† Slopes of less than −1 were obtained in the plot of log (x − 1) against pA$_x$ (250).

antagonists on the rabbit atria, aorta, stomach and trachea preparations (Table IV-72) by the dose-ratio plot of Arunlakshana and Schild (250). Their results indicate very clearly that the four agents have different spectra of β-antagonism and also that very significant differences exist in K_B values for a single antagonist in the various preparations.

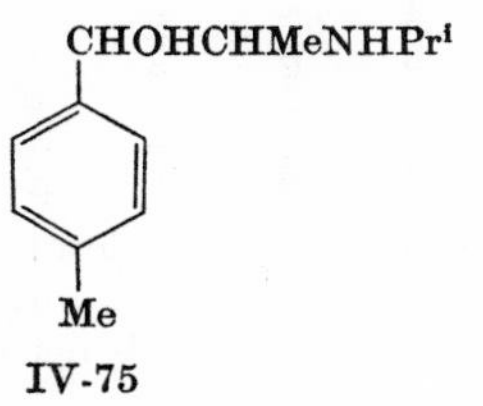

CHOHCHMeNHPr^i CHOHCH$_2$NHPr^i

Me   OH

IV-75 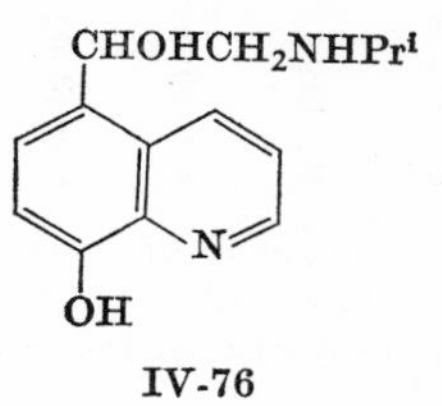   IV-76

Nonspecific Actions of Adrenergic β-Antagonists

It is important to note that many β-adrenergic antagonists interact at sites other than the β-receptor proper to produce effects that may be grossly and mechanistically similar to β-antagonism. In particular many of these agents possess antiarrhythmic activity against experimentally induced cardiac arrhythmias (409–411) which is attributable to a nonspecific "quinidine-like" activity (412) in depressing cardiac excitability.

Thus, both stereoisomers of DCI are capable of reversing digitalis-induced arrhythmias (411, 419) although there are pronounced differences in the β-antagonist activities of these isomers. Similarly, the fortyfold difference in the β-antagonist activities of the stereoisomers of pronethalol is not reflected in their ability to reverse digitalis-induced arrhythmias (416). Lucchesi *et al.* have also found that (+)-propranolol (417), ineffective in reducing catecholamine-induced arrhythmias, is equiactive to (±)-propranolol as a nonspecific antiarrhythmic agent.

Such nonspecific antiarrhythmic activities are not, however, common

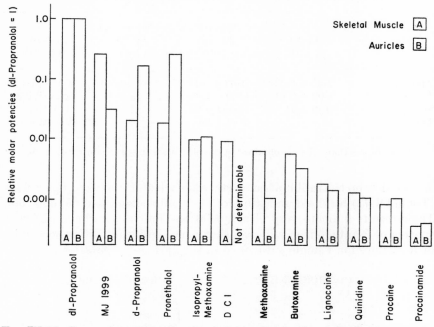

Fig. IV-52. Comparison of anti-epinephrine activities in skeletal (denervated soleus) and cardiac (rabbit auricles) muscles of a series of β-antagonists and anti-arrhythmic agents (*dl*-Propranolol = 1). Reproduced with permission from Raper and Jowett (429).

to all β-antagonists. Thus, INPEA (IV-67), MJ-1999 (IV-65) and 4-(2-hydroxy-3-isopropylaminopropoxy)acetanilide (IV-73) are effective against epinephrine-induced cardiac arrhythmias but ineffective against ouabain-induced arrhythmias: in contrast pronethalol is effective against both (375, 414, 415). It appears generally accepted that the effects of β-antagonists on epinephrine-induced arrhythmias are due to their specific effects at the β-adrenergic receptor since the duration of the β-antagonistic and antiarrhythmic (epinephrine-induced) effects of

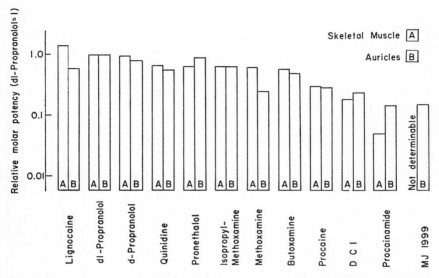

FIG. IV-53. Comparison of anti-fibrillatory activities in skeletal muscle (denervated soleus) and cardiac muscle (rabbit auricles). The same series of compounds was employed as in Fig. IV-52. Reproduced with permission from Raper and Jowett (429).

pronethalol are very similar and quite distinct from the duration of the nonspecific antiarrhythmic effects: furthermore, INPEA and MJ-1999 inhibit epinephrine-induced arrhythmias but not ouabain-induced arrhythmias. It is thus of particular interest that DCI, pronethalol and propranolol possess considerable local anesthetic activity (375, 419, 420) whilst INPEA (IV-67) and MJ-1999 (IV-65) are devoid of such activity (375, 421, 422). Accordingly, the quinidine-like antiarrhythmic properties of β-antagonists are probably exerted through a membrane stabilization process (Chapter II, see section, p. 175).

It is well recognized that changes in Na^+_{EXT} and Ca^{++}_{EXT} significantly alter the actions of quinidine (423–425) suggesting competition between Na^+, Ca^{++} and quinidine for Na^+ entry during depolarization. Together with

the findings (426–428) that quinidine, pronethalol (IV-63) and propranolol (IV-64) inhibit the transport of Ca^{++} across aqueous-membrane
lipid-solvent interfaces and the uptake of Ca^{++} by isolated cardiac
sarcoplasmic reticulum there is little doubt that a primary site of action
of some β-antagonists is concerned with Ca^{++} binding/mobilization.

Raper and Jowett (429) have extended these studies further in a
comparison of the β-antagonistic and quinidine-like actions of β-

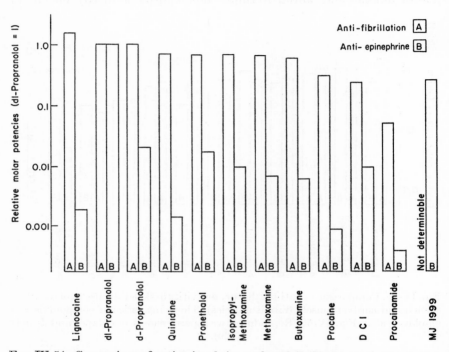

Fig. IV-54. Comparison of anti-epinephrine and anti-fibrillatory activities in the
denervated soleus preparation: listed in order of decreasing activity as anti-
fibrillary agents. Reproduced with permission from Raper and Jowett (429).

antagonists and other compounds in rabbit auricles and chronically
denervated skeletal muscle. Their data demonstrates a rather similar
order of activity as β-antagonists and quinidine-like agents in both
tissues (Figs IV-52 and IV-53) suggesting that the respective molecular
bases for these two processes are similar. Furthermore, the local
anesthetics, lignocaine and procaine, both have antifibrillatory effects
lending further support to the concept that membrane stabilization
forms the basis of the quinidine-like actions of β-antagonists. The data of
Figs IV-54 and IV-55 reveal no obvious correlation between the

structural requirements for β-antagonistic and quinidine-like actions: quite generally the quinidine-like activities are relatively constant and vary little with molecular structure in both the skeletal muscle and cardiac preparations and it is of interest that MJ-1999, the agent most structurally related to isopropylnorepinephrine, shows the least quinidine-like activity. Additionally, the quinidine-like actions are of significantly shorter duration than the β-antagonistic actions further

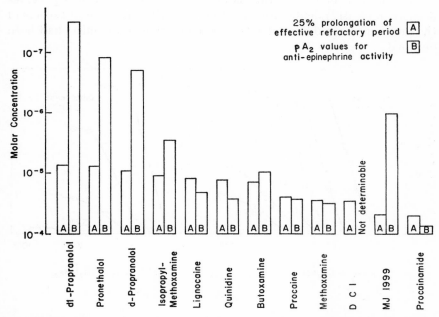

Fig. IV-55. Comparison of the molar concentrations of the agents listed in Fig. IV-52 to produce a 25 per cent prolongation of the effective refractory period and pA₂ values in isolated rabbit auricles: arranged in order of decreasing activity as antifibrillatory agents. Reproduced with permission from Raper and Jowett (429).

suggesting the separate character of these events. Finally, from Fig. IV-55 it is interesting to note that isopropylmethoxamine (IV-69) and tert-butylmethoxamine, agents described as devoid of β-activity on the heart do affect the heart but only at concentrations that produce quinidine-like effects also.

From the above comments it is clear that many β-antagonists possess the ability to produce membrane stabilization by a mechanism apparently independent of events at the β-adrenergic receptor. It appears probable, however, that both processes are intimately concerned with Ca^{++} (Chapter II, see section, p. 164 and Chapter VII): this is of great interest since there is evidence available (p. 336 and Chapter VII) that many α-adrenergic antagonists also share the dual function of interacting at the α-receptor site and at a site (or sites) concerned with Ca^{++} binding.

Antagonist Binding Sites and the Determination and Quantitation of Agonist–Receptor Interactions

The material of this section is actually an extension of a previous discussion (p. 212) deliberately postponed until some general aspects of the mechanisms and sites of action of irreversible antagonists had been outlined.

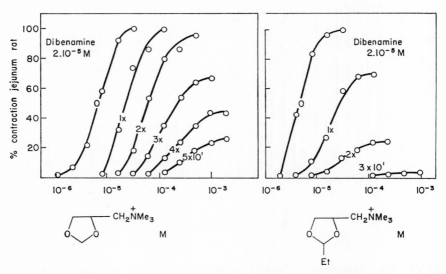

FIG. IV-56a. Cumulative concentration–response curves for two dioxolanes (as indicated) in rat jejunum following treatment with Dibenamine.

As irreversibly acting antagonists to the actions of acetylcholine, histamine, norepinephrine and 5-hydroxytryptamine the 2-halogeno-ethylamines, particularly Dibenamine and phenoxybenzamine, have been employed quite extensively in attempts to define the quantitative basis of agonist–receptor interactions and in particular, to determine agonist–receptor affinity constants and the relationship between receptor occupation and tissue response (p. 212). Nickerson, Stephenson, Ariëns, Furchgott and others have suggested that because the concentration–response curves for many agonists are initially shifted to the right by Dibenamine and related agents prior to declination in maximum response (Fig. IV-3) a "receptor reserve" is present which must be inactivated before an actual loss of agonist-induced response is observed. Such evidence lends support to the variously expressed hypotheses (p. 212) that agonists need not occupy all of the receptors to initiate maximum response and that different agonists may produce identical responses through interaction with different numbers of receptors. Quite generally, the extent of the parallel shift is dependent upon the agonist in question, partial agonists generally producing little or no shift compared with full agonists (Fig. IV-56; 6, 15, 16, 20) and the extent of the shift is, therefore, taken to be a measure of the effective receptor reserve, this being small or absent with partial agonists.

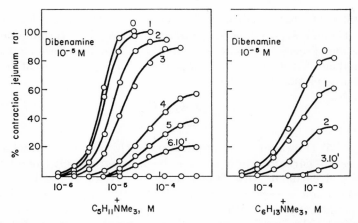

FIG. IV-56b. Cumulative concentration–response curves for two alkyltrimethyl-ammonium ligands (as indicated) in rat jejunum following treatment with Dibenamine. Reproduced with permission from Ariëns, van Rossum and Koopman (15).

Clearly, the above assumptions have extremely important consequences if correct, for they indicate rather forcibly that there is little significance in attempts to obtain K_A values directly from such curves and that more refined treatments will be necessary to generate "true" K_A values and to determine a parameter such as efficacy or intrinsic efficacy that will serve to characterize the ability of an agonist–receptor complex to initiate the response. In such treatments the irreversibly acting antagonists play a central role. Furchgott (14, 430) and Stephenson (431) have produced independently (see also Waud 432, 433) a method designed to generate values for K_A and efficacy. In their treatment the following relationship is assumed to be valid,

$$\frac{r_A}{r_{max}} = f(S) = f(\epsilon[RA]) = f\left\{\frac{\epsilon[R_{tot}][A]}{K_A + [A]}\right\} \qquad (XXXVII)$$

where the symbolism is as previously described (see section, p. 212). If a certain number of the receptors are inactivated by an irreversible antagonist leaving a fraction q still active,

$$\frac{r'_A}{r_{max}} = f(S') = f(\epsilon[RA'])$$
(XXXVIII)

and when $r'_A = r_{A'}$ then $S' = S$ and $[RA'] = [RA]$ so that

$$\frac{1}{[A]} = \frac{1-q}{qK_A} + \frac{1}{q[A']}$$
(XXXIX)

and a plot of $1/[A]$ against $1/[A']$ should yield a straight line with slope $= 1/q$ and $K_A = $ (slope $-$ 1)/intercept. If K_A is determinable then the fraction of receptors occupied, $[RA]/[R_{tot}]$, can be determined and r_A evaluated as a function of $[RA]/[R_{tot}]$ and with K_A for different agonists on the same preparation then

$$\frac{\epsilon_1}{\epsilon_2} = \frac{[RA_2]/[R_{tot}]}{[RA_1]/[R_{tot}]}$$
(XL)

Figure IV-57 shows a typical application of this approach in which the responses to carbamylcholine have been progressively modified by increasing treatment with Dibenamine to give a K_A value for the carbamylcholine–receptor complex of $1\cdot34 \times 10^{-5}$ M. Values obtained for other agonists together with efficacy data are presented in Table IV-73 and indicate the importance of dissociating the structural features which contribute to affinity and efficacy respectively (p. 212).

However, a number of assumptions are, of necessity, implicit in the Furchgott–Stephenson treatment; some of these, i.e., that the concentration of agonist in solution is equal to that at the receptor and that the agonist interacts at only one receptor, are not unique to this treatment. However, the fundamental assumption that "... the agent used to inactivate the receptors irreversibly, alters the sensitivity of the effector to the agonist only by reducing the concentration of active receptors for the agonist" (430), appears, viewed in the perspective of the previous discussion of the multiplicity of sites and mechanisms of action of the 2-halogenoethylamines, to be open to serious doubt: there is, in fact, considerable evidence that the antagonistic actions of many of these agents cannot be regarded as simply exerted through the irreversible inactivation of the agonist recognition site. Thus, procedures for quantitating agonist–receptor interactions which are based on the above assumption may well be invalid.

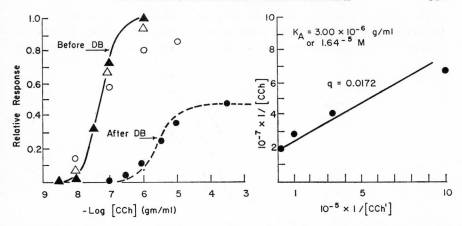

FIG. IV-57. Illustration of the Furchgott procedure for determining "true" affinity constants of ligands. Illustrated is carbamylcholine-Dibenamine antagonism in the rat stomach muscle. Left: concentration–response curves of carbamylcholine before and after Dibenamine ($\circ$, $\triangle$ and $\blacktriangle$ represent the first, second and third curves for carbamylcholine). On the right is the double reciprocal plot for obtaining values of K_A and q (see text). Reproduced with permission from Furchgott (101).

TABLE IV-73. Apparent K_a and Efficacy Values for Agonists Derived from the Furchgott Treatment (14)†

Agonist	Tissue	K_A moles^{-1} liter^{-1}	Efficacy
Carbamylcholine	Rabbit stomach fundus	$1 \cdot 1$–$1 \cdot 6 \times 10^{-5}$	190–266
	Rabbit aorta	$1 \cdot 1$–$1 \cdot 6 \times 10^{-5}$	0·5–10
Pilocarpine	Rabbit stomach fundus	$0 \cdot 7 \times 10^{-5}$	2·5
Histamine	Guinea-pig ileum	1×10^{-5}	21
Epinephrine	Rabbit aorta	3–5×10^{-6}	—

Agonists	Tissue	Affinity ratios	Efficacy ratios
Carbamylcholine/ acetylcholine	Rabbit stomach fundus	0·12	1·05
Acetyl-β-methyl-choline/acetyl-choline	Rabbit stomach fundus	0·7	0·73
Pilocarpine/ carbamylcholine	Rabbit stomach fundus	2·4	0·054
Pilocarpine/ acetylcholine	Rabbit stomach fundus	0·30	0·054

† Progressive inactivation by Dibenamine.

It is known that the extent of inactivation of an agonist response may be dependent upon the irreversible antagonist employed. In the α-adrenergic rat vas deferens preparation, for example, the modification

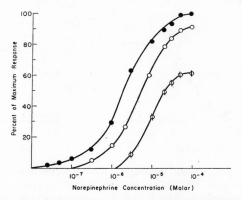

FIG. IV-58. Effect of N,N-dimethyl-2-bromo-phenylethylamine on concentration–response curve of norepinephrine in rat vas deferens: ●, control; ○ and ∅ progressive incubation with 5×10^{-6} M antagonist.

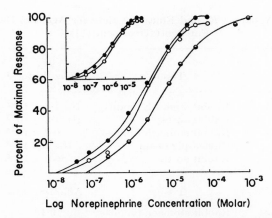

FIG. IV-59. Concentration–response curves of norepinephrine in rat vas deferens. Control, ●; after SY-28, ◕; after SY-28 and sodium thiosulfate, ○. Inset curve shows the effect of thiosulfate on norepinephrine alone.

of norepinephrine concentration–response curves produced by DMPEA and SY-28 are shown in Figs IV-58 and IV-59 respectively from which it is apparent that the characteristic parallel shift is produced only by SY-28. Furthermore, this parallel shift, which is not reversed by washing or with norepinephrine is almost entirely reversed by sodium thiosulfate

(Fig. IV-59; 351) suggesting that it is attributable to tightly bound SY-28 (or derived ethyleniminium ion) rather than to the irreversible inactivation of a receptor reserve. Comparison of DMPEA and SY-28 reveals that the latter structure (or its derived cyclic ion) has considerably more nonpolar character and may therefore be anticipated to bind more effectively in nonpolar areas and to be relatively resistant to desorption.

An interesting complexity is also observed in the actions of Dibenamine on the responses to a series of cholinergic agonists (Fig. IV-60) from which

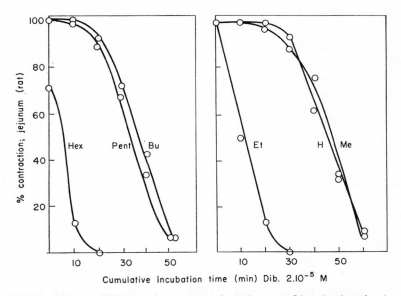

FIG. IV-60. Effects of Dibenamine (progressively increased incubation time) upon the responses of rat jejunum to a series of alkyltrimethylammonium ligands. Reproduced with permission from Ariëns (12).

it is apparent that less alkylation is required to abolish the responses to the poorer (partial) agonists than to the agonists which demonstrate the phenomena of a receptor reserve. On a simple basis, since the agonists are assumed to occupy the same receptors, it might be assumed that the same degree of alkylation would be required to eliminate the responses to both full and partial agonists. That this is very evidently not so may be explained by at least two mechanisms: according to the Stephenson–Furchgott treatment the efficacies of partial agonists are very low so that below a critical fraction of residual active receptors the term eY (eqn. XIII, p. 215) falls below a value sufficient to generate a significant stimulus, S, and hence no response is observed: alternatively, the findings represented in Fig. IV-60 could be quite simply explained by the assumption that the alkylation process produces differential inhibition of agonist binding, having an apparently greater effect upon the partial agonists. According to this latter mechanism the parallel shift of the agonist concentration–response curve produced by Diben-amine and related agents would be due, not to the elimination of a receptor reserve, but to an antagonist binding mechanism producing an allosterically modified binding site with reduced affinity for agonist ligands. Evidence to support this latter assumption derived both from receptor and enzyme systems will be presented in a subsequent section (p. 339).

The Quantitation of α-Adrenergic Responses. As noted previously (see section, p. 298) the use of Dibenamine analogs in the quantitation of adrenergic α-receptors is complicated by their apparent general lack of specificity and the absence of substantial evidence that their antagonism is exhibited only at the norepinephrine recognition site. In contrast, N,N-dimethyl-2-bromo-2-phenylethylamine and its analogs (see section, p. 308) appear to be substantially more specific in their actions and are more likely to have a major component of their antagonistic properties produced through interaction at the norepinephrine α-receptor site. Such agents should be more useful in quantitating agonist–receptor interactions.

In a detailed examination (94, 349–351) of the kinetics of recovery of α-adrenergic response following irreversible antagonism by N,N-dimethyl-2-bromo-2-phenylethylamine it has been observed that the agonist concentration–response curves obtained during the recovery period show no evidence for the parallel shift that would be anticipated if any significant receptor reserve existed in these systems (Fig. IV-58). Furthermore, the rates of recovery of response to a series of agonists are essentially identical (Table IV-74) suggesting that these agonists occupy the same number of receptors to produce the same fraction of their respective maximum responses. In addition the rate of loss of ^{3}H-label $(C_6H_5C^3HOHCH_2NMe_2)$ was found to follow first-order kinetics with a rate not distinguishable from the rates of recovery of response (Table IV-74). If this process does indeed reflect the loss of label from the α-receptor (p. 308) then, for rabbit aorta, rat aorta and vas deferens, the rate of recovery of response is identical to the rate of regeneration to free receptors and the response is therefore directly proportional to the number of α-receptors available for interaction with the agonist ligand and maximum response requires the availability of 100 per cent of the α-receptors. These are, of course, exactly the proposals originally advanced by A. J. Clark and they indicate that in the sequence of events (eqn. I, p. 211) initiated by the agonist–receptor interaction this primary interaction is determinant for the entire sequence. This conclusion is supported by the data of Fig. IV-61 which shows that the rate of recovery of response to Ca^{++} in a Ca^{++}-free media in the presence of a constant

TABLE IV-74. Half-lives of α-Receptor Blockade to Adrenergic Agonists following N,N-Dimethyl-2-bromo-2-phenylethylamine (350)

Agonist	$t_{1/2}$ (min) $\pm$ S.D.†
D(−)-Epinephrine	$19\cdot7 \pm 5\cdot8$
D(−)-Norepinephrine	$23\cdot0 \pm 2\cdot6$
DL-N-Ethylnorepinephrine	$26\cdot6 \pm 4\cdot4$
DL-N-Isopropylnorepinephrine	$27\cdot8 \pm 3\cdot2$
^{3}H-N,N-Dimethyl-2-bromo-2-phenylethylamine—appearance of ^{3}H-label	$20\cdot7 \pm 4\cdot1$

† Determined from first-order plots from rabbit aortic strips. Identical values were obtained from rat vas deferens preparation (351).

concentration of norepinephrine following antagonism by N,N-dimethyl-2-bromo-2-phenylethylamine is identical to the rate of recovery to norepinephrine in a normal Ca^{++} media: this indicates the existence of

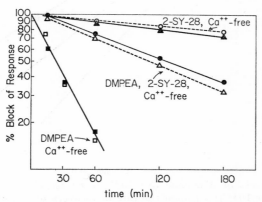

FIG. IV-61. Recoveries of response to norepinephrine and Ca^{++} following blockade of α-receptors in rat vas deferens by N,N-dimethyl-2-bromo-2-phenylethylamine (DMPEA) and N-ethyl-N-2-bromoethyl-2′-naphthylmethylamine(2-SY-28).

obligatorily linked norepinephrine recognition and Ca^{++} binding/ mobilization (434) sites (Fig. IV-62) such that Ca^{++} is not available for the contractile process until the norepinephrine site is activated (Chapter VII). Quite probably this represents a linked function in the sense defined by Wyman (Chapter I, see section, p. 71).

A number of lines of evidence indicate that the Ca^{++} involvement represented in Fig. IV-62 represents a major site of interaction at which α-adrenergic antagonism is produced by the Dibenamine class of

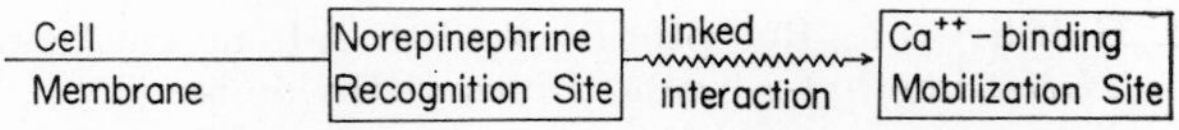

Cell	Norepinephrine	linked	Ca^{++}-binding
Membrane	Recognition Site	interaction	Mobilization Site

FIG. IV-62. Linked interaction of norepinephrine and Ca^{++} sites at the adrenergic α-receptor.

2-halogenoethylamines (see also Chapter VII, section on p. 535). In particular the characteristic prolonged duration of blockade produced by this class of compounds is drastically modified by a number of agents including diazoxide (435, 436) and local anesthetics (437; Chapter II, see

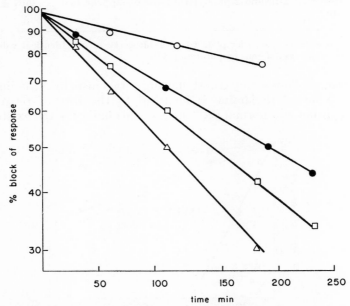

FIG. IV-63. Effects of diazoxide (5×10^{-5} M, ●) tetracaine (10^{-4} M, □) and cinchocaine (5×10^{-4}, M △) upon the rate of recovery of maximum response to norepinephrine in the rat vas deferens following blockade by N-2-bromoethyl-N-ethyl-2'-naphthylmethylamine.

section, p. 175) known to interfere with Ca^{++} binding-mobilization processes and which convert the prolonged antagonism to one of shorter duration without significant effect on the initial degree of blockade (Fig. IV-63). Many 2-halogenoethylamines apparently interact at least two sites, which are kinetically distinguishable, to produce α-adrenergic antagonism. The site of prolonged duration is concerned with Ca^{++}

function and that of shorter duration may be intimately concerned with the inactivation of the norepinephrine recognition site since the rate of recovery of response to norepinephrine following alkylation of this site only is identical to the rate of recovery of response to Ca^{++} (Fig. IV-61).

The Quantitation of Cholinergic (Muscarinic) Responses. The use of Dibenamine analogs in quantitating agonist–receptor interactions at muscarinic receptors in smooth muscle systems is complicated by factors essentially similar to those discussed under adrenergic α-receptor systems. However, the typical parallel shift of the full agonist concentration–response curves produced by these agents is generally significantly more prominent than with adrenergic α-receptor systems and has therefore been attributed to the existence of a large receptor reserve. The availability (94, 315, 438) of irreversible agents that have close structural analogy to known competitive reversible antagonists at muscarinic receptors (IV-77–IV-79) has served to offer alternative

$$(C_6H_5)_2COHCOOCH_2CH_2NMeCH_2CH_2Cl$$

IV-77

$$(C_6H_5)_2CHOCH_2CH_2NMeCH_2CH_2Cl$$

IV-78

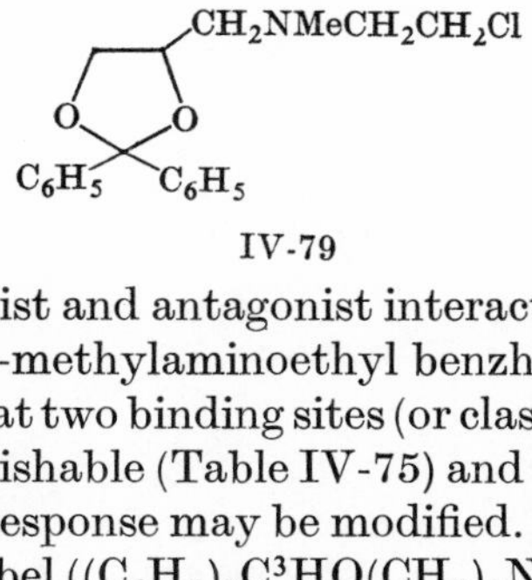

IV-79

interpretations of agonist and antagonist interactions at these receptors. 2-(N-2-Chloroethyl)-N-methylaminoethyl benzhydryl ether (IV-78) has been shown to interact at two binding sites (or classes of binding sites) that are kinetically distinguishable (Table IV-75) and at either of which modification of the agonist response may be modified. The biphasic kinetics of first-order loss of ^3H-label (($C_6H_5)_2C^3HO(CH_2)_2NMeCH_2CH_2OH$) accord with the two distinct rates of recovery of maximum response to a series of agonists in the rat jejunum (Table IV-75) such that alkylation of site A appears to determine the loss of maximum response to acetylcholine (Fig. IV-64) and other active compounds and alkylation of site B appears to determine the loss of maximum response to poor and partial agonists as hexyltrimethylammonium *and* the loss of sensitivity (as measured by the parallel shift without depression of maximum response) for acetylcholine and related polar ligands as carbamylcholine and *cis*-2-methyl-4-dimethylaminomethyl-1,3-dioxolane methiodide (Fig. IV-65). These

TABLE IV-75. Recovery of Maximum Response to Various Agonists following Blockade by $(C_6H_5)_2CHOCH_2CH_2NMeCH_2CH_2Cl$

Agonist		$t_{1/2}$ min	No. obs.
$CH_3COOCH_2CH_2\overset{+}{N}Me_3$		$32\cdot6 \pm 13\cdot6$	(10)
$H_2NCOOCH_2CH_2\overset{+}{N}Me_3$		$80 \pm 15\cdot0$	(10)
cis-2-Me-4-$CH_2\overset{+}{N}Me_3$-1,3-dioxolane		$74\cdot8 \pm 13\cdot5$	(10)
$C_3H_7\overset{+}{N}Me_3$		(215)	
$C_4H_9\overset{+}{N}Me_3$		$65 \pm 16\cdot0$	(10)
$C_5H_{11}\overset{+}{N}Me_3$		$75 \pm 11\cdot0$	(10)
$C_6H_{13}\overset{+}{N}Me_3$		$500 \pm 50\cdot0$	(10)
$C_4H_9\overset{+}{N}Me_2Et$		$245 \pm 15\cdot4$	(10)
$C_5H_{11}\overset{+}{N}Me_2Et$		$508 \pm 84\cdot0$	(10)
$(C_6H_5)_2C^3HOCH_2CH_2NMeCH_2CH_2Cl$	I:	$24\cdot7 \pm 6\cdot4$	(10)
	II:	602 ± 175	(10)

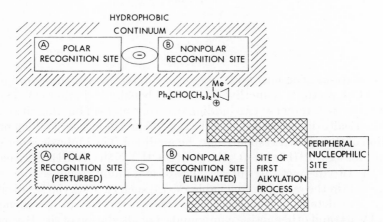

FIG. IV-64. A "two-site" representation of the muscarinic receptor site. Alkylation at a peripheral site eliminates binding at the nonpolar site and perturbs the polar binding area to reduce its affinity for polar ligands (see Fig. IV-65). Subsequent alkylation, perhaps at the receptor anionic site itself, eliminates all response. A generalized representation of the concentration–response curves is shown in Fig. IV-66.

observations suggest quite clearly that the interaction of IV-78 at site B is to be regarded as an allosteric modification of agonist binding site affinity rather than the elimination of a receptor reserve: the effect is generally least marked for the highly polar ligands (acetylcholine, carbamylcholine, *cis*-dioxolane, etc.), producing a reduction in affinity and most marked for the least active and least polar ligands (hexyl $\overset{+}{N}Me_3$, $Bu\overset{+}{N}Me_2Et$, etc.) producing a loss of response (Fig. IV-66). In

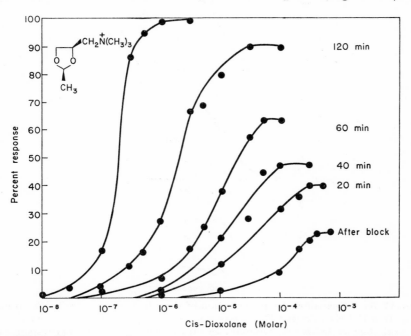

FIG. IV-65. Recovery of response of rat jejunum to *cis*-2-methyl-4-dimethylaminomethyl-1,3-dioxolane methiodide following exposure to $Ph_2CHOCH_2CH_2NMeCH_2CH_2Cl$. Curve on left is the control.

contrast, the alkylation of site A (which may be identical with the presumed anionic site of the acetylcholine recognition site of the receptor) produces loss of activity which is only apparent with the polar ligands.

The agreement between the rate of loss of ^3H-label from site A and the recovery of maximum response to acetylcholine suggests, according to the basically similar argument advanced for the adrenergic α-receptor (p. 336), that the response to acetylcholine in the rat jejunum is also directly proportional to the number of receptors available for interaction and that maximum response requires 100 per cent availability of the receptors. However, this situation at the muscarinic receptor is substantially more complex because of the existence of at least two binding sites for the antagonist ligand through which differential modification of the agonist-induced response may be achieved.

These observations relate very directly to the previous discussion of the structural requirements for cholinomimetic activity (see section, p.

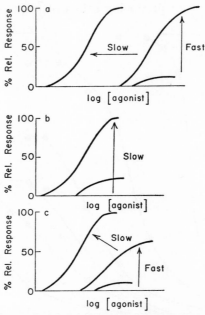

FIG. IV-66. A generalized representation of the effects of the alkylating species $Ph_2CHOCH_2CH_2NMeCH_2CH_2Cl$, upon concentration–response curves of cholinomimetic ligands in the rat jejunum. In (a) the recovery of original response to polar ligands (ACh etc.) is characterized by two discrete phases; in (b) the recovery of original response to nonpolar ligands ($hexN^+Me_3$ etc.) is characterized by one phase only; in (c) the recovery of original response to ligands of intermediate polarity is again a two phase process, but the relative importance of the two phases is markedly different to those in (a).

257) according to which the binding site for agonist ligands at the muscarinic receptor has discrete areas for binding of polar and nonpolar groups (Fig. IV-16): similar evidence is also available for acetylcholinesterase and other enzyme systems (see section, p. 257).

It is of some interest that similar differential effects of irreversible modification have been observed for substrate and inhibitor binding specificities to a number of enzyme systems. Thus, conversion of the two methionine residues of chymotrypsin, neither of which is essential to

TABLE IV-76. Effects of Methionine Oxidation upon Substrate Specificity of Chymotrypsin (439)

| | Relative hydrolysis rates | |
Substrate	Native/monosulfoxide	Native/disulfoxide
Acetyltyrosine ethyl ester	3	4
Acetyltyrosine hydroxamate	20	16
Acetyltyrosine amide	6	>400

activity, to the sulfoxide derivatives produces a change in the relative ability of the enzyme to hydrolyse ester and peptide substrates (439; Table IV-76): similarly, the oxidation of methionine-222 of subtilisin (Carlsberg) produces changes in K_m and k_{cat} that are substrate dependent (440; Table IV-77). Royer and Canady have demonstrated (441) that conversion of methionine-192 of chymotrypsin to $-\overset{+}{S}MeCH_2CONH-$ $C(Me)_2COO^-$ produces a decrease in the affinity of the enzyme for simple nonpolar inhibitors and decreases the affinity for the substrate methyl hippurate (Table IV-78). Of particular interest, of course, are studies with acetylcholinesterase (see section, p. 257) in which irreversible inhibition by aziridinium ions eliminates activity towards positively charged substrates and even increases activity towards some neutral substrates.

Finally, the evidence discussed above that irreversible antagonism to acetylcholine-induced responses can be exerted through an allosteric interaction is in accord with previous suggestions concerning the sites

TABLE IV-77. Effect of Methionine Oxidation upon Subtilisin Activity (440)

| | Subtilisin | | Oxidized subtilisin | |
Substrate	k_{cat} sec^{-1}	K_M (app.) M	k_{cat} sec^{-1}	K_M (app.) M
N-Acetyl-L-tyrosine ethyl ester	15×10^2	6.1×10^2	1.8×10^2	9.1×10^{-2}
N-Benzoyl-L-arginine ethyl ester	21	4.8×10^{-3}	1.7	9.5×10^{-2}
N-Benzyloxycarbonyl-glycine p-nitrophenyl ester	280	3.9×10^{-4}	79	2.8×10^{-4}
Cinnamoyl imidazole	22×10^{-3}	3.6×10^{-6}	9.4×10^{-3}	13×10^{-4}

and mechanisms of action of many adrenergic and cholinergic antagonists. In particular, the actions of atropine and related agents present a number of difficulties, from several points of view, with the concept that they compete directly with acetylcholine for the same binding site (see

TABLE IV-78. $\Delta F°$ Values for Formation of Enzyme-inhibitor Complexes in Chymotrypsin and Alkylated Chymotrypsin (441)

Inhibitor	K	$-\Delta F°$ kcal/mole
Benzene		
Control enzyme	96	2·71
Alkylated enzyme	59	2·42
Toluene		
Control enzyme	450	3·63
Alkylated enzyme	183	3·09
Naphthalene		
Control enzyme	10,500	5·50
Alkylated enzyme	5500	5·11
Methyl hippurate†		
Control enzyme	328	3·44
Alkylated enzyme	154	2·99

† Substrate values are for ES formation.

section, p. 365). However, by analogy with the mechanism of action proposed for IV-78 an allosteric interaction mechanism would appear to accommodate in a satisfactory manner the actions of atropine and related ligands.

Antagonists at the Skeletal Neuromuscular Junction

A representative selection of antagonists active at the skeletal neuromuscular junction is given in Fig. IV-67. Structural considerations lend some support to the original classification introduced by Bovet (442) of "leptocurares" (long, thin molecules) and "pachycurares" (fat molecules) a structural classification which parallels to a considerable extent the mechanistic classification of these agents into depolarizing and nondepolarizing categories. Several fairly comprehensive reviews of these agents are available (158, 443–450). There are fundamental differences in the mechanisms of action of agents belonging to these two classes which must indicate fundamentally different mechanisms of interaction.

Decamethonium and other depolarizing antagonists produce, like

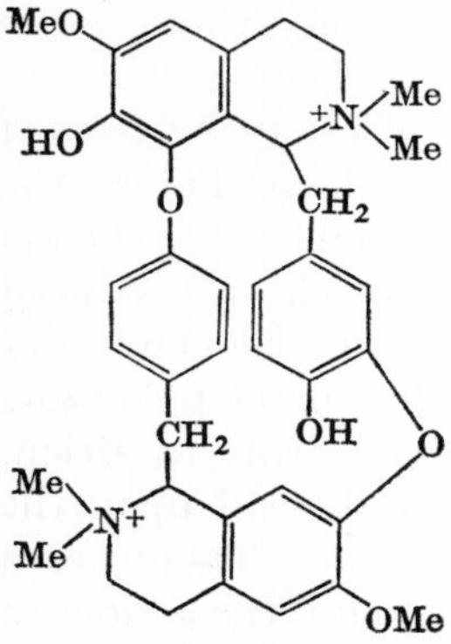

a d-Tubocurarine

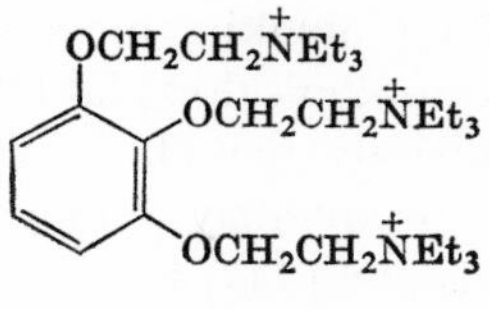

b Gallamine

$Me_3\overset{+}{N}(CH_2)_{10}\overset{+}{N}Me_3$

c Decamethonium

$Me_3\overset{+}{N}CH_2CH_2OOC(CH_2)_2COOCH_2CH_2\overset{+}{N}Me_3$

d Suxamethonium

FIG. IV-67. Structural formulae of antagonists effective at the skeletal neuro-muscular junction.

acetylcholine, an immediate depolarization of the muscle endplate (Chapter V, see sections on p. 407 and p. 413) and the closely adjacent muscle cell membrane which is often accompanied by initial signs of excitation-fasiculations, contractures, etc. (451–455). This depolarization is more prolonged (but see below) than that produced by acetylcholine and renders the endplate region insensitive to added acetylcholine. In contrast, tubocurarine and related nondepolarizing agents do not

TABLE IV-79. Differences in the Actions of Depolarizing (Decamethonium) and Nondepolarizing (d-Tubocurarine) Antagonists at the Skeletal Neuromuscular Junction

	d-Tubocurarine	Decamethonium
Prior addition of d-tubocurarine	Additive	Antagonistic
Effect of AChE inhibitors	Reversal	No effect
Effect on end plate	Elevated threshold to ACh	Partial depolarization
Initial effect on striated muscle	None	Transient excitation
Effect of K+	Transient reversal	No effect
Effect of current at end plate:		
Cathodal	Decreases block	Increases block
Anodal	Increases block	Decreases block
Effect of reduced temperature	Reversal and shortening of block	Increase and prolongation of block

depolarize the endplate and have been generally assumed to act quite simply as competitive antagonists.

In many respects, however, the division between these two classes of compounds is not as simple as that outlined above: the actions of the depolarizing blocking agents are highly species dependent and in certain species (monkey, dog, rabbit, rat) a so-called "dual block" is produced which initially has the characteristics of a depolarizing blockade but which subsequently changes to a blockade having nondepolarizing characteristics (447, 456, 457). There is some evidence that this transition, characteristic of depolarizing blocking agents, may depend upon the *intracellular* accumulation of the agents (447, 458–460). There are a number of other extremely significant differences between the actions of these two classes of blocking agents which are summarized in Table IV-79. It is clear that, at least in their initial effects, the depolarizing agents are to be regarded as agonists with persistent effects. Analysis of the structure–activity relationships of these two classes of antagonists lends further support to this assumption.

Depolarizing Blocking Agents. Following the discovery of the neuromuscular blocking activity of decamethonium (451, 461) a very large number of *bis*-onium compounds have been synthesized and evaluated (158, 443–450). In these compounds maximum depolarizing activity is, almost without exception, found with the $-\overset{+}{N}Me_3$ or $-\overset{+}{N}Me_2Et$ functions and a particularly marked decrease is observed with the transition from $-\overset{+}{N}Me_2Et$ to $-\overset{+}{N}MeEt_2$ (Table IV-17; cf. p. 236). This effect is entirely analogous to that observed with progressive substitution of the $-\overset{+}{N}Me_3$ group of acetylcholine and related agonists discussed earlier in this chapter (p. 236) and suggests a similar or identical binding site for the quaternary ammonium functions of *bis*-onium derivatives. Furthermore, the binding sites for both onium groups must be very similar since unsymmetrically substituted *bis*-onium ligands (i.e., $Et_3\overset{+}{N}-X-\overset{+}{N}Me_3$) are less active than the corresponding *bis*-trimethylammonium ligands. This is in marked contrast to the *bis*-onium ganglion blocking agents (pp. 356–365) where the same unsymmetrical substitution promotes activity and suggests that in the depolarizing blocking agents the two onium groups bind and function similarly or identically. Quite generally, the effects of *N*-substitution mark a division between the nondepolarizing and the depolarizing agents for in the former the ratio of activities, $-\overset{+}{N}Me_3/-\overset{+}{N}Et_3 < 1$ and for the latter the ratio $-\overset{+}{N}Me_3/-\overset{+}{N}Et_3 > 1$ is observed (445).

Several other lines of evidence are highly suggestive of common binding loci for the agonists and depolarizing blocking agents. In particular, the high blocking activity of succinylcholine (Table IV-80, $n = 2$), which is clearly two linked acetylcholine molecules, is of considerable interest (462, 463): the effects of progressive conversion of $-\overset{+}{N}Me_3$ to $-\overset{+}{N}Et_3$ in this series of compounds is closely similar to the

TABLE IV-80. Relative Neuromuscular Blocking Activity of Choline Esters of Aliphatic Dicarboxylic Acids (462, 463)

$$Me_3\overset{+}{N}CH_2CH_2OOC(CH_2)_nCOOCH_2CH_2\overset{+}{N}Me_3$$

n	Relative activity†	n	Relative activity
0	0·027	4	4·0
1	1·0	5	0·67
2	10·0	8	0·4
3	4·0		

† Rabbit head drop test, $n = 2 = 0.2$ mg/kg.

same substitutions in decamethonium (464). Succinyl-*bis*-α-methylcholine (IV-80) closely resembles succinylcholine (465) but, significantly, succinyl-*bis*-β-methylcholine (IV-81) is less potent and has at least some nondepolarizing properties (466). These results parallel the activities of acetyl α- and β-methylcholines at the skeletal neuromuscular junction (pp. 257–276). Furthermore, the (+) (+), (−) (−), and (−) (+) isomers of

$$Me_3\overset{+}{N}CH(Me)CH_2OOC(CH_2)_2COOCH_2CH(Me)CH_2\overset{+}{N}Me_3$$

IV-80

$$Me_3\overset{+}{N}CH_2CH(Me)OOC(CH_2)_2COOCH(Me)CH_2\overset{+}{N}Me_3$$

IV-81

succinyl-*bis*-α-methylcholine are approximately equieffective (467) again paralleling the results with the isomers of acetyl-α-methylcholine.

The effect of variation of the character and length of the chain separating the two onium functions has been extensively studied (445, 450). For many series of compounds including the polymethylene $(X(CH_2)_nX)$, dicarboxylic esters $(X(CH_2)_2OOC(CH_2)_nCOO(CH_2)_2X)$, ethers $(X(CH_2)_nO(CH_2)_nX, X(CH_2)_2O(CH_2)_nO(CH_2)_2X)$, monocarboxylic acids $(X(CH_2)_nCOO(CH_2)_mX)$ and several other series depolarizing activity rises sharply when the approximate equivalent of a C_{10} chain is

13

reached although this may represent only one area of a rather broad peak of activity.

These various findings support quite strongly the idea that decamethonium and related depolarizing blocking agents may actually interact simultaneously at two acetylcholine receptors. This suggestion, originally considered by Barlow (158), Stenlake (445) Rybolovlev (468)

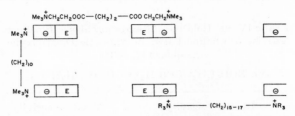

FIG. IV-68. A hypothetical lattice array of cholinergic receptors at the skeletal neuromuscular junction and the orientations of bisquaternary salts.

and Khromov-Boriso and Michelson (469) and other workers, must, if correct, require a regular lattice arrangement of acetylcholine receptors on the cell membrane to accommodate such interaction (Fig. IV-68). Several modes of ligand binding are possible according to the binding site scheme of Fig. IV-68 in which individual acetylcholine receptors are shown, for the sake of simplicity, as consisting of anionic ($\ominus$) and ester (E) binding sites. Decamethonium is represented as simply bridging two

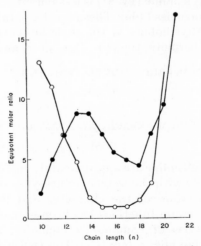

FIG. IV-69. Neuromuscular blocking activities of $Me_3\overset{+}{N}(CH_2)_n\overset{+}{N}Me_3$ ($\bullet$) and $Et_3\overset{+}{N}(CH_2)_n\overset{+}{N}Et_3$ ($\circ$) on cat tibialis preparation as a function of n. Reproduced with permission from Barlow and Zoller (470).

anionic sites, a possibility strengthened by arguments previously presented (pp. 243–247) that in monoquaternary agonists, $\overset{+}{R}NMe_3$, the polar/nonpolar balance of the R function will determine the relative orientation of the ligand around the anionic site: in contrast, succinylcholine may be visualized as occupying both anionic and ester binding sites of two adjacent receptors. Other binding interactions are also possible involving nonadjacent receptors and these may be important in accommodating a number of depolarizing antagonists in which the

TABLE IV-81. Relative Neuromuscular Blocking Activities of Polymethylene-*bis*-carbamylcholines (463, 471)

$$Me_3\overset{+}{N}CH_2CH_2OOCNH(CH_2)_nNHCOOCH_2CH_2\overset{+}{N}Me_3$$

n	Relative activity†	n	Relative activity
0	0·01	5	2·4
1	0·51	6	10·0
2	0·29	7	11·7
3	0·41	10	3·8
4	1·1		

† Rabbit head drop test, n = 6 = 0·034 mg/kg.

interonium distance is very significantly greater than the ten carbon equivalent of decamethonium and succinylcholine. Thus, in the polymethylene-*bis*-trimethylammonium series $(Me_3\overset{+}{N}(CH_2)_n\overset{+}{N}Me_3)$ a second peak of blocking activity is revealed at n = 15–17 and a similar peak is observed with the polymethylene-*bis*-triethylammonium series (Fig. IV-69). Similarly in the *bis*-carbamylcholines $(Me_3\overset{+}{N}(CH_2)_2OOCNH-(CH_2)_nNHCOO(CH_2)_2\overset{+}{N}Me_3)$ a peak of activity is observed at n = 6–7 (471, Table IV-81) these compounds being some twenty times more effective than the hexadecamethylene-*bis*-trimethylammonium structure: the *bis*-sulfonamido agent (IV-82) is as effective as succinylcholine

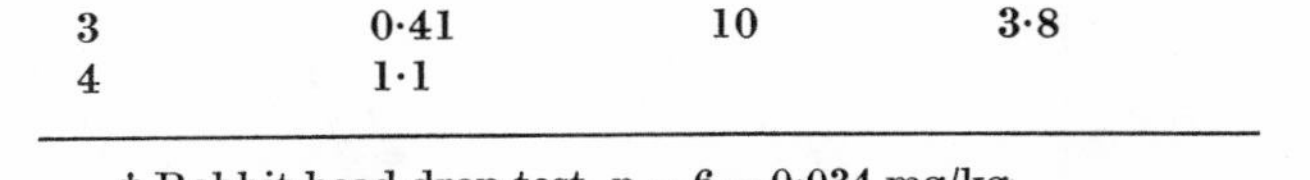

$$Me_3\overset{+}{N}CH_2CH_2NHO_2S-\!\!\!\!\bigcirc\!\!\!\!\bigcirc\!\!\!\!-SO_2NHCH_2CH_2\overset{+}{N}Me_3$$

IV-82

as a depolarizing antagonist. For those agents in which the onium functions are separated by a sixteen carbon chain, or its equivalent, binding across nonadjacent pairs of receptors is visualized as represented in Fig. IV-68.

The Geometry of Cholinergic Receptor Assemblies. This postulate of a lattice or repeating unit arrangement of acetylcholine receptors is also of extreme interest with regard to the actions of acetylcholine and related activator ligands at these receptors since it introduces the possibility of cooperativity of ligand binding (Chapter I, see section, p. 71: a discussion of cooperative membrane assemblies is presented in Chapter II, see section, p. 183). There are several lines of evidence to indicate that

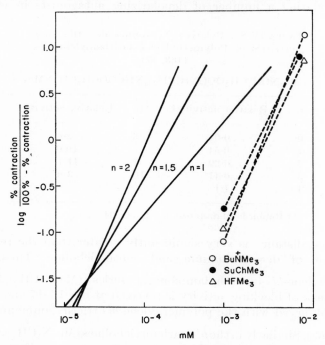

Fig. IV-70. Hill plots of concentration–response curves of cholinergic agonists on frog rectus (BuN̄Me$_3$ and SuChMe$_3$) and guinea-pig intestine (HFMe$_3$). Reproduced with permission from Ariëns (12).

such cooperative processes may indeed occur at the acetylcholine receptor.

The slopes of the concentration–response curves for cholinergic ligands obtained in a variety of tissues are often steeper than calculated theoretically so that plots (Fig. IV-70) of these curves according to the Hill procedure (472) (Chapter I, see section, p. 89) give values for n > 1. An analysis of the kinetics of acetylcholine action on the frog rectus muscle by Cavanaugh and Hearon (473) suggests that both the initial velocities of the contraction process and the extent of final contraction are best described in terms of a model in which two acetylcholine molecules participate in the determinant step. Furthermore, the response of the frog rectus muscle to acetylcholine is reported to be sensitized by the prior treatment of the muscle with small inactive concentrations of butyrylcholine or succinylcholine (474). One interpretation of these findings is clearly in terms of a ligand-induced shift of the allosteric equilibrium between the active and inactive forms of the acetylcholine protomer: there appears to be at least some analogy between the cholinergic receptor system and the allosteric proteins discussed in Chapter I.

However, interpretation of these findings in terms of cooperativity of ligand binding is not unambiguous (475). Thus, it can be argued that

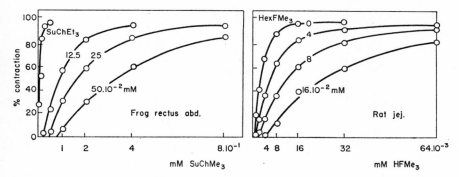

FIG. IV-71. Cumulative concentration–response curves for succinylcholine (SuChMe$_3$) on frog rectus and 4-dimethylaminomethyl-1,3-dioxolane methiodide (HFMe$_3$) on rat jejunum in the presence of increasing concentrations of competitive antagonists as indicated. Reproduced with permission from Ariëns (12).

since the muscle contraction is the net result of the responses of a large number of biological units, the biological variance in a series of objects reacting quantally but summating in graded fashion may be more or less steep than that predicted by theory (247, 476–478). The concept of a "threshold" where a certain number of receptors may have to be occupied before the output stimulus reaches a magnitude sufficient to produce a detectable response may also relate to the steepness of response curves: this may arise quite simply from inertial limitations of the muscle. This consideration has been developed by Kirschner and Stone (479) and Ariëns (472) who assume that the biological response is directly proportional to the input stimulus minus a constant, s, the threshold value. Thus, the extrapolation of the concentration–response curves of Fig. IV-71 results in an intersection point below zero which represents the threshold value, s. If the various threshold values obtained are incorporated into the Hill plot of Fig. IV-70 by plotting log %contraction + S/100-%contraction then the slopes of the plots become closer, although not equal, to unity (Fig. IV-72).

However, since evidence for cooperative ligand binding at cholinergic receptors can also be obtained from electrophysiological measurements using single end plates or single electroplax cells (Chapter V, see sections

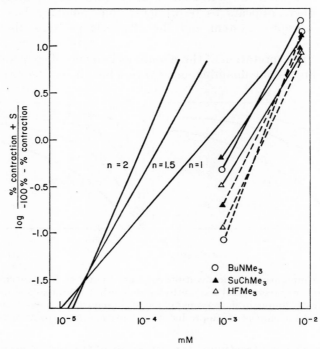

Fig. IV-72. Concentration–response curves of Fig. IV-70 (‑‑‑‑) replotted to include correction for threshold effect (——). Reproduced with permission from Ariëns (12).

on pp. 407 and 413) it seems probable that the various concentration–response curves discussed above do reveal at least some degree of cooperative ligand interaction.

Nondepolarizing Antagonists. The contrast in properties between decamethonium and *d*-tubocurarine which are representative of the two classes of neuromuscular blocking agents is actually not as abrupt as suggested by the data of Table IV-79 since there are many examples of compounds that have intermediate properties and share the activities of both decamethonium and *d*-tubocurarine. Quite generally the transition from depolarizing to nondepolarizing antagonists is accompanied by the progressive introduction of appropriately located hydrophobic groups into the depolarizing ligand. Several aspects of such substitution patterns have been reviewed by Stenlake (445). Thus the introduction of

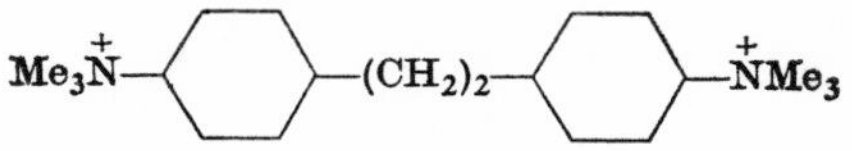

$$Me_3\overset{+}{N}-\langle\ \rangle-(CH_2)_2-\langle\ \rangle-\overset{+}{N}Me_3$$

IV-83

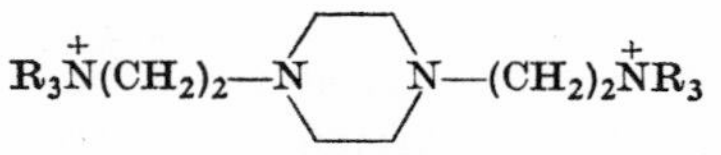

$$R_3\overset{+}{N}(CH_2)_2-N\langle\ \rangle N-(CH_2)_2\overset{+}{N}R_3$$

IV-84

$$R_3\overset{+}{N}(CH_2)_n NH-\langle\ \rangle-NH(CH_2)_n\overset{+}{N}R_3$$

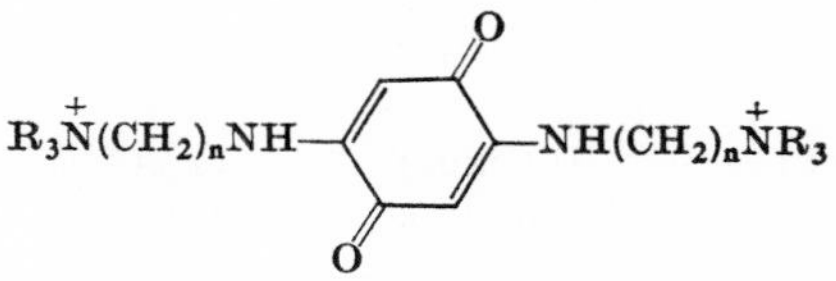

IV-85

cyclohexyl groups to give IV-83 results in the appearance of tubocurarine-like activity (480). Similarly, in the piperazine– (IV-84) and benzo-quinone– (IV-85) linked bisonium compounds tubocurarine-like activity is dominant and the $-\overset{+}{N}Me_3/-\overset{+}{N}Et_3$ activity ratio is <1 (481, 482). In succinylcholine the introduction of one phenyl substituent (IV-86) maintains depolarizing activity, but the diphenylsuccinylcholines

$$Me_3\overset{+}{N}CH_2CH(Ph)OOC(CH_2)_2COOCH_2CH_2\overset{+}{N}Me_3$$

IV-86

$$Me_3\overset{+}{N}CH_2CH(Ph)OOC(CH_2)_2COOCH(Ph)CH_2\overset{+}{N}Me_3$$

IV-87

$$Et_3\overset{+}{N}(CH_2)_{10}\overset{+}{N}Et_3$$

IV-88

(IV-87) are nondepolarizing antagonists (483, 484). Replacement of the terminal N-methyl groups in bisonium salts by ethyl or larger groups also produces the transition in neuromuscular blocking activities and decamethonium itself (IV-88) has weak nondepolarizing blocking activity (485). The decamethylene-*bis*-pyridinium (IV-89) and decamethylene-*bis*-quinolinium (IV-90) derivatives have reduced activity relative to decamethonium but are tubocurarine-like (486). Introduction of methoxy substituents produces, however, a marked increase in activity

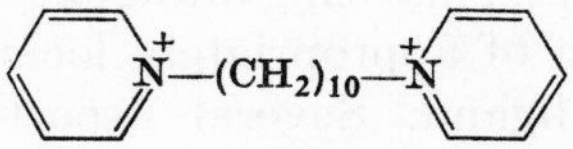

IV-89

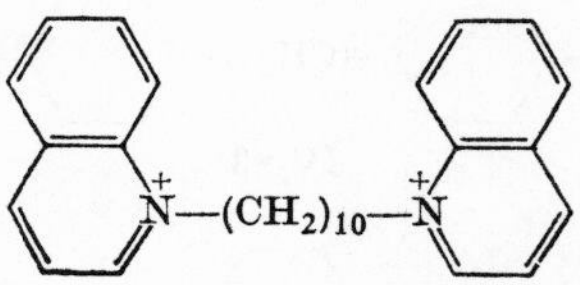

IV-90

(Table IV-82) and IV-90a is particularly active. Such compounds are approximating very closely to the structure of tubocurarine itself so that their potency and mode of action is not surprising. The activity of tubocurarine itself is increased approximately tenfold with methylation

TABLE IV-82. Neuromuscular Blocking Activity of Heterocyclic *bis*-Onium Compounds (486–488)

Structure	R	R'	R"	Rabbit ED_{50}† (mg/kg)
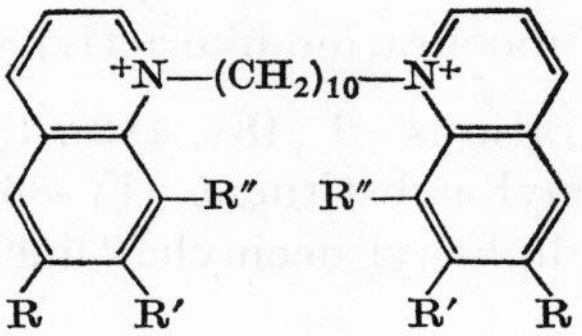	H	H	H	4·5
	MeO	H	H	4·4
	H	H	MeO	0·2
	H	H	EtO	0·3
	MeO	MeO	H	0·15
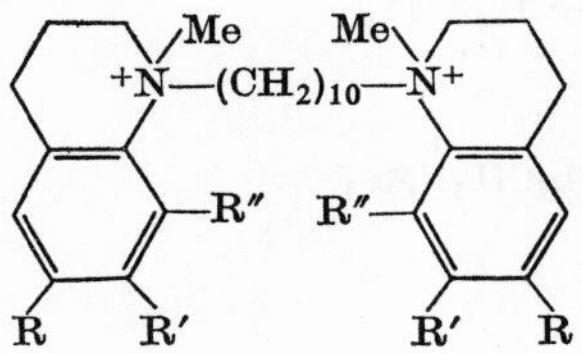	H	H	H	0·75
	MeO	H	H	0·2
	H	H	MeO	0·1
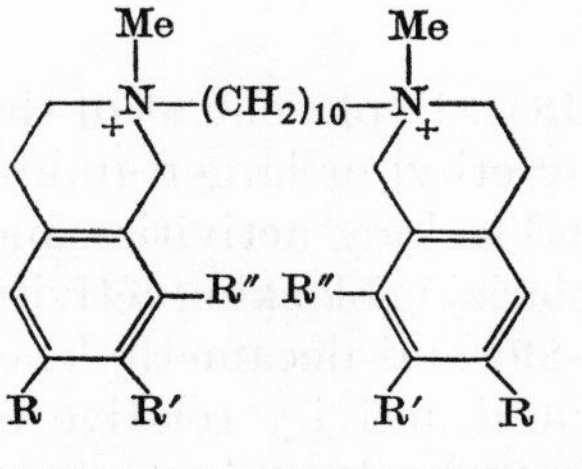	H	H	H	1·5
	MeO	H	H	0·2
	MeO	MeO	H	0·05
	MeO	MeO	MeO	0·02 (IV-90a)

† i.v. dose paralysing 50 per cent of rabbits.

PhCH$_2$COO $\diagdown$ $\overset{Me}{\underset{}{\overset{+}{N}}}$(CH$_2$)$_m$OOC(CH$_2$)$_n$COO(CH$_2$)$_m$$\overset{Me}{\underset{}{\overset{+}{N}}}$ $\diagup$ OOCCH$_2$Ph

IV-91

of the phenolic groups (445) in accord with the activities of the compounds listed in Table IV-82 and with a study of pH dependence of activity indicating that the unionized phenolic groups are important to activity.

Quite clearly a major structural difference between the depolarizing and nondepolarizing classes of neuromuscular blocking agents lies in the relative balance of polar and nonpolar groups in these structures—an increasing nonpolar:polar ratio favoring the dominance of nondepolarizing activity. Thus, the mechanisms of macromolecular interaction of these agents must be essentially that depolarizing agents bind through a mechanism that is dominantly ionic, and nondepolarizing agents through a mechanism that is dominantly nonpolar and hydrophobic. That this is so may be seen from the effects of temperature reduction upon neuromuscular blockade, that of decamethonium being increased and that of d-tubocurarine being decreased. These are precisely what is anticipated for dominantly ionic and hydrophobic interactions, respectively (Chapter I, see section, p. 16).

However, it is perhaps more than coincidental that the most active nondepolarizing blocking agents are *bis*(or poly)-onium salts and that, as with the depolarizing series, maximum activity is often associated with separation of the onium groups by the equivalent of a decamethylene chain. The well documented mutual antagonism of depolarizing and nondepolarizing agents (453, 457, 490, 491), whilst not conclusive proof that these agents act at a common site, is at least evidence that these agents bind at two mutually interacting sites.† Further evidence concerning the mode of action of these agents is derived from electrophysiological studies (Chapter V, see sections on p. 407 and p. 413): according to the evidence discussed so far, some basis exists to support the conclusion that acetylcholine receptors, at least of the skeletal neuromuscular junction, exist as a lattice array, that there may be some sort of cooperative binding (and hence response) of activator ligands and that the depolarizing and nondepolarizing antagonists may act through stabilization of the activated (depolarized) and nonactivated (polarized) forms respectively of the acetylcholine receptor. Whether this is achieved

---

† Our primary discussion has been in terms of these agents acting at the post-synaptic site, a concept which accords with many of the known facts (492). However, actions at other sites unquestionably occur and particular attention should be drawn to the work of Riker and his collaborators (493) on the *presynaptic* actions of many cholinergic ligands, together with the well established findings that many of these agents are inhibitors of cholinesterases.

13*

through interaction of the two classes of antagonist ligand at the same or different binding sites cannot be stated.

Finally, it is of some interest to note, in connection with the structural characterization of cholinergic receptors at various effector sites, that whilst atropine and related compounds are generally only weakly active at the skeletal neuromuscular junction (Chapter III) a number of bisquaternary tropine derivatives (IV-91) have nondepolarizing blocking activity comparable to that of d-tubocurarine (494–496).

Antagonists at Ganglionic Cholinergic Receptors

Because of interest in the use of ganglion blocking agents in the control of hypertension literally thousands of compounds have been examined and shown to exhibit ganglion blocking activity. Several general reviews of this area are available (158, 493–496) and in this section only a very brief outline of what appear to be the most salient points will be presented.

That there exist certain similarities in the structural requirements for stimulant activity at the ganglionic and skeletal neuromuscular junctions has already been noted (p. 236). Likewise, a number of antagonists exhibit activity at both of these sites: (+)-tubocurarine, although undoubtedly more active at the skeletal junction has, nonetheless, significant ganglion blocking activity. Similarly, a number of tropane derivatives (Table IV-93) exhibit antagonistic activities at both ganglionic and skeletal muscle junctions. A further similarity between these two sites exists in that at both sites classes of agents exist that block transmission through the production of a more or less prolonged depolarization.

Following Van Rossum (497) ganglion blocking agents may be conveniently divided into three classes.

(a) Depolarizing ganglionic blocking agents (nicotine, IV-92 (see Fig. IV-73); dimethylphenylpiperazinium, IV-93 (see Fig. IV-73)).

(b) Competitive ganglionic blocking agents (tetraethylammonium, IV-94 (see Fig. IV-73); hexamethonium, IV-95 (see Fig. IV-73)).

(c) Noncompetitive blocking agents (2-(2′-dimethylaminoethyl)-4,5, 6,7-tetrachloroisoindoline methiodide, IV-96 (see Fig. IV-73); 2,2-diphenyl-4-dimethylaminomethyl-1,3-dioxolane methiodide, IV-97 (see Fig. IV-73)). A representative selection of such agents is shown in Fig. IV-73. Of these agents, the greatest interest attaches to the bisquaternary salts related to hexamethonium (IV-95; see Fig. IV-73).

The characteristic actions of nicotine (IV-92; see Fig. IV-73), N,N-dimethyl-N^1-phenylpiperazinium (IV-93, DMPP; see Fig. IV-73) and pyridylalkylamines (IV-98; see Fig. IV-73) are to produce initial stimulation and subsequent block. Their concentration–response curves

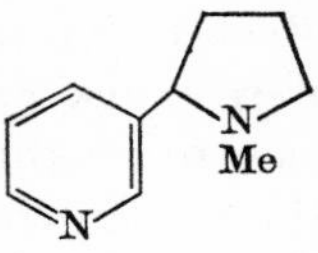

IV-92

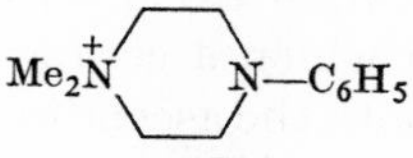

IV-93

Et_4N^+

IV-94

$Me_3\overset{+}{N}(CH_2)_6\overset{+}{N}Me_3$

IV-95

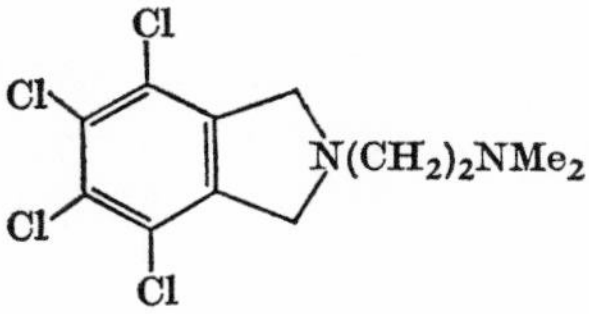

IV-96

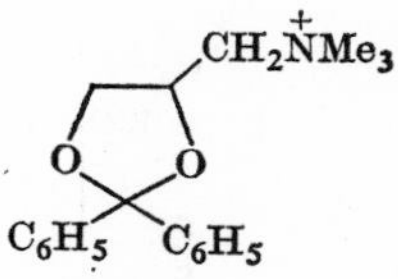

IV-97

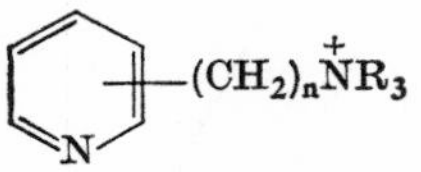

IV-98

Fig. IV-73. Structural formulae of ganglion blocking agents.

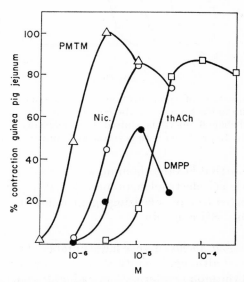

Fig. IV-74. Concentration–response curves of ganglion stimulants in the guinea-pig jejunum: note the bell-shaped curves. Reproduced with permission from van Rossum (497).

are, therefore, bell-shaped (Fig. IV-74), an effect which is not merely autoinhibition as shown by the concentration–response curves of Fig. IV-75 in which a competitive antagonist is seen to produce a parallel shift of both the ascending and descending portions of the concentration–response curve. It seems probable that, by analogy to their counterparts active at the skeletal neuromuscular junction, the depolarizing ganglion blocking agents act through stabilization of the depolarized state of the receptor and that the nondepolarizing antagonists act through stabilization of the polarized structure. In this connection it is extremely

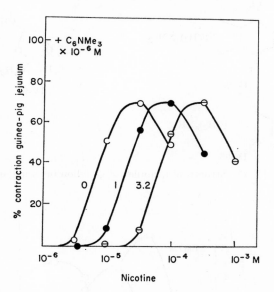

Fɪɢ. IV-75. Modification of concentration–response curves of nicotine in the guinea-pig jejunum in the presence of the competitive inhibitor hexamethonium. The original bell-shaped curve is shifted symmetrically by the competitive antagonist. Reproduced with permission from van Rossum (497).

interesting to note that hexamethonium which also serves as an antagonist in the electric eel electroplax preparation (Chapter V, see section, p. 420) is converted to a depolarizing agent following treatment of the electroplax with —SH reagents.

Competitive Blocking Agents. A very large number of agents probably fall into this category although quantitative data are often not available (495). Amongst the monoquaternary ions a highly generalized structure–activity rationalization can be derived that is essentially similar for that derived for antagonists active at other cholinergic junctions, namely that the addition of nonpolar function to the activator structure generally results in the development of antagonistic activity. As the simplest transition of this type, we note that tetramethylammonium and

TABLE IV-83. Effect of N-Substitution upon Activity at Ganglionic Junctions (498)

Activator	Antagonist
$CH_3CO_2CH_2CH_2\overset{+}{N}Me_3$	$CH_3CO_2CH_2CH_2\overset{+}{N}Et_3$
$Me_4\overset{+}{N}$	$Et_4\overset{+}{N}$
$C_6H_5OCH_2CH_2\overset{+}{N}Me_3$	$C_6H_5OCH_2CH_2\overset{+}{N}Et_3$
$Me_3\overset{+}{S}$	$Et_3\overset{+}{S}$
$C_2H_5OCH_2CH_2\overset{+}{N}Me_3$	$C_2H_5OCH_2CH_2\overset{+}{N}Et_3$

tetraethylammonium are activator and antagonist respectively (other examples are listed in Table IV-83). The activities of a number of simple quaternary ions are listed in Table IV-84: it is quite apparent that the binding site for these cations is of limited capacity and that there is a

TABLE IV-84. Ganglion Blocking Activities of Simple Quaternary Ammonium Ions (495, 499, 500)

$$R_1R_2R_3R_4\overset{+}{N}$$

No.	R_1	R_2	R_3	R_4	Equipotent molar activity (TEA = 1)
1	CH_2CH_3	CH_2CH_3	CH_2CH_3	CH_2CH_3	1·0
2	CH_2CH_3	CH_2CH_3	CH_2CH_3	CH_2CH_2OH	0·24
3	CH_2CH_2OH	CH_2CH_2OH	CH_2CH_2OH	CH_2CH_2OH	inactive
4	CH_2CH_3	CH_2CH_3	$(CH_2)_2CH_3$	$(CH_2)_2CH_3$	0·92
5	CH_2CH_3	CH_2CH_3	CH_2CH_3	$CH(CH_3)_2$	2·6
6	CH_2CH_3	CH_2CH_3	$CH(CH_3)_2$	$CH(CH_3)_2$	12·6
7	CH_2CH_3	CH_3	$CH(CH_3)_2$	$CH(CH_3)_2$	5·9
8	CH_3	CH_3	$CH(CH_3)_2$	$CH(CH_3)_2$	1·9
9	CH_3	CH_3	$CH_2CH(CH_3)_2$	$CH_2CH(CH_3)_2$	3·0
10	CH_2CH_3	CH_3	$CH_2CH(CH_3)_2$	$CH_2CH(CH_3)_2$	1·1
11	CH_2CH_3	CH_3	$(CH_2)_2CH(CH_3)_2$	$(CH_2)_2CH(CH_3)_2$	0·36
12	CH_2CH_3	CH_2CH_3	CH_2CH_3	$CH_2C_6H_5$	0·5
13	CH_2CH_3	CH_2CH_3	$CH_2C_6H_5$	$CH_2C_6H_5$	0·4
14	CH_2CH_3	CH_2CH_3	CH_2CH_3	$1\text{-}CH_2C_{10}H_7$	0·4

pronounced tendency for α-branching of N-alkyl substituents to enhance activity. This can be seen very clearly in the 2,6-dimethyl piperidine series (Table IV-85). A further point of interest from Tables IV-84 and

TABLE IV-85. Ganglion Blocking Activities of Cyclic Quaternary Ammonium Ions (495, 499, 500)

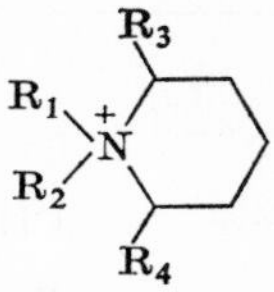

No.	R_1	R_2	R_3	R_4	Equipotent molar activity (TEA = 1)
1	CH_3	CH_3	H	H	<0·2
2	CH_2CH_3	CH_3	H	H	0·5
3	CH_2CH_3	CH_2CH_3	H	H	1·0
4	CH_3	CH_3	CH_3	CH_3	2·0
5	CH_2CH_3	CH_3	CH_3	CH_3	3·3
6	CH_2CH_3	CH_2CH_3	CH_3	CH_3	9·5
7	CH_2CH_3	CH_2CH_2OH	CH_3	CH_3	0·85

IV-85 is that replacement of N-ethyl by N-2-hydroxyethyl very greatly reduces antagonistic activity: this is probably relatable to the known detrimental influence of this structural change on the structure-making capacity of alkyl groups in water (Chapter I, p. 48).

TABLE IV-86. Ganglion Blocking Activities of Polymethylene-*bis*-onium Derivatives (501)

$$\overset{+}{R_3N}(CH_2)_n\overset{+}{NR_3}$$

	R_3			
n	Me$_3$	Me$_2$Et	MeEt$_2$	Et$_3$
	Equiactive molar ratios (HM = 1)†			
4	110	10	0·93	17
5	1·6	0·65	0·71	12
6	1·0 (HM)	0·62	1·1	>16
7	8·0	8·9	5·5	39

† Cat superior cervical ganglion (TEA = 30).

Of ganglion-blocking agents by far the greatest interest attaches to the bisquaternary ammonium salts, some members of which have already been discussed in connection with their role as antagonists at the skeletal neuromuscular junction. (pp. 344–356). The activities of the poly-methylene derivatives are listed in Table IV-86: activity can be seen to reach a maximum at the C_5 and C_6 members. Since, in the trimethyl-ammonium series, the corresponding monoquaternary derivatives are activators, it is evident that the presence of two quaternary ammonium groups is essential for antagonist activity. The presence of considerable ganglion blocking activity in many series of compounds where two quaternary ammonium groups are separated by the equivalence of 5 or 6

TABLE IV-87. Ganglion Blocking Activities
of Phenylalkane-*bis*-onium Salts (507)

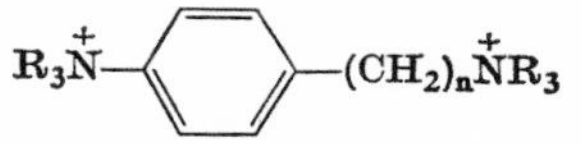

$$R_3\overset{+}{N}-\!\!\!\left\langle\!\!\!\bigcirc\!\!\!\right\rangle\!\!\!-(CH_2)_n\overset{+}{N}R_3$$

	R_3			
	Me_3	Me_2Et	$MeEt_2$	Et_3
n	Equiactive molar ratios (HM = 1)			
1	160	—	—	—
2	0·25	0·22	0·38	33
3	2·9	1·4	4·4	17
4	—	6	12	12

methylene groups has been noted by many workers (158, 451, 494–496, 502–507, Tables IV-87, IV-88). However, in a more extensive investigation of polymethylene-*bis*-trimethylammonium and polymethylene-*bis*-triethylammonium Barlow and Zoller (470) have found that a second maximum of ganglion blocking (Table IV-89) and neuromuscular blocking activities (Fig. IV-69, p. 348) occurs at the C_{15}–C_{17} interonium distance.

The two major features of interest in the *bis*-onium compounds are the influence of chain length and hence inter-onium group distance, and the effects of structural variation of the quaternary ammonium groups. Both Barlow and Ing (508) and Paton and Zaimis (451) in their original work on the polymethylene-*bis*-onium salts had argued that their effectiveness might be related to their ability to occupy simultaneously two receptor sites. Several workers, most notably Gill (509), have attempted to relate the dependency of activity upon inter-onium chain length with the probability of the *bis*-onium salt occupying simultaneously two anionic centers some 6·7–8 Å apart. Gill's treatment, which does generate quite fair agreement with experiment, does not, however, indicate the nature of the two anionic binding sites. That these

TABLE IV-88. Ganglion Blocking Activities of *bis*-Pyrollidinium, *bis*-Morpholinium and *bis*-Piperidinium Series (495)

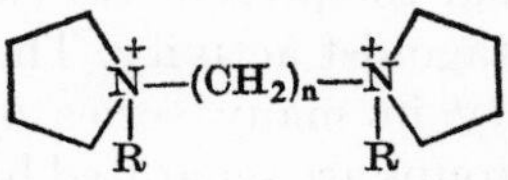

n	R	Equiactive molar ratio (HM = 1)
3	Me	20·0
4	Me	2·0
5	Me	0·2
6	Me	0·33
6	C_2H_5	1·8

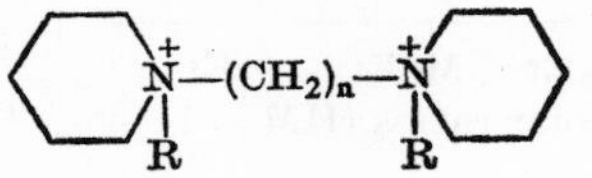

n	R	
3	Me	13·0
4	Me	1·2
5	Me	1·1
6	Me	1·2
6	C_2H_5	>10·0

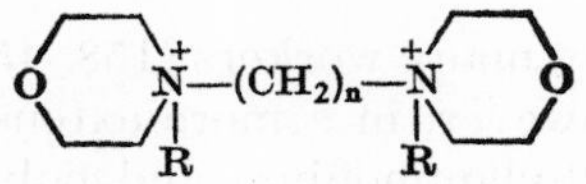

n	R	
4	Me	5·0
5	Me	1·0
6	Me	1·0
6	C_2H_5	16·0

are both receptor sites is, perhaps, unlikely for then it might have been anticipated that hexamethonium should act, by analogy with decamethonium at the skeletal junction, to produce an initial depolarization. It is more probable, as proposed by Gill and Ing (510), that the ganglion blocking *bis*-onium salts act through a cross-linking of the anionic sites of an acetylcholine receptor and a peripheral non-receptor site. Support for this suggestion is provided by the comparative effects of quaternary group substitution (Tables IV-86, IV-87): in addition to the effects of sequential N-ethyl substitution upon the optimum inter-onium chain distance and which may be related, according to the previously mentioned calculations of Gill, to the effect of charge shielding on chain terminus repulsion, it is of particular importance that complete replacement of $-\overset{+}{N}Me_3$ by $-\overset{+}{N}Et_3$ leads to a reduced level of activity approximating that of tetraethylammonium itself. Apparently the polymethylene-*bis*-triethylammonium salts may bind in a manner analogous to that of

TABLE IV-89. Ganglion Blocking Activity of Polymethylene-*bis*-onium Salts (Long-chain, 470)

$Me_3\overset{+}{N}(CH_2)_n\overset{+}{N}Me_3$	Equipotent molar† activity	$Et_3\overset{+}{N}(CH_2)_n\overset{+}{N}Et_3$	Equipotent molar activity
n = 10	11·5	n = 10	20·0
11	22·0	11	20·0
12	18·5	12	10·0
13	11·5	13	4·5
14	6·1	14	2·3
15	1·9	15	1·5
16	1·3	16	1·0
17	1·3	17	0·8
18	1·2	18	2·5
19	2·7	19	10·0
20	5·7	20	18·0
21	14·5	21	80·0
(6	5·0)		

† Cat superior cervical ganglion. Activities relative to $Et_3\overset{+}{N}(CH_2)_{16}\overset{+}{N}Et_3 = 1$.

tetraethylammonium itself with one onium group having no binding function. Furthermore, for a number of series of *bis*-onium derivatives it has been possible to study agents with unsymmetrical ammonium functions (Table IV-90): from such studies it is clear that the ammonium groups must interact differently since a number of compounds with one triethylammonium group are at least as active as their symmetrical *bis*-trimethylammonium analogs. Although this data is not as extensive as might be desired, it does appear that the structural requirements for the two onium binding sites are different—one site (Fig. IV-76, site A) binds effectively the series $-\overset{+}{N}Me_3 \rightarrow -\overset{+}{N}Et_3$ while the second site has a much more specific requirement for the smaller cationic group (Fig. IV-76, siteB) and approximates fairly closely the structural requirements previously discussed (pp. 236–247) for the onium group structure in activator ligands. Suggestive evidence that at least one of these anionic sites is at the receptor itself is derived from the finding (511) that hexa-

TABLE IV-90. Ganglion Blocking Activities of Ether Analogs of Polymethylene-*bis*-onium Salts (505, 506)

$$R_3\overset{+}{N}(CH_2)_mO(CH_2)_n\overset{+}{N}R_3'$$

No.	R	R′	m	n	Equiactive molar ratio† (HM = 1)
1	Me$_3$	Me$_3$	2	2	2·0
2	Me$_3$	Me$_3$	3	2	0·54
3	Me$_3$	Me$_3$	3	3	7·1
4	Et$_3$	Me$_2$Et	2	2	0·59
5	Et$_3$	MeEt$_2$	2	2	0·45
6	Et$_3$	Et$_3$	2	2	13·0
7	Me$_2$Et	Me$_2$Et	3	2	0·6
8	MeEt$_2$	MeEt$_2$	3	2	1·5
9	Me$_3$	MeEt$_2$	3	2	0·58
10	Me$_2$Et	Et$_3$	3	2	0·39

$$R_3\overset{+}{N}(CH_2)_mX(CH_2)_n\overset{+}{N}R_3'$$

No.	R	X	R′	m	n	
11	Me$_3$	O	Me$_3$	2	2	2·0
12	Me$_3$	S	Me$_3$	2	2	1·5
13	Et$_3$	O	Me$_2$Et	2	2	0·59
14	Et$_3$	S	Me$_2$Et	2	2	0·55

† Cat superior cervical ganglion.

methonium, normally an antagonist in the electric eel electroplax preparation, becomes an activator following treatment of the tissue with —SH reagents (Chapter V, see section, p. 420).

Since the *bis*-triethylammonium compounds of Tables IV-86, IV-87

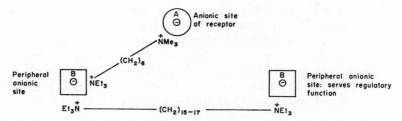

FIG. IV-76. Possible geometry of anionic sites at cholinergic receptors of ganglion indicating the difference in binding of hexamethonium-type agents and the longer chain *bis*-triethylammonium ligands.

and IV-90 are not significantly more active than tetraethylammonium itself, it may be concluded that in these compounds affinity for one binding site, presumably site A, has been lost. The interesting speculation is thus raised that the apparently competitive antagonism exhibited by tetraethylammonium and other related "hydrophobic" agents is due, not to their interaction at the receptor site proper, but to a regulatory-type interaction at a peripheral anionic site (Fig. IV-76). This conclusion, whilst speculative, accords nevertheless with other evidence discussed in this chapter concerning the general basis of interaction of cholinergic ligands.

The second peak of ganglion blocking activity observed at an inter-onium distance of C_{15}–C_{17} (Table IV-89) clearly reflects an interaction mechanism different from that operative for the C_5–C_6 peak, for with the longer series activity is maintained and even increased somewhat in the *bis*-triethylammonium compounds. This series of compounds may thus involve simultaneous interaction at two *peripheral* anionic sites (Fig. IV-76). In this respect antagonism at ganglionic junction appears super-ficially similar to antagonism at the skeletal neuromuscular junction.

Antagonists at the Parasympathetic Neuromuscular Junction

A large number of compounds show activity as antagonists at the parasympathetic neuromuscular junction and several general reviews of this activity are available (158, 512–515). Of these agents, atropine, the tropic acid ester of tropan-3-α-ol (IV-99) is one of the best known and

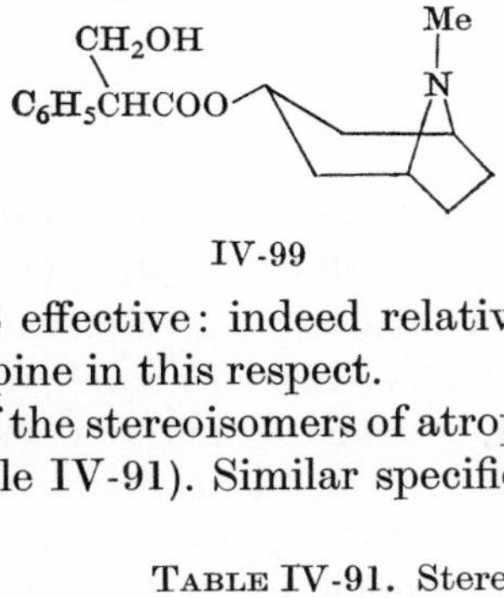

IV-99 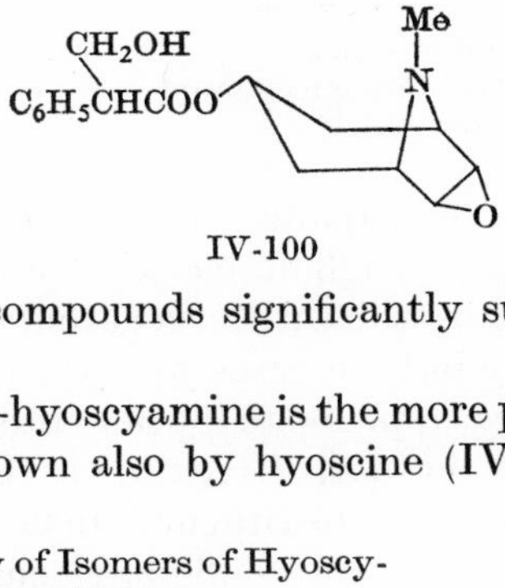   IV-100

most effective: indeed relatively few compounds significantly surpass atropine in this respect.

Of the stereoisomers of atropine, S(—)-hyoscyamine is the more potent (Table IV-91). Similar specificity is shown also by hyoscine (IV-100):

TABLE IV-91. Stereospecificity of Isomers of Hyoscy-
amine and Hyoscine (158)

Preparation		$S:R$ activity ratio
Guinea-pig ileum	Hyoscyamine	32
Rabbit ileum	Hyoscyamine	110
Rabbit intestine	Hyoscine	15

esters of tropan-3-β-ol (ψ-tropine) are consistently less active (512, 516) so that the configuration of the 3-ester group is important. The influence of quaternization of atropine and related agents has been studied by a number of workers (512, 517–519): conversion to N-methyl quaternary

TABLE IV-92. Effect of N-Methyl Quaternization upon Activities of Esters of Tropan-3α-ol (512)

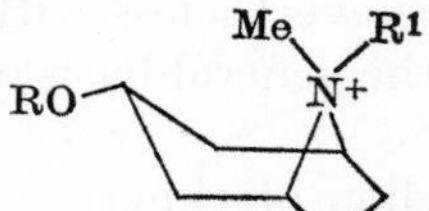

R	R^1	Atropine-like[†] activity (atropine = 1)	Ganglion[‡] blocking activity (TEA = 1)	Curare-like[§] activity (d-TC = 1)
C_6H_5CO-	H	0·006	0·1	—
C_6H_5CO-	Me	0·04	2·0	0·10
$C_6H_5CH(OH)CO-$	H	0·08	0·35	—
$C_6H_5CH(OH)CO-$	Me	0·3	4·5	0·07
$C_6H_5CH(CH_2OH)CO-$	H	1·0	0·35	—
$C_6H_5CH(CH_2OH)CO-$	Me	1·0	4·0	0·15
$(C_6H_5)_2CHCO-$	H	0·06	—	—
$(C_6H_5)_2CHCO-$	Me	0·08	5·3	0·05

† Rabbit intestine.
‡ Cat nictitating membrane.
§ Frog rectus.

salts increases parasympatholytic activity and at the same time markedly increases ganglion blocking and curare-like activity (Table IV-92): quaternization with larger groups generally decreases parasympatholytic activity but increases ganglion blocking activity (Table IV-93).

There appears to be an interesting dependence of activity in the quaternary derivatives upon the configuration at the nitrogen atom where unlike substituents can be in axial or equatorial positions (IV-101). According to the configurational assignments made by Fodor (520) for the N-methyl-N-ethyl quaternary derivatives (521) those with the

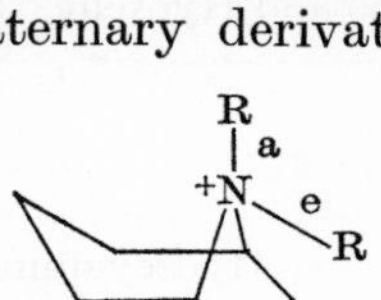

IV-101

TABLE IV-93. Cholinolytic Activities of N-Alkaryl-Quaternary Tropanes (512)

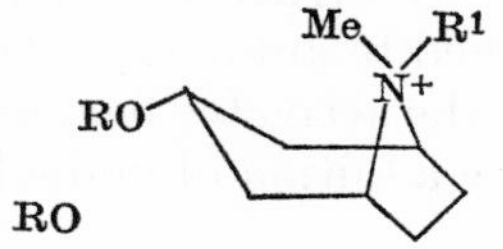

R	R^1	Atropine-like[†] activity (atropine = 1)	Ganglion[‡] blocking activity (TEA = 1)	Curare-like[§] activity (d-TC = 1)
C_6H_5CO—	$C_6H_5CH_2$	0·004	3·0	0·10
4-HNC_6H_5CO—	$C_6H_5CH_2$	0·005	8·0	0·20
$C_6H_5CH(OH)CO$—	C_6H_5	0·005	3·0	0·10
$C_6H_5CH(CH_2OH)CO$—	$C_6H_5CH_2$	0·10	2·1	0·18
$C_6H_5CH(CH_2OH)CO$—	$C_6H_5CH_2CH_2$	0·15	28·0	0·10

† Rabbit intestine.
‡ Cat nictitating membrane.
§ Frog rectus.

N-ethyl group axial are more active parasympatholytic by a two to sevenfold factor. (However, these configurational assignments may actually need to be reversed 522, 523.)

A very large number of esters of tropane-3α-ol have been examined to determine the effect of ester group substitution (158, 512, 524). Quite generally, only negligible activity is found with aliphatic esters and aromatic esters such as benzoic and phthalic acid but significant activity appears with mandelic, atrolactic, α-methylmandelic acids, etc., although these are all less active than atropine itself, thus suggesting a rather specific role for the interaction of the —OH group of the tropic acid.

TABLE IV-94. Parasympathomimetic and Parasympatholytic Activities of Acylcholines (525, 526)

$$RCOOCH_2CH_2\overset{+}{N}Me_3$$

R	i.a.	pD$_2$	pA$_2$
H—	1·0	5·2	—
Me—	1·0	7·0	—
Et—	1·0	5·3	—
Pr—	0·5	5·1	—
Bu—	0	—	4·7
$Me(CH_2)_{10}$—	0	—	5·4
$C_6H_5C(Me)CH_2OH$—	0	—	8·1
$(C_6H_5)_2C(OH)$—	0	—	8·6
$C_6H_5C(C_6H_{11})OH$—	0	—	9·1

Despite the great interest in compounds closely related to atropine, from the point of view of structure–activity relationships greater importance may be attached to antagonists that appear to bear greater structural resemblance to the activator ligands. Thus it has already been noted that the progressive addition of nonpolar groups to an activator

TABLE IV-95. Affinity Constants for Cholinergic Antagonists (529)

R—X

No.	R	log K (mean ± S.E.)			
		$\overset{+}{N}Me_3$	$\overset{+}{N}Me_2Et$	$\overset{+}{N}MeEt_2$	$\overset{+}{N}Et_3$
1	Ph(CH$_2$)$_5$—	5·180 (±0·016)	5·549 (±0·031)	5·735 (±0·013)	5·849 (±0·022)
2	Ph(CH$_2$)$_2$O(CH$_2$)$_2$—	4·702 (±0·016)	5·167 (±0·016)	5·415 (±0·022)	5·758 (±0·028)
3	PhCH$_2$COO(CH$_2$)$_2$—	4·533 (±0·012)	5·093 (±0·024)	5·379 (±0·022)	5·785 (±0·008)
4	C$_6$H$_{11}$(CH$_2$)$_5$—	5·387 (±0·032)	5·841 (±0·035)	5·878 (±0·033)	5·921 (±0·037)
5	C$_6$H$_{11}$(CH$_2$)$_2$O(CH$_2$)$_2$—	5·282 (±0·018)	5·657 (±0·015)	5·783 (±0·028)	5·912 (±0·024)
6	C$_6$H$_{11}$CH$_2$COO(CH$_2$)$_2$—	5·067 (±0·019)	5·517 (±0·017)	5·569 (±0·018)	5·630 (±0·017)
7	Ph$_2$CH(CH$_2$)$_4$—	7·015 (±0·021)	7·270 (±0·036)	7·091 (±0·025)	6·712 (±0·015)
8	Ph$_2$CHCH$_2$O(CH$_2$)$_2$—	6·413 (±0·020)	6·693 (±0·020)	6·543 (±0·018)	6·374 (±0·024)
9	Ph$_2$CHCOO(CH$_2$)$_2$—	7·159 (±0·025)	7·578 (±0·028)	7·584 (±0·045)	7·367 (±0·021)
10	(C$_6$H$_{11}$)$_2$CHCH$_2$O(CH$_2$)$_2$—	7·254 (±0·028)	7·615 (±0·034)	7·574 (±0·062)	7·354 (±0·030)
11	(C$_6$H$_{11}$)$_2$CHCOO(CH$_2$)$_2$—	7·686 (±0·024)	7·723 (±0·021)	8·083 (±0·025)	8·068 (±0·022)
12	Ph(C$_6$H$_{11}$)CHCOO(CH$_2$)$_2$—	8·438 (±0·046)	8·970 (±0·014)	8·699 (±0·014)	8·566 (±0·019)

ligand causes a gradual transition, through partial agonists, to antagonistic ligands. This can be seen for the dioxolanes (Table IV-15), the alkyltrimethylammonium (Table IV-16) and the acylcholine ligand (Table IV-94) and other series. Similar development of antagonistic activities can be realized through progressive replacement of N-methyl groups by larger substituents (Table IV-95). This pattern of nonpolar substitution is indeed quite common to the general development of antagonists. The great importance of the nonpolar groups to the production of antagonistic effects is particularly well illustrated by the finding (527) that the carbon isostere of benzilylcholine (IV-102) exhibits very significant parasympatholytic activity.

$$\overset{\displaystyle OH}{\underset{\displaystyle |}{(C_6H_5)_2CCOOCH_2CH_2C(CH_3)_3.}}$$

IV-102

A number of attempts have been made to define quantitatively those molecular parameters that appear important for the production of antagonistic activities. In particular, Barlow, Stephenson and their collaborators (528, 529) have investigated a rather extensive series of compounds (Table IV-95), all of which appear to act as competitive antagonists, and have attempted to define the relative contributions of the molecular components of these antagonists to the observed activity. A selection of their data is presented in Table IV-95. In their original work Barlow *et al.* (528) assumed that if a series of ligands interacted at the same site then it could be assumed that the total free energy of interaction is the sum of the constituent free energies,

$$\varDelta F = \sum \varDelta F$$

so that the effect of a given substituent change (i.e. $-\overset{+}{N}Me_3 \rightarrow \overset{+}{N}Et_3$) should be constant in all ligand series. The data of Table IV-95 (and the derived data of Table IV-96) reveal that this assumption is not generally valid: progressive substitution in the transition $-\overset{+}{N}Me_3 \rightarrow \overset{+}{N}Et_3$ has different effects upon the ligand affinity depending upon the remaining molecular structure. Thus, with the exception of the dicyclohexyl-acetate (No. 11, Table IV-95) the conversion, $-\overset{+}{N}Me_3 \rightarrow \overset{+}{N}Me_2Et$, significantly increases activity: the conversion, $-\overset{+}{N}Me_2Et \rightarrow \overset{+}{N}MeEt_2$, increases activity of most compounds (1–9, Table IV-95) but decreases others (10–12), Table IV-95) whilst the conversion $-\overset{+}{N}MeEt_2 \rightarrow -\overset{+}{N}Et_3$ increases activity (to a small extent) of some compounds (1–6, Table IV-95) and decreases activity of the remaining members (7–12, Table IV-95). In two cases the triethylammonium ligands are actually less active than the parent trimethylammonium ligands. These findings appear not to bear out any assumption of additivity of group contributions to the total interaction energy, but the apparent differences in onium group interaction amongst the various ligand series may relate to the total interaction mechanism of the ligands. Treatment of the ligand series $R\overset{+}{N}Me_3$ according to the Hansch π treatment (Chapter I, see section, p. 35) whereby $Ph(CH_2)_5\overset{+}{N}Me_3$ is assigned $\sum \pi = 0$ and the effects of varying modifications in R on $\sum \pi$ have been calculated (Table

TABLE IV-96. Contributions of N-Ethyl Groups to Affinity in Cholinergic Antagonists

No.	R	X				
		$\overset{+}{NMe_3} \to \overset{+}{NMe_2Et}$ $\log \Delta K$	$\overset{+}{NMe_2Et} \to \overset{+}{NMeEt_2}$ $\log \Delta K$	$\overset{+}{NMeEt_2} \to \overset{+}{NEt_3}$ $\log \Delta K$	$\overset{+}{NMe_3} \to \overset{+}{NEt_3}$ $\log \Delta K$
1	Ph(CH$_2$)$_5$—	0·369	0·184	0·114	0·669
2	Ph(CH$_2$)$_2$O(CH$_2$)$_2$—	0·465	0·248	0·343	1·056
3	PhCH$_2$COO(CH$_2$)$_2$—	0·560	0·286	0·406	1·252
4	C$_6$H$_{11}$(CH$_2$)$_5$—	0·454	0·037	0·043	0·534
5	C$_6$H$_{11}$(CH$_2$)$_2$O(CH$_2$)$_2$—	0·375	0·126	0·129	0·630
6	C$_6$H$_{11}$CH$_2$COO(CH$_2$)$_2$—	0·450	0·052	0·061	0·563
7	Ph$_2$CH(CH$_2$)$_4$—	0·255	0·179	−0·389	−0·303
8	Ph$_2$CHCH(CH$_2$)$_2$—	0·280	0·152	−0·169	−0·039
9	Ph$_2$CHCOO(CH$_2$)$_2$—	0·419	0·006	−0·217	0·208
10	(C$_6$H$_{11}$)$_2$CHO(CH$_2$)$_2$—	0·361	−0·041	−0·220	0·100
11	(C$_6$H$_{11}$)$_2$CHCOO(CH$_2$)$_2$—	0·037	0·360	−0·015	0·382
12	Ph(C$_6$H$_{11}$)CHCOO(CH$_2$)$_2$—	0·532	−0·271	−0·133	0·128

TABLE IV-97. π-Analysis for Cholinergic Antagonist Series

$$R—\overset{+}{N}Me_3$$

No.	R	$\sum\pi$	$\log K$
1	$Ph(CH_2)_5$—	0	5·180
2	$Ph(CH_2)_2O(CH_2)_2$—	−0·51	4·702
3	$PhCH_2COO(CH_2)_2$—	−1·28	4·533
4	$C_6H_{11}(CH_2)_5$—	+0·62	5·387
5	$C_6H_{11}(CH_2)_2O(CH_2)_2$—	+0·11	5·282
6	$C_6H_{11}CH_2COO(CH_2)_2$—	−0·66	5·067
7	$Ph_2CH(CH_2)_4$—	+1·89	7·015
8	$Ph_2CHCH_2O(CH_2)_2$—	+1·38	6·413
9	$Ph_2CHCOO(CH_2)_2$—	+0·31	7·159
10	$(C_6H_{11})_2CHCH_2O(CH_2)_2$—	+2·62	7·254
11	$(C_6H_{11})_2CHCOO(CH_2)_2$—	+1·85	7·686
12	$Ph(C_6H_{11})CHCOO(CH_2)_2$—	+1·23	8·438

IV-97) generates the $\log K$–π plot of Fig. IV-77. From Fig. IV-77 it is apparent, omitting the esters (3, 6, 9, 11, 12, Table IV-95) that the remaining compounds reveal an essentially linear dependence of activity upon π, so that antagonistic activity increases with increasing hydrophobic character of the ligand. The esters show a similar, but separate

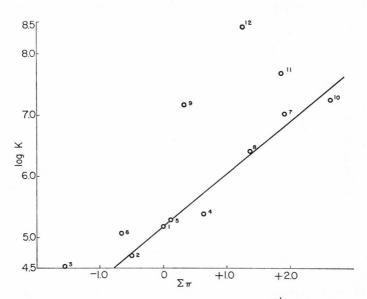

FIG. IV-77. $\log K$–π plot for the muscarinic antagonists ($—\overset{+}{N}Me_3$ ligands) listed in Table IV-97.

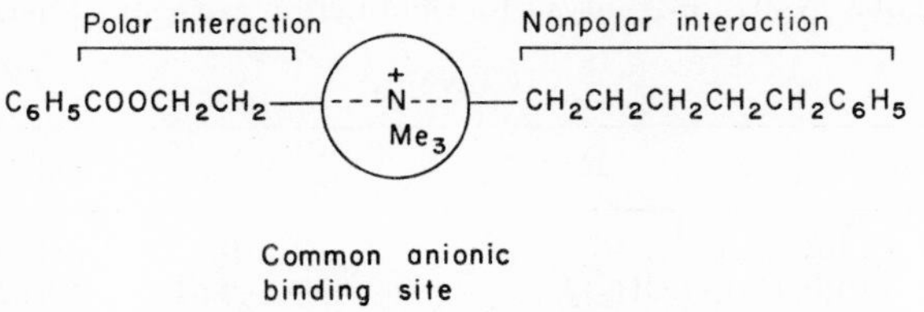

Polar interaction   Nonpolar interaction

$$C_6H_5COOCH_2CH_2 \overbrace{ \underset{Me_3}{\overset{+}{N}} ---}\ CH_2CH_2CH_2CH_2CH_2C_6H_5$$

Common anionic
binding site

FIG. IV-78. Partially overlapping binding sites for muscarinic antagonists.

and less well defined, dependence of activity upon π but in every instance activity is greater than indicated by $\sum \pi$ as based upon the non-ester series. Thus, it is possible that Fig. IV-77 reveals the existence of two separate interaction mechanisms, one dependent only upon the hydrophobic character of the R group in $R\overset{+}{N}Me_3$ and the other dependent upon both hydrophobic *and* polar character. Quite possibly these two interaction mechanisms may represent partially distinct binding sites (Fig. IV-78).

The differential effects of progressive N-ethylation in this antagonist series (Table IV-96) seem to be approximately related to the $\sum \pi$ values of the parent antagonist and a plot of $\sum \pi$ against $\log \varDelta K$ (Table IV-96, column IV) reveals (Fig. IV-79) that the effect of N-ethylation on $\log K$ becomes progressively less as $\sum \pi$ $(R\overset{+}{N}Me_3)$ becomes progressively more

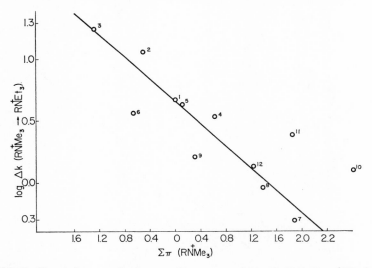

FIG. IV-79. Dependence of change in antagonist affinity $(\log \varDelta K)$ in the $R\overset{+}{N}Me_3 \rightarrow R\overset{+}{N}Et_3$ transition as a function of $\sum \pi$ of the $R\overset{+}{N}Me_3$ structure for the antagonist ligands listed in Table IV-97.

positive. This suggests that the hydrophobic bonding area for these antagonists is of limited dimensions and can tolerate ligands that contain up to a correspondingly limited hydrophobic component: beyond this point additional hydrophobic substitution results in loss of binding energy. Hansch has discussed (530) a number of situations where biological activity shows a parabolic dependence on π, decreasing above a certain critical π value.

A similar π-dependence of antagonist activity has been observed by Pratesi *et al.* (531) for a series of *N*-alkyl-*N*-phenyl-2-aminoethyl-(*N*-piperidino) ethiodides (IV-103) and a nicely linear relationship between

$$C_6H_5\underset{\underset{R}{|}}{N}CH_2CH_2\overset{+}{N}\!\!\!\overset{\displaystyle\diagup\!\!\diagdown}{\underset{\underset{Et}{|}}{\diagdown\!\!\diagup}}$$

IV-103

π and pA_2 is observed (Fig. IV-80) but showing progressive deviation with the *n*-hexyl, *n*-heptyl and *n*-octyl substituents suggesting that the steric limitations of the hydrophobic bonding area have been exceeded by these substituents.

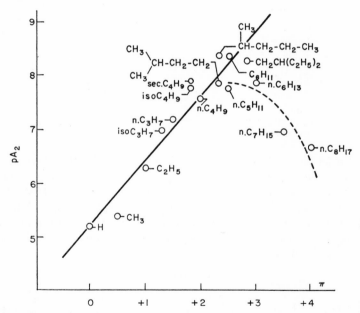

FIG. IV-80. Dependence of pA_2 (rat intestine) upon π for the series $C_6H_5N(R)CH_2CH_2\overset{+}{N}MeC_5H_{10}$. Reproduced with permission from Pratesi *et al.* (531).

TABLE IV-98. Stereospecificity of Parasympatholytic
Activity of 3-Cyclohexyl-3-phenylpropan-1-ols (534)

$$C_6H_5(C_6H_{11})COHCH_2CH_2R$$

R		Equipotent molar activity† (atropine = 1)	(+)/(−)
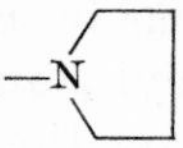	±	22	
	+	540	49
	−	11	
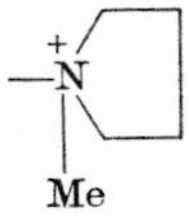 Me	±	1·2	
	+	81	160
	−	0·51	
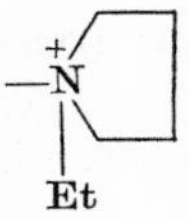 Et	±	2·0	
	+	230	290
	−	0·79	
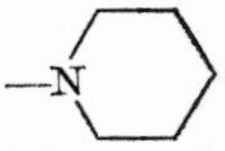	±	3·7	
	+	13·7	9·8
	−	1·4	
Me	±	1·4	
	+	45	48
	−	0·94	

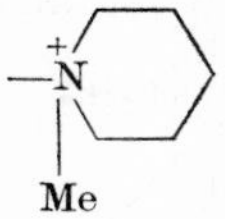

† Guinea-pig ileum.

The importance of hydrophobic interactions is also revealed in a
qualitative sense by the comparatively high parasympatholytic activity
of many derivatives of 2-diethylaminoethanol (IV-104, 158), 3-cyclo-
hexyl-3-phenyl-propan-1-ols (Table IV-98, 158, 532–534) high stereospecificity of interaction being observed with these compounds, and
2,2-diphenylbutyramides (IV-105; 158, 535) to cite but a few of the
compounds examined.

$$ROCH_2CH_2NEt_2$$

R = Ph₂CHCO ; ;

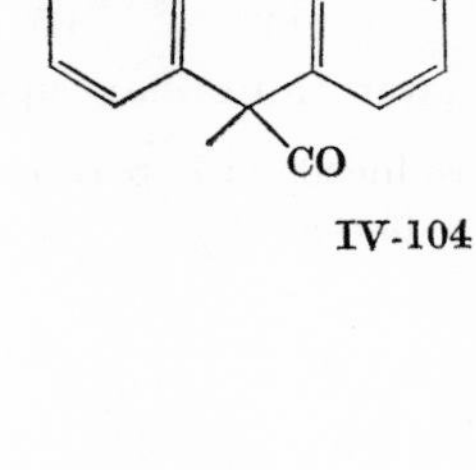

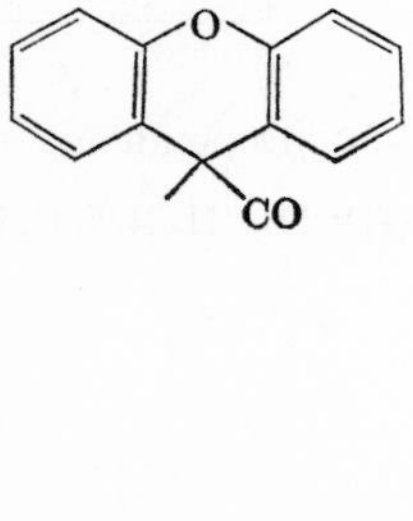

IV-104

The structured character of this proposed hydrophobic bonding site is revealed by the high stereoselectivity of the compounds listed in Table IV-98, indicating that the site shows substantial discriminating ability

$$\underset{\text{IV-105}}{(C_6H_5)_2\overset{\overset{\displaystyle CONH_2}{|}}{C}CH_2CH_2NR_2}$$

between the phenyl and cyclohexyl groups. Further subtleties of interaction are revealed by the substituted benzhydryl ethers of dimethylaminoethanol (IV-106) studied by Nauta and his co-workers (536) and which possess parasympatholytic, antihistamine and local anesthetic properties. Parasympatholytic activity is increased by 2-alkyl

$$Ar_2CHOCH_2CH_2NMe_2$$

IV-106

substitution and decreased by 4-alkyl substitution (Table IV-99). It appears probable that the effects of 2-alkyl substitution are to cause, through steric hindrance, progressive twisting of the phenyl rings away from coplanarity. This indicates that the nonpolar binding surfaces may be correspondingly aplanar. Some support for this view is provided by the data of Fig. IV-81 which shows a satisfactory correlation between parasympatholytic activity for the o-substituted compounds of Table IV-99 with the Taft steric parameter, E_s (537–540): no correlation exists between this activity and the π-values of the substituents.

TABLE IV-99. Parasympatholytic Activities of Alkyl Substituted Benzhydryl Ethers of 2-Dimethylaminoethanol (536)

$$Ar(C_6H_5)CHO(CH_2)_2NMe_2$$

No.	Ar	Parasympatholytic activity†
1	C_6H_5	100
2	2-MeC_6H_4	200
3	2-EtC_6H_4	270
4	$2\text{-Pr}^iC_6H_4$	650
5	$2\text{-Bu}^tC_6H_4$	3300
6	4-MeC_6H_4	25
7	4-EtC_6H_4	25
8	$4\text{-Pr}^iC_6H_4$	40
9	$4\text{-Bu}^tC_6H_4$	20

† Guinea-pig ileum.

The antagonists discussed in this section have generally been described as competitive antagonists of acetylcholine and related activator ligands. This conclusion is derived (12, 244–246, 249–251, 541) from observations that such antagonists produce parallel shifts of the agonist concentration–response curves and that this behavior can, in general, be quantitatively described by the equations for competitive antagonism (p. 283). However, as discussed previously, it is not an obligatory deduction from such observations that the activator and antagonist ligand compete at the same binding site: an appropriate interaction of the antagonist at an allosteric site serving to modify the affinity of the activator binding site (receptor) for the activator will, provided that the ability of the activator–receptor complex to initiate

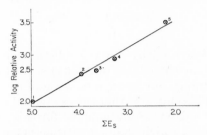

FIG. IV-81. Dependence of muscarinic antagonist activity in a series of *o*-substituted benzhydryl ethers of dimethylaminoethanol (Table IV-99) upon E_s.

the biological response is unimpaired, generate behavior characterized as competitive antagonism.

An early objection to the concept that acetylcholine and atropine interact at the same site was raised by Clark in 1926 (542), who noted the difficulty of reconciling the apparently very slow dissociation rate of atropine with the finding that acetylcholine can produce a prompt response in atropinized preparations and that large quantities of acetylcholine did not apparently facilitate the reversal of atropine antagonism. Similar objections may also be raised for a number of atropine-like agents where the offset of competitive antagonism appears relatively slow.

Three basic explanations would appear to be available to accommodate such discrepancies:† that atropine does not act at the activator–receptor site but acts through an indirect or regulatory mechanism; that activator ligands need only occupy a small fraction of the receptors to produce maximum response, and hence can achieve this even when a substantial

† We are concerned here with events at the cholinergic parasympathetic neuroeffector junction; however, essentially the same problem exists for competitive antagonists at other receptor systems, i.e., histamine (543–545).

fraction of the receptor is blocked by a slowly dissociating antagonist (13), and that the antagonists actually dissociate rapidly from the receptor but that access to and from the receptor from the aqueous phase is hindered by a biophase which does not, however, prevent the access of agonist (22, 546). Of these hypotheses the latter two have been most extensively discussed and some of the rather confusing evidence concerning them will be presented followed by some discussion of the first hypothesis.

Paton and Rang (17, 547, 548) have studied both the kinetics of establishment and reversal of atropine antagonism and the kinetics of atropine uptake into the smooth muscle of the guinea-pig ileum. According to Paton's treatment of antagonism (17), the equilibrium receptor occupancy, p_e, by an antagonist is described by an equation (compare eqn. VIII)† where x is antagonist concentration and K_e the equilibrium constant

$$p_e = \frac{x}{x + K_e} \qquad \text{(XLI)}$$

provided that diffusion delays are negligible, and the rate of rise of antagonism as measured by occupancy, p_t at time t, is given by

$$p_t = p_e[1 - \exp - (k_1 x + k_2) t] \qquad \text{(XLII)}$$

where k_1 is the association rate constant and k_2 the dissociation rate constant of antagonist from receptors. The rate of decline of antagonism, when $x = 0$ is given by,

$$p_t = p_0 \exp\{-k_2 t\} \qquad \text{(XLIII)}$$

The occupancy is assumed to be measured by the dose-ratio (DR) so that,

$$DR = \frac{1}{1 - p} \quad \text{and} \quad p = \frac{DR - 1}{DR} \qquad \text{(XLIV)}$$

Measurements of the rate of onset and offset of antagonism by methylatropinium determined by this method are presented in Table IV-100 and the equilibrium constants for antagonism in Table IV-101.

The uptake of atropine by guinea-pig longitudinal muscle (Table IV-102) clearly represents continuously increasing uptake and is difficult to

† The symbols used in this section differ from these employed previously (p. 212)—although conversion is obvious—in order to maintain consistency with the detailed treatments of Paton and Rang.

reconcile with a binding at a discrete receptor focus. The uptake can, however, be represented as the net result of binding at several sites and a partition factor (Table IV-103). It is interesting that the K_e (uptake, site I) and the K_e (antagonism)values for atropine and methylatropinium

TABLE IV-100. The Onset and Decline of Receptor Occupancy for Methylatropinium Acetylcholine Antagonism in Guinea-pig Longitudinal Muscle (547)

| Receptor | Time secs | |
occupancy	Onset*	Decline†
0·9	0	0
0·7	40	110
0·5	80	350
0·3	150	700
0·2	220	830

* From plot of $\ln p_e - p_t$ versus time (eqn. XLII).
† From plot of $\ln p_t$ versus time (eqn. XLIII).

are in good accord although the binding capacities of this site for the two antagonists differ by a factor of 2. Competitively acting antagonists, benzhexol (IV-107) and lachesine (IV-108) also act as competitive inhibitors of atropine uptake (Table IV-104) although the equilibrium

TABLE IV-101. Equilibrium Constants for Antagonist Interaction with Guinea-pig Ileum (547)

Antagonist	K_e (10^{-9} M)
Atropine	1·11 ± 0·03
Methylatropinium	0·47 ± 0·01
Lachesine	1·46 ± 0·04
Benzhexol	2·37 ± 0·05

constants for benzhexol as an antagonist and as an inhibitor of atropine uptake do not agree, but methylfurmethide (IV-109), a potent activator, is without affect. However, measurements of the kinetics of uptake of atropine at low concentrations ($0·4$–$5·0 \times 10^{-9}$ M) reveal no concentration dependence, in marked contrast to the rate for development of antagonism.

To circumvent the latter anomaly Paton and Rang propose a complex

TABLE IV-102. Uptake of Atropine into Guinea-pig
Longitudinal Muscle (547)

Atropine (nM)	Uptake (pmoles/g)
2·5	150
5·0	186
10·0	228
15·0	273
20·0	305
25·0	340
30·0	370
35·0	410

model, devised by analog computer simulation, in which it is assumed that atropine taken up by the receptor is sequentially transferred to additional sites,

$$D + R_a \underset{k_2}{\overset{k_1}{\rightleftharpoons}} DR_a, \qquad DR_a + R_b \underset{k_3}{\overset{k_3}{\rightleftharpoons}} R_a + DR_b,$$

$$DR_b + R_c \underset{k_3}{\overset{k_3}{\rightleftharpoons}} R_b + DR_c \qquad \text{(XLV)}$$

although there is no direct evidence for such a mechanism.

According to Paton and Rang the different rates of onset and offset of antagonism are not consistent with the simple biophase model (Fig.

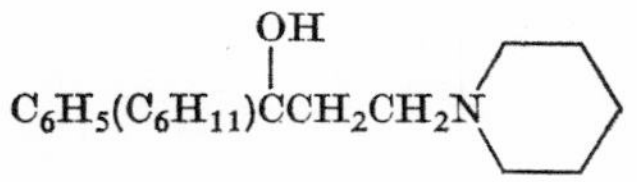

$$\overset{\text{OH}}{\underset{\text{IV-107}}{C_6H_5(C_6H_{11})CCH_2CH_2N}} \bigcirc \qquad \underset{\text{IV-108}}{(C_6H_5)_2CCOOCH_2CH_2\overset{+}{N}Me_2Et}$$

$$\underset{\text{IV-109}}{Me-\bigcirc\!\!\!\!\!\!O\!\!-CH_2\overset{+}{N}Me_3}$$

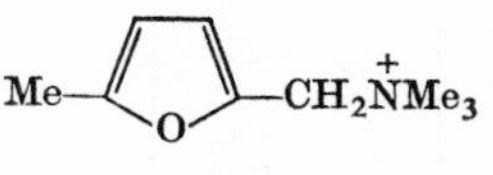

IV-82) which would appear to predict identical rates. Thron and Waud propose (549) however, that any access limited model (of which the

14

TABLE IV·103. Calculated Binding Parameters for Atropine and Methylatropinium Uptake (547)

Antagonist	Binding site I		Binding site II		Binding site III		Partition coefficient
	Capacity $(10^{-12}$ moles/g)	K_e $(10^{-9}$ M)	Capacity $(10^{-12}$ moles/g)	K_e $(10^{-9}$ M)	Capacity $(10^{-12}$ moles/g)	K_e $(10^{-9}$ M)	
Atropine	180	1·11	974	450	—	—	4·67
Methylatropinium	93	0·65	241	55	107,000	200,000	0·44

biophase description is but one case) will predict nonidentical rates simply because receptor occupancy rises initially faster than the antagonist concentration at the receptor environment. Rang (548) has also noted that modification of the biophase model to one in which the binding

TABLE IV-104. Equilibrium Constants for Competitive Antagonism of Acetylcholine Activity and Atropine Uptake (547)

Antagonist	K_e (uptake, 10^{-9} M)	K_e (acetylcholine, 10^{-9} M)
Benzhexol (IV-107)	7·1	2·4
Lachesine (IV-108)	1·4	1·4

capacity of the receptors is not negligible relative to the concentration of the agonist in the biophase can generate constants for onset and offset of antagonism in reasonable agreement with experimental data. It is also relevant that the decline of atropine antagonism is very much faster in the very thin longitudinal muscle of the guinea-pig ileum than in the intact ileum itself (548).

Rang has also argued that a distinction between the biophase and dissociation-limited models may be made by a study of the antagonism produced by combinations of fast and slow acting antagonists. According

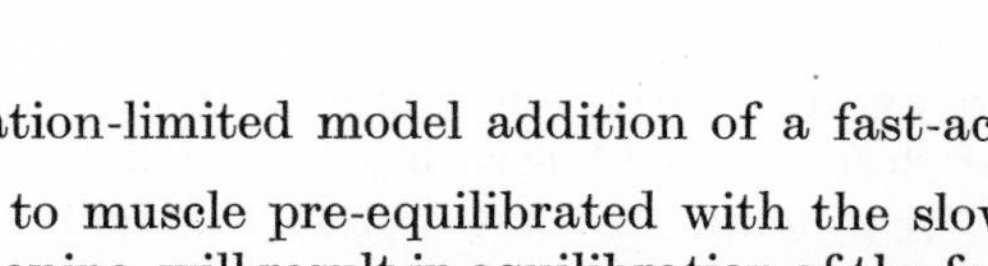

$$D_{EXT} \rightleftharpoons D_{BIO} \rightleftharpoons \text{Drug-Receptor complex}$$

FIG. IV-82. A simple biophase model in which drug at exterior enters into a biophase before forming a drug-receptor complex.

to the dissociation-limited model addition of a fast-acting antagonist ($C_{11}H_{23}\overset{+}{N}Me_3$) to muscle pre-equilibrated with the slowly dissociating antagonist, atropine, will result in equilibration of the former agent with that fraction of receptors $(1 - p)$ unoccupied by atropine *before* any shift in the equilibrium between the receptors and atropine has occurred. Consequently, there should exist an overshoot of antagonism that will decline to the new equilibrium occupancy at a rate determined by the dissociation constant of atropine. Similarly, when the fast acting antagonist is removed in the presence of atropine there will be an "undershoot" of antagonism that will be restored to the equilibrium level atropine at a rate determined by eqn. XLII. This phenomenon would not be anticipated to occur in the simple biophase model where antagonist–receptor kinetics are not the rate limiting step in the determination of antagonism.

A further notable feature of atropine antagonism noted by Stephenson (13) and by Rang (548) is that atropine behaves towards partial agonists as a noncompetitive antagonist and produces flattening of the concentration–response curves. Thus, hyoscine at concentrations of 0·16 nM and 0·3 nM produces only a parallel shift in the concentration–response relationship of 5-methyl-2-dimethylaminomethylfuran methiodide but a progressively marked nonparallel shift and decline in maximum response with the partial agonist, octyltrimethylammonium. (It will be recalled that entirely similar findings have been discussed with the use of irreversible antagonists (p. 330) which produce a parallel shift with full agonists but a decline in maximum response to partial agonists.) This finding is also consistent with the dissociation-limited hypothesis for, if it is accepted that higher receptor occupancy is required by partial agonists (p. 330) than by full agonists to produce a standard response, then that fraction of receptors available, following atropine equilibrium, may be insufficient to permit the production of the normal maximum response.

However, according to Thron and Waud (549) the phenomena of overshoot, undershoot and competitive antagonism are equally compatible with the limited access model (in which receptor binding capacity is significant relative to the binding capacity of adjacent space), for if the kinetics of onset or offset of a slow acting antagonist are access controlled then re-equilibration following addition or removal of a fast acting antagonist or addition of a partial agonist will be slow and generate the phenomena described above.

On the basis of the kinetic evidence thus far available a clear choice cannot be made between the limited access and reaction-rate controlled models of drug antagonism. It should be noted, however, that both treatments relate explicitly to the assumption of a receptor reserve, an assumption that deserves tight scrutiny (pp. 212 and 330) and that neither of the treatments discussed above actually generates any evidence that the antagonist species do compete with acetylcholine for the occupation of a common receptor site. Consideration of a third model, based upon the concept that antagonists may be considered to act at regulatory sites to control the affinity or transducing efficiency of the activator binding site, is thus desirable.

Some evidence that antagonists and agonist may not occupy the same binding site is derived from the studies of Ariëns et al. (550, 551). As noted previously (pp. 257–276) the activities of the isomers of acetyl-β-methylcholine differ markedly suggesting a specific role for the β-methyl group. Higher esters of β-methylcholine are, as anticipated, competitive antagonists (Table IV-105): however, the stereospecificity of interaction at the β-methyl asymmetric center is negligible. Quite clearly the binding environment of the β-methyl group of the β-methylcholine moiety is different in the agonist and antagonist series of compounds. This difference between the agonists and antagonist series is clearly seen in the phenylcyclohexylglycollic acid esters (Table IV-106): marked stereospecificity of interaction of the acyl group is clear, but again the

TABLE IV-105. Cholinergic Activities of Esters of β-Methylcholine (550)

$$\text{RCOOCH}_2\text{CH(Me)CH}_2\overset{+}{\text{N}}\text{Me}_3$$

R	i.a.†	pD$_2$	pA$_2$
Me—	1	6·3	—
Et—	1	5·1	—
Pr—	0·1	—	3·8
Am—	0	—	4·6
C$_6$H$_5$C(Me)CH$_2$OH—	0	—	7·4
(C$_6$H$_5$)$_2$COH—	0	—	8·3
C$_6$H$_5$C(C$_6$H$_{11}$)OH—	0	—	8·9

† Rat jejunum preparation.

configuration about the β-methyl group of choline plays little role in determining the activity of these compounds. The most plausible interpretation of these results is that the agonist and antagonist binding sites are topographically distinct or partially distinct (550, 551). Similar results are also available for the stereoisomers of 2,2-diphenyl-4-dimethylaminomethyl-1,3-dioxolane methiodide (IV-110) which are equally active as acetylcholine antagonists on the rat jejunum and guinea-pig longitudinal muscle preparations. Interestingly enough, there is no difference in activities of the cis- and trans-2-cyclohexyl-2-phenyl-4-dimethylaminomethyl-1,3-dioxolane methiodides (IV-111, IV-112): this stands in marked contrast to the date presented in Table IV-106 and suggests, as noted previously (p. 372) that there may exist at least partial differences in the binding sites and mechanisms of binding of antagonists (unpublished data of K. Chang and D. J. Triggle). That this is so is scarcely surprising if a comparison is made of the structural requirements for agonist and antagonistic activity: antagonistic activity increases and agonistic activity decreases as a general rule with

TABLE IV-106. Cholinergic Activities of Esters of β-Methylcholine with Centers of Assymmetry (550)

Compound	pD$_2$†	pA$_2$	Ratio
S_B—CH$_3$COOCHMeCH$_2\overset{+}{N}$Me$_3$	6·8	—	
R_B—CH$_3$COOCHMeCH$_2\overset{+}{N}$Me$_3$	4·1	—	320
S_B—(C$_6$H$_5$)$_2$C(OH)COOCHMeCH$_2\overset{+}{N}$Me$_3$	—	8·0	
R_B—(C$_6$H$_5$)$_2$C(OH)COOCHMeCH$_2\overset{+}{N}$Me$_3$	—	8·1	0·8
R_A—C$_6$H$_5$(C$_6$H$_{11}$)C(OH)COOCH$_2$CH$_2\overset{+}{N}$Me$_3$	—	9·6	
S_A—C$_6$H$_5$(C$_6$H$_{11}$)C(OH)COOCH$_2$CH$_2\overset{+}{N}$Me$_3$	—	8·2	25
R_AR_B—C$_6$H$_5$(C$_6$H$_{11}$)C(OH)COOCHMeCH$_2\overset{+}{N}$Me$_3$	—	8·9	
R_AS_B—C$_6$H$_5$(C$_6$H$_{11}$)C(OH)COOCHMeCH$_2\overset{+}{N}$Me$_3$	—	8·3	4
R_AR_B—C$_6$H$_5$(C$_6$H$_{11}$)C(OH)COOCHMeCH$_2\overset{+}{N}$Me$_3$	—	8·9	
S_AR_B—C$_6$H$_5$(C$_6$H$_{11}$)C(OH)COOCHMeCH$_2\overset{+}{N}$Me$_3$	—	6·9	100
R_AS_B—C$_6$H$_5$(C$_6$H$_{11}$)C(OH)COOCHMeCH$_2\overset{+}{N}$Me$_3$	—	8·3	
S_AS_B—C$_6$H$_5$(C$_6$H$_{11}$)C(OH)COOCHMeCH$_2\overset{+}{N}$Me$_3$	—	6·6	50
S_AR_B—C$_6$H$_5$(Me)C(CH$_2$OH)COOCHMeCH$_2\overset{+}{N}$Me$_3$	—	6·3	
S_AS_B—C$_6$H$_5$(Me)C(CH$_2$OH)COOCHMeCH$_2\overset{+}{N}$Me$_3$	—	6·9	0·25
R_AR_B—C$_6$H$_5$(Me)C(CH$_2$OH)COOCHMeCH$_2\overset{+}{N}$Me$_3$	—	4·7	
R_AS_B—C$_6$H$_5$(Me)C(CH$_2$OH)COOCHMeCH$_2\overset{+}{N}$Me$_3$	—	4·9	0·66

† Rat jejunum preparation.

increasing nonpolar character of the ligand. Whilst it could be argued that this represents the binding of antagonists to the agonist binding site *and* surrounding nonpolar areas, this appears unlikely in view of the data for the antagonists derived from β-methylcholine. Furthermore, extension to the reversible antagonists of the concepts derived from study of the irreversible antagonists (pp. 330–334) appears to argue very strongly in support of separate sites for agonist and antagonist interaction.

Finally, it should be noted that many of the suggestions and conclusions drawn from structure–activity analyses such as those discussed in this

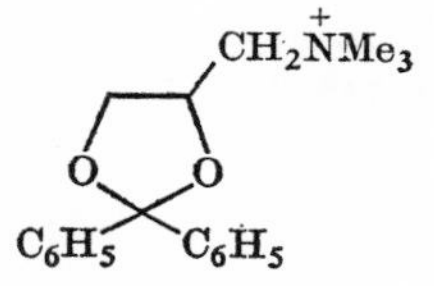

IV-110

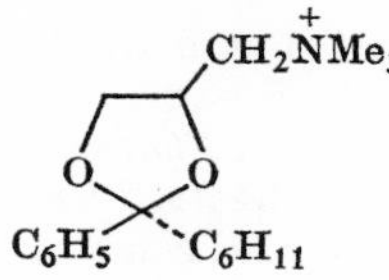

IV-111

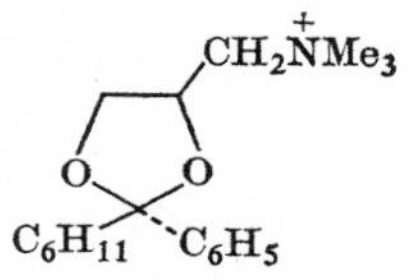

IV-112

chapter must of necessity be speculative. This is inevitable for until receptor isolation, purification and characterization procedures (Chapter VIII) reach the current level of sophistication of the study of ligand–enzyme complexes our information on ligand–receptor interactions will be that received through a glass darkly.

REFERENCES

1. J. B. Robinson, B. Belleau and B. Cox, *J. Med. Chem.* (1969) **12**, 848.
2. H. F. Ridley, S. S. Chatterjee, J. F. Moran and D. J. Triggle, *J. Med. Chem.* (1969) **12**, 931.
3. M. J. Greenberg, *Brit. J. Pharmacol. Chemother.* (1960) **15**, 375.
4. A. J. Clark, "The Mode of Action of Drugs on Cells", Chapters IV and VII (1933). Arnold, London.
5. A. J. Clark, "Handbuch der Experimentellen Pharmakologie" (eds A. Heffter and N. Heubner), Vol. 4 (1937). Springer, Berlin.
6. E. J. Ariëns, "Molecular Pharmacology", Vol. I, Chapter III, (1964). Academic Press, London and New York.
7. A. J. Clark, *J. Physiol. (London)* (1926) **61**, 530.
8. A. J. Clark, *J. Physiol. (London)* (1927) **64**, 123.
9. A. J. Clark, Ref. 4, pp. 60, 133.
10. J. Raventos, *Quart. J. Exp. Physiol.* (1937) **26**, 361.
11. E. J. Ariëns, *Arch. Int. Pharmacodyn.* (1954) **99**, 32.
12. E. J. Ariëns, "Molecular Pharmacology", Vol. I, Chapter IIA (1964). Academic Press, London and New York.
13. R. P. Stephenson, *Brit. J. Pharmacol.* (1956) **11**, 379.

14. R. F. Furchgott, *Advan. Drug. Res.* (1966) **3**, 21.
15. E. J. Ariëns, J. M. van Rossum and P. C. Koopman, *Arch. Int. Pharmacodyn,* (1960) **127**, 459.
16. J. M. van Rossum and E. J. Ariëns, *Arch. Int. Pharmacodyn.* (1962) **136**, 385.
17. W. D. M. Paton, *Proc. Roy. Soc. Ser. B.* (1961) **154**, 21.
18. D. Mackay *Advan. Drug. Res.* (1966) **3**, 1.
19. W. D. M. Paton and H. P. Rang, *Advan. Drug Res.* (1966) **3**, 57.
20. J. M. van Rossum, *Advan. Drug Res.* (1966) **3**, 189.
21. D. R. Waud, *Pharmacol. Rev.* (1968) **20**, 49.
22. R. F. Furchgott, *Pharmacol Rev.* (1955) **7**, 183.
23. M. Nickerson, *Nature (London)* (1956) **178**, 697.
24. W. H. Hartung, *Chem. Rev.* (1931) **9**, 389.
25. D. Bovet and F. Bovet-Nitti, "Medicaments du systeme nerveux et végetatif" (1948). Karger, Basle.
26. R. B. Barlow, "Introduction to Chemical Pharmacology", Ed. 2 (1964). Wiley, New York.
27. D. J. Triggle, "Chemical Aspects of the Autonomic Nervous System" (1965). Academic Press, London and New York.
28. D. J. Triggle, *in* "Medicinal Chemistry", Ed. 3 (ed. A. Burger), Ch. 46 (1970). Wiley, New York.
29. J. H. Burn, *J. Physiol. (London)* (1932) **75**, 144.
30. E. Bülbring and J. H. Burn, *J. Physiol. (London)* (1938) **91**, 459.
31. J. H. Gaddum and H. Kwiatkowski, *J. Physiol. (London)* (1938) **94**, 87.
32. A. Fleckenstein and J. H. Burn, *Brit. J. Pharmacol. Chemother.* (1953) **8**, 69.
33. A. Fleckenstein, *Verh. Deut. Ges. Inn. Med.* (1953) **17**.
34. J. H. Burn and M. J. Rand, *J. Physiol. (London)* (1958) **144**, 314.
35. R. A. Maxwell, H. Povalski and A. J. Plummer, *J. Pharmacol. Exp. Ther.* (1959) **125**, 178.
36. W. W. Fleming and U. Trendelenburg, *J. Pharmacol. Exp. Ther.* (1961) **133**, 41.
37. U. Trendelenburg and N. Weiner, *J. Pharmacol. Exp. Ther.* (1962) **136**, 152.
38. P. A. Shore, *Pharmacol. Rev.* (1962) **14**, 531.
39. J. L. Schmidt and W. W. Fleming, *J. Pharmacol. Exp. Ther.* (1963) **139**, 320.
40. U. Trendelenburg, *Pharmacol. Rev.* (1963) **15**, 225.
41. E. Marley, *Advan. Pharmacol.* (1964) **3**, 167.
42. U. Trendelenburg, *Pharmacol. Rev.* (1966) **18**, 629.
43. P. A. Shore, *Pharmacol. Rev.* (1966) **18**, 561.
44. L. L. Iversen, "The Uptake and Storage of Noradrenaline in Sympathetic Nerves" (1967). Cambridge University Press, Cambridge.
45. J. H. Burn and M. J. Rand, *Brit. J. Pharmacol. Chemother.* (1960) **15**, 47.
46. H. J. Schümann and A. Philippu, *Arch. Exp. Pathol. Pharmakol.* (1961) **241**, 273.
47. L. Stjärne, *Acta Physiol. Scand.* (1961) **51**, 224.
48. G. P. Burn and J. H. Burn, *Brit. J. Pharmacol. Chemother.* (1961) **16**, 344.
49. N. Weiner, P. R. Draskoézy and W. R. Burack, *J. Pharmacol. Exp. Ther.* (1962) **132**, 47.
50. M. J. Davey and J. B. Farmer, *J. Pharm. Pharmacol.* (1963) **15**, 178.
51. J. I. Moore and N. C. Moran, *J. Pharmacol. Exp. Ther.* (1962) **136**, 89.

52. J. R. Crout, A. J. Muskus and U. Trendelenburg, *Brit. J. Pharmacol.* (1962) 18, 600.

53. R. D. Green and J. W. Miller, *J. Pharmacol. Exp. Ther.* (1966) 152, 439.

54. C. A. Stone, J. M. Stavorski, C. J. Ludden, H. C. Wenger and M. L. Torchiana, *Arch. Int. Pharmacodyn.* (1966) 161, 49.

55. "Mechanisms of Release of Biogenic Amines" (eds U. S. von Euler, S. Rosell and B. Uvnas) (1966). Pergamon, New York.

56. P. Pratesi, A. LaManna, A. Campiglio and V. Ghislandi, *J. Chem. Soc.* (1958) 2069.

57. P. Pratesi, A. LaManna, A. Campiglio and G. Pagani, *J. Chem. Soc.* (1959) 4062.

58. P. Pratesi, A. LaManna, A. Campiglio and G. Pagani, *Farmaco, Ed. Sci.* (1960) 15, 3.

59. P. Pratesi, A. LaManna, G. Pagani and E. Grana, *Farmaco, Ed. Sci.* (1963) 18, 950.

60. A. LaManna and V. Ghislandi, *Farmaco, Ed. Sci.* (1964) 19, 377.

61. E. J. Ariëns, *in Proc. Int. Pharmacol Meet., 1st.* Vol. 7, p. 247, (1963). Pergamon, Oxford.

62. E. J. Ariëns and A. M. Simonis, *Acta Physiol. Pharmacol. Neerl.* (1962) 11, 151.

63. Y. Iwasawa and A. Kiyomoto, *Jap. J. Pharmacol.* (1967) 17, 143.

64. P. N. Patil, J. B. LaPidus, D. Campbell and A. Tye, *J. Pharmacol. Exp. Ther.* (1967) 155, 13.

65. L. H. Easson and E. Stedman, *Biochem. J.* (1933) 27, 1257.

66. P. Pratesi, E. Grana, L. Villa, A. LaManna and L. Lilla, *Farmaco, Ed. Sci.* (1963) 18, 920.

67. P. Pratesi, A. LaManna, L. Villa, E. Grana and L. Lilla, *Farmaco, Ed. Sci.* (1963) 18, 932.

68. P. Pratesi and E. Grana *Advan. Drug. Res.* (1965) 2, 127.

69. A. M. Lands and T. G. Brown, Jr., *in* "Drugs Affecting the Peripheral Nervous System" (ed. A. Burger), Vol. I, Chap. 8 (1967). Dekker, New York.

70. F. P. Luduena, U. S. von Euler, B. F. Tullar and A. M. Lands *Arch. Int. Pharmacodyn.* (1957) 111, 392.

71. A. M. Lands and M. L. Tainter *Arch. Exp. Pathol. Pharmakol.* (1953) 219, 76.

72. H. D. Moed, J. Van Dijk and H. Niewind, *Rec. Trav. Chim. Pays-Bas* (1955) 74, 919.

73. D. F. Marsh, M. H. Pelletier and C. A. Ross, *J. Pharmacol. Exp. Ther.* (1948) 92, 108.

74. L. Dertinger, H. R. Granger and H. M. McCarthy, *J. Pharmacol. Exp. Ther.* (1948) 92, 369.

75. A. M. Lands and T. G. Brown, Jr., *Proc. Soc. Exp. Biol. Med.* (1964) 116, 331.

76. P. A. Nuhfer, cited by J. H. Biel, E. G. Schwarz, E. P. Prengler, H. A. Zeiser and H. L. Friedman, *J. Amer. Chem. Soc.* (1954) 76, 3149.

77. K. Wiemers, *Arch. Exp. Pathol. Pharmakol.* (1951) 213, 283, 335.

78. C. G. Van Arman, L. M. Miller and M. P. O'Malley, *J. Pharmacol. Exp. Ther.* (1961) 133, 90.

79. G. P. Lewis, *Brit. J. Pharmacol.* (1954) 9, 488.

80. B. Belleau, *Can. J. Biochem. Physiol.* (1958) 36, 731.

81. B. Belleau, *in* "Adrenergic Mechanisms", Ciba Foundation Symposium (eds J. R. Vane, G. E. W. Wolstenholme and C. M. O'Connor) (1960). Churchill, London.

82. B. Belleau, *Advan. Drug Res.* (1965) 2, 89.

83. B. Belleau, *Ann. N.Y. Acad. Sci.* (1967) **139**, 580.
84. B. M. Bloom and J. M. Goldman, *Advan. Drug Res.* (1966) **3**, 121.
85. E. Grunwald and E. K. Ralph, III, *J. Amer. Chem. Soc.* (1967) **89**, 4405.
86. E. Grunwald, R. L. Lipnick and E. K. Ralph, *J. Amer. Chem. Soc.* (1969) **91**, 4333.
87. U. Trendelenburg, A. Muskus, W. W. Fleming and B. G. Alonso de la Sierra, *J. Pharmacol. Exp. Ther.* (1962) **138**, 170.
88. A. A. Larsen and P. M. Lish, *Nature (London)* (1964) **203**, 1283.
89. R. H. Uloth, J. R. Kirk, W. A. Gould and A. A. Larsen, *J. Med. Chem.* (1966) **9**, 88.
90. A. A. Larsen, W. A. Gould, H. R. Roth, W. T. Comer, R. H. Uloth, K. W. Dungan and P. M. Lish, *J. Med. Chem.* (1967) **10**, 462.
91. J. R. Knowles, *J. Theor. Biol.* (1965) **9**, 213.
92. B. R. Baker, "Design of Active-site-directed Irreversible Enzyme Inhibitors" (1967). Wiley, New York.
93. P. S. Portoghese, *J. Med. Chem.* (1965) **8**, 147.
94. J. F. Moran and D. J. Triggle, *in* "Fundamental Concepts in Drug-Receptor Interactions" (eds J. F. Danielli, J. F. Moran and D. J. Triggle) (1970). Academic Press, London and New York.
95. T. Kappe and M. D. Armstrong, *J. Med. Chem.* (1965) **8**, 369.
96. A. A. Larsen, *Nature (London)* (1969) **224**, 25.
97. A. B. Turner, *Quart. Rev. Chem. Soc.* (1964) **18**, 347.
98. A. Engelhardt, W. Hoefke and H. Wick, *Arzneim. Forsch.* (1961) **11**, 521.
99. N. C. Moran, *Pharmacol. Rev.* (1966) **18**, 503.
100. A. M. Lands, A. Arnold, J. P. McAuliff, F. P. Luduena and T. G. Brown, Jr., *Nature (London)* (1967) **214**, 597.
101. R. F. Furchgott, *Ann. N.Y. Acad. Sci.* (1967) **139**, 553.
102. J. M. van Rossum, *J. Pharm. Pharmacol.* (1965) **17**, 202.
103. P. N. Patil, *J. Pharm. Pharmacol.* (1969) **21**, 628.
104. J. J. Burns, K. I. Colville, L. A. Lindsay and R. A. Salvador, *J. Pharmacol. Exp. Ther.* (1964) **144**, 163.
105. B. Levy, *J. Pharmacol. Exp. Ther.* (1964) **146**, 129.
106. D. Hartley, D. Jack, L. H. C. Lunts and A. C. Ritchie, *Nature (London)* (1969) **219**, 861.
107. V. Bryson and H. J. Vogel (eds), "Evolving Genes and Proteins" (1965). Academic Press, New York and London.
108. C. Nolan and E. Margoliash, *Ann. Rev. Biochem.* (1968) **37**, 727.
109. R. R. Renshaw, D. Green and M. Ziff, *J. Pharmacol. Exp. Ther.* (1938) **62**, 430.
110. C. J. Cavallito, *in* "Curare and Curare-like Agents", p. 55 (1962). Little Brown, Boston.
111. K. Takagi and I. Takayanagi, *J. Pharm. Pharmacol.* (1966) **18**, 795.
112. K. Takagi, I. Takayanagi, T. Irikura and K. Nishino, *Jap. J. Pharmacol.* (1967) **17**, 115.
113. D. J. Triggle, "Chemical Aspects of the Autonomic Nervous System", p. 164 (1965). Academic Press, London and New York.
114. P. Holton and H. R. Ing, *Brit. J. Pharmacol.* (1949) **4**, 190.
115. H. L. Friedman, *in* "Drugs Affecting the Peripheral Nervous System", Vol. I (ed. A. Burger) (1967). Dekker, New York.
116. J. E. Gearien, *in* "Medicinal Chemistry", Ed. 3 (ed. A. Burger) (1970). Wiley, New York.
117. C. J. Cavalitto and A. P. Gray, *Progr. Drug. Res.* (1961) **2**, 135.

118. A. Bennington and R. W. Brimblecombe, *Advan. Drug Res.* (1966) **2**, 143.
119. A. S. V. Burgen, *Brit. J. Pharmacol.* (1965) **25**, 4.
120. C. J. Cavalitto, *Fed. Proc. Fed. Amer. Soc.* (1967) **26**, 1647.
121. R. B. Barlow and J. T. Hamilton, *Brit. J. Pharmacol.* (1962) **18**, 543.
122. J. T. Hamilton, *Can. J. Biochem.* (1963) **41**, 283.
123. I. Hanin, D. J. Jenden and A. K. Cho, *Mol. Pharmacol.* (1966) **2**, 352.
124. D. Pressman, A. L. Grossberg, L. H. Pence and L. Pauling, *J. Amer. Chem. Soc.* (1946) **68**, 250.
125. D. Pressman and M. Siegel, *J. Amer. Chem. Soc.* (1953) **75**, 686.
126. I. B. Wilson, *J. Biol. Chem.* (1952) **197**, 215.
127. S. A. Bernhard, *J. Amer. Chem. Soc.* (1955) **77**, 1966.
128. J. L. Webb, "Enzyme and Metabolic Inhibitors," Vol. I, p. 270 (1963). Academic Press, New York and London.
129. H. F. Marlow, J. C. Metcalfe and A. S. V. Burgen, *Mol. Pharmacol.* (1969) **5**, 166.
130. C. A. Kraus and R. M. Fuoss, *J. Amer. Chem. Soc.* (1933) **55**, 21, 1019.
131. L. M. Tucker and C. A. Kraus, *J. Amer. Chem. Soc.* (1947) **69**, 454.
132. W. E. Thompson and C. A. Kraus, *J. Amer. Chem. Soc.* (1947) **69**, 1017.
133. H. S. Frank and M. W. Evans, *J. Chem. Phys.* (1945) **13**, 507.
134. H. S. Frank and M.-Y. Wen, *Discuss. Faraday Soc.* (1957) **24**, 133.
135. T. S. Sarma, R. K. Mohanty and J. C. Ahluwalia, *Trans. Faraday Soc.* (1969) **65**, 2333.
136. R. L. Kay, T. Vituccio, C. Zawoyski and D. F. Evans, *J. Phys. Chem.* (1966) **70**, 2336.
137. W.-Y. Wen and S. Saito, *J. Phys. Chem.* (1964) **68**, 2639.
138. B. E. Conway, R. E. Verrall and J. E. Desnoyers, *Trans. Faraday Soc.* (1966) **62**, 2738.
139. W.-Y. Wen and K. Nara, *J. Phys. Chem.* (1967) **71**, 3907.
140. J. E. Desnoyers and M. Arel, *Can. J. Chem.* (1967) **45**, 359.
141. F. Franks and H. T. Smith, *Trans. Faraday Soc.* (1967) **63**, 2586.
142. F. J. Millero and W. Drost-Hansen, *J. Phys. Chem.* (1968) **72**, 1758.
143. S. Lindenbaum, *J. Phys. Chem.* (1966) **70**, 814.
144. R. H. Wood, H. L. Anderson, J. D. Beck, J. R. France, W. E. deVry and L. J. Soltzberg, *J. Phys. Chem.* (1967) **71**, 2149.
145. W.-Y. Wen and K. Nara, *J. Phys. Chem.* (1967) **71**, 3907.
146. R. L. Kay and D. F. Evans, *J. Phys. Chem.* (1966) **70**, 2325.
147. P. H. von Hippel and K.-Y. Wong, *J. Biol. Chem.* (1965) **240**, 3909.
148. P. H. von Hippel and T. Schleich, *in* "Structure and Stability of Biological Macromolecules" (eds S. N. Timasheff and G. D. Fasman) (1969). Dekker, New York.
149. H. J. Smith and H. Williams, *J. Theor. Biol.* (1967) **14**, 218.
150. H. C. Chang and J. H. Gaddum, *J. Physiol. (London)* (1933) **79**, 255.
151. G. L. Willey, *Brit. J. Pharmacol.* (1955) **10**, 466.
152. D. J. Triggle and K. Chang, unpublished data.
153. D. J. Triggle, unpublished data.
154. V. Erspamer and A. Glässer, *Brit. J. Pharmacol.* (1958) **13**, 378.
155. W. E. Ormerod, *Brit. J. Pharmacol.* (1956) **11**, 267.
156. P. Hey, *Brit. J. Pharmacol.* (1952) **7**, 117.
157. M. Wurzel, *Arch. Int. Pharmacodyn.* (1960) **124**, 330.
158. R. B. Barlow, "Introduction to Chemical Pharmacology", Chaps. V, VI and VII (1964). Methuen, London.
159. E. J. Ariëns and A. M. Simonis, *Arch. Int. Pharmacodyn.* (1960) **127**, 479.

160. L. Gyermek, *in* "Drugs Affecting the Peripheral Nervous System", Vol. I (ed. A. Burger) (1967). Dekker, New York.
161. H. R. Ing, P. Kordik and D. P. H. Tudor Williams, *Brit. J. Pharmacol.* (1952) **7**, 103.
162. C. Hansch, *in* "Drug Design", Vol. I (ed. E. J. Ariëns) (1971). Academic Press, New York and London.
163. F. Fukui, C. Nagata and A. Imamura, *Science, N.Y.* (1960) **132**, 87.
164. J. Crow, O. Wassermann and W. C. Holland, *J. Med. Chem.* (1969) **12**, 764.
165. M. Wurzel, *Experentia* (1959) **15**, 430.
166. K. A. Scott and H. G. Mautner, *Biochem. Pharmacol.* (1967) **16**, 1903.
167. E. J. Ariëns, "Molecular Pharmacology", Vol. I, Section IIA (1964). Academic Press, London and New York.
168. E. J. Ariëns, A. M. Simonis and W. M. DeGroot, *Arch. Int. Pharmacodyn.* (1954) **100**, 298.
169. G. A. Alles and P. K. Knoefel, *Univ. Calif. Publ. Pharmacol.* (1939) **I**, 187.
170. O. Schmiedeberg and R. Koppe, "Das Muscarine, das Giftige Alkaloid des Fliegenpilzes", (1869). Vogel, Leipzig.
171. S. Wilkinson, *Quart. Rev. Chem. Soc.* (1961) **15**, 153.
172. P. G. Waser, *Pharmacol. Rev.* (1961) **13**, 465.
173. L. Gyermek and K. R. Unna, *Proc. Soc. Exp. Biol. Med.* (1958) **98**, 882.
174. J. M. van Rossum, *Science, N.Y.* (1960) **132**, 954.
175. L. Gyermek and K. R. Unna, *J. Pharmacol. Exp. Ther.* (1960) **128**, 30, 37.
176. A. K. Armitage and H. R. Ing, *Brit. J. Pharmacol.* (1954) **9**, 376.
177. E. J. Fellows and A. E. Livingston, *J. Pharmacol. Exp. Ther.* (1940) **68**, 231.
178. A. H. Beckett, N. J. Harper and J. W. Clitherow, *J. Pharm. Pharmacol.* (1963) **15**, 362.
179. E. Fourneau, D. Bovet, F. Bovet and G. Montezin, *Bull. Soc. Chim. Biol.* (1944) **26**, 134, 516.
180. E. Fourneau, D. Bovet, G. Montezin, J. P. Fourneau and S. Chantalou, *Arch. Pharm. Fr.* (1945) **3**, 114.
181. E. Fourneau and S. Chantalou, *Bull. Soc. Chim. Fr.* (1945) **12**, 845.
182. J. P. Fourneau, C. Menin and A. Beauvillain, *Arch. Pharm. Fr.* (1958) **16**, 630.
183. D. J. Triggle and B. Belleau, *Can. J. Chem.* (1962) **40**, 1201.
184. B. Belleau and J. Puranen, *J. Med. Chem.* (1963) **6**, 325.
185. B. Belleau and J. L. Lavoie, *Can. J. Biochem.* (1968) **46**, 1397.
185a. A. H. Beckett, N. J. Harper, J. W. Clitherow and E. Lesser, *Nature (London)* (1961) **189**, 671.
186. A. H. Beckett, N. J. Harper and J. W. Clitherow, *J. Pharm. Pharmacol.* (1963) **15**, 349.
187. A. Simonart, *J. Pharmacol. Exp. Ther.* (1932) **46**, 157.
188. E. Lesser, *Brit. J. Pharmacol.* (1965) **25**, 213.
189. B. W. J. Ellenbroek, R. J. F. Nivard, J. M. van Rossum and E. J. Ariëns, *J. Pharm. Pharmacol.* (1965) **17**, 393.
190. A. H. Beckett, *Ann. N.Y. Acad. Sci.* (1967) **144**, 675.
191. L. Gyermek and K. R. Unna, *Proc. Soc. Exp. Biol. Med.* (1958) **98**, 882.
192. J. F. Moran and D. J. Triggle, unpublished data.
193. J. M. van Rossum and E. J. Ariëns, *Arch. Int. Pharmacodyn.* (1959) **118**, 447.
194. E. J. Ariëns, "Molecular Pharmacology", Vol. I, p. 163 (1964). Academic Press, New York and London.
195. B. L. Vallee, J. F. Riordan, J. L. Bethune, T. L. Coombs, D. S. Auld and M. Sokolovsky, *Biochemistry* (1968) **7**, 3547.
196. B. M. Sanborn and G. E. Hein, *Biochemistry* (1968) **7**, 3616.

197. B. R. Baker, "Design of Active-Site-Directed Irreversible Enzyme Inhibitors", Chap. 10 (1967). Wiley, New York.
198. M. A. Raftery, F. W. Dahlquist, S. M. Parsons and R. G. Wolcott, *Proc. Nat. Acad. Sci. USA* (1969) **62**, 44.
199. H. R. Ing, *Science, N.Y.* (1949) **109**, 264.
200. P. Pratesi, L. Villa and E. Grana, *Farmaco. Ed. Sci.* (1968) **23**, 1213.
201. F. W. Schueler, H. H. Keasling and R. M. Featherstone, *Science, N.Y.* (1951) **113**, 512.
202. W. B. Bass, F. W. Schueler, R. M. Featherstone and E. G. Gross, *J. Pharmacol. Exp. Ther.* (1950) **100**, 465.
203. M. Bergmann, J. S. Fruton and H. Pollok, *J. Biol. Chem.* (1939) **127**, 643.
204. H. Neurath and G. Schwert, *Chem. Rev.* (1950) **46**, 69.
205. J. E. Purdie and R. A. McIvor, *Biochim. Biophys. Acta* (1966) **128**, 590.
206. J. E. Purdie, *Biochim. Biophys. Acta* (1969) **185**, 122.
207. R. D. O'Brien, *Biochem. J.* (1969) **113**, 713.
208. B. Belleau, *in* "Fundamental Concepts in Drug-Receptor Interactions" (eds J. F. Danielli, J. F. Moran and D. J. Triggle) (1970). Academic Press, New York and London.
209. P. Bracha and R. D. O'Brien, *Biochemistry* (1968) **7**, 1545.
210. P. Bracha and R. D. O'Brien, *Biochemistry* (1968) **7**, 1555.
211. P. S. Portoghese, *J. Med. Chem.* (1965) **8**, 609.
212. P. Pauling, *in* "Structural Chemistry and Molecular Biology" (eds A. Rich and N. Davison) (1968). Freeman, San Francisco.
213. H. G. Mautner, *Ann. Rep. Med. Chem.* p. 230 (1968). Academic Press, New York and London.
214. F. P. Canepa, P. Pauling and H. Sörum, *Nature (London)* (1966) **210**, 907.
215. C. Chothia and P. Pauling, *Chem. Commun.* (1969) 626.
216. F. Jellinek, *Acta Crystallogr.* (1957) **10**, 277.
217. C. Chothia and P. Pauling, *Chem. Commun.* (1969) 746.
218. C. Chothia and P. Pauling, *Nature (London)* (1968) **219**, 1156.
219. E. Shefter and O. Kennard, *Science, N.Y.* (1966) **153**, 1389.
220. E. Shefter and H. G. Mautner, *Proc. Nat. Acad. Sci. USA* (1969) **63**, 1253.
221. P. Pauling and T. J. Petcher, *Chem. Commun.* (1969) 1258.
222. M. Sundaralingham, *Nature (London)* (1968) **217**, 35.
223. H. G. Mautner, E. Bartels and G. D. Webb, *Biochem. Pharmacol.* (1966) **15**, 187.
224. E. Bartels and H. G. Mautner, quoted in 220.
225. E. Eliel, N. Allinger, S. J. Angyal and G. A. Morrison, "Conformational Analysis", Chap. I (1965). Wiley, New York.
226. L. B. Kier, *Mol. Pharmacol.* (1967) **3**, 487.
227. A. M. Liquori, A. Damiani and G. Elefante, *J. Mol. Biol.* (1968) **33**, 439.
228. C. C. J. Culvenor and N. S. Hamm, *Chem. Commun.* (1966) 537.
229. R. J. Cushley and H. G. Mautner, unpublished data. Cited by H. G. Mautner in 213.
230. L. B. Kier, *in* "Fundamental Concepts in Drug-Receptor Interactions" (eds J. F. Danielli, J. F. Moran and D. J. Triggle) (1970). Academic Press, New York and London.
231. L. B. Kier, *in* "Quantum Biology" (L. B. Kier, ed.) (1970). Springer-Verlag, New York.
232. M. May and D. J. Triggle, *J. Pharm. Sci.* (1968) **57**, 511.
233. M. Martin-Smith, G. A. Smail and J. B. Stenlake, *J. Pharm. Pharmacol.* (1967) **19**, 561.

234. S. Archer, A. M. Lands and T. R. Lewis, *J. Med. Chem.* (1962) **5**, 423.
235. E. E. Smissman, W. L. Nelson, J. B. LaPidus and J. L. Day, *J. Med. Chem.* (1966) **9**, 458.
236. P. D. Armstrong, J. G. Cannon and J. P. Long, *Nature (London)* (1968) **220**, 65.
237. C. Y. Chiou, J. P. Long, J. G. Cannon and P. D. Armstrong, *J. Pharmacol. Exp. Ther.* (1969) **166**, 243.
238. D. R. Garrison, M. May, H. F. Ridley and D. J. Triggle, *J. Med. Chem.* (1969) **12**, 130.
239. B. Belleau, *J. Med. Chem.* (1964) **7**, 776.
240. B. Belleau, *Advan. Drug Res.* (1965) **2**, 89.
241. B. Belleau, *Ann. N.Y. Acad. Sci.* (1967) **144**, 705.
242. B. Belleau and J. L. Lavoie, *Can. J. Biochem.* (1968) **46**, 1397.
243. K. E. Neet and D. E. Koshland, *Proc. Nat. Acad. Sci. USA* (1966) **56**, 1606.
244. J. H. Gaddum, *J. Physiol. (London)* (1937) **89**, 7P.
245. J. H. Gaddum, *Trans. Faraday Soc.* (1943) **39**, 323.
246. J. H. Gaddum, K. A. Hameed, D. E. Hathway and F. F. Stephens, *Quart. J. Exp. Physiol.* (1955) **40**, 49.
247. J. H. Gaddum, *Pharmacol. Rev.* (1957) **9**, 211.
248. A. J. Clark and J. Raventos, *Quart. J. Exp. Physiol.* (1937) **26**, 375.
249. H. O. Schild, *Brit. J. Pharmacol.* (1947) **2**, 189.
250. O. Arunlakshana and H. O. Schild, *Brit. J. Pharmacol.* (1959) **14**, 48.
251. H. O. Schild, *Pharmacol. Res. Commun.* (1969) **1**, 1.
252. W. D. M. Paton, *Proc. Royal Soc. B* (1961) **154**, 21.
253. J. Monod, J.-P. Changeux and F. Jacob, *J. Mol. Biol.* (1963) **6**, 306.
254. R. B. Barlow, "Introduction to Chemical Pharmacology" Chap. IX (1964). Methuen, London.
255. D. J. Triggle, "Chemical Aspects of the Autonomic Nervous System", Chaps. XVII, XVIII (1965). Academic Press, London and New York.
256. N. B. Chapman and J. D. P. Graham, *in* "Drugs Affecting the Peripheral Nervous System", Vol. I (ed. A. Burger) (1967). Dekker, New York.
257. M. S. K. Ghouri and T. J. Haley, *J. Pharm. Sci.* (1969) **58**, 511.
258. W. T. Comer and A. W. Gomoll, *in* "Medicinal Chemistry", 3rd Ed. (ed. A. Burger) (1970). J. Wiley and Sons, Inc., New York.
259. E. Rothlin, *Bull. Schweiz. Akad. Med. Wiss.* (1947) **2**, 249.
260. M. Nickerson, *in* "The Pharmacological Basis of Therapeutics" (eds L. S. Goodman and A. Gilman) (1965). Macmillan, New York.
261. D. Bovet, A. Simon and J. Druey, *Arch. Int. Pharmacodyn.* (1937) **56**, 33.
262. D. Bovet and F. Bovet Nitti, "Medicaments du systeme nerveux et végatatif", Chap. 4 (1948). Karger, Basle.
263. D. Bovet and A. Simon, *Arch. Int. Pharmacodyn.* (1937) **55**, 15.
264. M. Nickerson, L. S. Goodman and G. Nomaguchi, *J. Pharmacol. Exp. Ther.* (1947) **89**, 167.
265. B. Belleau, R. Martel, G. Lacasse, M. Mennard, N. L. Weinberg and Y. Perron, *J. Amer. Chem. Soc.* (1968) **90**, 823.
266. L. W. Roth, *J. Pharmacol. Exp. Ther.* (1954) **110**, 157.
267. S. Hayao, H. J. Harvera, W. G. Strycker and T. J. Leipzig, *J. Med. Chem.* (1967) **10**, 400.
268. E. Urech, A. Marxer and K. Miescher, *Helv. Chim. Acta* (1950) **33**, 1386.
269. S. D. Gokhale, D. D. Gulati and H. M. Parikh, *Brit. J. Pharmacol.* (1964) **23**, 508.

270. E. J. Ariëns, "Molecular Pharmacology", Sect. IIA (1964). Academic Press, New York and London.
271. M. Nickerson and L. S. Goodman, *Fed. Proc. Fed. Amer. Soc.* (1945) **2**, 109.
272. P. D. Bartlett, J. W. Davis, S. D. Ross and C. G. Swain, *J. Amer. Chem. Soc.* (1947) **69**, 2977.
273. J. S. Fruton and M. Bergmann, *J. Org. Chem.* (1946) **11**, 559.
274. A. Streitweiser, "Solvolytic Displacement Reactions" (1962). McGraw Hill, New York.
275. M. Nickerson and W. S. Gump, *J. Pharmacol. Exp. Ther.* (1949) **97**, 25.
276. G. E. Ullyot and J. F. Kerwin, *in* "Medicinal Chemistry", **2** (eds F. F. Blicke and C. M. Suter) (1956). Wiley, New York.
277. J. D. P. Graham, *in* "Progress in Medicinal Chemistry", **2** (eds G. P. Ellis and G. B. West) (1962). Butterworth, London.
278. D. J. Triggle, *J. Theor. Biol.* (1964) **7**, 241.
279. T. A. Geissman, H. Hockman and R. T. Kukuto, *J. Amer. Chem. Soc.* (1952) **74**, 3313.
280. N. B. Chapman and J. W. James, *J. Chem. Soc.* (1954) 2103.
281. H. Bunte, *Chem. Ber.* (1874) **7**, 646.
282. J. S. Fruton, W. H. Stein, H. Stalman and G. M. Golumbic, *J. Org. Chem.* (1946) **11**, 571.
283. M. Nickerson and L. S. Goodman, *Fed. Proc. Fed. Amer. Soc.* (1948) **7**, 397.
284. F. C. Ferguson and W. C. Wescoe, *J. Pharmacol. Exp. Ther.* (1950) **100**, 100.
285. J. D. P. Graham and G. W. L. James, *J. Med. Pharm. Chem.* (1961) **3**, 489.
286. J. D. P. Graham, *Brit. J. Pharmacol.* (1957) **12**, 489.
287. J. F. Allen and N. B. Chapman, *J. Chem. Soc.* (1960) 1482.
288. J. F. Allen and N. B. Chapman, *J. Chem. Soc.* (1961) 1076.
289. N. B. Chapman and A. Tompsett, *J. Chem. Soc.* (1961) 1291.
290. R. A. McLean, J. F. Kerwin and E. J. Fellows, *J. Pharmacol. Exp. Ther.* (1957) **119**, 566.
291. R. Kitz and I. B. Wilson, *J. Biol. Chem.* (1962) **237**, 3245.
292. A. R. Main, *Science, N.Y.* (1964) **144**, 992.
293. A. R. Main and F. Iverson, *Biochem. J.* (1966) **100**, 525.
293a. R. D. O'Brien, B. D. Hilton and L. P. Gilmour, *Mol. Pharmacol.* (1966) **2**, 593.
293b. R. D. O'Brien, *Mol. Pharmacol.* (1968) **4**, 131.
294. H. J. Schaeffer, M. A. Schwartz and E. Odin, *J. Med. Chem.* (1967) **10**, 686.
295. H. J. Schaeffer and R. N. Johnson, *J. Med. Chem.* (1968) **11**, 21.
296. B. Belleau, *Can. J. Biochem. Physiol.* (1958) **36**, 731.
297. B. Cohen, E. R. Van Artsdalen and J. Harris, *J. Amer. Chem. Soc.* (1948) **70**, 281; **74**, 1875.
298. B. Belleau and P. Cooper, *J. Med. Chem.* (1963) **6**, 579.
299. B. M. Bloom and I. M. Goldman, *Advan. Drug. Res.* (1966) **3**, 121.
300. R. W. Butcher and F. H. Westheimer, *J. Amer. Chem. Soc.* (1955) **77**, 2420.
301. J. F. Cox, Jr. and O. B. Ramsay, *Chem. Rev.* (1964) **64**, 317.
302. W. P. Jencks, *in* "Enzyme Models and Enzyme Structure", Brookhaven Symposia in Biology, No. 15, p. 134, (1962). Brookhaven National Laboratory, Upton, New York.
303. T. C. Bruice and S. J. Benkovic, "Bioorganic Mechanisms", Chap. 5 (1966). Benjamin, New York.
304. C. A. Bunton, M. M. Mhala, K. G. Oldham and C. A. Vernon, *J. Chem. Soc.* (1960) 3293.
305. C. A. Bunton, *J. Chem. Educ.* (1968) **45**, 21.

306. W. E. Wehrli, D. L. M. Verheyden and J. G. Moffatt, *J. Amer. Chem. Soc.* (1964) **86**, 1254. .

307. E. R. Loew and A. Micetich, *J. Pharmacol. Exp. Ther.* (1949) **95**, 448.

308. J. D. P. Graham and G. P. Lewis, *Brit. J. Pharmacol.* (1953) **8**, 54.

309. J. D. P. Graham and M. A. Karrar, *J. Med. Chem.* (1963) **6**, 103.

310. J. D. P. Graham, *in* "5-Hydroxytryptamine", (ed. G. P. Lewis) (1957). Pergamon, London.

311. I. R. Innes, *Brit. J. Pharmacol.* (1962) **19**, 427.

311a. J. C. Winter and P. K. Gessner, *J. Pharmacol. Exp. Ther.* (1968) **162**, 286.

312. R. F. Furchgott, *J. Pharmacol. Exp. Ther.* (1954) **111**, 265.

313. H. Boyd, G. Burnstock, G. Campbell, A. Jowett, J. O'Shea and M. Wood, *Brit. J. Pharmacol.* (1963) **20**, 418.

314. B. G. Benfey and S. A. Grillo, *Brit. J. Pharmacol.* (1963) **20**, 528.

315. E. W. Gill and H. P. Rang, *Mol. Pharmacol.* (1966) **2**, 284.

316. J. F. Moran and D. J. Triggle, *in* "Fundamental Concepts in Drug-Receptor Interactions" (eds J. F. Danielli, J. F. Moran and D. J. Triggle) (1970). Academic Press, London and New York.

317. J. D. P. Graham and H. Al Katib, *Brit. J. Pharmacol.* (1966) **27**, 377.

318. J. A. Bevan, J. V. Osher and C. Su, *J. Pharmacol. Exp. Ther.* (1963) **139**, 216.

319. S. Shibata and O. Carrier, Jr., *Can. J. Physiol. Pharmacol.* (1967) **45**, 587.

320. S. Shibata, O. Carrier, Jr., and J. Frankenheim, *J. Pharmacol. Exp. Ther.* (1968) **160**, 106.

321. A. P. Somlyo and A. V. Somlyo, *Fed. Proc. Fed. Amer. Soc.* (1969) **28**, 1634.

322. J. D. P. Graham, *J. Med. Chem.* (1966) **9**, 499.

323. B. Belleau and H. Tani, *Mol. Pharmacol.* (1966) **2**, 411.

324. F. Beddoe and H. J. Smith, *Nature (London)* (1967) **216**, 706.

325. R. D. O'Brien, *Biochem. J.* (1969) **113**, 713.

326. B. D. Roufogalis and B. Belleau, *Life Sci.* (1969) **8** (I), 911.

327. G. L. Brown and L. S. Gillespie, *J. Physiol. (London)* (1957) **138**, 81.

328. J. Axelrod and R. Tomchick, *Nature (London)* (1959) **184**, 2027.

329. R. F. Furchgott and S. M. Kirkepar, *in Proc. Int. Pharmacol. Meet, 1st.* **7**, (ed. K. J. Brunings) (1963). Pergamon Press, London.

329a. H. Thoenen, A. Hurlimann and W. Hoefely, *Experientia* (1966) **20**, 272.

330. G. L. Brown, *Proc. Royal Soc. B* (1965) **162**, 1.

331. J. S. Gillespie, *Proc. Royal Soc. B* (1966) **166**, 1.

332. G. Hertting, J. Axelrod and L. G. Whitby, *J. Pharmacol. Exp. Ther.* (1961) **134**, 146.

333. J. Farrant, J. A. Harvey and J. N. Pennefather, *Brit. J. Pharmacol.* (1964) **22**, 104.

334. C. Matsumoto, *Life Sci.* (1966) **5**, 1963.

335. C. R. Ross, N. I. Pessah and A. Farah, *J. Pharmacol. Exp. Ther.* (1968) **160**, 375.

336. A. Reynard, *J. Pharmacol. Exp. Ther.* (1968) **163**, 461.

337. C. R. Ross, N. I. Pessah and A. Farah, *J. Pharmacol. Exp. Ther.* (1969) **167**, 235.

338. J. D. P. Graham and H. Al Katib, *Brit. J. Pharmacol.* (1967) **31**, 42.

339. D. R. Waud, *Nature (London)* (1962) **196**, 1107.

340. D. R. Waud, *Pharmacol. Rev.* (1968) **20**, 49.

341. J. E. Lewis and J. W. Miller, *J. Pharmacol. Exp. Ther.* (1966) **154**, 46.

342. P. N. Patil, A. Tye, C. May, S. Hetey and S. Miyagi, *J. Pharmacol. Exp. Ther.* (1968) **163**, 309.

343. J. F. Moran, M. May, H. Kimelberg and D. J. Triggle, *Mol. Pharmacol.* (1967) **3**, 15.
344. M. S. Yong and G. S. Marks, *Biochem. Pharmacol.* (1969) **18**, 1609.
345. M. Nickerson, *Arch. Int. Pharmacodyn.* (1962) **140**, 237.
346. D. J. Triggle, *Advan. Drug Res.* (1965) **2**, 173.
346a. B. Capon, *Quart. Rev. Chem. Soc.* (1964) **18**, 45.
347. T. C. Bruice and S. Benkovic, "Bioorganic Mechanisms", Vol. I, Chap. I, Vol. II, Chap. 5 (1966). Benjamin, New York.
348. B. Hansen, *Acta Chem. Scand.* (1962) **16**, 1927.
349. J. F. Moran, M. May, H. Kimelberg and D. J. Triggle, *Mol. Pharmacol.* (1967) **3**, 15.
350. M. May, J. F. Moran, H. Kimelberg and D. J. Triggle, *Mol. Pharmacol.* (1967) **3**, 28.
351. J. F. Moran, C. R. Triggle and D. J. Triggle, *J. Pharm. Pharmacol.* (1969) **21**, 30.
352. J. F. Moran and D. J. Triggle, unpublished data.
353. H. Kimelberg and D. J. Triggle, *J. Theor. Biol.* (1965) **9**, 313.
354. U. K. Pandit and T. C. Bruice, *J. Amer. Chem. Soc.* (1960) **82**, 3386.
355. D. M. Brown and G. O. Osborne, *J. Chem. Soc.* (1957) 2590.
356. D. M. Brown, D. A. Magrath and A. R. Todd, *J. Chem. Soc.* (1955) 4396.
357. T. R. Fukuto and E. M. Stafford, *J. Amer. Chem. Soc.* (1957) **79**, 6083.
358. E. Baer and J. Maurukas, *J. Biol. Chem.* (1955) **212**, 39.
359. D. M. Brown, *Ann. N.Y. Acad. Sci.* (1969) **165**, 687.
360. C. C. Hunt, *J. Pharmacol. Exp. Ther.* (1949) **95**, 177.
361. F. C. Ferguson and W. C. Wescoe, *J. Pharmacol. Exp. Ther.* (1950) **100**, 100.
362. F. C. Ferguson, *Proc. Soc. Exp. Biol. Med.* (1958) **99**, 362.
363. N. B. Chapman and D. J. Triggle, *J. Chem. Soc.* (1963) 1385, 4835.
364. N. B. Chapman, K. Clarke and R. D. Strickland, *Proc. Royal Soc. B* (1965) **163**, 116.
365. D. J. Triggle and B. Belleau, *J. Med. Pharm. Chem.* (1962) **5**, 636.
366. C. Hansch and E. J. Lien, *Biochem. Pharmacol.* (1968) **17**, 709.
367. E. Bülbring and I. Wajda, *J. Pharmacol. Exp. Ther.* (1945) **85**, 78.
368. C. E. Powell and I. H. Slater, *J. Pharmacol. Exp. Ther.* (1958) **122**, 480.
369. N. C. Moran and M. E. Perkins, *J. Pharmacol. Exp. Ther.* (1958) **124**, 223.
370. R. Howe, *Biochem. Pharmacol.* (1963) **12**, Suppl. 85.
371. J. W. Black and J. S. Stephenson, *Lancet* (1962) **2**, 311.
372. R. Howe and R. G. Shanks, *Nature (London)* (1966) **210**, 1336.
373. J. W. Black, A. F. Crowther, R. G. Shanks, L. H. Smith and A. C. Dornhurst, *Lancet* (1964) **1**, 1080.
374. D. C. Kvam, D. A. Riggilo and P. M. Lish, *J. Pharmacol. Exp. Ther.* (1965) **149**, 183.
375. P. Somani and B. K. B. Lum, *J. Pharmacol. Exp. Ther.* (1965) **147**, 194.
376. L. Almirante and W. Murmann, *J. Med. Chem.* (1966) **9**, 650.
377. C. Casagrande and G. Ferrari, *Farmaco Ed. Sci.* (1965) **21**, 229.
378. J. J. Burns, K. I. Colville, L. A. Lindsay and R. A. Salvador, *J. Pharmacol. Exp. Ther.* (1964) **144**, 163.
379. R. Howe, A. F. Crowther, J. S. Stephenson, B. S. Rao and L. H. Smith, *J. Med. Chem.* (1968) **11**, 1000.
380. A. F. Crowther and L. H. Smith, *J. Med. Chem.* (1968) **11**, 1009.
381. R. Howe, B. J. McLoughlin, B. S. Rao, L. H. Smith and M. S. Chodnekar, *J. Med. Chem.* (1969) **12**, 452.

382. H. Corrodi, H. Persson, A. Carlsson and J. Roberts, *J. Med. Chem.* (1963) **6**, 751.
383. A. F. Crowther, D. J. Gilman, B. J. McLoughlin, L. H. Smith, R. W. Turner and T. M. Wood, *J. Med. Chem.* (1969) **12**, 638.
384. R. Howe, *J. Med. Chem.* (1969) **12**, 642.
385. J. H. Biel and B. K. B. Lum, *Progr. Drug. Res.* (1966) **10**, 46.
386. E. J. Ariëns, *Ann. N.Y. Acad. Sci.* (1967) **139**, 606.
387. W. T. Comer, *in* "Medicinal Chemistry", 3rd Ed., (ed. A. Burger) (1970). Wiley and Sons, New York.
388. P. Pratesi, L. Villa and E. Grana, *Farmaco, Ed. Sci.* (1966) **21**, 409.
389. L. Villa, V. Ferri, E. Grana, O. C. Mastelli and D. Sossi, *Farmaco, Ed. Sci.* (1969) **24**, 329.
390. L. Villa and V. Ferri, *Farmaco, Ed. Sci.* (1969) **24**, 341.
391. L. Villa, E. Grana, C. Torlasco and P. Pratesi, *Farmaco, Ed. Sci.* (1969) **24**, 349.
392. P. Pratesi, E. Grana and L. Villa, *in Proc. Int. Pharmacol. Meet. 3rd.* **7**, 283, (ed. E. J. Ariëns) (1969). Pergamon Press, Oxford.
393. R. A. Salvador, K. I. Colville, S. A. April and J. J. Burns, *J. Pharmacol. Exp. Ther.* (1964) **144**, 172.
394. J. J. Burns, R. A. Salvador and L. Lemberger, *Ann. N.Y. Acad. Sci.* (1967) **139**, 833.
395. B. Levy, *J. Pharmacol. Exp. Ther.* (1964) **146**, 129.
396. B. Levy, *J. Pharmacol. Exp. Ther.* (1966) **151**, 413.
397. B. Levy, *Brit. J. Pharmacol.* (1966) **27**, 277.
398. N. C. Moran, *Ann. N.Y. Acad. Sci.* (1967) **139**, 649.
399. J. R. Blinks, *Ann. N.Y. Acad. Sci.* (1967) **139**, 673.
400. J. Cepelik, M. Cernohorsky, D. Lincova and M. Wenke, *Arch. Int. Pharmacodyn.* (1967) **165**, 37.
401. B. Levy, *J. Pharmacol. Exp. Ther.* (1967) **156**, 452.
402. B. Levy, *Arch. Int. Pharmacodyn.* (1967) **170**, 418.
403. D. R. Vanderipe, B. Åblad and N. C. Moran, *Fed. Proc. Fed. Amer. Soc.* (1964) **23**, 124.
404. N. C. Moran, *Pharmacol. Rev.* (1966) **18**, 503.
405. D. Dunlop and R. G. Shanks, *Brit. J. Pharmacol.* (1968) **32**, 201.
406. A. M. Barrett, A. F. Crowther, D. Dunlop, R. G. Shanks and L. H. Smith, *Naunyn-Schmiedebergs Arch. Pharmakol. Exp. Pathol.* (1968) **259**, 152.
407. B. Levy and B. E. Wilkenfeld, *Eur. J. Pharmacol.* (1969) **5**, 277.
408. M. Bristow, T. R. Sherrod and R. D. Green, *J. Pharmacol. Exp. Ther.* (1970) **171**, 52.
409. J. L. Gilbert, G. Lange and C. McC. Brooks, *Circ. Res.* (1959) **7**, 417.
410. B. R. Lucchesi and H. F. Hardman, *J. Pharmacol. Exp. Ther.* (1961) **132**, 372.
411. A. Sekiya and E. M. Vaughan Williams, *Brit. J. Pharmacol.* (1963) **21**, 462.
412. G. K. Moe and J. A. Abildskow, *in* "The Pharmacological Basis of Therapeutics", Chap. 32, Ed. 3, (eds L. S. Goodman and A. Gilman) (1965). Macmillan, New York.
413. W. Trautwein, *Pharmacol. Rev.* (1963) **15**, 277.
414. P. Somani, J. G. Fleming, G. K. Chan and B. K. B. Lum, *J. Pharmacol. Exp. Ther.* (1966) **151**, 32.
415. A. R. Laddu and P. Somani, *J. Pharmacol. Exp. Ther.* (1969) **170**, 79.
416. B. R. Lucchesi, *J. Pharmacol. Exp. Ther.* (1965) **148**, 94.
417. B. R. Lucchesi, L. S. Whitsitt and J. L. Stickney, *Ann. N.Y. Acad. Sci.* (1967) **139**, 940.
418. B. F. Hoffman and D. H. Singer, *Ann. N.Y. Acad. Sci.* (1967) **139**, 914.

419. B. R. Lucchesi, *J. Pharmacol. Exp. Ther.* (1964) **145**, 286.
420. E. W. Gill and E. M. Vaughan Williams, *Nature (London)* (1964) **20**, 199.
421. P. M. Lish, J. H. Weikel and K. W. Dungan, *J. Pharmacol. Exp. Ther.* (1965) **149**, 161.
422. G. Åberg and I. Welin, *Life Sci.* (1967) **6**, 975.
423. A. R. Cox and T. C. West, *J. Pharmacol. Exp. Ther.* (1961) **131**, 212.
424. S. Weidmann, *J. Physiol. (London)* (1955) **127**, 213.
425. B. L. Kennedy and T. C. West, *J. Pharmacol. Exp. Ther.* (1969) **168**, 47.
426. W. G. Nayler, *Amer. Heart J.* (1966) **71**, 363.
427. W. G. Nayler, *J. Pharmacol. Exp. Ther.* (1966) **153**, 479.
428. F. Fuchs, E. W. Gerta and F. N. Briggs, *Amer. J. Physiol.* (1968) **52**, 955.
429. C. Raper and A. Jowett, *Eur. J. Pharmacol.* (1967) **1**, 353.
430. R. F. Furchgott and P. Bursztyn, *Ann. N.Y. Acad. Sci.* (1967) **144**, 882.
431. R. P. Stephenson, Material Presented at Symposium on Drug-Receptor Interactions, Chelsea College of Science, London (1965). Quoted by Furchgott (**14**).
432. D. R. Waud, *Biochem. Pharmacol.* (1968) **17**, 649.
433. D. R. Waud, *J. Pharmacol. Exp. Ther.* (1969) **170**, 117.
434. J. F. Moran, V. C. Swamy and D. J. Triggle, *Life Sci.* (1970) **9** (I), 1303.
435. A. J. Wohl, L. M. Hausler and F. E. Roth, *Life Sci.* (1968) **7**, 381.
436. A. J. Wohl, L. M. Hausler and F. E. Roth, *J. Pharmacol. Exp. Ther.* (1967) **158**, 531.
437. B. J. Northover, *Brit. J. Pharmacol.* (1968) **34**, 417.
438. J. F. Moran and D. J. Triggle, unpublished data.
439. H. Weiner, C. W. Batt and D. E. Koshland, *J. Biol. Chem.* (1966) **241**, 2687.
440. C. E. Stauffer and D. Etson, *J. Biol. Chem.* (1969) **244**, 5333.
441. G. Royer and W. J. Canady, *Arch. Biochem. Biophys.* (1968) **124**, 530.
442. D. Bovet, *Ann. N.Y. Acad. Sci.* (1951) **54**, 407.
443. D. Bovet, F. Bovet-Nitti and G. B. Marini-Bettolo (eds) "Curare and Curare-like Agents" (1959). Elsevier, Amsterdam.
444. W. C. Bowman, *Progr. Med. Chem.* (1962) **2**, 88.
445. J. B. Stenlake, *Progr. Med. Chem.* (1963) **3**, 1.
446. D. J. Triggle, "Chemical Aspects of the Autonomic Nervous System", Chap. X (1965). Academic Press, London and New York.
447. D. B. Taylor and O. A. Nedergaard, *Physiol. Rev.* (1965) **45**, 523.
448. J. J. Lewis and T. C. Muir, *in* "Drugs Affecting the Peripheral Nervous System", Vol. I (ed. A. Burger) (1967). Dekker, New York.
449. D. Grob, *in* "Physiological Pharmacology", Vol. III (eds W. S. Root and F. G. Hoffmann) (1967). Academic Press, London and New York.
450. O. Carrier, Jr., *in* "Medicinal Chemistry", 3rd Ed. (ed. A. Burger) (1970). Wiley, New York.
451. W. D. M. Paton and E. Zaimis, *Brit. J. Pharmacol.* (1949) **4**, 381.
452. E. Zaimis, *J. Physiol. (London)* (1951) **112**, 176.
453. B. D. Bruns and W. D. M. Paton, *J. Physiol. (London)* (1951) **115**, 41.
454. S. Thesleff, *Acta Anaesthesiol. Scand.* (1958) **2**, 69.
455. B. L. Ginsborg and J. Warriner, *Brit. J. Pharmacol.* (1960) **15**, 410.
456. D. J. Jenden, K. Kamijo and D. B. Taylor, *J. Pharmacol. Exp. Ther.* (1951) **103**, 348.
457. E. Zaimis, *J. Physiol. (London)* (1953) **122**, 238.
458. R. Creese, D. B. Taylor and B. Tilton, *J. Pharmacol. Exp. Ther.* (1963) **139**, 8.
459. D. B. Taylor, *in* "Curare and Curare-like Agents", (ed. A. V. S. de Reuck) (Ciba Foundation Study Group No. 12) (1962). Churchill, London.

460. D. B. Taylor, R. Creese, O. A. Nedergaard and R. Case, *Nature* (*London*) (1965) **208**, 901.

461. R. B. Barlow and H. R. Ing, *Brit. J. Pharmacol.* (1948) **3**, 298.

462. D. Bovet, F. Bovet-Nitti, S. Guarino, V. G. Lango and R. Fusco, *Arch. Int. Pharmacodyn.* (1951) **88**, 1.

463. R. B. Barlow, *in* "Steric Aspects of the Chemistry and Biochemistry of Natural Products", Biochem. Soc. Symp. No. 19, (1960). Cambridge University Press, Cambridge.

464. E. J. Ariëns and J. M. van Rossum, *Arch. Int. Pharmacodyn.* (1957) **110**, 275.

465. V. Rosnati, *Gazz. Chim. Ital.* (1950) **80**, 663.

466. H. Vanderhaeghe, *Nature* (*London*) (1951) **167**, 527.

467. E. Lesser, *J. Pharm. Pharmacol.* (1961) **13**, 703.

468. R. S. Rybolovlev, cited in 28.

469. N. V. Khromov-Borisov and M. J. Michelson, *Pharmacol. Rev.* (1966) **18**, 1051.

470. R. B. Barlow and A. Zoller, *Brit. J. Pharmacol.* (1964) **23**, 131.

471. J. Cheymol, R. Delaby, P. Chabrier, H. Najer and F. Bourillet, *Arch. Int. Pharmacodyn.* (1954) **98**, 161.

472. E. J. Ariëns, "Molecular Pharmacology" Vol. I, p. 401 (1964). Academic Press, New York and London.

473. D. J. Cavanaugh and J. Z. Hearon, *Arch. Int. Pharmacodyn.* (1954) **100**, 68.

474. H. Lüllmann and W. Förster, *Arch. Exp. Path. Pharmakol.* (1953) **217**, 217.

475. E. J. Ariëns, "Molecular Pharmacology", Vol. I, pp. 144–148 (1964). Academic Press, New York and London.

476. J. H. Gaddum, *J. Physiol.* (*London*) (1962) **61**, 141.

477. A. J. Clark, "The Mode of Action of Drugs on Cells", Chaps. IV, VII (1933). Arnold, London.

478. P. S. Hewlett and R. L. Plackett, *Biometrics* (1956) **12**, 72.

479. L. B. Kirschner and W. E. Stone, *J. Gen. Physiol.* (1951) **34**, 821.

480. A. Mondon, *Ann. Chimie.* (1959) **628**, 123.

481. R. Hazard, J. Cheymol, P. Chabrier, E. Corteggiani and F. Nicolas, *Arch. Int. Pharmacodyn.* (1950) **84**, 237.

482. J. O. Hoppe, J. E. Funnell and H. Lape, *J. Pharmacol. Exp. Ther.* (1955) **115**, 106.

483. V. Rosnati, H. Angelini-Kothny and D. Bovet, *Gazz. Chim. Ital.* (1958) **88**, 1293.

484. V. Rosnati and H. Angelini-Kothny, *Gazz. Chim. Ital.* (1958) **88**, 1284.

485. S. Thesleff and K. R. Unna, *J. Pharmacol. Exp. Ther.* (1954) **111**, 99.

486. H. O. J. Collier and E. P. Taylor, *Nature* (*London*) (1949) **164**, 491.

487. E. P. Taylor, *J. Chem. Soc.* (1951) 1150.

488. H. O. J. Collier, *Brit. J. Pharmacol.* (1952) **7**, 392.

489. W. Kalow, *J. Pharmacol. Exp. Ther.* (1954) **110**, 433.

490. D. F. Hutter and J. E. Pascoe, *Brit. J. Pharmacol.* (1951) **6**, 691.

491. W. L. Nastuk and J. Karis, *J. Pharmacol. Exp. Ther.* (1964) **144**, 236.

492. A. G. Karczmar, *Ann. Rev. Pharmacol.* (1967) **7**, 241.

493. W. F. Riker, Jr. and M. Okamoto, *Ann. Rev. Pharmacol.* (1969) **9**, 173.

494. K. K. Kimura and K. R. Unna, *J. Pharmacol. Exp. Ther.* (1950) **98**, 286.

495. K. K. Kimura, K. R. Unna and C. C. Pfeiffer, *J. Pharmacol. Exp. Ther.* (1949) **95**, 149.

496. C. G. Haining, R. G. Johnston and J. M. Smith, *Brit. J. Pharmacol.* (1960) **15**, 71.

496a. D. J. Triggle, "Chemical Aspects of the Autonomic Nervous System", Chap. IX (1965). Academic Press, London and New York.

496b. L. Gyermek in "Drugs Affecting the Peripheral Nervous System" (ed. A. Burger) (1967). Dekker, New York.

496c. D. A. Kharkevich, "Ganglion-blocking and Ganglion-stimulating Agents" (1967). Pergamon, Oxford.

497. J. M. van Rossum, Int. J. Neuropharmacol. (1962) 1, 97, 403.

498. H. R. Ing, in "Hypotensive Drugs" (ed. M. Harington) (1957). Pergamon Press, Oxford.

499. M. M. Winbury, J. Pharmacol. Exp. Ther. (1952) 124, 25.

500. M. M. Winbury, D. L. Cook and W. E. Hambourger, J. Pharmacol. Exp. Ther. (1954) 111, 395.

501. R. Wien, D. F. J. Mason, N. D. Edge and G. T. Langston, Brit. J. Pharmacol. (1952) 7, 534.

502. R. Wien and D. F. J. Mason, Brit. J. Pharmacol. (1951) 6, 611.

503. J. Fakstorp and J. G. A. Pedersen, Acta Pharmacol. Toxicol. (1954) 10, 7.

504. D. F. J. Mason and R. Wien, Brit. J. Pharmacol. (1955) 10, 124.

505. J. Fakstorp and J. G. A. Pedersen, Acta Pharmacol. Toxicol. (1957) 13, 359.

506. J. Fakstorp, J. G. A. Pedersen, E. Poulsen and M. Schilling, Acta Pharmacol. Toxicol. (1957) 14, 148.

507. R. Wien and D. F. J. Mason, Brit. J. Pharmacol. (1953) 8, 306.

508. R. B. Barlow and H. R. Ing, Brit. J. Pharmacol. (1949) 3, 298.

509. E. W. Gill, Proc. Royal Soc. B (1959) 150, 381.

510. E. W. Gill and H. R. Ing, Farmaco., Ed. Sci. (1958) 13, 244.

511. A. Karlin and M. Winnik, Proc. Nat. Acad. Sci., U.S.A. (1968) 60, 668.

512. L. Gyermek and K. Nador, J. Pharm. Pharmacol. (1957) 9, 209.

513. D. J. Triggle, "Chemical Aspects of the Autonomic Nervous System", Chap. VIII (1965). Academic Press, London and New York.

514. H. Cullumbine, in "Physiological Pharmacology", Vol. III (eds N. S. Root and F. G. Hofmann) (1967). Academic Press, New York and London.

515. B. V. R. Sastry, in "Medicinal Chemistry", 3rd Ed. (ed. A. Burger) (1970). Wiley, New York.

516. L. Gyermek, Acta Phys. (1953) 4, 333.

517. H. R. Ing, G. S. Dawes and I. Wajda, J. Pharmacol. Exp. Ther. (1945) 85, 85.

518. A. Wick, Arch. Exp. Pathol. Pharmakol. (1957) 213, 485.

519. E. Rothlin, M. Taeschler, H. Konzett and A. Cerletti, Experientia (1954) 10, 142.

520. G. Fodor in "The Alkaloids," 9, 269 (1967). Academic Press, London and New York.

521. M. Dóda, L. György and K. Nador, Arch. Int. Pharmacodyn. (1963) 145, 264.

522. D. R. Brown, R. Lygo, J. McKenna, J. M. McKenna and B. G. Hutley, J. Chem. Soc. B (1967) 1184.

523. C. C. Thut and A. T. Bottini, J. Amer. Chem. Soc. (1968) 90, 4752.

524. F. L. Pyman, J. Chem. Soc. (1967) 1103.

525. J. M. van Rossum and J. A. Th. M. Hurkmans, Acta Physiol. Pharmacol. Neerl. (1962) 11, 173.

526. E. J. Ariëns and A. M. Simonis, Acta Physiol. Pharmacol. Neerl. (1962) 11, 151.

527. A. B. H. Funcke, R. F. Rekker, M. J. E. Ernsting, H. M. Tersteege and W. T. Nauta, Arzeim. Forsch. (1959) 9, 573.

528. R. B. Barlow, N. C. Scott and R. P. Stephenson, Brit. J. Pharmacol. (1963) 21, 509.

529. F. B. Abramson, R. B. Barlow, M. G. Mustafa and R. P. Stephenson, *Brit. J. Pharmacol.* (1969) **37**, 207.
530. C. Hansch, *Accounts. Chem. Res.* (1969) **2**, 232.
531. P. Pratesi, L. Villa, V. Ferri, E. Grana and D. Sossi, *Farmaco, Ed. Sci.* (1969) **24**, 313.
532. A. C. White, A. F. Green and A. Hudson, *Brit. J. Pharmacol.* (1951) **6**, 560.
533. A. M. Lands, *J. Pharmacol. Exp. Ther.* (1951) **102**, 219.
534. W. M. Duffin and A. F. Green, *Brit. J. Pharmacol.* (1955) **10**, 383.
535. A. Jageneau and P. Janssen, *Arch. Int. Pharmacodyn.* (1956) **106**, 199.
536. W. T. Nauta, R. F. Rekker and A. F. Harms, *in* "Physico-Chemical Aspects of Drug Action", (ed. E. J. Ariëns) *Proc. Int. Pharmacol. Meet., 3rd.* **7**, (1968). Pergamon Press, London.
537. R. W. Taft, *in* "Steric Effects in Organic Chemistry" (ed. M. S. Newman) (1956). Wiley, New York.
538. J. E. Leffler and R. W. Grunwald, "Rates and Equilibria of Organic Reactions" (1963). Wiley, New York.
539. M. Charton, *J. Amer. Chem. Soc.* (1969) **91**, 615.
540. E. Kutter and C. Hansch, *J. Med. Chem.* (1969) **12**, 647.
541. P. B. Marshall, *Brit. J. Pharmacol.* (1955) **10**, 354.
542. A. J. Clark, *J. Physiol. (London)* (1926) **61**, 547.
543. M. Rocha e Silva and W. T. Beraldo, *J. Pharmacol. Exp. Ther.* (1948) **93**, 457.
544. M. Rocha e Silva, *Pharmacol. Rev.* (1956) **9**, 259.
545. M. Rocha e Silva, *Eur. J. Pharmacol.* (1969) **6**, 294.
546. R. F. Furchgott, *Ann. Rev. Pharmacol.* (1964) 4, 21.
547. W. D. M. Paton and H. P. Rang, *Proc. Royal Soc. B* (1965) **163**, 1.
548. H. P. Rang, *Proc. Royal Soc. B* (1966) **165**, 488.
549. C. D. Thron and D. R. Waud, *J. Pharmacol. Exp. Ther.* (1968) **160**, 91.
550. B. W. J. Ellenbroeck, R. J. F. Nivard, J. M. van Rossum and E. J. Ariëns, *J. Pharm. Pharmacol.* (1965) **17**, 393.
551. E. J. Ariëns and A. M. Simonis, *Ann. N.Y. Acad. Sci.* (1967) **144**, 842.

Chapter V

MEMBRANE POTENTIALS, ION PERMEABILITIES AND NEUROTRANSMITTER ACTION

INTRODUCTION

A prominent feature of the action of neurotransmitters and related excitatory and inhibitory ligands at chemically excitable membranes is the production of changes in ion permeabilities often accompanied by alterations of membrane potential. Analysis of these events with respect to the involvement of various types of ligands may provide information concerning the initial actions of ligands, namely their interactions at the various receptors that are involved in transmitter action.

As described previously (Chapter II, p. 161) the action of acetylcholine at the end plate of "twitch fibers" of skeletal muscle,† a particularly well investigated example, is to produce an increased permeability to Na^+ and K^+ ions accompanied by depolarization (the end plate potential). Such analyses, of which the above is only one example, provide what is essentially a phenomenological description of neurotransmitter action, but the events described are obviously a consequence of a previous step— namely, the neurotransmitter-receptor interaction. Once this interaction is achieved, the changes in ion permeabilities and membrane potential may follow as a consequence of this primary event.‡ Furthermore, the

---

† It is necessary to make a division among various classes of skeletal muscle fibers since they differ very considerably in their junctional anatomy and their potential changes. The "twitch" fibers of vertebrate skeletal muscle resemble closely nerve axons in their ability to propagate action potentials. In the frog there also exist so called slow or tonic fibers which are characterized by a very slow development of tension in response to stimulation; these fibers, like many smooth and crustacean muscles, have a low resting potential (~60 mV), do not propagate an action potential and receive multiple innervation along the length of the fiber which responds to stimulation by a graded depolarization that resembles the end plate potential of twitch fibers. In many invertebrates propagated action potentials in muscle fibers are not found and the fiber receives multiple innervation through which it can generate graded responses.

‡ Actually this statement is true only if the neurotransmitters are acting to produce changes in ionic permeabilities through the selective "opening" or "closing" of ion-specific channels. Alternatively neurotransmitters might act to stimulate electrogenic ion pumps that selectively alter intracellular ionic concentrations and thus affect the membrane potential by processes dependent upon the utilization of metabolic energy. This second mechanism does not, however, appear to be as commonly operative.

relevance of the total sequence of observed ionic and potential changes to the end result of neurotransmitter action, i.e., muscle contraction and relaxation or alterations in secretory activity, etc., vary according to the tissue in question. For twitch skeletal muscle fibers the depolarization following the acetylcholine-stimulated increase in $Na^+ - K^+$ permeability is critical to the final contractile response for this depolarization initiates the propagated action potential which, in turn, initiates the contractile process (Chapter VIII). For other systems, most notably smooth muscle, it is possible to obtain contraction or relaxation in depolarized tissues where potential changes are impossible but where ligand-induced changes in ion permeabilities still occur. It will become clear that the immediate relevance of potential and permeability changes to neurotransmitter action is intimately concerned with the nature of the excitation-contraction coupling process: for smooth muscles the coupling is rather directly related to the events initiated at the receptor site proper, but for twitch skeletal muscle the linkage is less direct and requires the intermediacy of the propagated action potential.

Thus the major problem is to elucidate the changes in ion permeabilities, of which potential changes are a direct manifestation, because these should be relatable to, and interpretable in terms of, the primary neurotransmitter-receptor interaction, whether this be the essentially passive role of opening and closing ion channels or the stimulation of an electrogenic ion selective pump. As will become apparent calcium appears to be critically involved in this, and subsequent phases of neurotransmitter action.

THE IONIC CONSEQUENCES OF NEUROTRANSMITTER-RECEPTOR INTERACTIONS

Some brief reference has already been made to the actions of acetylcholine at the chemically sensitive endplate region of twitch skeletal muscles where the acetylcholine-receptor interaction generates a nonpropagating depolarization, the endplate potential, that in turn triggers the propagated action potential. This action may be represented by an equivalent circuit diagram (Fig. V-1a) in which the right hand circuit (E-R) represents the pathways through which ions interchange in the electrically excitable membrane and the left hand circuit (e-r) represents pathways that are utilized for ion transfer in the chemically sensitive area (1–3). If the switch S is regarded as the locus of transmitter action, then closing S will, provided that e < E, cause an inward flow of current and membrane depolarization. As a specific example, Fig. V-1b represents the equivalent circuit of the frog muscle fiber with a resting potential of 90 mV which, upon activation, generates a current flow of,

$$\frac{90 - 15 \text{ mV}}{(2 \times 10^5 + 2 \times 10^4) \text{ ohm}} = 3\cdot4 \times 10^{-7} \text{ amps}$$

thus producing an endplate depolarization of 68 mV : this is not normally seen since it is obscured by the rising phase of the action potential. From this diagram it is clear that if the membrane potential is set to 15 mV in the absence of neurotransmitter action, then there will be no induced current flow or alteration of membrane potential by subsequently added neurotransmitter. Thus e is that potential difference across the membrane

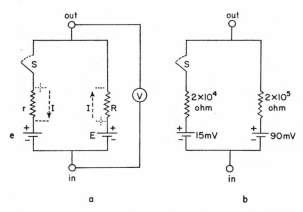

FIG. V-1. (a) Generalized equivalent circuit diagram showing pathway (er) opened by transmitter. (b) Equivalent circuit diagram for the action of acetylcholine at the skeletal muscle endplate. Reproduced with permission from Ginsborg (3).

at which the transmitter produces no potential change and is termed the transmitter equilibrium potential. There are now many examples available from vertebrate and invertebrate striated muscle and neurons (3) where such a circuit diagram serves to account satisfactorily for chemical excitation; however, smooth muscle in particular, appears to offer many peculiarities and may utilize rather different mechanisms (p. 430).

Evidence for the model proposed above has been obtained in a number of ways, reviewed fairly recently by Ginsborg (3), designed to obtain the transmitter equilibrium potentials and which are based on the prediction of Fig. V-1, that appropriate displacement of the membrane potential should not only abolish the transmitter-induced potential change, but when E > e, the potential change caused by the transmitter should be reversed.

Fatt and Katz (1) introduced the widely used method of displacing the membrane potential by a constant applied current and were able to show that the endplate potential would reach zero at a membrane potential of approximately −15 mV. Del Castillo and Katz (4) obtained essentially similar results using the so-called "collision" method in which an endplate potential is generated by nerve stimulation at various levels of the membrane potential (predetermined by the characteristics of the action potential). The powerful voltage clamp technique, in which the membrane potential is held constant at a predetermined level by a current supplying feedback amplifier has also been applied to the end-

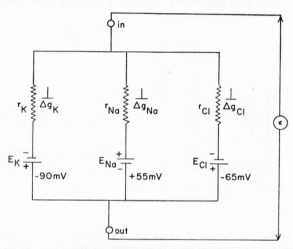

FIG. V-2. Equivalent circuit diagram for the ion channels opened during neurotransmitter action in nerve or skeletal muscle. The equilibrium potentials for K^+, Na^+ and Cl^- are (approximately) E_K, −70 to −100 mV; E_{Na}, +50 to +65 mV; and E_{Cl}, −40 to −90 mV. Reproduced with permission from Ginsborg (3).

plate (5). Clearly, the equilibrium potential will then be that value of the membrane potential at which no additional current is drawn from the feedback system. This method is particularly useful in studying transmitter action since it enables determination of the amplitude and time course of the current generated by the neurotransmitter.

It is apparent (3) that the equilibrium potentials for excitatory ligands (the values available refer primarily to skeletal muscle and neurons) lie between 0 and −20 mV. It follows that the action of these neurotransmitters is not confined to a change in permeability to a single ionic species but must be attributed to a permeability change to at least two ions, one of which must be Na^+ (Fig. V-2). Attention is specifically directed to Na^+, K^+ and Cl^- because these are the most common ionic species, but Ca^{++} may also play a role as a current carrying species. Thus the action of some (it should be noted that the model described above may not be applicable to all excitatory transmitters and their junctions) excitatory transmitters is to initiate the operation of ionic channels and the generation of ionic events that are quite distinct from those involved in the overall control of the membrane potential. In this regard, therefore, our visualization of the receptor sites at which these events are initiated must differ from that of the excitable cell membrane in general.

These preliminary considerations have so far involved only the action of excitatory ligands: at many synaptic junctions, however, the ligand action may be inhibitory and serve to increase or maintain the membrane potential at a level at which active responses are no longer generatable.

From Fig. V-2 it is clear that if the neurotransmitter is to maintain or increase membrane potential and stability then it cannot act by opening a Na^+ channel for this will inevitably lead to depolarization; however, opening of a K^+ or Cl^- channel will lead to the maintenance or increase of membrane potential depending upon the resting permeability to Na^+. With membranes that are highly permeable to Na^+ (notably smooth muscle) the action of the inhibitory transmitter is to cause hyper-polarization by, for instance, a selective increase in K^+ permeability so that the membrane potential moves closer to the equilibrium potential for K^+ (E_{K^+}). Where permeability to Na^+ is normally low the action of the inhibitory transmitter may not produce any change in membrane potential: this is the case with some crustacean muscles† (6) where, however, displacement of the resting membrane potential preceding inhibitory nerve stimulation reveals that the latter action does serve to restore membrane potential to its resting level.‡ Thus in this case, the transmitter equilibrium potential is identical with the resting membrane potential. The demonstration in a number of crustacean muscles that the equilibrium potential for inhibitory nerve stimulation is the same as that for applied GABA provides considerable support that this agent acts as an inhibitory transmitter (3, 8, 9). Studies of the effect of

---

† It is helpful here to consider very briefly some aspects of the innervation of crustacean muscles which, as noted previously, do not depend upon a self-propagating impulse mechanism. These muscles receive both excitatory and inhibitory axons; stimulation of the latter stops contraction induced by simultaneous repetitive excitatory stimulation and the muscle relaxes. There is good evidence (7–9) that this inhibitory transmitter is γ-aminobutyric acid (GABA). Actually because of the multiple excitatory and inhibitory innervation of the crustacean muscle and the fact that the final response is the product of these interacting antagonistic impulses this system is rather similar to the central neuron where the final output signal is the net product of the various input signals (7).

‡ The action of the inhibitory stimulus is not, however, confined to the postsynaptic membrane but also occurs presynaptically serving to decrease the liberation of excitatory transmitter (10): this phenomenon is termed presynaptic inhibition and assumes great importance in the vertebrate central nervous system (11).

variation of the concentrations of K_{ext}^+ and Cl_{ext}^- support the idea that GABA functions primarily by increasing Cl^- permeability (3, 8); this is perhaps not surprising since GABA possesses a formal negative charge and is thus more likely to be concerned with the modification of anion transport and binding than transmitters such as acetylcholine and noradrenaline which possess only a positive charge.

In cardiac muscle Trautwein and Dodd (12) have shown that the equilibrium potential for the action of acetylcholine on the dog atrium is identical with E_{K^+}: the channels opened by acetylcholine are the K^+ channels. In smooth muscle (taenia coli) it is now evident that the inhibitory action of adrenaline at the α-receptor is due to an increased K^+ permeability with perhaps some contribution from an increased Cl^- permeability (13).

In addition to the mechanisms of synaptic transmission outlined above and in which ion transfers occur down concentration gradients without the involvement of metabolic energy, there is also evidence for a second type of synaptic transmission process which involves the utilization of metabolic energy and ion transfer through the stimulation of an electrogenic ion pump. Pinsker and Kandel (14) have reported that an interneuron of the abdominal ganglion of *Aplysia california* mediates four synaptic processes at different receptor cells through the action of a single transmitter, acetylcholine. Three of these processes—excitation, inhibition and excitation-inhibition—involve changes in permeability to Na^+, Cl^- and Na^+ and Cl^- ions respectively, but the fourth process manifests itself as a slow component of the inhibitory postsynaptic potential (IPSP) and was argued by Pinsker and Kandel (14) to involve an acetylcholine-stimulated Na^+/K^+ ATPase. It should be noted, however, that Kehoe and Ascher (15) conclude from a similar investigation that activation of an electrogenic Na^+ pump is not involved but rather an increased K^+ inductance.

Libet and co-workers (16–19) have proposed that the slow inhibitory and excitatory postsynaptic potential observed in sympathetic ganglia which appear to occur without any increase in membrane conductance and which are closely mimicked by exogenous norepinephrine and acetylcholine respectively also arise from stimulation of electrogenic mechanisms. The nature of the ion pump(s) involved is not known but ouabain is ineffective in inhibiting the hyperpolarizing response to norepinephrine. It seems possible that electrogenic mechanisms may prove to be an important feature of transmitter action at least as far as slowly generated events are concerned although considerable caution may be needed (15) to make an unambiguous characterization of these mechanisms.

It is clear from the brief outline of neurotransmitter-induced ionic and potential changes involved in junctional transmission that a complex array of events have to be interpreted. The key question to be solved is *how* the neurotransmitter generates the observed ionic and potential events.

Ionic Events at the Skeletal Neuromuscular Junction

The actions of acetylcholine in generating the endplate potential in skeletal muscle have already been noted previously (Chapter II, p. 161). In brief, interaction of acetylcholine at the skeletal muscle endplate causes a simultaneous increase in permeability to Na^+ and K^+ ions. These changes in ionic permeability operate over a wide range of membrane potential.

The relatively detailed knowledge available of the ionic and chemical events at this junction is due, in large part, to the relative ease with which single fiber preparations can be set up, to the use of micropipettes, pioneered by Nastuk (20), by which carefully controlled quantities of agonists and antagonists can be applied to the endplate and to the use of microelectrodes to record potential changes occurring at the endplate itself. The use of intracellular electrodes to record the epp is described in the classic paper of Fatt and Katz (1).

By the micropipette technique it has been established that the minimum effective quantity of acetylcholine (to initiate an action potential) is of the order of 10^{-17}–10^{-16} moles (21, 22). This same technique has also permitted localization of the site of action of acetylcholine as the external membrane surface (21), injection into the interior of the endplate region proving completely ineffective.† Analysis of the time course of the events of the epp reveals (23, 24) the extreme rapidity of the ionic changes which are complete in approximately 1·5 msec with a latency period, following administration of acetylcholine, of some 150 μsec (24, 25). Any attempt to describe the molecular basis of stimulant ligand action at the endplate must consider the following factors (24):

   (a) the mechanism operates over a wide range of membrane potential,

   (b) the mechanism operates at high speed, and,

   (c) the mechanism is clearly distinguishable from that involved in maintaining propagated potential changes.

The work of Takeuchi (26) on the influence of Ca_{ext}^{++} on the endplate potential sheds some light on the problem. An increase in Ca_{ext}^{++} from 2 to 30 mM reduces the amplitude of the endplate current and the

---

† It is essentially this work that has led to general conclusions that all neurotransmitters act similarly. Whilst neurotransmitter action at the membrane surface appears to be most probable it cannot be said to have been established for all agents.

conductance change produced by acetylcholine in the frog sartorius preparation to about 72 and 84% respectively. The effect of Ca^{++}_{ext} is primarily due to a reduction in Na^+ conductance—the mutual interaction between Na^+ and Ca^{++} ions has been discussed previously (Chapter II, p. 164). The apparent interaction between acetylcholine and Ca^{++} is confirmed by the work of Nastuk and Liu (24, 27) who have demonstrated the competitive antagonism between Ca^{++} and (Mg^{++}) and carbamylcholine in generating the endplate potential (Fig. V-3). Additionally,

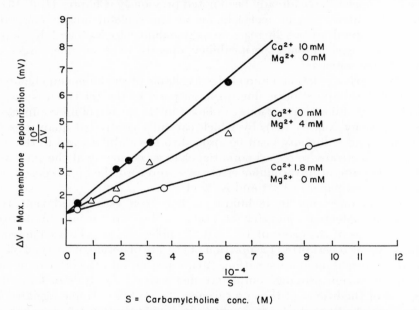

FIG. V-3. Lineweaver-Burk plot showing the influence of Ca^{++} (and Mg^{++}) on the generation by carbamylcholine of the epp in the frog sartorius muscle. Reproduced with permission from Nastuk (24).

the uranyl cation, UO_2^{++}, known to have a high affinity for phosphate groups (Chapter II, p. 175), acts similarly to Ca^{++} and Mg^{++} (Fig. V-4) and the suggestion was made by Nastuk that the anionic sites controlling cation permeability at the endplate are phosphate species. Cavalitto (28) has also discussed this possibility. Presumably cationic excitatory ligands may act to displace, directly, or indirectly, Ca^{++} from these anionic sites and thus initiate the increased ionic permeabilities of the endplate potential. How this increase is achieved is not known but the extreme rapidity of the process suggests a rapid alteration of membrane structure and possibly a phase change controlled by the M^+/M^{++} ratio of bound cations at the membrane surface is involved (Chapter II,

p. 183). This suggestion finds support from observations made by Katz and Thesleff (29) on the slope of the concentration-depolarization curves for epp generation: application of equal, separate and simultaneous amounts of carbachol from a twin-barreled pipette to the endplate region revealed a positive deviation from additivity (Fig. V-5). Apparently, low concentrations of carbachol facilitate the depolarizing effects of a second quantity of carbachol: one explanation of this finding is that the stimulant ligand binds in a cooperative manner (Chapter I, p. 71: this

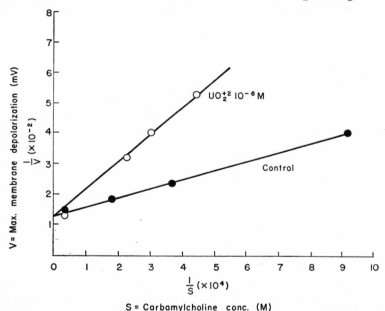

FIG. V-4. Lineweaver–Burk plot showing the competitive interaction between carbamylcholine and the uranyl cation at the endplate of the frog sartorius muscle. Reproduced with permission from Nastuk (24).

Chapter, p. 413) each interaction facilitating a subsequent interaction. It seems possible that low concentrations of carbachol displace a number of Ca^{++} ions thereby creating a localized phase change and exposing or creating sites of increased affinity for the simultaneously applied second quantity of carbachol. Similarly S-shaped concentration-response curves have been observed by Jenkinson (30) at single endplates of frog skeletal muscle.

The relative ease of recording potential changes at the endplate region of skeletal muscle has facilitated quantitative analyses of the actions of a variety of stimulant and inhibitory ligands on the endplate potential (i.e., 1, 24, 30, 31). Thus tubocurarine, a classically described antagonist of neuromuscular transmission (Chapter IV, p. 344), has long been recognized to interfere with the generation of the epp (1, 32, 33) but not to interfere with the resting or action potential. This effect of tubocurarine is very clearly seen in Fig. V-6, taken from the work of Kuffler (33), and in which progressive increases in tubocurarine concentration cause a progressive lowering of the endplate potential until it falls below the level necessary to initiate the propagated action potential. It is important to note that transmission block may be obtained without complete abolition of the endplate potential: the curarized preparation is thus

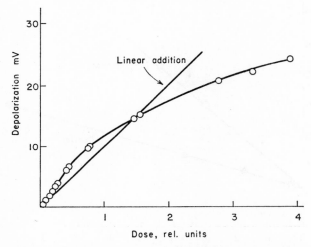

FIG. V-5. Concentration-response relationship for the effect of carbamylcholine on the frog sartorius endplate. The 45° line indicates linear addition of effects produced by twin pulses of carbamylcholine: the experimental curve, produced by the addition of equal, separate and simultaneous amounts of stimulant shows initially a more than additive effect. Reproduced with permission from Katz and Thesleff (29).

very convenient for study of the epp in the absence of complicating propagated potentials (32).

   The antagonism by tubocurarine of skeletal muscle contraction induced by acetylcholine has been described as competitive by several groups of workers (i.e., 34, 35). Jenkinson (30) has extended these studies to a quantitative analysis of the antagonism between acetylcholine, carbachol and tubocurarine in endplate potential generation. The antagonism obeys (Fig. V-7) the relationship, (Chapter IV, p. 283)

$$\frac{(A)}{(A')} - 1 = K(I) \qquad \text{V-I}$$

where (A) and (A') are the concentrations of stimulant producing the same effect in the presence and absence respectively of a concentration (I) of the antagonist. The affinity constant for tubocurarine with acetylcholine as stimulant was found to be $2 \cdot 20 \times 10^6$ M^{-1}, and with carbamylcholine as stimulant, $2 \cdot 40 \times 10^6$ M^{-1}. Studies of the antagonism between carbamylcholine and tubocurarine obtained through intra-

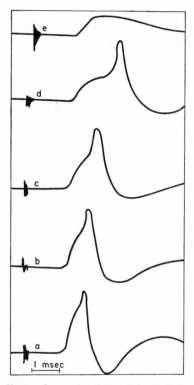

FIG. V-6. Progressive effects of curarization on the endplate potential: a, control; b, c, d, progressive curarization; e, total curarization, endplate potential only. Reproduced with permission from Kuffler (33).

cellular recording yielded a value of $1 \cdot 37 \times 10^6$ M^{-1} for the affinity constant of tubocurarine: of particular interest is the finding that the affinity constant of tubocurarine determined by measuring the contracture–concentration relationship in the "slow" frog rectus abdominus muscle, $3 \cdot 15 \times 10^6$ M^{-1}, is in excellent agreement with that obtained from the concentration depolarization relationship in "twitch" muscle. The affinity of tubocurarine for the endplate is modified by external cations, an increase of Ca^{++}_{ext} increasing the affinity and a reduction of

15

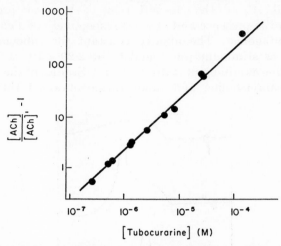

FIG. V-7. Plot of the antagonism by tubocurarine, according to equation V-1, towards the depolarizing effects of carbamylcholine in the ext. long. dig muscle of the frog. Reproduced with permission from Jenkinson (30).

TABLE V-1. Affinity Constants for Tubocurarine in
Modified Ringer's Solution (30)

Modified Ringer's Solution	$K \times 10^6 \ \mathrm{M}^{-1}$
None	$2 \cdot 3 \pm 0 \cdot 05$
$+6 \cdot 3$ mM K^+	$2 \cdot 4$
$+5 \cdot 4$ mM Ca^{++}	$1 \cdot 7$
$+8 \cdot 6$ mM Mg^{++}	$1 \cdot 35$
Containing 66% Na^+ (of normal)	$2 \cdot 5$
Containing 33% Na^+ (of normal)	$5 \cdot 5$

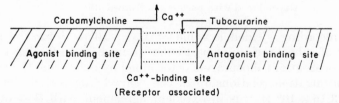

FIG. V-8. Schematic representation showing how, in receptors at the skeletal muscle endplate, agonists (carbamylcholine) and antagonists (tubocurarine) might act by labilizing and stabilizing respectively a specific membrane-bound Ca^{++} ion (or ions).

Na^{++}_{ext} reducing the affinity (Table V-1). Since increased Ca^{++}_{ext} reduces the depolarizing action of carbachol (p. 175) it seems possible that the apparent competitive interaction between tubocurarine and stimulant ligands in this preparation is mediated through opposing effects on Ca^{++}-binding at the endplate region (Fig. V-8).

IONIC EVENTS IN ELECTRIC ORGANS

The electric organ found in a variety of fishes and eels represents a specialized derivation of skeletal muscle (36) in which contractile ability has been lost but where the ability to generate electric potentials is extremely well developed. The electroplax, the individual cellular unit of the electric organ, can be isolated and studied with relative ease according to the basic procedures originally described by Schoffeniels (37, 38; also 39, 40) for *Electrophorous electricus*. This preparation has formed the basis of a considerable number of investigations in which the effects of various ligands upon the electrical characteristics of the cell may be studied in the absence of such complicating factors as muscle contraction: the chemical sensitivity of the electroplax is essentially that of the skeletal neuromuscular junction. The individual cell contains both innervated and non-innervated surface membranes: the former is sensitive to both electrical and chemical stimuli and is best regarded as containing areas sensitive to acetylcholine and related ligands coupled to electrically sensitive areas in which action potentials may be generated either directly or through the spread of a sufficient depolarization ($\sim$30 mV) from the adjacent chemosensitive areas (36, 39, 40). During the latter process the electrically excitable areas of the innervated membrane undergo a transition from a low to a high resistance state (41).

In its resting state the electroplax maintains a potential of, some -80 mV and upon exposure to acetylcholine and other excitatory ligands a graded depolarization occurs (Figs V-9, V-10), with a maximum depolarization characteristic of the ligand employed (42–44). As with the skeletal neuromuscular junction these changes in potential involve increased permeabilities to Na^+ and K^+ (42, 45–48) and, in common with other excitable membranes, these appear relatable to a critical role played by Ca^{++}. Higman and Bartels (39; also 49) noted, that tetracaine ($2 \cdot 5 \times 10^{-5}$ M) reverses the depolarizing action of acetylcholine ($2 \cdot 5 \times 10^{-6}$ M) behaving, in this regard, essentially similarly to tubocurarine: a similar antagonism was noted between carbachol and tetracaine (however, tetracaine differs from tubocurarine in that its action is not confined to the chemically sensitive membrane area). Since tetracaine, in common with a number of other local anesthetics is known to compete with Ca^{++} for Ca^{++} binding sites in membranes and model systems

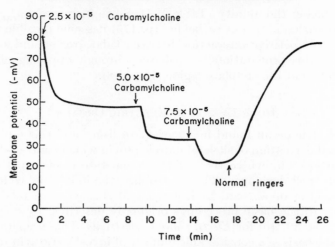

FIG. V-9. The graded depolarization (ordinate) produced by carbamylcholine in the monocellular electroplax preparation. Reproduced with permission from Higman, Podleski and Bartel (42).

(Chapter II, p. 175), it seems possible that in the electroplax, as in the skeletal neuromuscular junction (p. 407), excitatory ligand action may cause increased Na^+/K^+ permeabilities through mobilization of bound Ca^{++} at, or in the vicinity of, the receptor site. However, as for the other receptor systems, the nature of the molecular processes involved in the

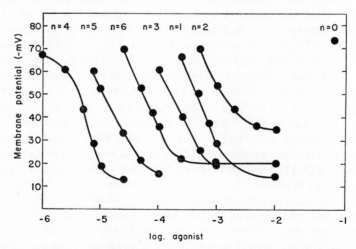

FIG. V-10. The graded depolarization (ordinate) produced by the alkylammonium series $C_nH_{2n+1}N^+Me_3$ in the monocellular electroplax preparation. Reproduced with permission from Podleski (43).

TABLE V-2. Characteristics of the Concentration-depolarization Curves of Activator Ligands (50)

Activator	n_H†	$C_{1/2}$‡ M	$E_{Max} - E_0$§ mV	E_0‖ mV
Carbamylcholine	1.9 ± 0.1	2.8×10^{-5}	65	-75
Carbamylcholine				
$+1.5 \times 10^{-7}$ decamethonium	1.6 ± 0.1	(1.5×10^{-5})	58.5	-80
$+7.5 \times 10^{-7}$ decamethonium	1.0 ± 0.1	(4.0×10^{-6})	50	-85
Carbamylcholine				
$+1.0 \times 10^{-6}$ M gallamine	2.1 ± 0.1	1.2×10^{-4}	60	-77
Decamethonium	1.63 ± 0.02	1.2×10^{-6}	50	-85
Phenyltrimethylammonium	1.72 ± 0.05	1.2×10^{-5}	50	-80

† Hill coefficient.
‡ Concentration producing 1/2 max. depolarization.
§ Decrease of potential from resting value.
‖ Resting value.

linkage between ligand binding and permeability change remain to be established.

Nevertheless, with the assumption that the characteristics of the ligand dose-response curve for depolarization are a quantitative reflection of the primary ligand binding event (see, however, 43, 44 and 48)

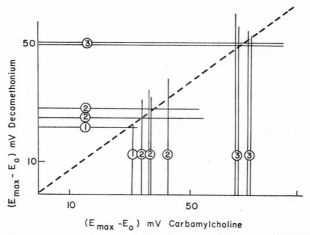

$(E_{max} - E_0)$ mV Carbamylcholine

FIG. V-11. Effect of the ionic composition of the medium on the maximum responses to carbamylcholine and decamethonium in the isolated electroplax. In addition to 0·3 mM NaH_2PO_4, 1·2 mM Na_2HPO_4, 2 mM $MgCl_2$ and 2 mM $CaCl_2$ the medium contained: (1), high K^+ medium, 150 mM NaCl, 15 mM KCl; (2), low Na^+ medium, 50 mM NaCl, 5 mM KCl, 220 mM sucrose; (3), Ringer's medium, 160 mM NaCl, 5 mM KCl. E_0 was: (1), -63 ± 5 mV; (2), -85 ± 10 mV; and (3), -75 ± 10 mV. Reproduced with permission from Changeux and Podleski (50).

and, *a priori*, this may be a more plausible assumption than can be made for concentration-response curves for muscle contraction or relaxation where more intermediate steps between initial and final events may be involved, then some extremely valuable inferences may be drawn concerning the general nature of the ligand interaction at this receptor system.

For this purpose the two important characteristics of the ligand dose-response curves are a), the maximum depolarizations produced by different agonists and b), the shape of the curve. Different ligands

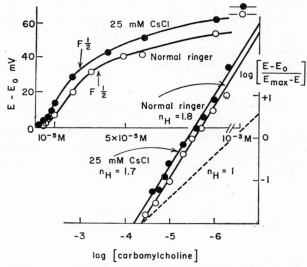

FIG. V-12. Effect of cesium chloride (25 mM) on the position and slope of the concentration-response curve to decamethonium in the isolated electroplax. Ordinate (left), $E - E_0$ (mV), depolarization produced by decamethonium; ordinate (right), log depolarization/relative depolarization at given ligand concentration. Reproduced with permission from Podleski and Changeux (44).

produce different depolarizations (Fig. V-10; Table V-2): that this reflects a property of the ligand-receptor interaction rather than the stimulation of different ionic mechanisms was indicated by Changeux and Podleski (44, 50) who observed that a membrane driven to a maximum depolarization with a given agonist (decamethonium, ~—40 mV) could be depolarized further with a second agonist (carbamylcholine) to the maximum depolarization (~—15 mV) normally attained with the second agent alone. Substantiating evidence that the two ligands activate the same ionic processes, although to different extents, is obtained from Fig. V-11 which shows that the extent of depolarization is, as anticipated, dependent upon the ionic composition of the external medium but that the difference between the maximum depolarizations produced by carbamylcholine and decamethonium remains constant. Thus, with some assurance it may be concluded that the differential effects of ligands upon the depolarization are dependent upon the ligand-receptor interaction and not upon the involvement of different ionic mechanisms (that agonists may produce different maximum responses has, of course, long been recognized from classical studies employing muscle contraction as the measured response (Chapter IV), however, arguments that such efforts reflect a primary-drug receptor interaction, although common, are difficult to establish).

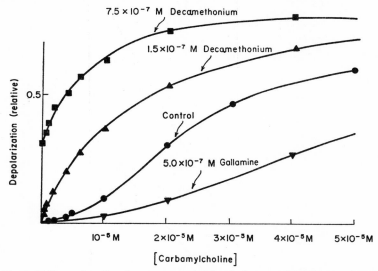

FIG. V-13. Effect of gallamine (antagonist) and decamethonium (activator) on the concentration-response curves of carbamylcholine. Ordinate expressed as relative depolarization, $E - E_0/E_{max} - E_0$ between the limits of 0 and 1. Reproduced with permission from Changeux and Podleski (50).

The second important characteristic of the concentration-depolarization curves—the sigmoid deviation from a regular hyperbola—was first observed by Higman, Podleski and Bartels (42) with carbamylcholine as the activator ligand. These workers drew attention to the analogy between this curve and the oxygen-hemoglobin saturation curve. The significance of these observations has been considerably elaborated by Karlin (51) and Changeux and Podleski (44, 50). The latter workers noted that the three ligands, carbamylcholine, phenyltrimethylammonium and decamethonium, all yielded sigmoid concentration-depolarization curves and generated Hill coefficients (n_H) close to 2 (Table V-2). That the sigmoid relationship is also an integral feature of the ligand-receptor interaction and not derived from a secondary consequence in the complex membrane systems seems to have been established by Changeux and Podleski (*loc. cit.*): the slope of the curve is independent of membrane potential (unaffected by K^+_{ext}) and is not affected by tetrodotoxin which abolished the electrical excitability of the membrane. Furthermore, cesium chloride (25 mM) which completely abolishes the potential-dependent conversion of low to high resistance states has no effect on the position and slope of the dose-response curve to carbamylcholine (Fig. V-12).

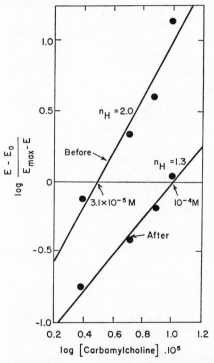

FIG. V-14. The Hill plot of the response of the isolated electroplax to carbamylcholine before and after treatment with *p*-hydroxymercuribenzoate. Reproduced with permission from Karlin (48).

Substantial further evidence that the ligand-receptor interaction in the electroplax preparation may be treated according to the various considerations applied to the cooperative protein systems previously discussed (Chapter I, p. 82) comes from studies to the modification of activator dose-response curves by other ligands. Thus, gallamine (Chapter IV, p. 344), a nondepolarizing skeletal neuromuscular blocking agent, acts as a competitive inhibitor of carbamylcholine shifting the concentration response curve to the right *without* a significant change of slope (Table V-2; Fig. V-13). On the other hand "partial" receptor activators, such as phenyltrimethylammonium and decamethonium, cause a leftward shift of the carbamylcholine dose-response curve *together* with a change of slope (Table V-2) towards a hyperbola ($n_H = 1$). As was first

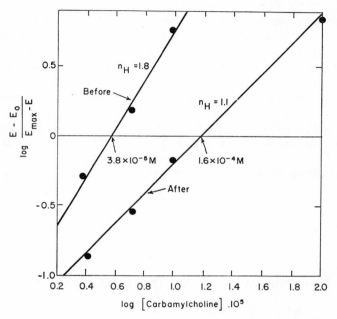

FIG. V-15. The Hill plot of the response of the isolated electroplax to carbamylcholine before and after treatment with dithiothreitol (1 mM, 10 min). Reproduced with permission from Karlin (48).

described by Karlin and Bartels (52) it is possible to abolish the sigmoid characteristics of activator binding by sulfhydryl reagents, including p-hydroxymercuribenzoate (Fig. V-14) and dithiothreitol (Fig. V-15), which reduce the affinity but do not significantly alter the maximum response. Furthermore the inhibition by dithiothreitol can be reversed by —SH oxidizing agents a process which can be prevented by interaction with N-ethylmaleimide (V-1) in concentrations that, prior to

V-1

reduction, have no effect on the electroplax preparation. That the effect of these —SH reagents is in all probability exerted in the vicinity of but not directly at the ligand binding area is indicated by a number of lines of evidence including the lack of protection by tubocurarine against p-hydroxymercuribenzoate and the particularly striking observation that hexamethonium, normally a competitive inhibitor, becomes an activator following dithiothreitol treatment (53). Presumably the —SH reagents act as "desensitizers" abolishing or altering the macromolecular interactions necessary for cooperative binding: in this respect their actions are entirely analogous to the effects of similar agents in other cooperative protein systems (ATCase, hemoglobin, etc.).

Further evidence concerning the disposition of the susceptible disulfide relative to the acetylcholine recognition site was obtained by Karlin and Winnik (53, 54) in a study of maleimide derivatives containing a quaternary ammonium function designed with the intent that such agents might act as affinity labels. In a study of a series of such agents (V-2 a-e) the rates of their reactions with the reduced disulfide linkage

$R = $ (a) C_2H_5; (b) $4\text{-}Me_2NC_6H_4$; (c) $3\text{-}Me_3\overset{+}{N}C_6H_4$; (d) $4\text{-}Me_3\overset{+}{N}C_6H_4$;

(e) $4\text{-}Me_3\overset{+}{N}CH_2C_6H_4$.

V-2 a–e

were estimated (Table V-3) and compared to their relative reactivities with cysteine to obtain an approximation to the enhancement in reaction rate produced by the quaternary ammonium function. It will be noted that all three quaternary ammonium maleimides show a substantial enhancement factor. Furthermore, these compounds do not react covalently with the unreduced receptor but act as competitive antagonists and hexamethonium, which affords partial protection against V-2a, does not protect against N-ethylmaleimide. Thus, there appears reasonable evidence for a reducible disulfide bridge at a distance of some 10–12 Å from a trimethylammonium recognition site, presumably that involved in activator ligand binding: in its oxidized state the disulfide bridge is presumably responsible, in part, for the cooperative ligand activation processes previously discussed. It is also of great interest that dithiothreitol and dithiothreitol + N-ethylmaleimide treatments of the electroplax produce *differential* changes in the activity of ligands: one spectacular change, the conversion of hexamethonium from an antagonist to an agonist has already been noted and others are listed in Table V-4. From these data it can be observed that the responses to acetylcholine, butyltrimethylammonium and carbamylcholine are affected to approximately the same extent by either treatment, but that

TABLE V-3. Kinetic Constants for the Reaction of Maleimide Derivatives with Cysteine and the Reduced Acetylcholine Receptor (53, 54)

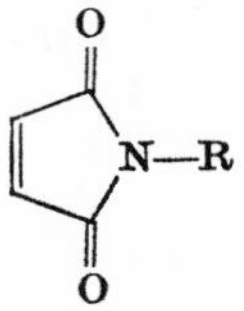

R =	k_{cysteine} liter/mole sec	k_{Rec} liter/mole sec	$k_{\text{Rec/cys}}$	Enhancement factor
—C_2H_5	1620 ± 130	60	0·037	1·0
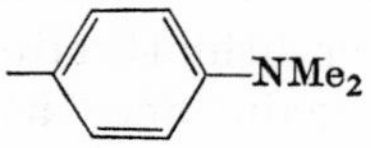 —⟨⟩—NMe_2	3920 ± 80	90	0·023	0·065
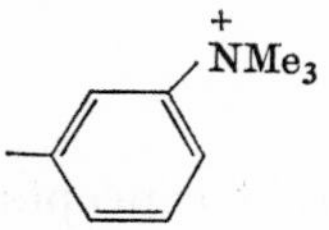 —⟨⟩$\overset{+}{N}Me_3$	9710 ± 390	$\sim 1 \times 10^5$	10	270
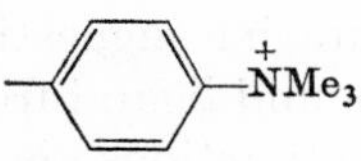 —⟨⟩—$\overset{+}{N}Me_3$	8850 ± 700	$1·5 \times 10^5$	17	460
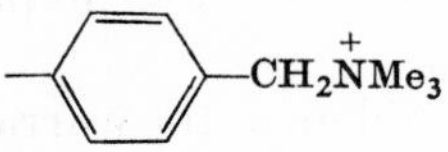 —⟨⟩—$CH_2\overset{+}{N}Me_3$	6950 ± 340	$2·8 \times 10^5$	40	1100

the reduction in response of tetramethylammonium is very significantly less and the activity of decamethonium is *increased* after dithiothreitol treatment but inhibited following dithiothreitol + N-ethylmaleimide. These differences clearly reflect the existence of differences in ligand binding and may be usefully compared to similar conclusions drawn from the action of irreversible antagonists on the activities of cholinomimetic ligands in smooth muscle preparations (Chapter IV; p. 339).

TABLE V-4. Ligand Activity at Reduced and Alkylated Electroplax
Preparation (54)

Ligand	Activity $(ACh = 1)$	Change in activity after DTT† %	DTT + NEM‡ %
$CH_3COOCH_2CH_2N^+Me_3$	1	−80	−96
$CH_3(CH_2)_3N^+Me_3$	0·3	−75	—
$H_2NCOOCH_2CH_2N^+Me_3$	0·1	−81	−92
Me_4N^+	0·001	−55	−70
$Me_3N^+(CH_2)_{10}N^+Me_3$	1	+44	−94
$Me_3N^+(CH_2)_6N^+Me_3$	0	Depolarizes	
		14 mV	0 mV

† DDT, dithiothreitol.
‡ NEM, N-ethylmaleimide.

Finally, the activity of bromoacetylcholine (V-3) in this preparation is of considerable interest (55) since it acts as a reversible receptor activator but, following dithiothreitol treatment, appears to become an irreversible receptor activator (Fig. V-16). That this is due to reaction with an adjacent —SH group is demonstrated since after dithiothreitol + N-ethylmaleimide treatment, bromoacetylcholine again acts as a

$$BrCH_2COOCH_2CH_2\overset{+}{N}Me_3$$

V-3

reversible receptor activator. Of great interest to current concepts of activator-inhibitor binding is the finding that the irreversible activation produced by bromoacetylcholine is reversed by tubocurarine suggesting either that tubocurarine can displace the covalently bound ligand from the receptor or, and equally probably, the tubocurarine functions via an allosteric mechanism to produce its competitive inhibition (see Chapter IV, pp. 344–356, Chapter VI, p. 460).

There appears, therefore, to be substantial evidence to warrant consideration of the ligand sensitive areas of the electroplax membrane (and probably also the skeletal NMJ) as similar to other, but better defined, cooperative ligand binding systems. Both Karlin (51) and Changeux and Podleski (44, 50) have advanced formal models to accommodate the above findings: these models are based essentially on the Monod-Wyman-Changeux treatment of cooperative proteins (Chapter I, p. 83) although the Changeux-Podleski model is encompassed within the larger boundaries of a general description of cooperative membrane phenomena (Chapter II, p. 183). In brief, the ligand recognition unit of the membrane is presumed to pre-exist in (at least) two states in reversible equilibrium,

$$R \rightleftharpoons S$$

In the resting polarized state the protomers exist in the S conformation and activators (acetylcholine, carbamylcholine, decamethonium etc.) stabilize the alternative R (depolarized) conformation: this state is highly permeable to cations. Inhibitors, such as tubocurarine will, in contrast, stabilize the S conformation. The ability of structurally related ligands to produce different maximum depolarizations (that is, different intrinsic activities in the terminology of Ariëns, Chapter IV, p. 214), is

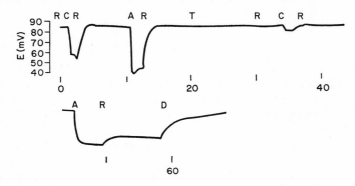

Time (min)

FIG. V-16. The effect of bromoacetylcholine on the dithiothreitol-treated electroplax. Ordinate, membrane potential. R, Ringer's solution; C, carbamylcholine, 4×10^{-5} M; A, bromoacetylcholine, 2×10^{-6} M; T, dithiothreitol, 10^{-3} M; D, tubocurarine, 1×10^{-4} M. Reproduced with permission from Silman and Karlin, *Science, N.Y.* (1969) **164**, 1420. Copyright, 1969 by the American Association for the Advancement of Science.

rationalized according to the non-exclusive binding concept of Rubin and Changeux (Chapter I, p. 83) so that the final response will be determined by the R/S ratio determined in turn by the ratio of the microscopic dissociation constants of the ligand for the R and S states. However, the actual cooperativity of the system is rather low ($n_H \sim 2$) suggesting, according to Changeux and Podleski, two possible arrangements of receptor sites on the membrane surfaces: an oligomeric arrangement of clusters of small numbers of acetylcholine receptors interacting within a unit or a lattice arrangement with a uniform receptor distribution but with weak interprotomer interactions.

Whilst a formal description has not been offered it is clear that the cooperative events at the electroplax membrane may also be accommodated on the "induced fit" model of cooperative binding advanced by

Koshland and his co-workers (Chapter I, p. 95) whereby the relative actions of activators and inhibitors may be ascribed to their abilities to induce a new permeable conformation or to stabilize an existing non-permeable conformation. Present evidence simply does not permit a decision to be made between these models or between other, less widely described models of ligand binding that also generate cooperative phenomena (Chapter I, p. 82). However, it should be noted here that Belleau has offered (56) a treatment of ligand-receptor interactions, directed primarily at agonists active at the postganglionic parasympathetic junction, in which induced conformational changes, both productive and nonproductive, are proposed to accommodate parameters of agonist and antagonist action.

Ionic Events in Cardiac Muscle

In this section an attempt is made to present the briefest possible outline of ionic events in cardiac muscle and their alteration by autonomic agents. A number of excellent reviews and symposia are available that discuss the general problems of ionic influences and cardiac excitability (57–61).

Understanding of cardiac excitability is complicated, relative to skeletal muscle, by the automaticity and rhythmicity of the organ, factors which are controlled through pacemaker activity. Normally, the sinoatrial node is the dominant locus of pacemaker activity but there are other areas, i.e., Purkinje fibers, that can also function as a pacemaker. External influences such as varying ionic concentrations and the neurotransmitters, their analogs and antagonists can modify cardiac function through effects on pacemaker loci as well as by acting directly on the cardiac muscle cells. Despite the many differences in cardiac and skeletal muscle it is reasonably well established that there are fundamental similarities in the nature of the ionic events in the two tissues and, as will be noted in Chapter VII, the mechanisms of excitation-contraction coupling also have much in common.

The basic cyclic potential changes in the heart are shown in Fig. V-17. The resting potential in the heart is approximately −90 mV (although this is species dependent): at the sinotrial node a slow diastolic depolarization occurs (marked by upward shift of the potential-time curve of Fig. V-17) and when this has reduced the resting potential to a critical level (−60 mV) an action potential is initiated in the atrium and is propagated, with delay, into the conductile Purkinje fiber system (which also has pacemaker activity) and the ventricular myocardium. It will be observed that the action potentials in cardiac tissue have, in contrast to skeletal muscle and nerve, a large plateau or area of delayed recti-

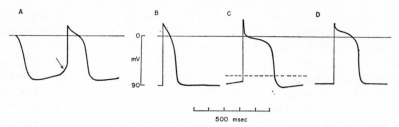

FIG. V-17. Membrane potential changes in the canine heart: A, sinotrial (SA) node; B, atrium; C, Purkinje fibers; D, Ventricular myocardium. Note the slow depolarization phases in A and C. Reproduced with permission from Trautwein (57).

fication in which repolarization of the cardiac cell membrane is relatively slow. Since the shapes of action potentials can be altered substantially by changes in heart rate (61, 62) some care has to be taken in interpreting data from experiments in which constant rate electrically driven preparations were not used.

The ionic mechanisms underlying both the action potentials and the pacemaker potentials have been intensively investigated (57, 63, 64). In the action potential there is very considerable evidence to indicate that the initial depolarization occurs through a large increase in Na^+ permeability. As in other excitable systems (Chapter II, p. 164) Ca^{++}_{ext} can have a profound effect on this depolarization process: increased

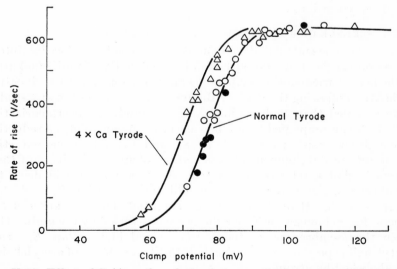

FIG. V-18. Effect of Ca^{++} on the relation between membrane potential and rate of rise of the action potential in sheep Purkinje fibers. Reproduced with permission from Weidmann (65).

Ca_{ext}^{++} raises the threshold for excitation and produces a shift of the curve relating membrane potential to the rate of rise of the action potential (availability of Na^+ channels) as shown in Fig. V-18.

However, in contrast to action potentials in nerve and skeletal muscle the restorative increase in K^+ permeability is delayed and the membrane remains in a depolarized state. This phase of prolonged depolarization has important physiological consequences for it renders the heart nonsusceptible to rapid trains of impulses (66) and, as will be discussed elsewhere, represents the time period during which activation of the contractile process can occur. The ionic events underlying the generation of the pacemaker potential have been established (67) as a slow decrease in K^+ conductance which causes a slow reduction in membrane potential until a critical threshold is reached at which time an action potential is generated. In addition to the variations in Na^+ and K^+ conductances there is an increasing amount of evidence to substantiate a very important role for an inward Ca^{++} current: several workers (68–72) have proposed that associated with the rapid Na^+ current of the depolarization phase there is a slower Ca^{++} current. Reuter (69) has observed (in sheep Purkinje fibers) that in Na^+-free solutions there is a net inward current with a threshold of -50 mV: this is dependent on the concentrations of Ca_{ext}^{++} and the reversal potential observed indicates very clearly that this is a Ca^{++} current. Reuter and Beeler (70) and Mascher and Peper (71) have described similar slow currents in dog and sheep ventricular myocardium.

THE INFLUENCE OF ACETYLCHOLINE ON IONIC EXCHANGES

Acetylcholine and related compounds are known to produce inhibitory effects on cardiac function, although the sensitivity of individual areas of the heart varies considerably, being most pronounced at the sinoatrial node (57). Following the work of Burgen and Terroux (72) many studies have revealed that cholinomimetic agents produce hyperpolarization (57, 73–76) accompanied by an increase in K^+ permeability, a reduction in membrane resistance (57, 73, 77, 81) and a simultaneous reduction in the rate of development of pacemaker potential. The basis of these effects is that a selective increase in K^+ conductance will drive the membrane potential towards the equilibrium potential, E_{K^+}, which is generally higher than the membrane potential. The specificity of this process for an increase in K^+ conductance is revealed by the finding that when the membrane potential is maintained higher than E_{K^+} then acetylcholine produces depolarization (73). These effects of acetylcholine are abolished by atropine.

Van Zwieten has employed ^{86}Rb as a substitute for K^+ (82) and has demonstrated that acetylcholine and carbachol both cause concentration-dependent effluxes of ^{86}Rb in electrically driven guinea-pig atria and that these effects are abolished by atropine.

Of equal importance to the hyperpolarization produced by cholinominetic ligands is their reduction in the duration of the action potential (72, 76, 83–86). This may reflect the opening of an acetylcholine-sensitive "shunt" for K$^+$ ions and has very important consequences for the excitation-coupling process in cardiac muscle (Chapter VII, p. 514): reduction of duration of the plateau phase of the action potential reduces the slow inward Ca^{++} current known to be critically involved in the activation of the contractile process.

THE INFLUENCE OF ADRENERGIC AGENTS ON IONIC EXCHANGES

A number of studies have revealed that epinephrine and allied catecholamines have several important effects on ion transfer and potential changes in the heart (57, 61, 87, 88).

A particularly clear effect of catecholamines is upon pacemaker cells in which an increase in the rate of spontaneous depolarization is produced. This results in a more rapid discharge of action potentials or the activation of discharge in quiescent systems (57, 87–90). This effect of catecholamines on the pacemaker potential arises from an increased sodium conductance, although the mechanism of control by the catecholamines is not understood (87). In contrast to its effects on the slope of the pacemaker potential in Purkinje fibers epinephrine does not alter the relationship between membrane potential and the ability of the cell to generate an action potential (Fig. V-19). β-Adrenergic blocking agents have been shown to decrease the rate of rise of the generator potential (88) and also to reset the relationship between membrane potential and electrical responsiveness (Fig. V-20) so that membrane response is depressed. It is particularly interesting in connection with proposed interrelationships between adrenergic agents and calcium (Chapter VII, p. 520) that these effects of propranolol are exactly the opposite of those produced by increased Ca$_{ext}^{++}$ (Fig. V-18) but are similar to those produced by local anesthetics (30) believed to act through competition with Ca^{++} and Ca^{++}-binding sites.

In addition to their effects on the rate of pacemaker potential generation catecholamines have important effects on the plateau phase of the cardiac action potential. Reuter (91) has demonstrated, in bovine Purkinje fibers, that epinephrine increases the inward Ca^{++} current of the depolarization and shifts the plateau itself to more positive levels (Fig. V-21; note similarity in effects to increased Ca$_{ext}^{++}$). Epinephrine also affects the slow repolarizing K$^+$ current flow of the action potential, shifting the degree of activation to the depolarizing direction (92), an effect prevented by pronethalol (Fig. V-22).

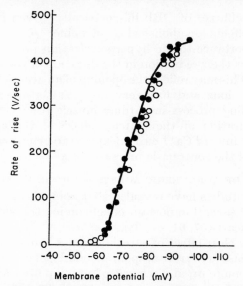

FIG. V-19. Relationship between membrane potential and rate of rise of the action potential in Canine Purkinje fibers: ●, determinations made under control conditions; ○, determinations made in the presence of norepinephrine. Reproduced with permission from Hoffman and Singer (88).

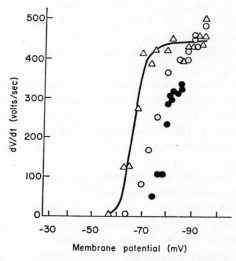

FIG. V-20. Relationship between membrane potential and rate of rise of the action potential in canine Purkinje fibers: △, control conditions; ○ and ●, with prone-thalol, 1 and 2 mg/liter respectively. Reproduced with permission from Hoffman and Singer (88).

The studies by Carmeliet and Vereecke (93) have also demonstrated an important role of epinephrine in increasing the inward Ca^{++} current flow. This inward current is linearly dependent upon $\log Ca_{ext}^{++}$ and is

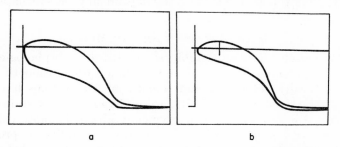

a   b

Fig. V-21. Superimposed action potentials of two sheep Purkinje fibers: (a) lower trace at $Ca_{ext}^{++} = 0\cdot45$ mM, upper trace at $7\cdot2$ mM. (b) Lower trace—control; upper trace—showing effect of epinephrine (5×10^{-7} g/ml). Reproduced with permission from Reuter (91).

abolished when the Ca_{ext}^{++} level falls below $0\cdot1$ mM: Mn^{++}, believed from other studies (this Chapter, p. 435) to inhibit Ca^{++} flow, completely abolishes the slow current in the presence or absence of epinephrine. The stimulation of the Ca^{++} current appears to be a β-receptor process since it is blocked by propranolol but unaffected by phentolamine. Of

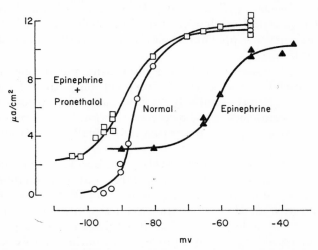

Fig. V-22. Relationship between membrane potential and current (measured as current (ordinate) immediately following return to -80 mV) in presence of epinephrine (5×10^{-7} g/ml) and pronethalol (10^{-6} g/ml). Reproduced with permission from Hauswirth, Noble and Tsien (*Science, N.Y.* (1968) **162**, 916). Copyright, 1968 by the American Association for the Advancement of Science.

particular interest is the finding that caffeine (1–5 mM) produces similar results to epinephrine: since caffeine is known to increase the concentration of cyclic AMP (Chapter VI, p. 470) the very real possibility exists that the Ca^{++} flow may be a cyclic AMP-dependent process (Chapter VII, p. 539).

IONIC EVENTS IN SMOOTH MUSCLE

Smooth muscle systems exhibit a number of morphological and functional differences to skeletal and cardiac muscle. Smooth muscle cells are typically very short and smooth muscle systems have, as a general characteristic, the ability to undergo slow, sustained and spontaneous contractions that are typically absent in most voluntary muscles. Smooth muscle shows an extreme variability of properties according to species, age, sex, hormonal influences etc., and, as Bozler has noted (94), this "has at least the advantage that it protects us from premature generalization." Because of the continuing pertinence of this observation the following treatment of smooth muscle systems will present a brief general introduction to smooth muscle electrophysiology followed by more detailed treatments of the effects of ligands on ionic events in a few selected smooth muscle systems for which sufficient data are available. Several comprehensive reviews of smooth muscle physiology are available for further references (94–100).

The pioneering studies of Bozler (101–105) form a convenient starting point for this discussion. Bozler (105) classified smooth muscles according to their electrical and mechanical behavior, their degree of dependence upon intrinsic nerve supply and their ability to respond in an all-or-none fashion to stimuli:

(a) Multiunit muscles (including nictitating membrane, iris, some vascular muscle)—these normally respond only to extrinsic nerve stimulation and behave similarly to voluntary skeletal muscle in that their electrical and mechanical responses to stimulation can be regarded as originating from separate fibers that individually respond in an all-or-none fashion.

(b) Single unit muscles (most visceral and vascular smooth muscles)—in contrast such muscles behave as one large unit (or assemblies of large units)—a syncitium—in which the individual fibers make functional contact one with another. These muscles frequently show spontaneous rhythmic activity independent of their extrinsic nerve supply which is, however, of considerable importance in regulating the excitability of these systems.

It appears doubtful whether all smooth muscles are thus classifiable and more probably this classification should be regarded as representing two extremes of smooth muscle behavior.

In addition to the syncitial character and spontaneous activity of much smooth muscle, a number of other extremely important differences exist relative to skeletal muscle and which relate very directly to an understanding of the mechanisms of action of neurotransmitters and related molecules. Among the more important of these differences are the high resting permeability to Na^+ (many leading citations are presented in references 95–99) and the ability of the muscle to respond to ligands when in a totally depolarized state (106; Chapter VII, p. 520).

Studies of the ionic composition of smooth muscle reveal, despite a level of uncertainty introduced by the lack of precise knowledge of the extracellular space in these systems, high levels of intracellular Na^+ and it is now quite generally agreed that smooth muscles do have a high resting permeability to Na^+: from the data of Table V-5 it appears that

TABLE V-5. Ionic Concentrations in Smooth Muscles

Muscle	K^+ mEq/Kg/wet wt	Na^+ mEq/Kg/wet wt	Cl^- mEq/Kg/wet wt
Guinea-pig taenia coli	90	90	65
Guinea-pig uterus	74	78	61
Rat stomach	72–80	65–91	46–53
Rat uterus (estrogen)	94	59	37
Rabbit uterus (estrogen)	76	71	—
Cat uterus (estrogen)	62	92	—
Cat intestine	77	61	67

Data selected from the collection by Burnstock, Holman and Prosser (95).

the intracellular concentrations of Na^+, K^+ and Cl^- tend to be rather similar (95) but are, in any event, relatively quite distinct from the corresponding levels in skeletal muscle or nerve axons (p. 407 and Chapter II, p. 153). These ionic levels relate directly to the low and often unstable resting potential in smooth muscle (Table V-6).

As pointed out by Bozler (101, 105), the contractile process in smooth muscle may be initiated by action (spike) potentials generated by external stimuli (neural stimulation, addition of transmitter analogs) or, as in spontaneously active smooth muscle, from the so called "slow wave" potential, a generally rhythmic small depolarization originating from an electrogenic sodium pump (105, 105a, 105b) which, at critical levels, will initiate the firing of spike potentials. The shape and duration of spike potentials in smooth muscles may be extremely varied but in general the rate of depolarization is slower and the duration of the spike is longer than in skeletal muscle. Certain smooth muscles (notably the ureter (95, 107) generate a "plateau" spike in which the rate of re-polarization is very slow. This prolonged phase of repolarization is actually not unique to smooth muscle but can be duplicated in a variety of excitable systems by the action of appropriate ligands such as Ba^{++} and quaternary ammonium ions (108, 109). A general characteristic of the smooth muscle spikes is that their generation is relatively indepen-dent of the concentration of Na^+_{ext} (98, 110–116. Chapter II, p. 165).

TABLE V-6. Membrane Potentials in Smooth Muscles

Muscle	Spont. activity	Resting potential mV	Action potential (mV) and type
Rat uterus (estrogen)	+	50–66	54–73 (spike)
Rat ureter	0	57	68 (plateau)
Rabbit uterus (estrogen)		43–48	—
Rabbit taenia coli	+	25–50	5–20 (spike)
Guinea-pig taenia coli	+	54–70	50–75 (spike)
Guinea-pig vas deferens	0	50–80	57–90 (spike)
Guinea-pig ureter	0	60	75 (plateau)
Guinea-pig mesenteric arterioles	+	26–59	—
Rat mesenteric arterioles	+	30–50	—
Rabbit pulmonary artery	—	52	—

Data selected from the collections by Burnstock, Holman and Prosser (95) and Somlyo and Somlyo (99).

This may reflect the existence of only a relatively small number of Na^+ binding (or entry) sites on the smooth muscle cell membrane so that they are normally saturated until very low levels of Na^+_{ext} are reached (115, 116): alternatively it seems probable that for at least some systems, the inward current of the spike may be carried totally or to a significant extent by Ca^{++}_{ext}. Such findings relate very directly to the undoubtedly critical role of Ca^{++} in excitation-contraction coupling in all types of muscle systems: whilst this question proper will form the subject matter of Chapter VII it is pertinent to point out that for smooth muscle systems the excitation-contraction (relaxation) coupling process shows a rather direct dependence upon Ca^{++}-mobilization processes.

It appears unlikely, however, that the association of spike potentials with contraction is a universal property of smooth muscle. The findings that drugs can produce responses in depolarized smooth muscle (106; Chapter VII, p. 520) indicates an action independent of potential changes although not, of course, of changes in ion permeability. Somlyo and Somlyo (99, 117, 118) consider that in some vascular smooth muscles (i.e., rabbit and canine pulmonary artery and aorta) stimulants (acetylcholine, norepinephrine, histamine, etc.) may elicit contractile responses by mechanisms that are independent of spike electrogenesis (see also 119, 120). The first mechanism is that of graded depolarization which precedes and is roughly proportional to the observed graded mechanical response. It was also observed for mesenteric vein strips that the spike potentials that were the normal response to external stimuli could be reversibly abolished by caffeine, while the mechanical response, although reduced, persisted. Additionally, the differential in the responses to epinephrine, histamine and angiotension observed in the polarized preparations is also maintained in the depolarized preparations: thus the actions of these stimulants cannot be ascribed simply to their ability to produce spike potentials or potential changes. Somylo and Somylo propose that there exists a third type of mechanism through which stimulant ligands may affect mechanical activity, in both polarized and depolarized tissues, without intervention of electrical events; this mechanism has been termed pharmacomechanical coupling (117).

Thus in any discussion attempting to relate drug action, ionic and potential changes across the membrane and the final tissue response (i.e., contraction/relaxation, secretion, etc.) in smooth muscle systems, it seems probable that there are three discrete pathways through which excitation-contraction (or inhibition-relaxation) coupling may occur: (1) variable frequency spike generation, (2) graded depolarization and (3) graded pharmacomechanical coupling; most smooth muscles may be capable of utilizing all three pathways although their relative importance will depend upon the tissue in question and various modulating external factors. As will become increasingly apparent, Ca^{++} unquestionably plays a central role in all of these processes and the actions of stimulant and inhibitory ligands in smooth muscle are very directly related to the roles played by Ca^{++} both at the cell membrane and in intracellularly located sites.

INTESTINAL SMOOTH MUSCLE

The taenia coli of guinea-pig, a tissue exhibiting spontaneous electrical and mechanical activity, shows a complex pattern of electrical activity. Essentially, there appears to be a slow fluctuation in the resting potential which, in common with many other smooth muscles, is distinctly lower than that observed with nerve and skeletal muscle and which is probably generated, at least in part, by pacemaker activity. Superimposed upon this slow fluctuation are spontaneous spikes (121–123) the occurrence of which appear to be only loosely related to the slow wave fluctuations (Fig. V-23). Presumably the pacemaker activity will generate spikes provided that a critical threshold of depolarization is attained; lack of total correspondence between the slow wave fluctuations and the spikes may well be due to the proximity of the cell to the pacemaker generator and also upon the electronic spread of excitation from neighboring cells.

The spike potentials of taenia coli, in common with those of other mammalian smooth muscles and crustacean muscle (Chapter II, p. 165), show a much lower dependence on the concentration of Na^+_{ext} than skeletal muscle or nerve fibers and it has been suspected for some time that ionic species other than Na^+ may be involved in the spike potential. Thus, Holman noted (110, 111) that spontaneous spike generation proceeded indefinitely when Na^+_{ext} was reduced to 5 mM, although the

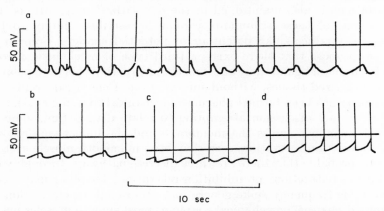

FIG. V-23. Intracellular recordings of potential changes in the guinea-pig taenia coli: (a) the relation between slow changes and spikes does not appear constant; (b)–(d), the slow changes and spikes are synchronous but in (b) the spikes occur on the rising phase of the slow potential change and in (c) much later: (d) the spikes appear to eliminate the slow potential changes. Reproduced with permission from Bülbring, Burnstock and Holman (123).

rates of rise and decline of the spike were reduced and eventually abolished in 2 mM Na^+_{ext}. Similar observations were made by Bülbring and Kuriyama (115, 124) who observed that spikes were generated for some 45 min in Na^+-free media but were then abolished; at approximately this time Na^+_{int} has fallen to almost zero concentration (124, 126). Even though spike potentials are produced in Na^+-free media the slow wave (generator) potential is abolished (115). In additional contrast to the spike potential the amplitude and duration of the slow wave potentials are markedly increased at high concentration of Na^+_{ext} suggesting that the slow wave potential is brought about by a Na^+-dependent mechanism.

There are actually several lines of evidence to indicate that the spike is a Ca^{++}-mediated process: the critical role of Ca^{++} for spike generation in Na^+-free media has been recognized by several workers (13, 115, 127–131a) and, furthermore, tetrodotoxin has no effect on the spontaneous spike generation which is, however, abolished by Mn^{++} (127). These findings are entirely analogous to those with crustacean muscle for which a fairly well defined role of Ca^{++} as a current carrying species has been developed (Chapter II, p. 164). Some further clarification of the mechanisms of slow wave and spike potentials have been provided by the work of Brading *et al.* (131) who observed that in reduced Na^+ media spontaneous spikes cease but that spikes can still be evoked by a depolarizing current. Furthermore, at low concentrations of Na^+_{ext} the evoked spike amplitude and overshoot are larger and the rate of rise faster than in normal media, findings in marked contrast to the effects of low Na^+_{ext} on spontaneous spike characteristics. The effects of increased Ca^{++}_{ext} are to produce hyperpolarization and to increase the amplitude and rate of rise of the evoked spike similarly to its effects on spontaneous spikes (111, 115). However, the effects of reduced Ca^{++}_{ext} were found to be dependent upon the level of Na^+_{ext}; thus, the depolarization and spike reduction found with reduced Ca^{++}_{ext} could be counteracted by a reduction in Na^+_{ext}. Mn^{++} was also observed to block evoked spike activity although higher concentrations were needed (2·0 mM) than required (0·5 mM) to block spontaneous spike activity.

Apparently both the spontaneous and evoked spikes in taenia coli utilize Ca^{++}_{ext} as the current carrying species. Nevertheless, the differences in their characteristics briefly outlined above suggest that the spontaneous spikes arise from a Na^+-dependent pacemaker activity manifesting itself as the slow wave potential.

The Effects of Adrenergic Agents on Taenia Coli

The early studies of Bülbring (115, 122, 132) revealed that epinephrine abolishes the spontaneous spike activity, hyperpolarizes the membrane and brings about a reduction in tension. However, the two electrical events are not, apparently, related one to another but are independent phenomena. A variety of ionic mechanisms may be proposed to account for epinephrine-induced hyperpolarization:

(a) Reduction in Na^+ permeability—attractive in view of the known high resting permeability to Na^+ (115).

(b) Stimulation of an electrogenic Na^+ pump (133)—attractive because of the known involvement (134) of catecholamines in metabolic pathways (Chapter VI, p. 470).

(c) Increased K^+ permeability.

Several distinct lines of evidence indicate that the hyperpolarizing influence of epinephrine on taenia coli is due to its increasing K^+ permeability and thus resembles other inhibitory processes such as the action

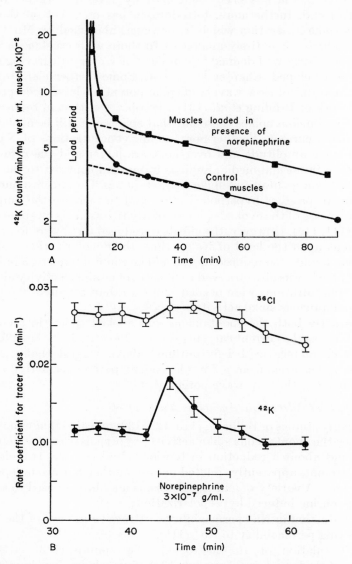

FIG. V-24. Effects of norepinephrine (3×10^{-7} g/ml) on the uptake and efflux of
$^{42}K^+$ in depolarized guinea-pig taenia coli. A, effect on $^{42}K^+$ uptake: tissues were
incubated in $^{42}K^+$ media in the presence and absence of norepinephrine. B, effect
of norepinephrine on the rate of loss of $^{42}K^+$ (●) and $^{35}Cl^-$ (o) in preloaded tissues.
Reproduced with permission from Jenkinson and Morton (138).

of acetylcholine on pacemaker and atrial tissue of the heart (72, 135). An increased K^+ permeability is not readily demonstrated in polarized tissue (136, 137) because the hyperpolarization resulting from K^+ influx will hinder K^+ efflux. In depolarized preparations, however, norepinephrine-induced increases in K^+ influx and efflux have been demonstrated (Fig. V-24) by Jenkinson and Morton (138) without effects on Na^+ or Cl^- exchange. Furthermore, since the norepinephrine-induced increases in K^+ influx and efflux are essentially identical it seems probable that norepinephrine is not involved in accelerating active transport of K^+ ions. The order of effectiveness of the catecholamines is NE > ISO and the effects on K^+ permeability are blocked by phentolamine (10^{-7} g/ml) but not by pronethalol: apparently the hyperpolarizing effect of catecholamines brought about by increased K^+ permeability is to be classified as an α-receptor mechanism.

Bülbring and Tomita (139), using the sucrose gap technique for measuring membrane resistance, showed that epinephrine abolishes both spontaneous and evoked (in response to current pulses) spikes, hyperpolarizes the membrane, reduces the size of the electrotonic potential and tension response (Fig. V-25). The potential change produced by epinephrine is actually dependent upon the membrane potential: in a hyperpolarized membrane epinephrine produces depolarization and in a normal or depolarized membrane produces hyperpolarization. Thus the effect of a given pulse of epinephrine is to drive the membrane potential to a given level. The effects of variation in concentration of K^+_{ext} on the epinephrine-induced potential changes are marked and quite consistent with the hypothesis that an increase in K^+ permeability results: the epinephrine-induced hyperpolarization is reduced in elevated K^+_{ext} and increased in reduced K^+_{ext}. Increased permeability to Cl^- also appears to play a role in epinephrine-induced hyperpolarization since replacement of Cl^-_{ext} by the impermeable benzenesulfonate anion produced a marked reduction in the effect of epinephrine.

The order of effectiveness of catecholamines in producing hypolarization and blocking evoked spikes is typical of α-receptor activity, epinephrine > norepinephrine ⩾ isopropylnorepinephrine; however, isopropylnorepinephrine is uniquely effective in blocking the *spontaneous* spike activity without producing significant hyperpolarization or electrotonic potential reduction.† The effects of isopropylnorepinephrine differ in that they are also significantly more long lasting than norepinephrine or epinephrine.

The effects of these three catecholamines on the electrical responses of

† Since all three catecholamines abolish spontaneous spikes and since spontaneous mechanical activity is correlated with such spikes, mere observation of mechanical responses would not indicate any difference, apart from potency, in these three agonists.

the taenia coli are further distinguished by the use of α- and β-blocking agents (140). Phentolamine† converts the effects of epinephrine to essentially those of isopropylnorepinephrine, i.e., a reduction in spontaneous spike activity with little change in membrane or electronic potential (Fig. V-26b) and in the presence of both phentolamine and propranolol the total effect of epinephrine is virtually abolished (Fig. V-26). Propranolol alone reduces the spontaneous activity (Fig. V-26d) and thus acts similarly to ISO: this effect of propranolol is abolished by phentolamine (Fig. V-26c). The observed antagonism between α- and

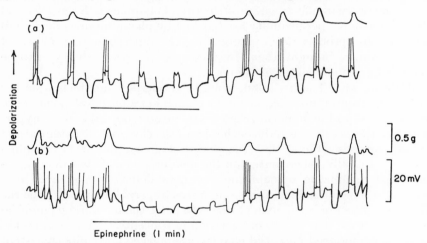

Epinephrine (1 min)

FIG. V-25. Effects of epinephrine on the mechanical and electrical responses of guinea-pig taenia coli. Mechanical changes and electrical changes evoked by current pulses alternately depolarizing and hyperpolarizing. Epinephrine was applied at 5×10^{-8} g/ml in (a) and 1×10^{-7} g/ml in (b) and reduces mechanical activity and electrotonic potential and suppresses the spontaneous and evoked activity. Reproduced with permission from Bülbring and Tomita (139).

β-blocking agents is of considerable interest and strengthens previous conclusions suggesting a mutual interaction of α- and β-blocking agents (Chapter IV, p. 319).

The studies discussed above clearly reveal the duality of the ionic contributions of the α- and β-receptor activation mechanisms in taenia coli: an α-effect (increased K^+ permeability) which hyperpolarizes the membrane thus reducing spontaneous and evoked spikes and producing a reduction in mechanical activity and a β-effect which is concerned only with the suppression of spontaneous spike activity.

† Phentolamine alone produces depolarization, increased spontaneous activity and increased electrotonic potential, effects which are strikingly similar to those of reduced Ca_{ext}^{++} concentration. This important observation will be discussed later in this chapter.

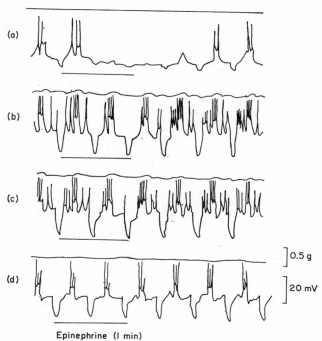

(a)

(b)

(c)

]0.5 g

(d)

]20 mV

Epinephrine (I min)

FIG. V-26. The effects of phentolamine and propranolol on the actions of epinephrine in guinea-pig taenia coli. (a) Control; (b) 33 min after phentolamine (1×10^{-5} g/ml); (c) after further addition of propranolol (1×10^{-5} g/ml); (d) after increasing the concentration of propranolol to 5×10^{-5} g/ml. Reproduced with permission from Bülbring and Tomita (140).

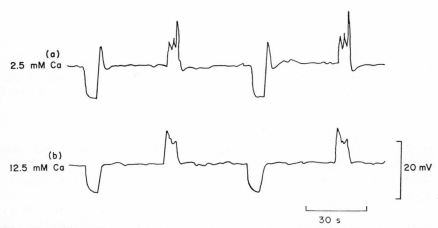

(a)
2.5 mM Ca

(b)
12.5 mM Ca

20 mV

30 s

FIG. V-27. The effects of Ca_{ext}^{++} concentration upon electrical parameters of the guinea-pig taenia coli. Reproduced with permission from Bülbring and Tomita (13).

Further elucidation of the linkage between receptor activation and ionic events comes from studies on the interrelationship between Ca^{++} and the actions of catecholamines. In the polarized taenia coli preparation (13) an increased concentration of Ca_{ext}^{++} produces hyperpolarization, abolishes the spontaneous spike discharge (115), reduces the amplitude

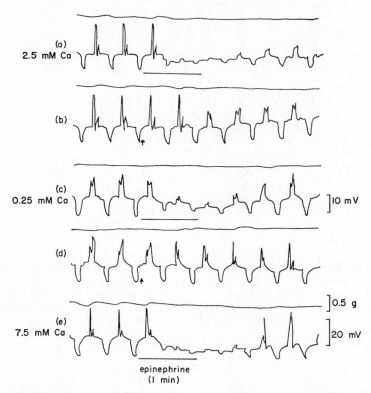

FIG. V-28. The effects of Ca_{ext}^{++} upon the effects of epinephrine on the guinea-pig taenia coli. (a) Control; (b) at $\uparrow Ca_{ext}^{++}$ reduced to 0·25 mM. (c) Effect of epinephrine after 8 min exposure of tissue to 0·25 mM Ca^{++}; (d) at $\uparrow Ca_{ext}^{++}$ increased to 7·5 mM. (e) Effect of epinephrine after 18 min exposure of tissue to 7·5 mM Ca^{++}. Reproduced with permission from Bülbring and Tomita (13).

of the evoked spike discharge and reduces the electrotonic potential (Fig. V-27b). These effects may be produced through an increased K^+ conductance. A reduction in Ca_{ext}^{++} has the opposite effect, leading to depolarization, reduced spike amplitude and abolition of the mechanical response. The resemblance between the effects of epinephrine and an increased concentration of Ca_{ext}^{++} is clear and it may be that the effects of epinephrine on the K^+ conductance are mediated through an increase in the concentration of membrane bound Ca^{++}. In this connection the effects of variation of the concentration Ca^{++}_{ext} on the actions of epinephrine (Fig. V-28) are of interest; Fig. V-28c shows that a 10-fold reduction in Ca^{++}_{ext} greatly reduces the ability of epinephrine to hyperpolarize and reduce the electrotonic potential and, in contrast, an increase in Ca^{++}_{ext} significantly potentiates the effects of epinephrine (Fig. V-28e). It is noteworthy that Ba^{++}_{ext} (at a low concentration of 0.25 mM), which can substitute for Ca^{++}_{ext} in the maintenance of membrane potential and both spontaneous and evoked spike activity (13), abolishes all the effects of epinephrine. This probably indicates that Ca^{++}_{ext} has a number of sites of action and that those involved in spike generation and maintenance of membrane potential and at which Ba^{++}_{ext} can replace Ca^{++}_{ext} are either independent of epinephrine or involve highly specific epinephrine-Ca^{++}_{ext} interactions (Chapter VII, p. 531) for which Ba^{++} is not an effective substitute. Further division of these sites is indicated by the finding (13) that Mn^{++}_{ext} (0·5 mM) in the presence of normal concentrations of Ca^{++}_{ext} abolishes the spontaneous spikes but not the evoked spikes; however, at higher concentrations Mn^{++} (2·5 mM) also abolishes the evoked spikes. The effect of Mn^{++}_{ext} at a concentration of 0·5 mM is to produce a marked reduction in the activity of adrenaline.

Since the removal of Ca^{++}_{ext} and its replacement by either Ba^{++} or Mn^{++} abolishes both the α- and β-effects of adrenaline and since these effects are distinguishable according to their electrical characteristics it must also be that there are specific Ca^{++} involvements at the α- and β-receptor sites. At the α-receptor a mutual effect of Ca^{++} and epinephrine in increasing K^+ conductance seems plausible and at the β-receptor an interaction with Ca^{++} at a stage between the generator potential and the spontaneous spike seems probable.

Further evidence concerning the mutual interactions of Ca^{++}_{ext} and catecholamines at the β-receptor may be obtained from studies of depolarized taenia coli where Jenkinson and Morton (138) have shown that isopropylnorepinephrine is some 30–100 times more effective than norepinephrine in inhibiting Ca^{++} contractures, and that these effects on the contractures are antagonized by pronethalol but not by phentolamine.

If it can be accepted that events in polarized and depolarized tissue do indeed relate to one another and that there is a very close relationship between membrane and contractile events in smooth muscle (105) then comparison of the studies by Bülbring and Tomita and Jenkinson and Morton of the adrenergic β-receptors in taenia coli indicate that the catecholamine-receptor interaction specifically abolishes a Ca^{++} mobilization process involved in both the spontaneous spike and tension development. The molecular basis of this interaction remains uncertain but its high specificity is evidenced by the fact that epinephrine does not abolish the spontaneous spikes produced by Ba^{++}_{ext}. The relationship between adrenergic agents and Ca^{++} is discussed more fully in Chapter VII.

The Effects of Cholinergic Agents on Intestinal Smooth Muscle

Acetylcholine and related cholinomimetic molecules increase the permeability of intestinal smooth muscle to inorganic ions. In contrast to norepinephrine, acetylcholine depolarizes the membrane, increases spike frequency and prolongs spike duration in single cell taenia coli preparations (122, 132). Bülbring and Kuriyama, from studies of the dependence of acetylcholine-induced electrical changes on the ionic composition of the external medium, observed that acetylcholine fails to accelerate spike discharge, although still producing some depolarization, in the absence of Na^+_{ext} and that an increased concentration of Na^+_{ext} causes a marked potentiation of the effects of acetylcholine on both depolarization and spike acceleration. In the absence of Ca^{++}_{ext} acetylcholine is totally ineffective while increased Ca^{++}_{ext} potentiates the actions of acetylcholine in a manner very similar to that observed with increased Na^+_{ext}. These results suggest a relatively non-selective increase of membrane permeability induced by acetylcholine, the permeabilities to both Na^+ and Ca^{++} ions being increased. It is of interest to compare the potentiating effects of increased Ca^{++}_{ext} in this preparation with events at the sekeletal neuro-muscular junction, at which Nastuk has shown (p. 174) that an increased concentration of Ca^{++}_{ext} competitively *reduces* the magnitude of the endplate potential produced by carbamylcholine: in the latter system it seems doubtful that Ca^{++} has a *major* role as a current carrying species.

Changes in K^+ permeability are also involved in the response of intestinal smooth muscle to cholinergic agents and have been documented by a number of workers (141–146). Durbin and Jenkinson (147) have studied the actions of carbamylcholine on K^+-depolarized taenia coli in which ion fluxes caused by depolarization and secondary to the agonist-induced permeability changes may be avoided. Carbamylcholine increases permeability to both K^+ and Cl^- in both influx and efflux experiments (Table V-7). The effects on $^{42}K^+$ efflux together with the simultaneously developing tension induced by carbamylcholine are shown in Fig. V-29: these effects are reversibly abolished by atropine $(3 \times 10^{-8}$ g/ml). Permeability changes to Na^+ and Ca^{++} ions were less easy to determine quantitatively although it is clear that they were affected by the agonist. The carbamylcholine-induced increase in K^+ efflux is a Ca^{++}-dependent process and in Ca^{++}-free solution carbamylcholine produces neither a change in permeability nor an increase in

TABLE V-7. The effects of carbamylcholine on potassium and chloride fluxes in depolarized taenia coli (147)

Ion†	Efflux ratio‡	Uptake ratio§
K⁺	2·32 ± 0·35	1·88 ± 0·12
Cl⁻	1·33 ± 0·08	1·38 ± 0·10

† Carbamylcholine $(3 \times 10^{-7}$ g/ml) applied for 7 min.

‡ Obtained by dividing the quantity of tracer lost during carbamylcholine treatment with the amount estimated to be exchanged in the absence of carbamylcholine.

§ Calculated as above using tracer uptake.

tension. Clearly Ca^{++}_{ext} is involved in both processes (the association of Ca^{++} with muscle contraction is further discussed in Chapter VII) but probably at different levels for it is possible (147) to reduce the concentration of Ca^{++}_{ext} to a level at which tension development is abolished but at which appreciable permeability changes still occur. It appears probable, therefore, that the effects of carbamylcholine and, presumably, other

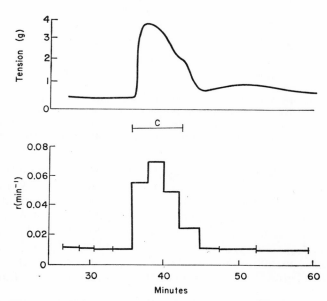

FIG. V-29. The effects of carbamylcholine $(3 \times 10^{-7}$ g/ml) on tension development (upper plot) and the rate (r) of loss of $^{42}K^+$ (lower plot) in depolarized guinea-pig taenia coli. Reproduced with permission from Durbin and Jenkinson (147).

16

cholinergic agents are associated with Ca^{++} which has a role in maintaining the integrity of the receptive area and the membrane in general. Displacement of the Ca^{++}, perhaps directly by the agonist, initiates the ion fluxes and contraction, but the latter *only* if the Ca^{++}-concentration gradient across the cell membrane is large enough.

Most analyses of the relationship between structure and pharmacological activity are described in terms of the final tissue response (contraction/relaxation) but it is clearly desirable to extend such analyses to include quantitative studies of agonist-induced permeability

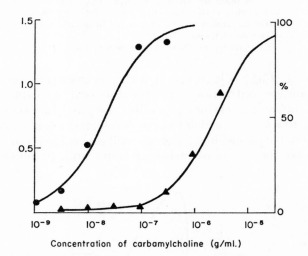

Concentration of carbamylcholine (g/ml.)

Fig. V-30. Comparison of carbamylcholine concentration-response curves for contraction and Rb^+ efflux in guinea-pig ileum: ordinate (left), rate constant for efflux, min^{-1}; ordinate (right), contraction (●—●) as percentage of maximum response. Reproduced with permission from Burgen and Spero (148).

changes. A notable attempt in this direction has been made by Burgen and Spero (148) who have studied the effects of a series of cholinergic agonists on $^{42}K^+$ and $^{86}Rb^+$ efflux† in guinea-pig intestinal smooth muscle. From concentration-response curves obtained for both agonist induced $^{86}Rb^+$ efflux and muscle contraction (Fig. V-30) the maximum efflux rate, f_{max}, and apparent affinity constants, K_f and K_c, of the agonist for the efflux and contraction processes respectively were determined (Table V-8). From this data a number of important points

† $^{86}Rb^+$ was employed as a substitute for $^{42}K^+$ because of its longer half-life. In the guinea-pig intestine efflux rates for K^+ and Rb^+ were found to be identical suggesting a compatible substitution. It is not certain, however, whether Rb^+ can substitute for K^+ in all tissues (82, 149, 150).

TABLE V-8. Parameters of Agonist-induced Contraction and Rubidium Efflux in Guinea-Pig Ileum (148)

No.	Compound	K_f (M^{-1})	K_c (M^{-1})	f_{max}	K_c/K_f
1.	Acetylcholine $CH_3COOCH_2CH_2\overset{+}{N}Me_3$	$3\cdot60 \times 10^3$	$3\cdot67 \times 10^6$	$0\cdot91$	1020
2.	Acetyl-β-methylcholine $CH_3COOCH(Me)CH_2\overset{+}{N}Me_3$	$5\cdot50 \times 10^3$	$3\cdot79 \times 10^6$	$1\cdot15$	683
3.	Carbamylcholine $H_2NCOOCH_2CH_2\overset{+}{N}Me_3$	$7\cdot70 \times 10^4$	$2\cdot56 \times 10^7$	$0\cdot91$	332
4.	Carbamyl-β-methylcholine $H_2NCOOCH(Me)CH_2\overset{+}{N}Me_3$	$7\cdot52 \times 10^3$	$4\cdot74 \times 10^5$	$1\cdot21$	63
5.	(1,3-dioxolane, 2-Me, 4-$CH_2\overset{+}{N}Me_3$)	$1\cdot05 \times 10^3$	$5\cdot29 \times 10^5$	$0\cdot78$	51
6.	(tetrahydrofuran, HO-, Me-, 2-$CH_2\overset{+}{N}Me_3$)	$5\cdot53 \times 10^4$	$8\cdot03 \times 10^5$	$1\cdot00$	14
7.	(pyrrolidinone $NCH_2C{\equiv}CCH_2\overset{+}{N}Me_3$)	$7\cdot68 \times 10^5$	$9\cdot81 \times 10^6$	$1\cdot47$	12
8.	(pyrrolidinone $NCH_2C{\equiv}CCH_2N$ pyrrolidine)	$6\cdot91 \times 10^4$	$6\cdot07 \times 10^6$	$1\cdot41$	9
9.	(Me-tetrahydrofuran-$CH_2\overset{+}{N}Me_3$)	$1\cdot63 \times 10^5$	$8\cdot01 \times 10^5$	$1\cdot67$	5
10.	(tetrahydrofuran-$CH_2\overset{+}{N}Me_3$)	$7\cdot17 \times 10^3$	$1\cdot70 \times 10^4$	$1\cdot57$	$2\cdot5$
11.	$CH_3CH_2CH_2CH_2CH_2\overset{+}{N}Me_3$	$2\cdot39 \times 10^3$	$7\cdot10 \times 10^3$	$1\cdot37$	$3\cdot0$
12.	$\overset{+}{N}Me_4$	$1\cdot60 \times 10^3$	$5\cdot06 \times 10^3$	$0\cdot80$	$3\cdot2$
13.	$CH_3(CH_2)_5\overset{+}{N}Me_3$	$3\cdot73 \times 10^2$	$5\cdot44 \times 10^2$	$0\cdot53$	$1\cdot5$
14.	$CH_3(CH_2)_6\overset{+}{N}Me_3$	$3\cdot50 \times 10^2$	$7\cdot19 \times 10^2$	$0\cdot23$	$2\cdot0$
15.	$CH_3(CH_2)_7\overset{+}{N}Me_3$	$1\cdot49 \times 10^2$	—	$0\cdot04$	—
16.	$CH_3(CH_2)_4\overset{+}{N}Me_2Et$	$5\cdot53 \times 10^2$	$2\cdot83 \times 10^2$	$0\cdot05$	$5\cdot1$

arise: for many agonists listed in Table V-8 it is clear that the concentration-response curves for efflux and contraction are substantially non-coincident $(K_c/K_f \gg 1)$: this is most pronounced with acetylcholine itself. A number of compounds reveal themselves as classifiable as partial agonists in that f_{max} lies substantially below that of other agonists: this is particularly well seen in the alkyltrimethylammonium series (Fig. V-32), in which the relative abilities to increase $^{86}Rb^+$ flux parallel quite well the activities as measured by contraction. It also appears as

TABLE V-9. Affinity Constants of Reversible Antagonists for Efflux and Contraction Processes (148)

Agent	K_A M^{-1} efflux	K_A M^{-1} contraction	Significance of difference (P)
Atropine	7.53×10^8	6.54×10^8	>0.5
Lachesine (V-4)	3.90×10^8	4.09×10^8	>0.6
Tricyclamol (V-5)	1.32×10^9	1.64×10^9	>0.9
Benzilyldimethylbutanol (V-6)	2.10×10^6	4.14×10^6	>0.1
Benzhexol (V-7)	6.6×10^{10}	7.7×10^9	<0.001

$$Ph_2COHCOOCH_2CH_2\overset{+}{N}Me_2Et$$
V-4

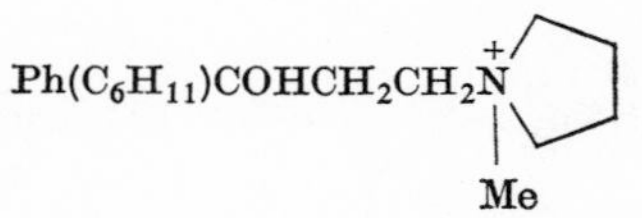

$$Ph(C_6H_{11})COHCH_2CH_2\overset{+}{N}$$
Me

V-5

$$Ph_2COHCOOCH_2CH_2CMe_3$$
V-6

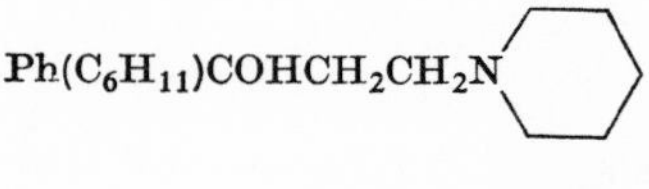

$$Ph(C_6H_{11})COHCH_2CH_2N$$

V-7

a rough generalization that the greatest coincidence of efflux and contraction concentration-response curves is observed with the weakest agonists (Nos. 10–17, Table V-8). Finally, the data of Table V-8, considering only the most potent agonists, show two very distinct orders of potency for producing contraction $(3 > 1 > 2 > 8 > 7 > 4 > 5 > 9 > 6)$ and increasing $^{86}Rb^+$ efflux $(9 > 7 > 6 > 8 > 3 > 5 > 1 > 2 > 3)$. Since both the efflux and contractile responses to these agonists are unaffected by hexamethonium and are reversibly antagonized to the same extent (with one exception) by atropine and related agents (Table V-9) the corresponding receptors are formally classifiable as muscarinic. These findings are of very considerable relevance to interpretations of cholinergic ligand-receptor interactions.

Because of the non-coincidence of the efflux and contraction dose-response curves and which is so marked with acetylcholine, acetyl β-methycholine and carbamylcholine it seems improbable that, for these compounds at least, the observed $^{86}Rb^+$ efflux is relatable to the contractile response. Thus in the concentration-response curves to carbachol (Fig. V-31) $^{86}Rb^+$ efflux has only reached 15% of its maximum when the contraction height is 100%: for acetylcholine and acetyl-β-methyl-

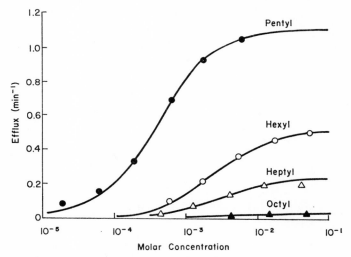

FIG. V-31. Efflux rates of Rb^+ from guinea-pig ileum upon exposure to alkyl-trimethylammonium ligands. Reproduced with permission from Burgen and Spero (148).

choline, the disparity in effects is even larger. This conclusion is compatible with the work of Bass, Hurwitz and Smith (146) who found that pilocarpine produces near maximal contraction of the longitudinal smooth muscle of guinea-pig ileum in the presence of desoxycorticosterone acetate, an inhibitor of K^+ efflux.

Nevertheless, for a number of the agonists listed in Table V-8 there is substantial coincidence of the efflux and contraction dose-response curves. One interpretation of these findings is that two distinct ligand-macromolecular interactions are being observed, an interaction at the acetylcholine receptor proper producing contraction accompanied by negligible to small changes in $^{86}Rb^+$ efflux and a second less specific process, occurring at sites where contraction and $^{86}Rb^+$ efflux are related (it should be emphasized here that permeability changes to ions other than $^{86}Rb^+$ are also involved). It is to be anticipated that recognition processes for neurotransmitters are highly specific (Chapter IV) and thus it is probable that the receptor site for acetylcholine can only accommodate a small number of close structural analogs of acetylcholine

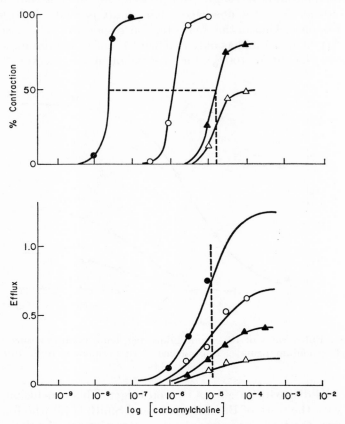

FIG. V-32. Effects of Dibenamine on contractions and Rb^+ efflux produced by carbamylcholine: ●—●, control; ○—○, Dibenamine, 10^{-6} g/ml for 4 min; ▲—▲, 10 min and △—△, 18 min. Reproduced with permission from Burgen and Spero (148).

(i.e., acetyl-β-methylcholine and carbamylcholine). Progressive molecular deviation from the structure of acetylcholine will thus reduce affinity for the acetylcholine binding site yet leave the possibility of interaction at a receptor subsite or even an entirely distinct membrane site at which ion exchange processes concomitant with contraction may be initiated. Superficially, the lack of discrimination shown by the reversible antagonists listed in Table V-9 between the efflux and contraction processes may appear to argue against a two site hypothesis. However, since quite convincing arguments may be advanced (Chapter IV, p. 343) that such antagonists do not act at the receptor site proper but rather through an allosteric mechanism, this is probably not a serious objection. In any event other types of antagonist do discriminate between these two processes: thus, the irreversible antagonist Dibenamine produces a displacement of the contraction concentration-response curve prior to reduction of the maximum but produces an immediate reduction in the maximum of the efflux curve (Fig. V-32). The local anesthetics cinchocaine (dibucaine) and lignocaine also produce similar effects. It is to be noted that the concept of the two distinct classes of muscarinic receptors advances by Burgen and Spero on the basis of the work outlined above finds support from several independent lines of evidence that are discussed elsewhere (Chapter IV, p. 343).

A final, and extremely important, conclusion to be drawn from the above work is that it indicates the great caution necessary when agonist-receptor interactions are interpreted solely according to the analysis of one type of biological response. Further studies on the above lines are urgently needed.

UTERINE SMOOTH MUSCLE

The actions of catecholamines on uterine tissues remain but poorly understood and present a remarkably complex situation in the light of the hormonal dependence of the responses to catecholamines (151). Unfortunately, complete electrophysiological data are not available to warrant generalization about uterine tissue, although progress is being made (151–154); hence the following discussion is essentially limited to uterine tissue of the rat which, pregnant or non-pregnant, shows spontaneous electrical and mechanical activity and where the dominant effects of catecholamines are exerted through a β-receptor process.

As is the case with intestinal smooth muscle uterine tissue shows slow depolarizations that generate spike discharge: this pacemaker activity may be a general feature of all uterine smooth muscle cells. There appears to be some controversy concerning the ionic basis of the spikes (152) but the recent studies of Anderson (154) indicate very strongly that a regenerative sodium-dependent excitation phenomenon is involved: however, a contribution by Ca^{++} is not ruled out.

Diamond and Marshall have studied the effects of catecholamines and adrenergic blocking agents on the resting membrane potential (RMP) of the pregnant rat uterus. Table V-10 reveals that, in concentrations that completely abolish spontaneous contractile activity, norepinephrine, epinephrine and isopropylnorepinephrine all hyperpolarize the

TABLE V-10. The Effects of Catecholamines on Resting Membrane Potential of Isolated Rat Uterus (135)

Agent	Conc. M	Resting membrane potential (RMP) mV	Change RMP mV
Control	—	$46 \cdot 0 \pm 0 \cdot 9$	
Epinephrine	6×10^{-7}	$56 \cdot 7 \pm 0 \cdot 7$	$+10 \cdot 7$
Control	—	$46 \cdot 0 \pm 1 \cdot 0$	
Norepinephrine	10^{-6}	$53 \cdot 4 \pm 1 \cdot 0$	$+7 \cdot 4$
Control	—	$47 \cdot 6 \pm 1 \cdot 4$	
Isopropylnorepinephrine	3×10^{-7}	$59 \cdot 3 \pm 1 \cdot 2$	$+11 \cdot 7$

membrane. Similar findings have been reported by Burnstock and Holman (98) and by Kumar (156) working with human uterus. This hyperpolarization is quite evidently a β-receptor process for it is unaffected by phentolamine (10^{-7} M) and abolished by propranolol (10^{-7} M). Whilst concentrations of epinephrine (6×10^{-7} M) that produce complete relaxation also produce hyperpolarization, at lower concentrations (2×10^{-8} M) epinephrine produces partial relaxation unaccompanied by hyperpolarization, thus suggesting, as noted for other smooth muscle systems, a partial dissociation of electrical and mechanical events. This is also revealed by the data of Table V-11, which show that non-adrenergic relaxants, at concentrations that produce complete relaxation, have no effect on the resting membrane potential. The independence of the relaxant and electrical events is also strongly supported by the work of Schild (8, 9) on rat uterus depolarized in high K^+ media where epinephrine and isopropylnorepinephrine still produce relaxant effects.

TABLE V-11. The Effects of Non-Adrenergic Relaxants on Resting Membrane Potential of Rat Uterus (155)

Agent	Conc. M	Resting membrane potential (RMP) mV	Change in RMP mV
Control		$46 \cdot 7 \pm 0 \cdot 5$	
Papaverine†	10^{-5}	$47 \cdot 0 \pm 0 \cdot 7$	$+0 \cdot 3$
Control		$46 \cdot 0 \pm 1 \cdot 1$	
Nitroglycerin†	10^{-3}	$50 \cdot 6 \pm 1 \cdot 6$	$+4 \cdot 6$
Control		$47 \cdot 7 \pm 0 \cdot 7$	
Tetracaine†	10^{-4}	$48 \cdot 1 \pm 0 \cdot 6$	$+0 \cdot 4$

† These concentrations completely inhibited spontaneous contractions.

The actions of the relaxant agents listed in Table V-11 of which epinephrine is by far the most potent, are actually achieved through decreasing the rate of spontaneous discharge of spike potentials initiated by the pacemaker cells (Table V-12). There are, however, significant differences revealed in the mechanisms of actions of these four agents since papaverine, tetracaine and nitroglycerin reduce the rate of rise of the action potential whilst epinephrine increases the rate of rise, effects that were not accompanied by significant changes in the resting potential or spike potential amplitude. Thus, the actions of epinephrine are exerted primarily on the pace-maker potential generating mechanism (compare with studies on taenia coli, p. 435). From the work of Diamond

TABLE V-12. Effects of Relaxants on Pacemaker Frequency and Tension Development in Rat Uterus (155)

Agent	Conc. M	AP/min	Change in AP %	Tension g/cm²	Change in tension %
Control	—	211 ± 20		179 ± 18	
Epinephrine	2×10^{-8}	95 ± 11	-55	87 ± 19	-51
Control	—	231 ± 13		251 ± 21	
Papaverine	10^{-5}	149 ± 16	-36	159 ± 21	-37
Control	—	185 ± 12		241 ± 26	
Nitroglycerine	6×10^{-4}	108 ± 10	-42	128 ± 19	-47
Control	—	197 ± 11		263 ± 28	
Tetracaine	10^{-4}	108 ± 13	-45	130 ± 19	-51

and Marshall (loc. cit.) it is noteworthy that epinephrine and the non-adrenergic agents act as relaxants in AC-field stimulated and K⁺-depolarized preparations but that epinephrine is significantly less effective than the other agents relative to its effects on spontaneous contractions. Feinstein et al. have also noted that isopropylnorepinephrine is *very much* less effective in relaxing field-stimulated preparations, providing further evidence for a pacemaker locus of action of catecholamines. Differences between the relaxant agents discussed above are also revealed by a study of the effects of increased concentrations of Ca_{ext}^{++} (5·4 mM), a concentration which markedly antagonizes the effects of tetracaine, papaverine and nitroglycerine in normal and field stimulated preparations but only antagonizes the actions of epinephrine in the normal preparations.

The data of Marshall, Feinstein and their co-workers thus suggests very strongly that the primary site of action of catecholamines is at the pacemaker potential generator, that relaxation can be produced without

16*

change of RMP and that local anesthetics, papaverine and other relaxants probably produce their effects at the level of the excitation-contraction coupling process (Chapter VII) by interfering in the Ca^{++} mobilization/storage events so critical to this process. It is particularly pertinent to note that propranolol, a β-antagonist, was found (159) to be particularly effective in antagonizing AC-field induced contractions of the rat uterus, suggesting that adrenergic β-receptor antagonists have an important component of action exerted at the Ca^{++} mobilization level.[†] The involvement of these and related agents with Ca^{++} will be discussed further in Chapter VII.

VASCULAR SMOOTH MUSCLE

In contrast to visceral smooth muscle (p. 430), the actions of neurotransmitters, their analogs and antagonists on vascular smooth muscle have been little investigated (99, 160, 161), and detailed studies of the passive and excitable electrical properties and ionic events involved in these actions are not yet available. Nevertheless, there appear to be a number of similarities existing between the events in vascular and visceral smooth muscle although as recently re-emphasized by Holman (161), great care is needed in extrapolating data from one smooth muscle system to another.

A number of studies (162–166) have reported the stimulant effects of norepinephrine to be accompanied by increased action potential frequency in various arterial and venous preparations. Johansson et al. (164, 167) have studied the effects of epinephrine and isopropylnorepinephrine on simultaneously measured electrical and mechanical activity of the rat portal vein under a variety of ionic conditions. Under normal conditions this preparation is spontaneously active showing bursts of action potentials accompanied by simultaneous contractions: addition of norepinephrine produces a pattern of continuous electrical discharge accompanied by greatly increased mechanical activity. Very high concentrations of norepinephrine produce a continuous discharge accompanied by a prolonged contracture. In high K^+ depolarizing media, the cells are depolarized and spike activity abolished but norepinephrine produces an increased tension without change in membrane potential: however, higher concentrations of norepinephrine were required than in media of normal composition. Elimination of Ca^{++}_{ext} leads to partial depolarization and elimination of electrical and mechanical activity: however, high concentrations of norepinephrine result in the reappearance of both activities. The ability of norepinephrine to restore mechanical activity gradually disappears with increasing time of exposure

[†] It must not be forgotten, however, that β-antagonists have important sites of action in addition to the β-receptor (Chapter IV, p. 326).

to Ca^{++}-free media although electrical activity is maintained. Phenoxy-benzamine abolishes the responses to norepinephrine which are, therefore, presumably of the α-class. In contrast, isopropylnorepinephrine, produces a decrease in the force of individual contractions accompanied by an increase in frequency of contraction and these effects are paralleled by decreased spike amplitude and increased frequency. These latter effects stand in interesting contrast to events in taenia coli (p. 435) where adrenergic inhibition produces hyperpolarization and reduced frequency of action potentials.

In high K^+ medium which produces sustained contracture and abolition of electrical activity, isopropylnorepinephrine produces relaxation in the rat portal vein without any apparent change in electrical activity. Propranolol abolishes the electrical and mechanical responses to isopropylnorepinephrine and the relaxant effect of iso-propylnorephrine in high K^+ medium but has no effect on the contracture produced by high K^+ media. From these studies it may be concluded that although the major effects of norepinephrine on tension in polarizing media are mediated through changes in electrical activity, some evidence exists that norepinephrine can influence tension without accompanying potential changes. This effect is particularly obvious in the K^+-depolarized preparation. Similar conclusions may be drawn for the action of isopropylnorepinephrine. It is particularly interesting that exposure of the portal vein to Ca^{++}-free media results in the abolition of spontaneous electrical and mechanical activity and that norepinephrine is capable of restoring both activities, presumably by liberating tightly bound Ca^{++} from a membranal or internal store (Chapter VII, p. 531). The effects of norepinephrine in Ca^{++}-free, polarizing and depolarizing media are all abolished by phenoxybenzamine and are thus formally classifiable as α-receptor mediated processes, which are apparently capable of operating under a variety of ionic conditions and varying membrane potentials.

It is clear that a great deal remains to be learned about ligand-induced ionic and potential changes in vascular smooth muscle. It is important to note that attempts to correlate electrical and mechanical events are probably an oversimplification, the electrical events being merely epiphenomena of the basic underlying activation process which is unquestionably concerned with Ca^{++} mobilization (reference has previously been made to "pharmacomechanical" coupling (p. 432)). Cuthbert and Suter (166) have also provided evidence that in, for example, the rabbit anterior mesenteric vein strip norepinephrine produces contraction *both* via electrical processes and by a more direct pathway. The relative importance of these two pathways may, as suggested previously differ between tissues: thus ouabain abolishes epinephrine-linked electrical changes in the guinea-pig taenia coli and the rabbit anterior mesenteric vein but only abolishes the contractile effect in the former tissue, leading Matthews and Suter (168) to conclude that in the vascular tissue contraction may be produced by a mechanism relatively independent of electrical events at the cell membrane.

REFERENCES

1. P. Fatt and B. Katz, *J. Physiol. (London)* (1951) **115**, 320.
2. J. Del Castillo and B. Katz, *J. Physiol. (London)* (1955) **128**, 157.
3. B. L. Ginsborg, *Pharmacol. Rev.* (1967) **19**, 289.
4. J. Del Castillo and B. Katz, *J. Physiol. (London)* (1954) **125**, 546.
5. A. Takeuchi and N. Takeuchi, *J. Neurophysiol.* (1959) **22**, 395.
6. P. Fatt and B. Katz, *J. Physiol. (London)* (1953) **121**, 374.
7. B. Katz, "Nerve, Muscle and Synapse", p. 144 (1966). McGraw-Hill, New York.
8. D. R. Curtis and J. C. Watkins, *Annu. Rev. Pharmacol.* (1965) **17**, 347.
9. A. Takeuchi and N. Takeuchi, *J. Physiol. (London)* (1965) **177**, 225.
10. J. C. Dudel and S. W. Kuffler, *J. Physiol. (London)* (1961) **155**, 543.
11. J. C. Eccles, "The Physiology of Synapses", p. 316 (1964). Springer-Verlag, New York.
12. W. Trautwein and J. Dudel, *Pflügers Arch. Gesamte Physiol. Menschen.* (1958) **266**, 324.
13. E. Bülbring and T. Tomita, *Proc. Roy. Soc. London Ser. B.* (1969) **172**, 121.
14. H. Pinsker and E. R. Kandel, *Science, N.Y.* (1969) **163**, 931.
15. J. Kehoe and P. Ascher, *Nature (London)* (1970) **225**, 820.
16. B. Libet and T. Tosaka, *J. Neurophysiol.* (1969) **32**, 43.
17. H. Kobayashi and B. Libet, *Proc. Nat. Acad. Sci. U.S.A.* (1968) **60**, 1304.
18. R. M. Eccles and B. Libet, *J. Physiol. (London)* (1961) **157**, 484.
19. B. Libet, *J. Neurophysiol.* (1967) **30**, 494.
20. W. L. Nastuk, *Fed. Proc. Fed. Amer. Soc.* (1953) **12**, 102.
21. J. Del Castillo and B. Katz, *J. Physiol. (London)* (1955) **128**, 157.
22. K. Krnjević and R. Miledi, *Nature (London)* (1958), **182**, 805.
23. A. Takeuchi and N. Takeuchi, *J. Neurophysiol.* (1959) **22**, 395.
24. W. L. Nastuk, *Fed. Proc. Fed. Amer. Soc.* (1967) **26**, 1639.
25. B. Katz and R. Miledi, *Proc. Roy. Soc. London Ser. B.* (1965) **161**, 483.
26. N. Takeuchi, *J. Physiol. (London)* (1963) **167**, 141.
27. W. L. Nastuk and J. Liu, *Science, N.Y.* (1966) **154**, 266.
28. C. J. Cavallito, *Fed. Proc. Fed. Amer. Soc.* (1967) **26**, 1647.
29. B. Katz and S. Thesleff, *J. Physiol. (London)* (1957) **138**, 63.
30. D. H. Jenkinson, *J. Physiol. (London)* (1960) **152**, 309.
31. J. Del Castillo and B. Katz, *Proc. Roy. Soc. London Ser. B.* (1957) **146**, 369.
32. J. C. Eccles, B. Katz and S. W. Kuffler, *J. Neurophysiol.* (1941) **5**, 211.
33. S. W. Kuffler, *J. Neurophysiol.* (1945) **8**, 75.
34. L. B. Kirschner and W. E. Stone, *J. Gen. Physiol.* (1951) **34**, 821.
35. E. J. Ariëns, Molecular Pharmacology, Vol. 1. (1964). Academic Press, New York and London.
36. R. D. Keynes and H. Martins-Ferreira, *J. Physiol. (London)* (1953) **119**, 315.
37. E. Schoffeniels, *Biochim. Biophys. Acta* (1957) **26**, 585.
38. E. Schoffeniels and D. Nachmanson, *Biochim. Biophys. Acta.* (1957) **26**, 1.

39. H. B. Higman and E. Bartels, *Biochim. Biophys. Acta* (1962) **54**, 543.
40. H. B. Higman and E. Bartels, *Biochim. Biophys. Acta* (1962) **57**, 77.
41. Y. Nakamura, S. Nakajima and H. Grundfest, *J. Gen. Physiol.* (1965) **49**, 321.
42. H. B. Higman, T. R. Podleski and E. Bartels, *Biochim. Biophys. Acta* (1963) **75**, 187.
43. T. R. Podleski, *Biochem. Pharmacol.* (1969) **18**, 211.
44. T. R. Podleski and J.-P. Changeux, *in* "Fundamental Concepts in Drug-Receptor Interactions" (eds J. F. Danielli, J. F. Moran and D. J. Triggle) (1970). Academic Press, London and New York.
45. R. Whittam and M. Guinnebault, *Biochim. Biophys. Acta* (1960) **45**, 336.
46. R. Whittam and M. Guinnebault, *J. Gen. Physiol.* (1960) **43**, 1171.
47. E. Schoffeniels, *Ann. N.Y. Acad. Sci.* (1959) **81**, 285.
48. A. Karlin, *Proc. Nat. Acad. Sci. U.S.A.* (1967) **57**, 1162.
49. T. R. Podleski and E. Bartels, *Biochim. Biophys. Acta* (1963) **75**, 387.
50. J.-P. Changeux and T. R. Podleski, *Proc. Nat. Acad. Sci. U.S.A.* (1968) **59**, 944.
51. A. Karlin, *J. Theor. Biol.* (1967) **16**, 306.
52. A. Karlin and E. Bartels, *Biochim. Biophys. Acta* (1966) **126**, 525.
53. A. Karlin and M. Winnik, *Proc. Nat. Acad. Sci. U.S.A.* (1968) **60**, 668.
54. A. Karlin, *J. Gen. Physiol.* (1969) **54**, 2455.
55. I. Silman and A. Karlin, *Science, N.Y.* (1969) **164**, 1420.
56. B. Belleau, *J. Med. Chem.* (1964) **7**, 776.
57. W. Trautwein, *Pharmacol. Rev.* (1963) **15**, 277.
58. "Pharmacology of Cardiac Function", (ed. O. Krayer) (1964). Macmillan, New York.
59. "Structure and Function of Heart Muscle", *Circ. Res.* (1964) **14, 15**, Suppl. II.
60. G. A. Langer, *Physiol Rev.* (1968) **48**, 708.
61. A. M. Shanes, *Pharmacol Rev.* (1958) **10**, 59, 165.
62. B. F. Hoffman and E. E. Suckling, *Amer. J. Physiol.* (1954) **179**, 123.
63. R. E. McAllister and D. Noble, *J. Physiol. (London)* (1966) **186**, 632.
64. R. E. McAllister and D. Noble, *J. Physiol. (London)* (1967) **190**, 381.
65. S. Weidmann, *J. Physiol. (London)* (1955) **129**, 568.
66. E. M. Vaughan Williams, Ref. 58, p. 119.
67. D. Noble and R. W. Tsien, *J. Physiol. (London)* (1968) **195**, 185.
68. H. Reuter, *Pflügers Arch. Gesamte Physiol. Menschen* (1966) **287**, 357.
69. H. Reuter, *J. Physiol. (London)* (1968) **197**, 233.
70. H. Reuter and G. W. Beeler, Jr., *Science, N.Y.* (1969) **163**, 399.
71. D. Mascher and K. Peper, *Pflügers Arch. Gesemte Physiol. Menschen* (1969) **307**, 190.
72. A. S. V. Burgen and K. G. Terroux, *J. Physiol. (London)* (1953) **120**, 449.
73. W. Trautwein and J. Dudel, *Pflügers Arch. Gesemte Physiol. Menschen* (1958) **266**, 324.
74. T. C. West, L. D. Turner and T. A. Loomis, *J. Pharmacol. Exp. Ther.* (1954) **111**, 475.
75. R. F. Furchgott, W. Sleator, Jr. and T. De Gubareff, *J. Pharmacol. Exp. Ther.* (1960) **129**, 405.
76. O. F. Hutter, Ref. 58, p. 87.
77. E. J. Harris and O. F. Hutter, *J. Physiol. (London)* (1956) **133**, 58.
78. B. Rayner and M. Weatherall, *J. Physiol. (London)* (1959) **146**, 392.
79. O. F. Hutter, *in* "Nervous Inhibition" (ed. E. Florey) (1961). Pergamon, London.

80. W. C. Holland, R. L. Klein and A. H. Briggs, *Amer. J. Physiol.* (1959) **196**, 478.
81. J. Dudel and W. Trautwein, *Pflügers Arch. Gesemte Physiol. Menschen* (1958) **267**, 553.
82. P. A. Van Zwieten, *Eur. J. Pharmacol.* (1968) **5**, 49.
83. B. F. Hoffman and E. E. Suckling, *Amer. J. Physiol.* (1953) **73**, 312.
84. J. L. Webb and B. Hollander, *Circ. Res.* (1956) **4**, 332.
85. O. F. Hutter and W. Trautwein, *J. Gen. Physiol.* (1956) **39**, 715.
86. B. F. Hoffman, *Bull. N.Y. Acad. Med.* (1967) **43**, 1087.
87. D. G. Kassebaum, Ref. 58, p. 95.
88. B. F. Hoffman and D. H. Singer, *Ann. N.Y. Acad. Sci.* (1967) **139**, 914.
89. W. Trautwein, *Pflügers Arch. Gesemte Physiol. Menschen* (1960) **271**, 715.
90. D. G. Kassebaum and A. R. Van Dyke, *Circ. Res.* (1966) **19**, 940.
91. H. Reuter, *J. Physiol. (London)* (1967) **192**, 479.
92. O. Hauswirth, D. Noble and R. W. Tsein, *Science, N.Y.* (1968) **162**, 916.
93. E. Carmeliet and J. Vereecke, *Pflügers Arch. Gesemte Physiol. Menschen* (1969) **313**, 300.
94. E. Bozler, *Physiol. Rev.* (1962) **42**, Suppl. 5, 179.
95. G. Burnstock, M. E. Holman and C. L. Prosser, *Physiol. Rev.* (1963) **43**, 482.
96. D. F. Bohr, *Pharmacol. Rev.* (1964) **16**, 85.
97. E. E. Daniel, *Ann. Rev. Pharmacol.* (1964) **4**, 189.
98. G. Burnstock and M. E. Holman, *Annu. Rev. Pharmacol.* (1966) **6**, 129.
99. A. P. Somlyo and A. V. Somlyo, *Pharmacol. Rev.* (1968) **20**, 197.
100. J. W. Lewis and J. E. Miller, *Annu. Rev. Pharmacol.* (1969) **9**, 147.
101. E. Bozler, *Amer. J. Physiol.* (1938) **122**, 614.
102. E. Bozler, *Amer. J. Physiol.* (1939) **127**, 301.
103. E. Bozler, *Amer. J. Physiol.* (1942) **136**, 553.
104. E. Bozler, *Amer. J. Physiol.* (1946) **146**, 496.
105. E. Bozler, *Experentia* (1948) **4**, 213.
105a. E. E. Daniel, *Can. J. Physiol. Pharmacol.* (1965) **43**, 551.
105b. D. D. Job, *Amer. J. Physiol.* (1969) **217**, 1534.
106. D. H. L. Evans, H. O. Schild and S. Thesleff, *J. Physiol. (London)* (1958) **143**, 474.
107. C. L. Prosser, C. E. Smith and C. E. Melton, *Amer. J. Physiol.* (1955) **181**, 651.
108. A. M. Shanes, *Pharmacol. Rev.* (1958) **10**, 59.
109. H. Takahashi, T. Murai and T. Sasaki, *Jap. J. Physiol.* **10**, 280.
110. M. E. Holman, *J. Physiol. (London)* (1957) **136**, 569.
111. M. E. Holman, *J. Physiol. (London)* (1958) **141**, 464.
112. E. E. Daniel and H. Singh, *Can. J. Biochem. Physiol.* (1958) **36**, 959.
113. H. K. Kuriyama, Ciba Foundation Study Group No. 9, "Progesterone and the Defence Mechanism of Pregnancy", p. 51 (1961). Churchill, London.
114. R. L. Kolodny and W. G. Van der Kloot, *Nature (London)* (1961) **190**, 786.
115. E. Bülbring and H. Kuriyama, *J. Physiol. Lond.* (1963) **166**, 29, 59.
116. A. Csapo and H. Kuriyama, *J. Physiol. (London)* (1963) **165**, 575.
117. A. V. Somlyo and A. P. Somlyo, *J. Pharmacol. Exp. Ther.* (1968) **159**, 129.
118. A. P. Somlyo and A. V. Somlyo, *Fed. Proc. Fed. Amer. Soc.* (1969) **28**, 1634.
119. C. Su, J. A. Bevan and R. C. Ursillo, *Circ. Res.* (1964) **15**, 20.
120. C. Su and J. A. Bevan, *Life Sci.* (1965) **4**, 1025.
121. E. Bülbring, *J. Physiol. (London)* (1954) **125**, 302.
122. E. Bülbring, *J. Physiol. (London)* (1955) **128**, 200.
123. E. Bülbring, G. Burnstock and M. E. Holman, *J. Physiol. (London)* (1958) **142**, 420.

124. E. Bülbring and H. Kuriyama, *Biochem. Pharmacol.* (1961) **8**, 154 (1st Int. Congr. Pharmacol.).

125. P. J. Goodford, *J. Physiol.* (*London*) (1962) **163**, 411.

126. E. Bozler, M. E. Calvin and D. W. Watson, *Amer. J. Physiol.* (1958) **195**, 38.

127. Y. Nonomura, Y. Hotta and H. Ohashi, *Science, N.Y.* (1966) **152**, 97.

128. Y. Hotta and R. Tsukiu, *Nature* (*London*) (1968) **217**, 867.

129. P. J. Goodford, *J. Physiol.* (*London*) (1967) **192**, 145.

130. A. Brading, E. Bülbring and T. Tomita, *J. Physiol.* (*London*) (1969) **200**, 621.

131. A. Brading, E. Bülbring and T. Tomita, *J. Physiol.* (*London*) (1969) **200**, 637.

131a. J. Liu, C. L. Prosser and D. D. Job, *Amer. J. Physiol.* (1969) **217**, 1542.

132. E. Bülbring, *J. Physiol.* (*London*) (1957) **135**, 412.

133. G. Burnstock, *J. Physiol.* (*London*) (1958) **143**, 183.

134. E. Bueding, E. Bülbring, G. Grecken, J. T. Hawkins and H. Kuriyama, *J. Physiol.* (*London*) (1967) **193**, 187.

135. O. F. Hutter, *Brit. Med. Bull.* (1957) **13**, 176.

136. G. V. R. Born and E. Bülbring, *J. Physiol.* (*London*) (1956) **131**, 690.

137. J. Huter, H. Bauer and P. J. Goodford, *Arch. Exp. Pathol. Pharmakol.* (1963) **246**, 75.

138. D. H. Jenkinson and I. K. Morton, *J. Physiol.* (*London*) (1967) **188**, 373, 387.

139. E. Bülbring and T. Tomita, *Proc. Roy. Soc. London, Ser. B.* (1969) **172**, 89.

140. E. Bülbring and T. Tomita, *Proc. Roy. Soc. London, Ser. B.* (1969) **172**, 103.

141. G. Burnstock, *J. Physiol.* (*London*) (1953) **143**, 165.

142. E. Bülbring and G. Burnstock, *Brit. J. Pharmacol.* (1960) **15**, 611.

143. L. Hurwitz, *Amer. J. Physiol.* (1960) **198**, 94.

144. G. B. Weiss, R. E. Coalson and L. Hurwitz, *Amer. J. Physiol.* (1961) **200**, 789.

145. L. Hurwitz, *in* "Biophysics of Physiological and Pharmacological Actions" (ed. A. M. Shanes) (1961). American Physiological Society, Washington, D.C.

146. A. D. Bass, L. Hurwitz and B. Smith, *Amer. J. Physiol.* (1964) **206**, 1021.

147. R. P. Durbin and D. H. Jenkinson, *J. Physiol.* (*London*) (1961) **157**, 74.

148. A. S. V. Burgen and L. Spero, *Brit. J. Pharmacol.* (1968) **34**, 99.

149. P. Müller, *J. Physiol.* (*London*) (1965) **177**, 453.

150. P. A. VanZwieten, *Pflügers Arch. Gesemte Physiol. Menschen* (1968) **303**, 81.

151. J. W. Miller, *Ann. N.Y. Acad. Sci.* (1967) **139**, 788.

152. C. Y. Kao, *in* "Cellular Biology of the Uterus" (ed. R. M. Wynn) (1967). Appleton-Century-Crofts, New York.

153. E. Bülbring, R. Casteels and H. Kuriyama, *Brit. J. Pharmacol.* (1968) **34**, 388.

154. N. C. Anderson, Jr., *J. Gen. Physiol.* (1969) **54**, 145.

155. J. Diamond and J. M. Marshall, *J. Pharmacol. Exp. Ther.* (1969) **168**, 13, 21.

156. D. Kumar, T. Wagatsuma and A. C. Barnes, *Amer. J. Obstet. Gynecol.* (1965) **91**, 575.

157. K. A. P. Edman and H. O. Schild, *J. Physiol.* (*London*) (1962), **169**, 404.

158. H. O. Schild, *Brit. J. Pharmacol.* (1967) **31**, 579.

159. M. B. Feinstein, M. Paimre and M. Lee, *Trans. N.Y. Acad. Sci.* (1968) **30**, 1073.

160. R. F. Furchgott, *Pharmacol. Rev.* (1955) **7**, 183.

161. M. E. Holman, *Ergeb. Physiol.* (1969) **61**, 137.

162. W. M. Steedman, *J. Physiol.* (*London*) (1966) **186**, 382.

163. S. Funaki, *Bibl. Anat.* (1967) **8**, 5.
164. B. Johansson, O. Jonsson, J. Axelsson and B. Wahlström, *Circ. Res.* (1967) **21**, 619.
165. M. E. Holman and J. A. F. Wilson, *J. Physiol.* (*London*) (1968) **196**, 111.
166. A. W. Cuthbert, and M. C. Suter, *Brit. J. Pharmacol.* (1965) **25**, 592.
167. J. Axelsson, B. Wahlström, B. Johansson and O. Jonsson, *Circ. Res.* (1967) **21**, 609.
168. E. K. Matthews and M. C. Suter, *Can. J. Physiol.* (1967) **45**, 509.

Chapter VI

ENZYME MEDIATED PROCESSES AND NEUROTRANSMITTER ACTION

A recurrent theme in neurotransmitter literature concerns the possibility of equating the neurotransmitter receptors with enzymes. Among the various possibilities that have been discussed is that the receptors are identical with those enzymes responsible for the metabolic destruction of the neurotransmitter, i.e., monoamine oxidase and the receptors for phenyl- and indolyl-ethylamines, catechol-O-methyl transferase and the receptors for catecholamines and acetylcholinesterase and the receptors for acetylcholine (*inter alia*, 1–11). It is clear, however, that this possibility is not correct in the sense that the initiation of the physiological response is dependent upon the neurotransmitters serving as substrates of these enzymes since inhibition of the latter does not produce corresponding inhibition of the neurotransmitter-induced processes. Nevertheless, the possibility does remain that interaction of the neurotransmitter with the enzyme, independent of the catalytic processes, could be involved in the initiation of responses to neuro-transmitters: this may be particularly true for acetylcholinesterase. Whether or not the general hypothesis expressed above is proved correct the use of the more readily characterizable enzyme systems such as acetylcholinesterase can serve, at the very least, as valuable model systems for the understanding of neurotransmitter-receptor interactions.

A second possibility is that the neurotransmitters serve as regulatory ligands (Chapter I, p. 62) modifying the catalytic activity of enzymes and hence the responses to neurotransmitters. In this category of events may be considered the involvement of acetylcholine in phospholipid metabolism leading to local alterations of membrane structure, the modification of ATPase ion pumps leading to changes in membrane potential and pacemaker activity (Chapter V, p. 402 and p. 430) and, particularly for the catecholamines, an involvement with the ubiquitous adenyl cyclase.

Of the various possibilities suggested the greatest attention has been given to the involvement of cholinergic ligands with acetylcholinesterase and phospholipid turnover and the involvement of adrenergic ligands with adenyl cyclase. The following discussion will be confined essentially to these systems.

CHOLINERGIC LIGANDS, ACETYLCHOLINESTERASE AND THE CHOLINERGIC RECEPTOR

In 1937 Roepke (1), describing certain analogies in the interaction of cholinergic ligands with acetylcholinesterase and the cholinergic receptor, advanced the suggestion that the possibility of the identity of the two systems warranted further investigation. Despite continued interest in the potential interrelationship of these systems the question of their identity, partial identity or non-identity has simply not been solved. However, a steadily increasing amount of evidence indicates very clearly a number of intriguing similarities. Thus, in a previous chapter (Chapter IV, p. 276) a fairly detailed account was presented of Belleau's thermodynamic analysis of ligand binding to acetylcholinesterase and the possible extensions of the underlying physical events to the acetylcholine receptor.

It is to be recognized, however, that there are significant problems in the way of generating legitimate comparisons between ligand-induced events in the two systems. Belleau (8, 9, 12–14) has explicitly emphasized the difficulties in comparing the measurements of affinity constants (and derived thermodynamic data) that are readily available from acetylcholinesterase studies with the abilities of the same ligands to produce contractions, depolarizations or other physiological events in tissue systems: some discussion of the general problem of quantitating ligand-receptor interactions has already been presented (Chapter IV, p. 209). Furthermore, critical differences may well exist between events occurring at the membrane-bound receptor and those at solubilized acetylcholinesterase preparations even if both are identical: Ehrenpreis (6) has commented on differences existing between membrane bound and soluble acetylcholinesterase. With these difficulties in mind a number of comparative studies of acetylcholinesterase and the cholinergic receptors may be discussed.

The active site of acetylcholinesterase is usually regarded (15) as consisting of an anionic site and an esteratic site (Chapter I, p. 66). It is clear that the latter site can have little connection in any involvement of acetylcholinesterase and receptor function for the majority of agonists are not substrates and, although many are inhibitors of the enzyme they appear not to bind to the esteratic site as judged by their ability to protect the enzyme against mesylation at this site (9, 13). That inhibitors of acetylcholinesterase (carbamylating, mesylating and phosphorylating species) leave unchanged or potentiate the responses to agonists does not argue very well against a possible involvement of acetylcholinesterase and cholinergic receptor function for these agents leave the anionic site available for ligand interaction.

A number of comparisons have been made of the structural features of cholinergic ligands determining affinity (as substrates or inhibitors) for acetylcholinesterase and for the cholinergic receptor (*inter alia*, 1, 5, 8, 12–14, 16–20; Chapter IV, p. 276). Because of the previously noted difficulties of relating quantitatively events in the two systems many of these studies have led to rather indefinite conclusions. A significant advance in such analyses has been made by Belleau (8, 12) in his thermodynamic analysis of ligand binding to acetylcholinesterase which attempts to utilize changes in ΔH and ΔS as descriptive of a physical model for events initiated by the ligand-receptor interaction. These studies, which have been discussed previously (Chapter IV, p. 276) indicate that abrupt changes in ΔH and ΔS, obscured by relatively invariant changes in ΔF, often parallel alterations in agonist activity or transitions from agonist to antagonist activity at the muscarinic receptors.

As discussed previously Kitz and Wilson (Chapter I, p. 66) noted that certain quaternary ions accelerated the reaction of methanesulfonyl fluoride with acetylcholinesterase. In an extension of these studies Belleau (9, 13, 14) has found some intriguing similarities between the effects of quaternary ligands upon this mesylation process and their effects at cholinergic receptors. As anticipated acetylcholine inhibits but the alkyltrimethylammonium ligands accelerate the reaction (Fig. VI-1). The two immediate points of interest are that there are different binding orientations for these agonist ligands, a conclusion also derived, from entirely independent lines of evidence, for the interaction of these ligands with cholinergic receptors (Chapter IV, p. 257): a second point of interest is the finding that the optimum activating effect of the alkyl series occurs at the hexyl member, paralleling the transition (at C_6-C_7 from agonist to antagonist activities in this series (Chapter IV, p. 247). An extension of this study to include a number of antagonists active at the skeletal neuromuscular junction (9, 14) reveals further striking parallels between acetylcholinesterase and the cholinergic receptor. The polymethylenebistrimethylammonium series ($Me_3\overset{+}{N}$-$(CH_2)_n\overset{+}{N}Me_3$, Chapter IV, p. 346) also accelerate the mesylation reaction with a maximum at C_9-C_{11} (Fig. VI-2); succinylcholine has been found to be particularly effective in this regard (acceleration factor 42). In contrast, tubocurarine and gallamine, representatives of the nondepolarizing class of antagonists (Chapter IV, p. 352), offer protection against inactivation by methanesulfonyl fluoride through a mechanism

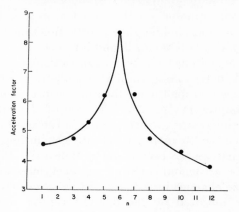

FIG. VI-1. Accelerative effects of alkyltrimethylammonium ligands, $C_nH_{2n+1}\overset{+}{N}$-$Me_3$, upon mesylation of acetylcholinesterase. Reproduced with permission from Belleau (3).

that is only partially competitive, suggesting that they interact allosterically at a site (or sites) topographically distinct from the active site and the sites occupied by the depolarizing antagonists (Fig. VI-3). Again, structure-activity studies of these two classes of antagonists also suggest the existence of distinct binding sites (Chapter IV, p. 339). However, it should be noted that in the above studies very high concentrations of tubocurarine and gallamine were employed.

The interaction of curare-like agents with acetylcholinesterase (from

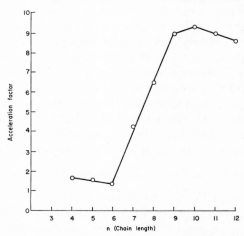

FIG. VI-2. Accelerative effects of bisquaternary ligands, $Me_3\overset{+}{N}(CH_2)_n\overset{+}{N}Me_3$, upon mesylation of acetylcholinesterase. Reproduced with permission from Belleau, DiTullio and Tsai (14).

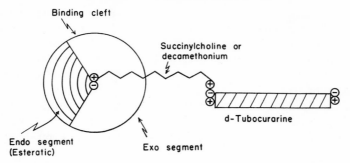

FIG. VI-3. Representation of arrangement of cholinergic ligand binding sites at acetylcholinesterase. Only ester ligands (acetylcholine) can occupy the endo binding site. Reproduced with permission from Belleau, DiTullio and Tsai (14).

electric eel) has also been studied in some detail by Changeux (21): this study revealed the aggregation of acetylcholinesterase† under low salt concentrations, conditions which promoted the binding of gallamine and tubocurarine which are inhibitors normally described as having low affinity for the enzyme (15). Furthermore, the inhibition produced by these agents towards acetylcholine hydrolysis is only partially competitive (Fig. VI-4), a plateau being reached at a level which is dependent

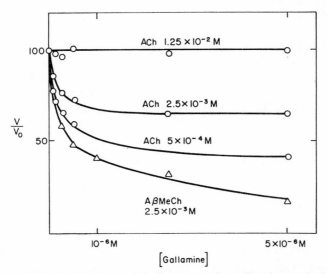

FIG. VI-4. The inhibition of acetylcholinesterase by gallamine: only incomplete inhibition of the hydrolysis of either acetylcholine or acetyl-β-methylcholine can be observed. Reproduced with permission from Changeux (21).

† This phenomenon is observed with acetylcholinesterase from electric organs and erythrocytes but not with pseudocholinesterase (21).

upon the substrate and its concentration and at which further increases in antagonist concentration do not lead to further inhibition. In contrast the inhibition by decamethonium and related depolarizing agents follows a simple competitive pattern. The analogy between this finding and Belleau's later data (p. 462) on the effect of these agents on the mesylation of acetylcholinesterase is very apparent.

A further analogy between the interaction of these agents with acetylcholinesterase and the cholinergic receptor is revealed by Changeux's findings of a competitive interaction between depolarizing

TABLE VI-1. Antagonism between Gallamine and Depolarizing Antagonists at Acetylcholinesterase (21)

Ligand	I_{50}, Control M	I_{50}, Gallamine† M	I_{50} (G)/I_{50}
$\overset{+}{Me_3N}(CH_2)_{10}\overset{+}{N}Me_3$	3.5×10^{-8}	2.3×10^{-6}	64
$[3\text{-}\overset{+}{Me_3N}C_6H_4O(CH_2)_3]_2$	1.7×10^{-8}	1.5×10^{-6}	88‡
$[3\text{-}\overset{+}{Me_3N}C_6H_4O(CH_2)_{1.5}]_2$	3.0×10^{-8}	3.0×10^{-6}	100

† Gallamine, 5×10^{-5} M.
‡ With tubocurarine (5×10^{-5} M) this ratio was 7.4.

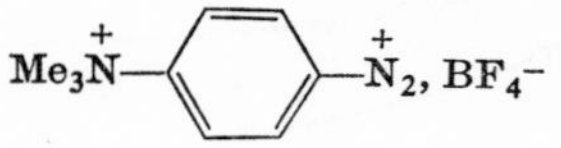

and nondepolarizing antagonists at acetylcholinesterase whereby at low ionic strengths gallamine and tubocurarine overcome the inhibition produced by depolarizing agents (Table VI-1). Several studies employing irreversible inhibitors have also revealed similarities in the interactions of these agents with acetylcholinesterase and the cholinergic receptor. p-Trimethylammoniumbenzenediazonium fluoborate (VI-1, TDF) has

$$Me_3\overset{+}{N}-\langle\bigcirc\rangle-\overset{+}{N}_2, BF_4^-$$

VI-1

been shown to irreversibly inactivate acetylcholinesterase and the cholinergic receptor of the electroplax (22, 23), although acetylcholinesterase is significantly more sensitive (Table VI-2). Protection against inactivation was afforded by tetramethylammonium for acetylcholinesterase and gallamine and tubocurarine for the receptor; however, no protection was afforded by the acetylcholinesterase inhibitors (phosphocholine and DFP) which occupy the esteratic site. From comparative studies of the abilities of TDF-acetylcholinesterase (compare with work of Purdie, Belleau and O'Brien, Chapter IV, p. 267), to hydrolyse polar and neutral substrates Meunier and Changeux (24) have concluded that TDF interacts with at least two distinct sites on the enzyme: one site is presumably the anionic area of the active site proper and the other a "peripheral" anionic site.

In a previous chapter (Chapter V, p. 419) the effects of the disulfide-sulfhydryl reagent dithiothreitol upon the responses of the electroplax preparation of the electric organ were documented. It is noteworthy

TABLE VI-2. Irreversible Inactivation of Acetyl-cholinesterase and the Cholinergic Receptor by TDF (22, 23)

TDF Conc. M	Enzymatic activity remaining (%)†	Receptor activity remaining (%)‡
0	100	100
2×10^{-7}	71·3	—
10^{-6}	40·5	—
5×10^{-6}	14·4	—
10^{-5}	7·2	106
10^{-4}	—	0

† Bovine erythrocyte enzyme, pH 6·0, incubation time 30 min.

‡ *Electrophorus* electroplax, pH 5·9, incubation time 20 min.

that exposure of acetylcholinesterase to dithiothreitol has no effect on the maximum velocity or affinity for the hydrolysis of polar and neutral substrates (25, 26). However, the effects of TDF on the enzyme are dramatically modified: following dithiothreitol treatment TDF acts as a *reversible* inhibitor towards the hydrolysis of neutral substrates (26). Apparently the modification produced by dithiothreitol of the mechanism of interaction of TDF is upon the reactivity of the amino acid residue normally coupled for the affinity of TDF for the control and dithiothreitol-treated enzyme is identical ($K_I = 2\cdot5 \times 10^{-5}$ M). This finding with the enzyme is paralleled by the effect of dithiothreitol on the electroplax preparation where a similar conversion from irreversible to reversible antagonism by TDF (at significantly lower concentrations than required for irreversible action) is found. (There is a certain analogy between these results and the finding by Karlin and Winnick (Chapter V, p. 419) that the actions of hexamethonium are converted from antagonism to agonism by dithiothreitol treatment.)

These studies indicate that both acetylcholinesterase and the cholinergic receptor[†] contain disulfide linkages which upon conversion to sulfhydryl groups affect the interactions of some cholinergic ligands in similar fashion. However, there are also apparent differences in the two preparations: acetylcholinesterase requires, in comparison to the receptor preparation, very prolonged exposure to dithiothreitol to affect the interaction of TDF. Furthermore, while dithiothreitol abolishes the sensitivity of the receptor preparation to agonists it has no effect upon substrate susceptibility to hydrolysis by acetylcholinesterase. This suggests differences in the two systems at least with respect to the relationship of the reducible disulfide linkage to the active site and recognition site of the enzyme and receptor respectively.

Podleski (29) has examined the responses of the *Electrophorus* electroplax preparation to cholinergic ligands following accelerated inactivation of the esteratic site by methanesulfonyl fluoride in the presence of tetraethylammonium. The depolarizing action of tetramethylammonium was, not surprisingly, unaffected by this treatment; also unaffected by this treatment, however, was the depolarizing activity of 3-hydroxyphenyltrimethylammonium an agent for which some evidence exists (30) that it interacts with both anionic and esteratic sites. Similarly it has been observed that the activity of the N-methyl-7-hydroxyquinolinium ion, one of a series of quinolinium derivatives showing parallel dependence of inhibitory activity upon structure towards both acetylcholinesterase and the cholinergic receptor (31), was unaffected by the mesylation procedure.

As noted previously there are likely to be significant differences existing between free and membrane-bound acetylcholinesterase. del Castillo and his co-workers (28) have examined the ligand sensitivity of bimolecular lipid membranes (Chapter II, p. 151) formed from bovine brain lipids in the presence of bovine erythrocyte acetylcholinesterase. The ligands studied were found to produce either impedance changes or to block the impedance changes produced by acetylcholine: a summary of these effects together with a classification of the actions of these ligands at cholinergic receptors is presented in Table VI-3. It is clear that the analogy between the two systems is not complete: nevertheless, this general approach would appear to offer very distinct possibilities for the examination of receptor material *in vitro*.

From the preceding discussion it is apparent that a number of very intriguing resemblances exist between patterns of ligand binding at acetylcholinesterase and the cholinergic receptors (nicotinic and

† Similar effects of dithiothreitol upon ligand action at the cholinergic receptor of the chick biventer cervicis muscle have been reported by Rang and Ritter (27) and for rat and frog skeletal muscle by Albuquerque *et al.* (28).

muscarinic). However, on the basis of the evidence thus far available it would be most presumptuous to advance definitive claims for either the identity or nonidentity of the two systems. Although it is fairly certain that the catalytic function of the acetylcholinesterase active site is not necessary for receptor activity, this by no means rules out the possibility that acetylcholinesterase has the dual function of serving both as

TABLE VI-3. Comparison of Effects of Cholinergic Ligands on Bimolecular Lipid Membranes and Cholinergic Receptors (28)

Ligand	BLM + ACh E Impedance change	Block†	Receptor Depolarization	Block†
Acetylcholine	+	−	+	−
Carbamylcholine	−	+	+	−
Hexamethonium	−	+	−	+
Decamethonium	−	+	+	+
Nicotine	+	−	+	+
Tubocurarine	+	−	−	+
Neostigmine	+	+	+	−

† Block to acetylcholine-induced events.

enzyme and receptor. Such function is not inconsistent with the work by Leuzinger *et al.* (32, 33) who have purified the enzyme from *Electrophorus* and have found it to be a dimeric hybrid structure with two α and two β chains. There are only two active sites per molecule (M. Wt. = 260,000) and hence two chains may have a regulatory function (34) and/or be associated with receptor function. Further speculation must await the results of more detailed studies of the enzyme and of current attempts to isolate receptor material (Chapter VIII).

CHOLINERGIC LIGANDS AND PHOSPHOLIPID METABOLISM

In the light of both direct and circumstantial evidence that the receptors for neurotransmitters are an integral component of the cell membrane the demonstrated involvement of these agents with increased phospholipid turnover in several systems including both neural and secretory tissues takes on a special significance (35, 36). It is also worthy of note that two of the most recent attempts to isolate cholinergic ligand binding materials from neural tissues have resulted in the isolation of lipoproteins (Chapter VIII). Much of the work in the area of phospholipid turnover has been reported by the Hokins who, in 1955 (37), reported that acetylcholine, a physiological stimulant of protein secretion from the pigeon pancreas, stimulated incorporation of ^{32}P into the phospholipid fraction. Maximum incorporation was observed with phosphatidic acid, phosphatidylinositol and phosphatidylethanolamine (38–40). Similar stimulatory effects of acetylcholine have been observed in rabbit parotid and submaxillary glands (41, 42), guinea-pig brain (38), adrenal medulla (43, 43a), the albatross salt gland (44) and cat brain synaptosomes (46). Furthermore, Larrabee *et al.* have shown that electrical stimulation of sympathetic ganglia through the preganglionic fiber also increases the rate of labelling of phosphatidylinositol by ^{32}P from inorganic phosphate (47, 48).

The problem to be solved is whether these effects of acetylcholine on phospholipid turnover bear a *direct* relationship to the acetylcholine-induced physiological response, be it depolarization or secretion. In this connection it should be noted that such cholinergic antagonists as

1. Diglyceride—P—X $\xrightarrow[\text{stimulated}]{\text{ACh}}$ Diglyceride + P—X
2. Diglyceride + ATP $\rightarrow$ Diglyceride—P + ADP
3. Diglyceride—P – CTP $\rightarrow$ Diglyceride—P—P—C + P—P
4. Diglyceride—P—P—C + In $\rightarrow$ Diglyceride—P—In + CMP

Diglyceride—P $\equiv$ phosphatidic acid; diglyceride—P—In $\equiv$ phosphatidylinositol; diglyceride—P—X $\not\equiv$ phosphatidic acid

FIG. VI-5. Sequence of reactions in phospholipid hydrolysis stimulated by acetylcholine.

atropine have an inhibitory effect on phospholipid turnover in the secretory systems while tubocurarine inhibits turnover in the ganglionic preparations.

Durell, Garland and Friedel have advanced an hypothesis (49, 50) to directly link the phospholipid effects outlined above with the known effects of acetylcholine on the ionic permeability of cell membranes. According to this hypothesis the effects of acetylcholine are actually to promote phosphodiesteratic cleavage of phospholipids (Reaction 1, Fig. VI-5): in turn the diglyceride, which is assumed to remain attached to the cell membrane (49, 51), is converted to phosphatidic acid (Reaction 2) and thence to phosphatidylinositol (Reactions 3 and 4): clearly if phosphatidylinositol is also the substrate for phosphodiesterase then a closed system exists. It is postulated, according to this sequence of reactions, that the effects of acetylcholine are to promote cleavage, through activation of a membrane-bound phosphodiesterase, of one or more phospholipid components of the cell membrane. In turn this is envisaged to lead to changes in cation permeability.

Whether polyphosphoinositides, species with rapid turnover (52, 53) and believed to be of substantial physiological significance in neural tissues (54, 55), are involved in acetylcholine-mediated reactions is not clear; Hokin (56) has reported that the turnover of phosphate in di-phosphoinositide and triphosphoinositide is not increased. It is of interest, however, that polyphosphoinositides have high affinity for Ca^{++}, forming insoluble salts (35, 55, 57, 58) which, when present in membranes will generate hydrophobic patches; hydrolysis will release this tightly bound Ca^{++} *and* generate a hydrophilic area (Fig. VI-6) that could be involved in increased ion permeability (55).

Primary emphasis has thus far been placed upon the interrelationship of acetylcholine and phospholipid metabolism. However, Durell and

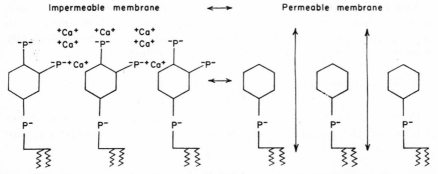

FIG. VI-6. Hypothetic mechanism by which polyphosphoinositide might control membrane permeability. Reproduced with permission from Kai and Hawthorne (55).

Garland have shown (50) that norepinephrine and dopamine can also stimulate the hydrolysis of phosphoinositides. Hokin (59) has also described an accelerated incorporation of ^{32}P into phosphatidic acid and phosphatidylinositol in several areas of the guinea-pig brain by norepinephrine at concentrations of 10^{-3} to 10^{-4} M. Thus, the possibility exists that increased turnover of phospholipids is a phenomenon of general relevance to the actions of neurotransmitters.

The suggestions outlined above are clearly very speculative and much further work is needed to demonstrate the true interrelationship of the observed events and ligand-receptor interactions. Furthermore, there is some evidence which appears to be inconsistent with the proposals outlined above. In particular, the concentrations of acetylcholine (and norepinephrine) that are required to demonstrate effects on phospho-lipid turnover are very significantly higher than those required for the production of the physiological effects. Thus, Hokin has demonstrated (60) that amylase secretion from pigeon pancreas can be very signi-ficantly stimulated by concentrations of pancreozymin or acetylcholine that have little or no effect on phospholipid turnover. She concludes that the phospholipid response may represent an adaptive response of the cell to meet greatly increased demands for secretion imposed by the high hormone or neurohormone levels. Similarly, Trifaró's studies (43a) of the effects of acetylcholine upon catecholamine release and ^{32}P-incorporation in the adrenal medulla indicate that the latter process becomes observable only *after* catecholamine secretion has reached a maximum level: Trifaró suggests that this may reflect the formation of new membranes. Additionally, L. E. Hokin has demonstrated, from radioautography with sympathetic ganglia incubated with ^{3}H-inositol, that the acetylcholine-induced phosphatidylinositol turnover is not confined to the cell membrane but occurs throughout the cell (61). Basically, it appears necessary to develop methods that are sensitive to any changes in phospholipid turnover produced by physiologically effective concentrations of hormones and neurohormones.

NEUROTRANSMITTERS AND THEIR RELATIONSHIP TO ADENYL CYCLASE

Following the original discovery by Sutherland and his colleagues (62–64) of the intermediary role of adenosine-3′-5′-monophosphate

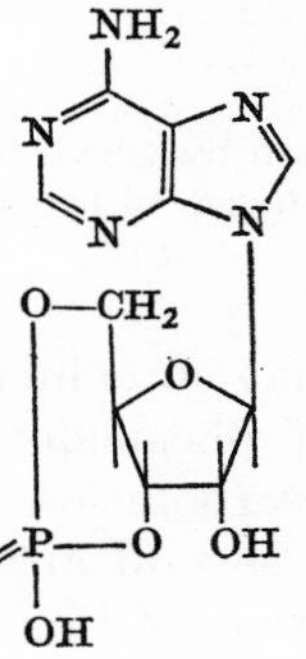

VI-2

(VI-2, cyclic AMP) in epinephrine- and glucagon-mediated hepatic glycogenolysis, cyclic AMP has been reported as a mediator of the physiological effects of a large number of hormones of diverse structure

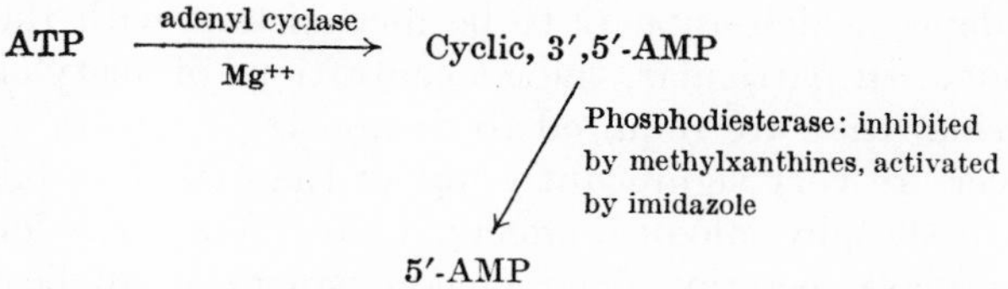

FIG. VI-7. Formation and destruction of cyclic AMP.

TABLE VI-4. Some Hormones whose Activities may be Mediated by Cyclic AMP

Hormone	Tissues	Reference
Catecholamines	Various	67–70, 79–81
Glucagon	Liver, adipose, cardiac	82–87
ACTH	Adrenal cortex, adipose	73, 83, 86–89
Vasopressin	Toad bladder, kidney, frog skin	91–94
Luteinizing hormone	Corpus luteum	87, 95, 96
Thyroid stimulating hormone	Thyroid, adipose, cardiac	87, 97–103
Insulin	Adipose, muscle	83, 104–106
Prostaglandins	Smooth muscle, adipose	67, 81, 103, 107–109
Melanocyte stimulating hormone	Frog skin	110, 111
Oxytocin	Frog bladder, skin	112, 113
Histamine	Brain, gastric mucosa	114, 115
Serotonin	Fluke	116
Acetylcholine	Heart	117
Estradiol	Uterus	118

and type. Several excellent reviews covering one or more aspects of cyclic AMP function are available (65–70). Cyclic AMP is formed from ATP in the presence of Mg^{++} through the enzyme adenyl cyclase (Fig. VI-7) and is hydrolysed to adenosine-5′-monophosphate through

TABLE VI-5. Some Cellular Processes Affected by Cyclic AMP

Process or enzyme affected	Change in activity or rate	Reference
Phosphorylase	Increased	79, 119–123
Glycogen synthetase	Decreased	120
Phosphofructokinase	Increased	124
Tyrosine aminotransferase	Increased	125, 126
Lipolysis	Increased	80, 127, 128
Glucose oxidation	Increased	129
Gluconeogenesis	Increased	130
β-Galactosidase synthesis	Increased	131, 132
Amino acid uptake (uterus)	Increased	133
Melatonin and serotonin synthesis (pineal)	Increased	134, 135
Amylase secretion	Increased	136
Iodine binding (thyroid)	Increased	137
Thyrotropin release	Increased	138
Relaxation of rat ileum	Increased	139
Melanophore dispersion	Increased	140, 141
Steroidogenesis	Increased	89, 96, 142

the actions of the widely distributed enzyme phosphodiesterase (71, 72). This enzyme is inhibited by a number of agents, particularly the methyl-xanthines (71–74); many of the pharmacological activities of the latter agents may be due to their ability to raise the levels of cyclic AMP. In contrast, imidazole appears to stimulate the enzyme system (71, 74–78).

A partial listing of the hormones whose actions are believed, partially or totally, to involve cyclic AMP is given in Table VI-4, and in Table VI-5 is presented some of the physiological processes affected by cyclic AMP. The diversity of the hormones and the physiological responses

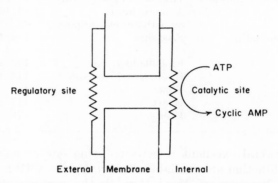

FIG. VI-8. Representation of organization of adenyl cyclase in cell membrane with intracellular cyclic AMP serving as the "second messenger".

thus mediated has given rise to the concept that cyclic AMP acts as a second messenger transmitting the information input of the primary hormone (Fig. VI-8; 143).

SOME GENERAL ASPECTS OF CYCLIC AMP AND ADENYL CYCLASE

Considering first some general aspects of adenyl cyclase relating to hormone-induced processes there is, despite the resistance of this enzyme system to any significant degree of purification, substantial evidence that it is a cell membrane component (68, 69, 86, 93, 144–152) and it is distinctly possible that localization in intracellular membrane structures is also involved. From the data of Table VI-4 it is clear that the hormonal sensitivity of adenyl cyclase differs from tissue to tissue. Some cells appear to be responsive to only one hormone while for other cellular systems a number of hormones can activate the enzyme system. Renal adenyl cyclase, which is sensitive to both parathyroid hormone and vasopressin, is actually located in two distinct cell types: the para-thyroid hormone sensitive fraction being confined to the cortex and the vasopressin sensitive fraction to the medulla (93).

An important question to be answered is whether there exists more than one enzyme for those tissues that respond to two or more hormones. This is not always a simple question to answer because of the heterogeneity of cell types in most tissues. Robison and Sutherland have argued, for the rat liver, that there is but a single cyclase, since the effects of the two stimulating agents, epinephrine and glucagon, were not additive. However, Bitensky *et al.* (85) and Pohl *et al.* (149) have

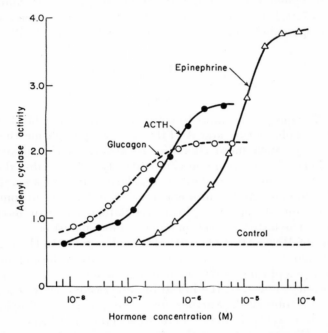

FIG. VI-9. Concentration-response curves for glucagon, ACTH and epinephrine in activating adenyl cyclase in fat cells. Reproduced with permission from Birnbaumer and Rodbell (87).

both described the isolation of adenyl cyclase from rat liver cell membranes that is sensitive only to glucagon: either the epinephrine regulatory site is more readily destroyed (85) or there exist two different cell types each with adenyl cyclase of different sensitivity. For the rat fat cell, which can readily be obtained free from other cell types, there appears substantial evidence for the existence of a single cyclase: Birnbaumer and Rodbell (87) and Bär and Hechter (86) have shown that several lipolytic agents including adrenocorticotropin (ACTH), epinephrine, glucagon, luteinizing hormone and thyroid stimulating hormone all stimulate adenyl cyclase activity, but to different extents (Fig.

VI-9) and that the effects of combinations of these agents given simultaneously at maximally activating doses are not additive. Apparently there is a single active site that is allosterically linked to different and specific hormone recognition sites. This latter point has been demonstrated on a number of occasions by showing that antagonists of one hormone do not affect the activation of adenyl cyclase by unrelated hormones. Thus in fat cells β-adrenergic antagonists antagonize the response to epinephrine but not to ACTH or glucagon: similarly an antagonist of ACTH (containing a number of D-amino residues) does not antagonize epinephrine or glucagon (87). The 2-, 3- and 4-nitro isomers

$$O_2N-\text{(phenyl)}-CHOHCH_2NHCHMe_2$$

VI-3

(VI-3) of N-isopropyl-2-amino-1-(x-nitrophenyl)ethanol block lipolysis activated by epinephrine and ACTH: against epinephrine the 4-nitro isomer is very much more effective. However, all three isomers are equally effective in blocking non-competitively ACTH-induced lipolysis (153–155), suggesting either that the regulatory units of adenyl cyclase for epinephrine and ACTH interact have some features in common, or that occupation of the epinephrine regulatory site can modify the ACTH sites. The latter suggestion appears more plausible.

The data of Marinetti et al. (151) also lend support to the concept of separate recognition sites for hormones distinct from the enzyme active site itself. Epinephrine binds to rat liver cell membranes with adenyl cyclase activity; however, the initial binding occurs before the enzyme stimulation is observed. Furthermore, the processes of epinephrine binding and enzyme activity were dissociable by heat or p-HMB treatments. We may note also that the activating influences of various hormones upon adenyl cyclase seem to vary in their requirements for extrinsic factors such as Ca^{++}. In the rat liver cell preparation activation by epinephrine requires at least 10^{-5} M Ca^{++} whereas this concentration reduces the effect of glucagon (151). In fat cells the activating influence of ACTH is lost in the absence of Ca^{++} while the effects of epinephrine and glucagon remain unchanged (87). The apparent interrelationships between Ca^{++} and cyclic AMP are being increasingly studied and will be discussed further in relationship to excitation-contraction coupling, in Chapter VII.

According to the concept that cyclic AMP acts as a second messenger it should be possible to reproduce the effects of hormones through the addition of exogenous cyclic AMP to the system under study. This has, in fact, been achieved in a number of systems (66–70, 143). Thus, the effects of glucagon and epinephrine in the liver can be duplicated by high concentrations of cyclic AMP (156). The effects of epinephrine and glucagon in stimulating the release of polysome bound proteins are duplicated by cyclic AMP (157) as are the effects of epinephrine upon the induction of tyrosine-α-ketoglutarate transaminase.

Cyclic AMP mimics MSH in darkening frog skin (141) and similarly mimics the enzyme-inducing effects of testosterone in rat seminal vesicles (158) and accelerates, as does ACTH, the formation of cytosol protein in cultured adrenocortical tumor cells (159); the effects of oxytocin and vasopressin in increasing the permeability of frog skin are also reproduced by cyclic AMP (113). Furthermore, in those instances where the experiments have been carried out the hormone specific antagonists are, as anticipated from the second messenger concept, ineffective against cyclic AMP. In many of the experiments just discussed the concentrations of exogenous cyclic AMP employed appear inordinately high and in some preparations extracellular cyclic AMP is without effect. These features of cyclic AMP action probably derive from its low permeability through cell membranes. It is, therefore, of interest that dibutyryl cyclic AMP (VI-4; 160) an agent that permeates

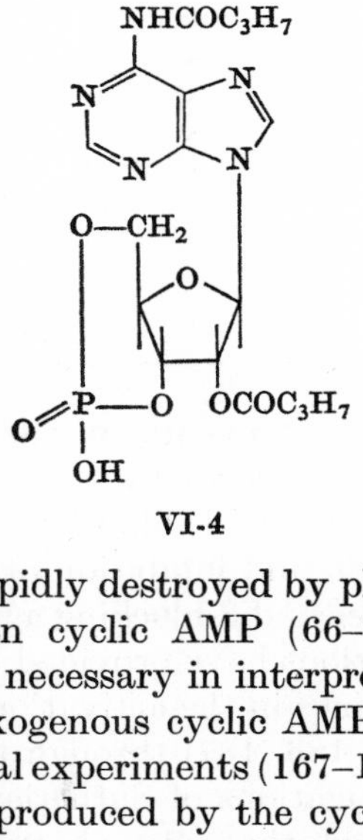

$$NHCOC_3H_7$$

VI-4

more rapidly and is less rapidly destroyed by phosphodiesterase is often much more effective than cyclic AMP (66–70, 135, 141, 161–170). However, some caution is necessary in interpreting the results of those experiments employing exogenous cyclic AMP or its analogs for, particularly in pharmacological experiments (167–170), there is considerable evidence that the effects produced by the cyclic nucleotides may also be produced by ATP, AMP, etc. (171–173) and the nucleotides are, in general, known to have powerful pharmacological actions (171, 174). Similarly, caution is necessary in the interpretation of the effects of the xanthine inhibitors of phosphodiesterase for, while they unquestionably prevent the destruction of cyclic AMP (66–70) they are also known to

17

have well established effects on Ca^{++} binding and mobilization in muscle tissues (175–178; Chapter VII).

ADENYL CYCLASE, CYCLIC AMP AND NEUROTRANSMITTER ACTION

In considering the relationship between adenyl cyclase, cyclic AMP and the physiological effects of the neurotransmitters it is clear that the greatest number of studies have been carried out with the catecholamines and have led to the development of a functional association of adenyl cyclase and the adrenergic β-receptor. This association derives from findings that, quite generally, the relative activity of the catecholamines in initiating the physiological process *and* in activating adenyl cyclase lies in the order, isopropylnorepinephrine > epinephrine > nore-

TABLE VI-6. Some Tissues in which Adenyl Cyclase Activation is Affected by Catecholamines and β-Blocking Agents (70)

Tissue	Stimulation by catecholamines	Antagonism by β-blockers	Reference
Liver	√	√	117
Cardiac muscle	√	√	122, 179
Smooth muscle	√	√	163
Adipose tissue	√	√	127
Brain cerebellum and cortex	√	√	70, 180, 181
Pineal gland	√	√	182, 183
Avian and amphibian erythrocytes	√	√	144, 150
Pancreatic islets	√		184
Frog skin	√	√	113

pinephrine, characteristic of events at the β-receptor (Chapter IV, p. 224). Furthermore, the activation by catecholamines can be prevented by adrenergic β-blocking agents. Table VI-6 contains a selection of some tissues in which activation and inhibition of adenyl cyclase have been found with catecholamines and β-blocking agents respectively.

A number of investigations have provided impressive documentation of the role of catecholamines in the activation of glycogenolysis in liver and muscle systems (65, 186, 187) through the intermediacy of cyclic AMP. In liver the investigations of Sutherland and his colleagues (65, 188–191) have established that phosphorylase, which catalyses the transformation of glycogen to glucose-1-phosphate and exists as an inactive dephosphorylated form is, in the presence of dephosphophosphorylase kinase and cyclic AMP, converted to the active form. The phosphorylase found in muscle differs in several respects from liver phosphorylase although it is activated also by a cyclic AMP dependent process. In skeletal muscle (192, 193) inactive dimeric phosphorylase b is converted to active tetrameric phosphorylase a by phosphorylase b kinase (194, 195) which itself is activated, in a cyclic AMP-dependent reaction, by phosphorylase b kinase kinase (186, 196):

$$\text{inactive phosphorylase b kinase} \xrightarrow[\text{ATP}]{\substack{\text{kinase, kinase} \\ \text{cyclic AMP}}} \text{active phosphorylase b kinase}$$

$$\text{phosphorylase b} + 4\,\text{ATP} \xrightarrow[\text{b kinase}]{\text{phosphorylase}} \text{phosphorylase a} + 4\,\text{ADP}$$

Studies on the phosphorylase enzymes from cardiac and smooth muscle reveal fundamental similarities in properties with those from skeletal muscle (122, 185, 197–206).

However, there is also substantial evidence for a mechanism of

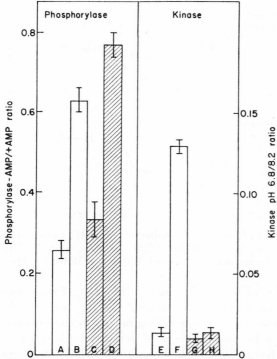

FIG. VI-10. The effects of electrical stimulation and epinephrine on phosphorylase and phosphorylase kinase activities in rat gastroenemius muscle—A and E control; B and F 5 μg epinephrine/Kg/40 sec; C and G, elec. stimulation 8 pulses/sec 5 sec; D and H, stimulation at 20 pulses/sec 5 sec. Reproduced with permission from Drummond, Harwood and Powell (123).

phosphorylase activation that is independent of the cyclic AMP-requiring route, but requires the presence of Ca^{++} (194). Ca^{++} (in mM concentrations) is known to convert inactive phosphorylase b kinase to the active form in the presence of a kinase-activating factor, a proteolytic enzyme with Ca^{++} requirements (207–209). This process seems unlikely to be of physiological significance in view of the normally very low concentrations of free intracellular Ca^{++} (Chapter VII). However, at much lower concentrations Ca^{++} can also stimulate the catalytic activity

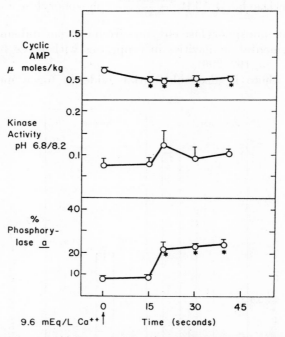

Fɪɢ. VI-11. Effect of Ca^{++} upon cardiac cyclic AMP, kinase activity and phosphorylase a levels (* = significant difference from control). Reproduced with permission from Namm, Mayer and Maltbie (205).

of inactive phosphorylase b kinase (208, 210). Drummond *et al.* have found (123) that in electrically stimulated frog and rat skeletal muscle the phosphorylase b → a conversion occurs in the absence of increased cyclic AMP or increased levels of activated phosphorylase b kinase (Fig. VI-10). Namm (205) and Friesen (211) have also reported similar findings in the isolated rat heart: perfusion of the heart with a high Ca^{++} medium produced an increased level of phosphorylase a accompanied by *decreased* cyclic AMP levels and an unchanged level (Fig. VI-11) of catalytic activity of phosphorylase b kinase (as measured by the ratio of activities measured at pH 6·8 and 8·2: the nonactivated enzyme has minimal activity at pH 6·8 and maximal activity at pH 8·2).†

In view of the importance of the phosphorylase enzymes in the energy yielding glycogenolytic pathway and the involvement of catecholamines in the initial step of this sequence substantial effort has been devoted to the elucidation of the possible linkage between these metabolic effects and the mechanical events induced by catecholamines in smooth and cardiac muscle.

Cardiac Muscle

Despite the findings that in cardiac muscle phosphorylase activation is induced by catecholamines with an order of effectiveness paralleling their effectiveness in producing positive inotropic effects and that both the metabolic and mechanical effects are abolished by β-blocking agents it is quite clear that the catecholamine-induced activation of phosphorylase a is irrelevant to the immediate mechanical events. This has been demonstrated by several groups of workers including Mayer et al. (212), Øye (213), Williamson and Jamieson (214), Cheung and Williamson (215), Robison et al. (179) and Drummond et al. (216, 217) who have shown a clear dissociation of the rise in phosphorylase a levels and the positive inotropic response. This is clearly shown in Fig. VI-12. Since the increase in cyclic AMP rises rapidly in parallel and precedes the increased force of contraction the concept of a cause and effect relationship between cyclic AMP and the mechanical events is very attractive. Furthermore, catecholamines are known to stimulate adenyl cyclase activity in particulate fractions of the dog heart, the relative potencies of these agents being rather similar to their potencies in vivo: DCI and pronethalol antagonize these effects at the concentrations required to block in vivo the inotropic responses to catecholamines, and the latter responses are potentiated by the phosphodiesterase inhibitor, theophylline (76, 218). However, cyclic AMP itself does not reproduce the inotropic effects of catecholamines (81, 179, 218), but this is very probably due to its impermeability (179). In contrast, dibutyryl cyclic AMP has been shown (219) to produce concentration-dependent increases in tension and rate of tension in cat ventricular papillary muscles (Fig. VI-13): the maximum effects produced by dibutyryl cyclic AMP (at 3×10^{-3} M) were found to be similar to the peak responses produced by norepinephrine (at 10^{-5} M). There are, however, certain differences between

† It should be noted here that the methylxanthines, presumed to increase cyclic AMP and hence phosphorylase a levels through their inhibitory actions on phosphodiesterase could also, through their effects on Ca^{++} binding mobilization processes, affect the activation of phosphorylase through this cyclic AMP-independent process.

dibutyryl cyclic AMP and norepinephrine; in particular, dibutyryl cyclic AMP requires some 30–40 min to exert its full effect. This may relate to the necessity for deacylation of the intracellular dibutyryl cyclic AMP to give the active cyclic AMP. A further association of cyclic AMP and the positive inotropic effects of catecholamines is suggested by the studies of Sobel *et al.* (220) who have determined that in guinea-pig

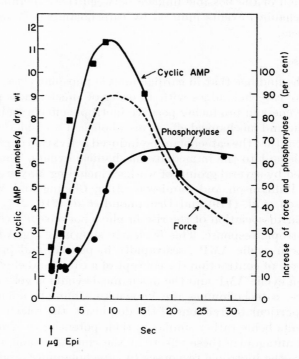

Fig. VI-12. Effects of epinephrine on cardiac (rat) contractile force, cyclic AMP and phosphorylase a levels. Reproduced with permission from Cheung and Williamson (215).

hearts with experimentally induced congestive heart failure there is a 36% reduction in the level of adenyl cyclase.

Standing in *apparent* contradiction to previous findings, however, is the work of Shanfeld *et al.* (221, 222) who have claimed the dissociation of the norepinephrine increased inotropic response and cyclic AMP levels in the rat heart. Using isopropylmethoxamine (IV-69), a β-antagonist whose spectrum of activity differs from many other agents in that it is more effective against metabolic responses (Chapter IV, p. 319), it was found that isopropylmethoxamine (4×10^{-5} M) abolished the rise in cyclic AMP without significantly affecting the increase in contractility produced (Fig. VI-14) by norepinephrine (0·03 μg). These results stand in marked contrast to the earlier studies of Robison *et al.* (179) who reported that isopropylmethoxamine (5×10^{-5} M) affected neither the positive inotropic responses nor the increased cyclic AMP levels produced by epinephrine in the rat heart. However, there are very important

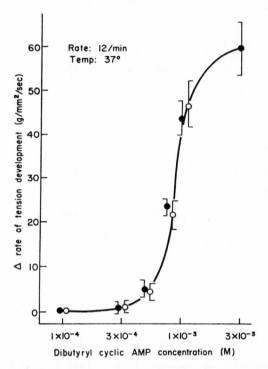

FIG. VI-13. Concentration-response curve for dibutyryl cyclic AMP in cat papillary muscles in the presence (o) and absence (●) of propranolol. Reproduced from Skelton, Levey and Epstein (219) with permission of the authors and the American Heart Association, Inc.

differences in the two studies which may be responsible for the disparate conclusions: Robison employed epinephrine at a concentration some 700 times that of the norepinephrine employed by Shanfeld. Extension of these findings is urgently required. That dissociation of mechanical and biochemical events can occur is afforded support by the findings of Namm *et al.* (205) that in Ca^{++}-free media the contractile responses to epinephrine are lost but that increases in cyclic AMP still occur: the latter observation indicate that Ca^{++} is as important as cyclic AMP in the production of the positive inotropic response but do not necessarily eliminate the intermediary role of cyclic AMP in the inotropic response.

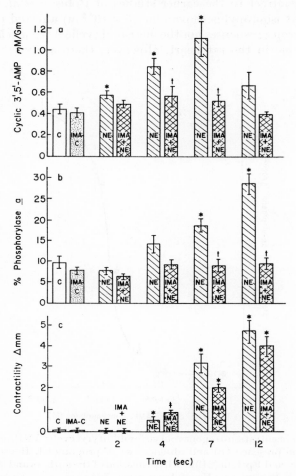

FIG. VI-14. Effects of norepinephrine (NE, 0·03 μg) on cyclic AMP levels, phosphorylase a activity and force of contraction in isolated rat hearts in the presence and absence of isopropylmethoxamine (IMA, 10 μg/ml). *, significant difference from buffer or IMA control; †, significant difference from NE alone; ‡, significant difference from IMA control and from NE alone. Reproduced with permission from Shanfeld, Frazier and Hess (221).

(A more detailed discussion of the role of Ca⁺⁺ is presented in Chapter VII, together with some comments on possible interrelationships between Ca⁺⁺ and cyclic AMP.)

Smooth Muscle

Early experiments appeared to indicate that there might exist a relationship between the catecholamine-induced relaxation of smooth muscle and phosphorylase a levels (223), in apparent accord with a prior proposal by Bülbring (224) that smooth muscle relaxation is an energy demanding process. Later work (225) showed that increased levels of phosphorylase a were artifactual and Bueding *et al.* were able to show (226) unaltered levels of phosphorylase a during the epinephrine-induced relaxation of guinea-pig taenia coli.

However, intestinal smooth muscle is unusual in that it contains both α- and β-adrenergic receptors mediating a relaxation process (Chapter III, p. 207); complete inhibition of the relaxation normally requires both α- and β-blocking agents. Diamond and Brody (227, 228) have attempted to correlate the time courses of catecholamine-induced relaxation and phosphorylase activation with the α- and β-receptor activation processes. Their results, which are summarized in Table VI-7, show that there are early and late components of the relaxation process, these being associated with α- and β-receptor events respectively. Quite clearly, phosphorylase a activation is not involved with the α-receptor induced relaxation since the latter precedes the former. However, at 30 and 120 sec when the β-component of relaxation is observed there are significant increases in the levels of phosphorylase a. Nevertheless, it is improbable that the elevated phosphorylase a levels contribute to the relaxation process; in fact, the reverse situation appears to be the case since increased phosphorylase a levels are found in spontaneously contracting taenia coli (Table VI-8). Bueding and his co-workers have demonstrated (230) changes (40% increase) in cyclic AMP in taenia coli induced by epinephrine at a concentration (2.5×10^{-8} M) that produces effective relaxation: no changes in phosphorylase a levels could be detected at the time of measurement (7–15 sec after addition of epinephrine).

In the estrogen-primed rat uterus which contains essentially β-receptors and relaxes in response to catecholamines epinephrine is more effective than norepinephrine in producing relaxation and elevating phosphorylase a levels, both effects being blocked by β-antagonists (227). However, as with the taenia coli, the levels of phosphorylase a are elevated during spontaneous contraction and there is a clear cut temporal dissociation between the mechanical and biochemical events (Fig. VI-15). A similar dissociation has been observed with serotonin-induced changes (227).

Apart from the work of Bueding showing that cyclic AMP levels in the guinea-pig taenia coli precede the β-receptor relaxation component

17*

TABLE VI-7. Effects of Catecholamines on the Physiological and Biochemical Responses of Guinea-Pig Taenia Coli (227, 228)

Agent	Relaxation onset time (sec)	% Phosphorylase a			Effect of propranolol† on response phosphorylase		Effect of phentolamine‡ on response phosphorylase	
		15 sec	30 sec	120 sec				
Epinephrine (3 × 10⁻⁶ M)	11·0	2·5	10	10	Partial§ block	Block	Slight block	None
Norepinephrine (6 × 10⁻⁷ M)	—	—	—	—	Partial block	—	None	—
Isopropylnorepinephrine (6 × 10⁻⁷ M)	28	—	—	—	Block	—	—	—
Epinephrine (3 × 10⁻⁶ M) after phentolamine (1 × 10⁻⁴ M)	25	—	—	—	—	—	—	—

† 10⁻⁵ M.
‡ 10⁻⁴ M.
§ Complete block requires propranolol and phentolamine.

TABLE VI-8. Changes in Phosphorylase Activity
Induced by Spontaneous Contraction of Taenia
Coli (227)

	% Phosphorylase a
Control	0·8 ± 0·5
Spontaneous contraction	3·8 ± 0·6†

† Significantly different, P < ·01.

there appear to be no other studies of the temporal relationships of
tension and cyclic AMP levels in smooth muscle. There have, however,
been a number of reports of the effects of cyclic AMP and its dibutyryl
analog on smooth muscle systems.

In the rat uterus the relaxing β-adrenergic effect of isopropylnorepinephrine is mimicked by dibutyryl cyclic AMP (70, 163) and the effects of

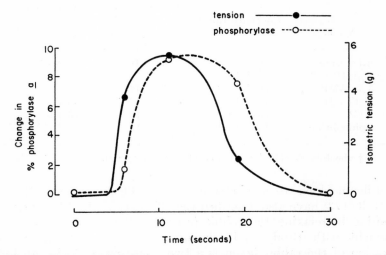

FIG. VI-15. Tension and phosphorylase a changes in spontaneous contractions of
rat uterus. Reproduced with permission from Diamond and Brody (227).

both agents are potentiated by theophylline. In the guinea-pig tracheal
chain β-receptor preparation dibutyryl cyclic AMP causes relaxation
although cyclic AMP is ineffective (167): it is worth noting that the
equieffective concentrations of dibutyryl cyclic AMP and isopropylnorepinephrine are in the ratio of 104:1. As anticipated the relaxant effects
of isopropylnorepinephrine were antagonized by propranolol but those
of dibutyryl cyclic AMP were unchanged. In rat and rabbit intestine

relaxant effects of cyclic AMP and its dibutyryl analog have been noted (168, 173) effects that are potentiated by theophylline and antagonized by imidazole. Of some interest is the finding that glucagon also causes relaxation of rabbit ileum (230).

While the above data on the effects of exogenous cyclic AMP are consistent with the proposed role of cyclic AMP as the second messenger in β-receptor mediated processes it cannot be ignored that other explanations may also be available. As noted previously (p. 475) adenine nucleotides, other than cyclic AMP, have long been known to exert effects on smooth muscle systems. This is clearly illustrated from the data of Table VI-9 showing the inhibitory effects of several nucleotides on the

TABLE VI-9. Effects of Nucleotides and Epinephrine on Rabbit Ileum (230)

Agent	Concentration M	Mean inhibitory response	
		Preadrenergic Postadrenergic[†] blockade % Control	
Adenosine	10^{-4}	65 ± 16	58 ± 17
5'-AMP	10^{-4}–10^{-5}	93 ± 5	85 ± 14
3',5'-AMP	10^{-4}–10^{-6}	51 ± 12	41 ± 13
2',3'-AMP	10^{-4}–10^{-6}	56 ± 14	48 ± 21
ATP	10^{-4}–10^{-5}	64 ± 13	76 ± 9
Epinephrine	10^{-7}–10^{-8}	88 ± 12	0

† Phentolamine (10^{-4} g/ml) plus MJ 1999 (10^{-6} g/ml).

rabbit ileum which are unaffected by α- and β-blocking agents. Bowman and Hall (173) have also described the effects of ATP, ADP AMP and adenosine in relaxing the rabbit intestine. These authors noted, in agreement with Brody and Diamond, that catecholamine-induced relaxation of the rabbit ileum is a two phase process with an initial α-receptor mediated relaxation: the relaxant effects of cyclic AMP were found generally consistent with an α-process while those of the dibutyryl analog were consistent with a β-relaxation process. Obviously some caution is necessary before the effects of exogenous cyclic AMP can be specifically attributed to any role in the second messenger hypothesis of adrenergic β-receptor processes.

To this point the discussion of cyclic AMP has been essentially in relation to its proposed role as an intermediate in adrenergic β-receptor mediated processes. Since α-adrenergic receptor stimulation produces

TABLE VI-10. Effects of Adrenergic Agents on Cyclic AMP Levels and Responses in Pancreatic Islets, Fat Cells and Toad Bladder (184)

Experimental conditions	Theophylline (180 μg/ml)	Cyclic AMP concentration in pancreatic islets μmoles/g	Insulin secretion μ units/min/ml
Control	−	355 ± 50	0
Epinephrine (10 μg/ml)	+	5570 ± 302	487 ± 42
	+	415 ± 12	208 ± 29
Epinephrine + phentolamine (10 μg/ml)	+	4450 ± 363	1272 ± 36
Epinephrine + propranolol	+	305 ± 20	0

Experimental conditions	Theophylline	Cyclic AMP concentration μmoles/10^{12} cells	FFA release mmoles/10^{12} cells/30 min
Control	−	23.3 ± 3	11.4 ± 0.8
Epinephrine (0.05 μg/ml)	−	95 ± 5	200
Epinephrine + propranolol (5 μg/ml)	−	13 ± 2	8.0 ± 0.2
Epinephrine + phentolamine (5 μg/ml)	−	70.8	200

Experimental conditions	Theophylline 180 μg/ml	Cyclic AMP concentration mμmoles/g	Permeability of toad bladder to water % of control
Control	−	1.40 ± 0.07	100
Epinephrine (1 μg/ml)	+	9.30 ± 0.5	+950
Epinephrine (1 μg/ml)	−	2.0 ± 0.1	−78
	+	2.38 ± 0.3	—
Epinephrine + phentolamine (10 μg/ml)	+	21.95 ± 3.6	+47

effects that are generally opposed to β-receptor stimulation it would be satisfying, from the standpoint of biological symmetry, if α-receptor processes were mediated by decreases in cyclic AMP levels. There are, in fact, several pieces of evidence that offer some support to this speculation: Turtle and Kipnis (184) have documented three separate systems in which α- and β-receptor stimulation have opposing effects on the physiological response and cyclic AMP levels (Table VI-10).

In frog skin MSH causes melanophore dispersion and darkening accompanied by increased cyclic AMP levels, effects that are antagonized by norepinephrine. These effects of norepinephrine are blocked by

TABLE VI-11. The Effects of MSH and Adrenergic Agents
on Cyclic AMP in Frog Skin (70)

Experimental conditions	Cyclic AMP mmoles $\times$ 10^{-7}/g
Control	$4 \cdot 2 \pm 0 \cdot 2$
α-MSH ($1 \cdot 25 \times 10^{-7}$ g/ml)	$41 \cdot 3 \pm 7 \cdot 8$
α-MSH + NE (10 μg/ml)	$15 \cdot 7 \pm 1 \cdot 6$
α-MSH + phentolamine (100 μg/ml)	$46 \cdot 9 \pm 6 \cdot 5$
α-MSH, phentolamine + NE	$32 \cdot 6 \pm 4 \cdot 7$
α-MSH ($0 \cdot 5 \times 10^{-7}$ g/ml)	$27 \cdot 1 \pm 3 \cdot 3$
α-MSH + NE (10 μg/ml)	$10 \cdot 8 \pm 1 \cdot 9$
α-MSH + propranolol (100 μg/ml)	$23 \cdot 3 \pm 3 \cdot 8$
α-MSH, propranolol + NE	$7 \cdot 5 \pm 1 \cdot 8$

α-antagonists but unaffected by β-antagonists (Table VI-11). Catecholamines also produce changes in Na^+ transport across frog skin (231): β-adrenergic stimulation increases Na^+ transport and cyclic AMP levels. In a test of the hypothesis that α-adrenergic stimulation decreases Na^+ transport and cyclic AMP levels, phenylephrine in the presence of propranolol was shown to block the permeability increase caused by vasopressin but to be ineffective against added cyclic AMP (232).

There have also been reports that elevated levels of cyclic AMP may be associated with adrenergic α-receptor mediated processes. Thus, potentiating and inhibiting effects of theophylline and imidazole have been reported for the contractile responses to norepinephrine in the rabbit uterus and aortic strip (169) and cyclic AMP has been reported to potentiate, although in highly variable fashion, the response of the aortic strip. Similarly, catecholamines appear to relax rat ileum by an α-mediated process and the effects of catecholamines have been shown to be potentiated by theophylline (233).

ADENYL CYCLASE, CYCLIC AMP AND NON-ADRENERGIC PERIPHERAL NEUROTRANSMITTERS

There have been regrettably few studies of the possible interrelationships between cyclic AMP and neurotransmitters other than the catecholamines. An early study by Murad et al. (117) showed that carbamylcholine, acetylcholine and acetyl-β-methylcholine produced an approximately 30% reduction of cyclic AMP levels in heart adenyl cyclase and that these effects were antagonized by the parasympatholytic agent, atropine. Further studies of this type are urgently needed.

CYCLIC AMP AND NEUROTRANSMITTERS: SOME GENERAL COMMENTS

Despite the very considerable efforts outlined in the previous section it cannot be said that the linkage between neurotransmitters, primarily the catecholamines, and cyclic AMP is understood. There is no doubt that catecholamines do affect the activity of adenyl cyclase but it has not been established unambiguously that there is a causal relationship between cyclic AMP levels and the mechanical activity of cardiac and smooth muscle. Thus, despite the several experiments in cardiac tissue showing that cyclic AMP levels increase prior to or together with the increased contractility the work of Shanfeld et al. (222) apparently suggesting, through the action of isopropylmethoxamine, an apparent dissociation of the biochemical and mechanical events indicates that there may not be an obligatory linkage between cyclic AMP and the mechanical events. Furthermore, as previously noted, the effects of methylxanthines or exogenous cyclic AMP are not free from ambiguity of interpretation in view of the known locus of action of the former agents at Ca^{++}-binding mobilization sites and of the wide variety of actions of adenosine and adenosine phosphates on mechanical events.

Nonetheless, it is quite clear that catecholamines do activate adenyl cyclase in particulate enzyme preparations from a variety of tissues and that this is an adrenergic β-receptor event as judged by the activity ratios of catecholamines and the effect of β-antagonists. If cyclic AMP is not a necessary intermediate in catecholamine-induced mechanical events in cardiac and smooth muscle some consideration must be given to why mechanical events and regulation of adenyl cyclase activity are normally associated and are not apparently distinguished by agonist ligands.

A possible solution is afforded through consideration of the general role of adenine nucleotides as regulatory agents in the control of the cellular metabolic processes. Atkinson and his colleagues (234–237) have advanced a general hypothesis according to which the relative concentrations of adenine nucleotides constitute a regulatory mechanism effective at those points in the metabolic sequence where a metabolite may be directed to energy-yielding or energy-demanding processes: more specifically, this hypothesis has been expressed in terms of the adenylate charge which is defined by $(ATP + 1/2\ ADP)/(ATP + ADP + AMP)$, varies between 0 and 1 and is numerically equivalent to half the number of anhydride-bound phosphate groups per adenosine. According to this concept, Fig. VI-16 depicts a generalized response to the energy charge level of ATP-utilizing (U) and ATP-regenerating (R) reactions so that the rate of ATP-utilizing enzymes will increase steeply as the adenylate charge increases and the rate of ATP-regenerating enzymes will decrease steeply. Examples of both classes include phosphofructokinase (R), isocitrate dehydrogenase (R), phosphoribosyl pyrophosphate

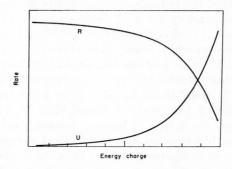

FIG. VI-16. Generalized scheme for response of ATP-regenerating (R) and ATP-utilizing (U) enzymes as a function of adenylate charge. Reproduced with permission from Atkinson (236).

synthetase (U) and pyrophosphorylase (U). An important feature of this concept is that the steep velocity curves so produced, and characteristic of cooperative binding processes (Chapter I, p. 71), are obtained in the absence of multiple substrate sites.

Atkinson views the role of cyclic AMP as that of overriding the regulatory control exerted by the adenylate charge. This can be seen quite clearly in the responses of phosphofructokinase which is inhibited by ATP and activated by cyclic AMP (124, 237, 238). Figure VI-17 shows that the enzyme is strongly inhibited by high adenylate charge and that this inhibition is relieved by cyclic AMP.

Accordingly, the actions of epinephrine and perhaps also of other hormones that appear to regulate cyclic AMP levels may be viewed, at least in part, as a mechanism for bypassing the adenylate charge regulatory mechanism (237). It may be that the actions of catecholamines in modifying mechanical events and cyclic AMP levels should be

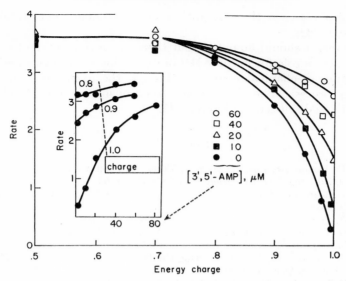

FIG. VI-17. Effect of energy charge on the rate of reaction catalysed by rabbit muscle phosphofructokinase. Energy charge determined by levels of AMP and ATP: cyclic AMP was added at the concentrations shown. The inset figure is a replot of rate against cyclic AMP levels at energy charges of 0·8, 0·9 and 1·0. Reproduced with permission from Shen, Fall, Walton and Atkinson (237).

regarded as exerted at two distinct receptors, one initiating the mechanical events and the other, a regulatory component of adenyl cyclase (Fig. VI-18). These sites are apparently very similar and both have the structural characteristics of adrenergic β-receptors. In response to agonist ligands both pathways will be activated, the function of the generated cyclic AMP being to override charge control for the energy demanding mechanical events in smooth and cardiac muscle. Because of their close structural similarities, or perhaps identity as far as agonist binding sites are concerned, these sites may not be readily distinguished, although isopropylmethoxamine, a β-antagonist, can apparently

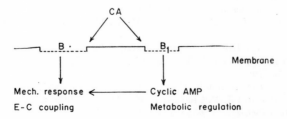

FIG. VI-18. Dual receptor concept for catecholamine (CA) interaction.

distinguish between the recognition sites on adenyl cyclase and the β-receptor (222).

However, it should be noted that there are several lines of evidence that suggest a role for cyclic AMP in regulating Ca^{++} levels and hence modulating mechanical responses through the excitation-contraction coupling process. The possible interrelationship of Ca^{++} and cyclic AMP will be discussed in Chapter VII.

REFERENCES

1. M. H. Roepke, *J. Pharmacol. Exp. Ther.* (1937) **59**, 264.
2. A. O. Župančič, *Acta Physiol. Scand.* (1953) **29**, 63.
3. B. Belleau, *in "Proc. 1st. Int. Pharmacol. Meet."* **7**, 75 (1963). Pergamon, London.
4. A. O. Župančič, *Ann. N.Y. Acad. Sci.* (1967) **144**, 689.
5. A. H. Beckett, *Ann. N.Y. Acad. Sci.* (1967) **144**, 675.
6. S. Ehrenpreis, *Ann. N.Y. Acad. Sci.* (1967) **144**, 720.
7. S. Ehrenpreis, *in* "Drugs Affecting the Peripheral Nervous System", Vol. I (1968). M. Dekker, New York.
8. B. Belleau, *Ann. N.Y. Acad. Sci.* (1967) **144**, 705.
9. B. Belleau, *in* "Fundamental Concepts in Drug-Receptor Interactions" (eds J. F. Danielli, J. F. Moran and D. J. Triggle) (1970). Academic Press, New York and London.
10. D. Nachmanson, "Chemical and Molecular Basis of Nerve Activity" (1959). Academic Press, New York and London.
11. J. P. Changeux, T. R. Podleski and J. C. Meunier, *in* "Membrane Proteins" (1969). Little Brown, Boston.
12. B. Belleau and J. L. Lavoie, *Can. J. Biochem.* (1968) **46**, 1397.
13. B. Belleau, *in "Proc. 3rd. Int. Pharmacol. Meet."* **7**, 207 (1968). Pergamon, London.
14. B. Belleau, V. DiTullio and Y.-H. Tsai, *Mol. Pharmacol.* (1970) **6**, 41.
15. J. A. Cohen and R. A. Oosterbaan, *in* "Handbuch der Experimentellen Pharmakologie", Vol. 15, "Cholinesterases and Anticholinesterase Agents" (ed. G. B. Koelle) (1963). Springer-Verlag, Heidelberg.
16. L. Gyermek and K. R. Unna, *Proc. Soc. Exp. Biol. Med.* (1958) **98**, 802.
17. A. H. Beckett, N. J. Harper and J. W. Clitherow, *J. Pharm. Pharmacol.* (1963) **15**, 362.
18. T. R. Podleski and D. Nachmanson, *Proc. Nat. Acad. Sci. U.S.A.* (1966) **56**, 1034.
19. E. Bartels, *Biochem. Pharmacol.* (1968) **17**, 945.
20. G. H. Cocolas, E. C. Robinson and W. L. Dewey (1970) *J. Med. Chem.* **13**, 299.
21. J.-P. Changeux, *Mol. Pharmacol.* (1966) **2**, 369.
22. J.-P. Changeux, T. R. Podleski and L. Wofsy, *Proc. Nat. Acad. Sci. U.S.A.* (1967) **58**, 2063.
23. L. Wofsy and D. Michaeli, *Proc. Nat. Acad. Sci. U.S.A.* (1967) **58**, 2296.
24. J.-C. Meunier and J.-P. Changeux, *FEBS Let.* (1969) **2**, 224.
25. A. Karlin, *Biochim. Biophys. Acta* (1967) **137**, 358.
26. T. R. Podleski, J.-C. Meunier and J.-P. Changeux, *Proc. Nat. Acad. Sci. U.S.A.* (1969) **63**, 1239.

27. H. P. Rang and M. J. Ritter, *Brit. J. Pharmacol.* (1969) **37**, 538P.
28. E. X. Albuquerque, M. D. Sokoll, B. Sonesson and S. Thesleff, *Eur. J. Pharmacol.* (1968) **4**, 40.
29. T. R. Podleski, *Proc. Nat. Acad. Sci. U.S.A.* (1967) **58**, 268.
30. R. M. Krupka, *Biochemistry* (1965) **4**, 429.
31. T. R. Podleski and D. Nachmanson, *Proc. Nat. Acad. Sci. U.S.A.* (1966) **56**, 1034.
32. W. Leuzinger and A. L. Baker, *Proc. Nat. Acad. Sci. U.S.A.* (1967) **57**, 446.
33. W. Leuzinger, M. Goldberg and E. Cauvin, *J. Mol. Biol.* (1969) **40**, 217.
34. R. J. Kitz, L. M. Braswell and S. Ginsburg, *Mol. Pharmacol.* (1970) **6**, 108.
35. G. B. Ansell and J. N. Hawthorne, "Phospholipids", B. B. A. Library, Vol. 3, Chap. 13 (1964). Elsevier, Amsterdam.
36. L. E. Hokin, *in* "Structure and Function of The Nervous System", Vol. 2 (ed. G. H. Bourne) (1969). Academic Press, New York and London.
37. M. R. Hokin and L. E. Hokin, *J. Biol. Chem.* (1953) **203**, 967.
38. L. E. Hokin and M. R. Hokin, *Biochim. Biophys. Acta* (1955) **18**, 102.
39. L. E. Hokin and M. R. Hokin, *J. Biol. Chem.* (1958) **233**, 805.
40. M. R. Hokin, *Arch. Biochem. Biophys.* (1968) **124**, 271.
41. L. E. Hokin and M. R. Hokin, *Can. J. Biochem. Physiol.* (1956) **34**, 349.
42. L. E. Hokin and A. L. Sherwin, *J. Physiol. (London)* (1957) **135**, 18.
43. M. R. Hokin, B. G. Benfey and L. E. Hokin, *J. Biol. Chem.* (1958) **233**, 814.
43a. J. M. Trifaro, *Mol. Pharmacol.* (1969) **5**, 382, 424.
44. L. E. Hokin and M. R. Hokin, *J. Gen. Physiol.* (1960) **44**, 61.
45. L. E. Hokin, *J. Neurochem.* (1966) **13**, 179.
46. J. Durell and M. A. Sodd, *J. Neurochem.* (1966) **13**, 487.
47. M. G. Larrabee, J. D. Klingman and W. S. Leicht, *J. Neurochem.* (1963) **10**, 549.
48. M. G. Larrabee and W. S. Leicht, *J. Neurochem.* (1965) **12**, 1.
49. J. Durell, J. T. Garland and R. O. Friedel, *Science, N.Y.* (1969) **165**, 861.
50. J. Durell and J. T. Garland, *Ann. N.Y. Acad. Sci.* (1969) **165**, 743.
51. L. E. Hokin and M. R. Hokin, *J. Biol. Chem.* (1958) **233**, 818.
52. H. Brockerhoff and C. E. Ballou, *J. Biol. Chem.* (1962) **237**, 49.
53. R. M. C. Dawson, *Ann. N.Y. Acad. Sci.* (1969) **165**, 774.
54. E. P. Kennedy, *in* "The Neurosciences", (eds G. C. Quarton, T. Melnechuk and F. O. Schmitt) (1967). Rockefeller University Press, New York.
55. M. Kai and J. N. Hawthorne, *Ann. N.Y. Acad. Sci.* (1969) **165**, 761.
56. M. R. Hokin, quoted by L. E. Hokin, *Ann. N.Y. Acad. Sci.* (1969) **165**, 695.
57. J. N. Hawthorne and P. Kemp, *Advan. Lipid Res.* (1964) **2**, 127.
58. H. S. Hendrickson, *Ann. N.Y. Acad. Sci.* (1969) **165**, 668.
59. M. R. Hokin, *J. Neurochem.* (1969) **16**, 127.
60. M. R. Hokin, *Arch. Biochem. Biophys.* (1968) **124**, 280.
61. L. E. Hokin, *Ann. N.Y. Acad. Sci.* (1969) **165**, 695.
62. T. W. Rall, E. W. Sutherland and J. Berthet, *J. Biol. Chem.* (1957) **224**, 463.
63. T. W. Rall and E. W. Sutherland, *J. Biol. Chem.* (1958) **232**, 1065.
64. E. W. Sutherland and T. W. Rall, *J. Biol. Chem.* (1958) **232**, 1077.
65. E. W. Sutherland and T. W. Rall, *Pharmacol. Rev.* (1960) **12**, 265.
66. E. W. Sutherland, G. A. Robison and R. W. Butcher, *Circulation* (1968) **37**, 279.
67. R. W. Butcher, G. A. Robison, J. G. Hardman and E. W. Sutherland, *Advan. Enzyme Regul.* (1968) **6**, 357.
68. G. A. Robison, R. W. Butcher and E. W. Sutherland, *Ann. Rev. Biochem.* (1968) **37**, 149.

69. B. McL. Breckenridge, *Ann. Rev. Pharmacol.* (1970) **10**, 19.
70. G. A. Robison, R. W. Butcher and E. W. Sutherland, *in* "Fundamental Concepts in Drug-Receptor Interactions" (eds J. F. Danielli, J. F. Moran and D. J. Triggle) (1970). Academic Press, New York and London.
71. R. W. Butcher and E. W. Sutherland, *J. Biol. Chem.* (1962) **237**, 1244.
72. W. Y. Cheung, *Biochemistry* (1967) **6**, 1079.
73. L. Birnbaumer, S. L. Pohl and M. Rodbell, *J. Biol. Chem.* (1969) **244**, 3468.
74. L. A. Menahan, K. D. Hepp and O. Wieland, *Eur. J. Biochem.* (1969) **8**, 435.
75. E. Bueding, E. Bülbring, G. Gercken, J. T. Hawkins and H. Kuriyama, *J. Physiol. (London)* (1967) **193**, 187.
76. W. R. Kukovetz and G. Pöch, *J. Pharmacol. Exp. Ther.* (1967) **156**, 514.
77. E. Bülbring and T. Tomita, *Proc. Roy. Soc. Ser. B.* (1969) **172**, 103.
78. B. McL. Breckenridge and R. E. Johnston, *J. Histochem. Cytochem.* (1969) **17**, 505.
79. N. Haugaard and M. E. Hess, *Pharmacol. Rev.* (1965) **17**, 27.
80. E. W. Sutherland and G. A. Robison, *Pharmacol. Rev.* (1966) **18**, 145.
81. G. A. Robison, R. W. Butcher and E. W. Sutherland, *Ann. N.Y. Acad. Sci.* (1967) **139**, 703.
82. M. H. Makman and E. W. Sutherland, *Endocrinology* (1964) **75**, 127.
83. R. W. Butcher, J. G. T. Sneyd, C. R. Park and E. W. Sutherland, *J. Biol. Chem.* (1966) **241**, 1652.
84. F. Murad and M. Vaughan, *Biochem. Pharmacol.* (1968) **18**, 1053.
85. M. W. Bitensky, V. Russell and W. Robertson, *Biochem. Biophys. Res. Commun.* (1968) **31**, 706.
86. H. P. Bär and O. Hechter, *Proc. Nat. Acad. Sci. U.S.A.* (1969) **63**, 350.
87. L. Birnbaumer and M. Rodbell, *J. Biol. Chem.* (1969) **241**, 3477.
88. G. C. Karaboyas and S. B. Koritz, *Biochemistry* (1965) **4**, 462.
89. D. G. Grahame-Smith, R. W. Butcher, R. L. Ney and E. W. Sutherland, *J. Biol. Chem.* (1967) **242**, 5535.
90. G. N. Gill and L. D. Garren, *Proc. Nat. Acad. Sci. U.S.A.* (1969) **63**, 512.
91. E. Browne, D. L. Clarke, V. Roux and G. H. Sherman, *J. Biol. Chem.* (1963) **238**, PC 852.
92. J. Orloss and J. S. Handler, *Amer. J. Med.* (1967) **42**, 757.
93. L. R. Chase and G. D. Aurbach, *Science, N.Y.* (1968) **159**, 545.
94. C. O. Watlington, *Biochim. Biophys. Acta* (1969) **193**, 394.
95. P. F. Hall and S. B. Koritz, *Biochemistry* (1965) **4**, 1037.
96. J. M. Marsh, R. W. Butcher, K. Savard and E. W. Sutherland, *J. Biol. Chem.* (1966) **241**, 5436.
97. S. Tarui, K. Nonaka, Y. Ikurga and K. Shima, *Biochem. Biophys. Res. Commun.* (1963) **13**, 329.
98. I. Pastan, *Biochem. Biophys. Res. Commun.* (1966) **25**, 617.
99. I. Pastan and R. Katzen, *Biochem. Biophys. Res. Commun.* (1967) **29**, 792.
100. G. Krishna, S. Hynie and B. B. Brodie, *Proc. Nat. Acad. Sci. U.S.A.* (1968) **59**, 884.
101. I. Pastan and V. Macchia, *J. Biol. Chem.* (1967) **242**, 5757.
102. G. S. Levey and S. E. Epstein, *Biochem. Biophys. Res. Commun.* (1968) **33**, 990.
103. V. Zor, T. Kaneko, I. P. Lowe, G. Bloom and J. B. Field, *J. Biol. Chem.* (1969) **244**, 5189.
104. R. L. Jungas, *Proc. Nat. Acad. Sci. U.S.A.* (1966) **56**, 757.
105. N. D. Goldberg, C. Villar-Palasi, H. Sasko and J. Larner, *Biochim. Biophys. Acta* (1967) **148**, 665.

106. M. Rodbell, *J. Biol. Chem.* (1967) **242**, 5751.
107. R. W. Butcher and E. W. Sutherland, *Ann. N.Y. Acad. Sci.* (1967) **139**, 849.
108. R. W. Butcher and C. E. Baird, *J. Biol. Chem.* (1968) **243**, 1713.
109. E. W. Horton, *Physiol. Rev.* (1969) **49**, 122.
110. M. W. Bitensky and S. R. Burstein, *Nature (London)* (1965) **208**, 1282.
111. K. Abe, R. W. Butcher, C. E. Baird, W. E. Nicholson, R. A. Liddle and G. W. Liddle, quoted by Robison in ref. 70.
112. J. Bourget, *Biochim. Biophys. Acta* (1968) **150**, 104.
113. F. Bastide and S. Jard, *Biochim. Biophys. Acta* (1968) **150**, 113.
114. J. B. Harris and D. Alonso, *Fed. Proc. Fed. Amer. Soc.* (1965) **24**, 1368.
115. S. Kakiuchi and T. W. Rall, *Fed. Proc. Fed. Amer. Soc.* (1965) **24**, 150.
116. D. B. Stone and T. E. Mansour, *Mol. Pharmacol.* (1967) **3**, 161.
117. F. Murad, Y.-M. Chi, T. W. Rall and E. W. Sutherland, *J. Biol. Chem.* (1962) **237**, 1233.
118. C. M. Szego and J. S. Davis, *Proc. Nat. Acad. Sci. U.S.A.* (1967) **58**, 1711.
119. E. G. Krebs, R. J. DeLange, R. G. Kemp and W. D. Riley, *Pharmacol. Rev.* (1966) **18**, 163.
120. J. Larner, *Trans. N.Y. Acad. Sci.* (1967) **29**, 192.
121. K. E. Hammermeister, A. A. Yunis and E. G. Krebs, *J. Biol. Chem.* (1965) **240**, 986.
122. D. H. Namm and S. E. Mayer, *Mol. Pharmacol.* (1968) **4**, 61.
123. G. I. Drummond, J. P. Harwood and C. A. Powell, *J. Biol. Chem.* (1969) **244**, 4235.
124. D. B. Stone and T. E. Mansour, *Mol. Pharmacol.* (1967) **3**, 177.
125. W. D. Wicks, *J. Biol. Chem.* (1968) **243**, 900.
126. W. D. Wicks, *Science, N.Y.* (1968) **160**, 997.
127. R. W. Butcher, C. E. Baird and E. W. Sutherland, *J. Biol. Chem.* (1968) **243**, 1705.
128. M. Blecher, N. S. Merlino and J. T. Roane, *J. Biol. Chem.* (1968) **243**, 3973.
129. M. Blecher, *Biochem. Biophys. Res. Commun.* (1967) **27**, 560.
130. J. H. Exton, L. S. Jefferson, R. W. Butcher and C. R. Park, *Amer. J. Med.* (1966) **40**, 709.
131. I. Pastan and R. L. Perlman, *Proc. Nat. Acad. Sci. U.S.A.* (1968) **61**, 1336.
132. D. A. Chambers and G. Zubay, *Proc. Nat. Acad. Sci. U.S.A.* (1969) **63**, 118.
133. D. M. Griffin and C. M. Szego, *Life Sci.* (1968) **7** (II), 1017.
134. H. M. Shein and R. J. Wurtman, *Science, N.Y.* (1969) **166**, 519.
135. D. C. Klein, G. R. Berg, J. Weller and W. Glinsmann, *Science, N.Y.* (1970) **167**, 1738.
136. R. J. Grand and P. R. Gross, *J. Biol. Chem.* (1969) **244**, 5608.
137. C.-S. Ahn and I. N. Rosenberg, *Proc. Nat. Acad. Sci. U.S.A.* (1968) **60**, 830.
138. J. F. Wilber, G. T. Peake and R. D. Utiger, *Endocrinology* (1969) **84**, 758.
139. A. Kawasaki, T. Kashimoto and H. Yoshida, *Jap. J. Pharmacol.* (1969) **19**, 494.
140. R. R. Novales and W. T. Davis, *Endocrinology* (1967) **81**, 283.
141. M. E. Hadley and J. M. Goldman, *Brit. J. Pharmacol.* (1969) **37**, 650.
142. J. Kowal, *Biochemistry* (1969) **8**, 1821.
143. E. W. Sutherland, I. Øye and R. W. Butcher, *Recent Progr. Horm. Res.* (1965) **21**, 623.
144. P. R. Davoren and E. W. Sutherland, *J. Biol. Chem.* (1963) **238**, 3016.
145. M. Rabinowitz, L. DeSalles, J. Meisler and L. Lorand, *Biochim. Biophys. Acta* (1965) **97**, 29.
146. K. Seraydarian and W. F. H. M. Mommaerts, *J. Cell Biol.* (1965) **26**, 641.

147. M. Castaneda and A. Tyler, *Biochem. Biophys. Res. Commun.* (1968) **33**, 782.
148. B. P. Schimmer, K. Veda and G. H. Sato, *Biochem. Biophys. Res. Commun.* (1968) **32**, 806.
149. S. L. Pohl, L. Birnbaumer and M. Rodbell, *Science, N.Y.* (1969) **164**, 566.
150. O. M. Rosen and S. M. Rosen, *Arch. Biochem. Biophys.* (1969) **131**, 449.
151. G. V. Marinetti, T. K. Ray and V. Tomasi, *Biochem. Biophys. Res. Commun.* (1969) **36**, 185.
152. L. Reik, G. L. Petzold, J. A. Higgins, P. Greengard and R. J. Barnett, *Science, N.Y.* (1970) **168**, 382.
153. K. Stock and E. Westermann, *Life Sci.* (1965) **4**, 1115.
154. K. Stock and E. Westermann, *Life Sci.* (1966) **5**, 1667.
155. J. J. Lech, P. Somani and D. N. Calvert, *Mol. Pharmacol.* (1966) **2**, 501.
156. W. F. Henion, E. W. Sutherland and T. Posternak, *Biochim. Biophys. Acta* (1967) **148**, 106.
157. E. A. Khairallah and H. C. Pitot, *Biochem. Biophys. Res. Commun.* (1967) **29**, 269.
158. R. L. Singhal, R. Vijayvargiya and G. M. Ling, *Science, N.Y.* (1970) **168**, 261.
159. M. F. Grower and E. D. Bransome, *Science, N.Y.* (1970) **168**, 483.
160. T. Posternak, E. W. Sutherland and W. F. Henion, *Biochim. Biophys. Acta* (1962) **65**, 558.
161. I. Pastan, *Biochem. Biophys. Res. Commun.* (1966) **25**, 14.
162. A. Aulich, K. Stock and E. Westermann, *Life Sci.* (1967) **6**, 929.
163. J. W. Dobbs and G. A. Robison, *Fed. Proc. Fed. Amer. Soc.* (1968) **27**, 352.
164. R. A. Levine and S. E. Lewis, *Biochem. Pharmacol.* (1969) **18**, 15.
165. M. Heimberg, I. Weinstein and M. Kohout, *J. Biol. Chem.* (1969) **244**, 5131.
166. R. J. Grand and P. R. Gross, *J. Biol. Chem.* (1969) **244**, 5608.
167. P. F. Moore, L. C. Iorio and J. M. McManus, *J. Pharm. Pharmacol.* (1969) **20**, 368.
168. A. Kawasaki, T. Kashimoto and H. Yoshida, *Jap. J. Pharmacol.* (1969) **19**, 494.
169. H. J. Bartelstone, P. A. Nasmyth and J. M. Telford, *J. Physiol.* (*London*) (1967) **188**, 159.
170. J. W. Lambe, *Life Sci.* (1970) **9** (I), 463.
171. A. N. Drury, *Physiol. Rev.* (1936) **16**, 292.
172. E. Bueding, E. Bülbring, G. Gercken, J. Hawkins and H. Kuriyama, *J. Physiol.* (*London*) (1967) **193**, 187.
173. W. C. Bowman and M. T. Hall, *Brit. J. Pharmacol.* (1970) **38**, 399.
174. E. E. Daniel and J. Irwin, *Can. J. Physiol. Pharmacol.* (1965) **43**, 89.
175. A. Sandow, *Pharmacol. Rev.* (1965) **17**, 265.
176. C. P. Bianchi, "Cell Calcium" (1968). Butterworth, London.
177. A. Weber, *J. Gen. Physiol.* (1968) **52**, 760.
178. P. N. Johnson and G. Inesi, *J. Pharmacol. Exp. Ther.* (1969) **169**, 308.
179. G. A. Robison, R. W. Butcher, I. Øye, H. E. Morgan and E. W. Sutherland, *Mol. Pharmacol.* (1965) **1**, 168.
180. T. W. Rall and S. Kakiuchi, *in* "Molecular Basis of Some Aspects of Mental Activity", (ed. O. Walaas) (1966). Academic Press, London and New York.
181. S. Kakiuchi and T. W. Rall, *Mol. Pharmacol.* (1968) **4**, 367.
182. B. Weiss and E. Costa, *J. Pharmacol. Exp. Ther.* (1968) **161**, 310.
183. B. Weiss, *J. Pharmacol. Exp. Ther.* (1969) **166**, 330.
184. J. R. Turtle and D. M. Kipnis, *Biochem. Biophys. Res. Commun.* (1967) **28**, 797.

185. N. Haugaard and M. E. Hess, *Pharmacol. Rev.* (1965) 17, 27.
186. E. G. Krebs, R. J. DeLange, R. G. Kemp and W. D. Riley, *Pharmacol. Rev.* (1966) 18, 163.
187. E. Helmreich and C. F. Cori, *Pharmacol. Rev.* (1966) 18, 189.
188. E. W. Sutherland and W. D. Wosilait, *J. Biol. Chem.* (1956) 218, 459, 469.
189. T. W. Rall, E. W. Sutherland and W. D. Wosilait, *J. Biol. Chem.* (1956) 218, 483.
190. T. W. Rall, E. W. Sutherland and J. Berthet, *J. Biol. Chem.* (1957) 224, 463.
191. E. W. Sutherland and T. W. Rall, *J. Biol. Chem.* (1958) 232, 1065.
192. D. H. Brown and C. F. Cori, *in* "The Enzymes", Vol. 5 (eds P. D. Boyer, H. Lardy and K. Myrback) (1961). Academic Press, New York and London.
193. E. H. Fischer and E. G. Krebs, *Fed. Proc. Fed. Amer. Soc.* (1966) 25, 1511.
194. R. Caputto, H. S. Barra and F. A. Cumar, *Ann. Rev. Biochem.* (1967) 36, 213.
195. E. G. Krebs, A. B. Kent and E. H. Fischer, *J. Biol. Chem.* (1958) 231, 73.
196. D. A. Walsh, J. P. Perkins and E. G. Krebs, *J. Biol. Chem.* (1968) 243, 3763.
197. G. T. Cori and B. Illingworth, *Biochim. Biophys. Acta* (1956) 21, 105.
198. C. H. Davies, R. B. Olsgaard, E. H. Fischer and E. G. Krebs, *Fed. Proc. Fed. Amer. Proc.* (1964) 23, 488.
199. A. A. Yunis, E. H. Fischer and E. G. Krebs, *J. Biol. Chem.* (1962) 237, 2809.
200. E. Mohme-Lundholm, *Acta Physiol. Scand.* (1962) 54, 200.
201. E. Bueding, N. Kent and J. Fisher, *J. Biol. Chem.* (1964) 239, 2099.
202. E. Mohme-Lundholm, *Acta Physiol. Scand.* (1963) 59, 74.
203. G. I. Drummond, J. R. E. Valadares and L. Duncan, *in* "Muscle" (eds W. M. Paul, E. E. Daniel, C. M. Kay and G. Monckton) (1965). Pergamon Press, New York.
204. G. I. Drummond and L. Duncan, *J. Biol. Chem.* (1966) 241, 5893.
205. D. H. Namm, S. E. Mayer and M. Maltbie, *Mol. Pharmacol.* (1968) 4, 522.
206. S. E. Mayer, D. H. Namm and L. Rice, *Circ. Res.* (1970) 26, 225.
207. E. G. Krebs, D. J. Graves and E. H. Fischer, *J. Biol. Chem.* (1959) 234, 2807.
208. W. L. Meyer, E. H. Fischer and E. G. Krebs, *Biochemistry* (1964) 3, 1033.
209. R. B. Huston and E. G. Krebs, *J. Biol. Chem.* (1968) 7, 2116.
210. E. Ozawa, K. Hosoi and S. Ebashi, *J. Biochem.* (*Tokyo*) (1967) 61, 531.
211. A. J. D. Friesen, G. Allen and J. R. E. Valadares, *Science, N.Y.* (1967) 155, 1108.
212. S. E. Mayer, M. deV. Cotten and N. C. Moran, *J. Pharmacol. Exp. Ther.* (1963) 139, 275.
213. I. Øye, *Acta Physiol. Scand.* (1965) 65, 251.
214. J. R. Williamson and D. Jamieson, *Nature* (*London*) (1965) 206, 364.
215. W. Y. Cheung and J. R. Williamson, *Nature* (*London*) (1965) 207, 979.
216. G. I. Drummond, J. R. E. Valadares and L. Duncan, *Proc. Soc. Exp. Biol. Med.* (1964) 117, 307.
217. G. I. Drummond, L. Duncan and E. Hertzman, *J. Biol. Chem.* (1966) 241, 5899.
218. T. W. Rall and T. C. West, *J. Pharmacol. Exp. Ther.* (1963) 139, 269.
219. C. L. Skelton, G. S. Levey and S. E. Epstein, *Circ. Res.* (1970) 26, 35.
220. B. E. Sobel, P. D. Henry, A. Robison, C. Bloor and J. Ross, *Circ. Res.* (1969) 24, 507.
221. J. Shanfeld, A. Frazer and M. E. Hess, *Fed. Proc. Fed. Amer. Soc.* (1968) 27, 352.
222. J. Shanfeld, A. Frazer and M. E. Hess, *J. Pharmacol. Exp. Ther.* (1969) 169, 315.

223. J. Axelsson, E. Bueding and E. Bülbring, *J. Physiol.* (*London*) (1961) **156**, 357.
224. E. Bülbring, *in* "Adrenergic Mechanisms", a Ciba Foundation Symposium, (eds J. R. Vane, G. E. W. Wolstenholme and M. O'Connor) (1960). Little Brown, Boston.
225. A. R. Timms, E. Bueding, J. T. Hawkins and J. Fisher, *Biochem. J.* (1962) **84**, 80P.
226. E. Bueding, E. Bülbring, H. Kuriyama and G. Gercken, *Nature* (*London*) (1962) **196**, 944.
227. J. Diamond and T. M. Brody, *J. Pharmacol. Exp. Ther.* (1966) **152**, 202, 212.
228. T. M. Brody and J. Diamond, *Ann. N.Y. Acad. Sci.* (1967) **139**, 772.
229. E. Bueding, R. W. Butcher, J. Hawkins, A. R. Timms and E. W. Sutherland, *Biochim. Biophys. Acta* (1966) **115**, 173.
230. T. S. Kim, J. Shulman and R. A. Levine, *J. Pharmacol. Exp. Ther.* (1968) **163**, 36.
231. C. O. Watlington, *Comp. Biochem. Physiol.* (1968) **24**, 965.
232. C. O. Watlington, *Biochim. Biophys. Acta* (1969) **193**, 394.
233. J. Smith and J. Ireson, *Pharmacology* (1970) **3**, 155.
234. J. A. Hathaway and D. E. Atkinson, *J. Biol. Chem.* (1963) **238**, 2875.
235. D. E. Atkinson and G. M. Walton, *J. Biol. Chem.* (1967) **242**, 3239.
236. D. E. Atkinson, *Biochemistry* (1968) **7**, 4030.
237. L. C. Shen, L. Fall, G. M. Walton and D. E. Atkinson, *Biochemistry* (1968) **7**, 4041.
238. D. B. Stone and T. E. Mansour, *Mol. Pharmacol.* (1967) **3**, 177.

Chapter VII

THE NEUROTRANSMITTER—Ca++ LINKAGE IN MUSCLE CONTRACTION AND RELAXATION

INTRODUCTION

Previous chapters have presented fragmentary discussions of the various aspects of neurotransmitter action including the general relationships existing between chemical structure and biological activity, the various changes in membrane permeability and potential and the biochemical events initiated or modified by neurotransmitters, their analogs and antagonists. In this penultimate chapter it is necessary to consider the possible linkages existing between these events and the actual contractile or relaxant response of the muscle. However, in attempting such a synthesis several problems become immediately apparent: the molecular basis of the contractile process has been established primarily for skeletal muscle and, whilst they are probably fundamentally similar processes, the corresponding events in cardiac and smooth muscle are certainly less well defined. Furthermore, the nature of the linkage between the initial receptor interaction and the initiation of the contractile response appears to be significantly different in various muscle systems. Nevertheless, it is quite apparent that calcium represents the key component of this linkage in all muscle systems so far investigated.

In the following discussions the assumption will be made that the contractile machinery is basically identical in skeletal and vertebrate cardiac and smooth muscles and will thus be described first followed by separate discussions of the various mechanisms through which the neurotransmitters may regulate the activity of the contractile process. Several excellent reviews and symposia are available (1–11) of the contractile process and its regulation and these have been extensively employed in the preparation of this chapter.

THE CONTRACTILE SYSTEM

The structural organization of striated skeletal muscle reveals an array of partially overlapping actin and myosin filaments (Fig. VII-1).

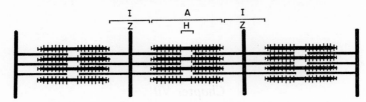

FIG. VII-1. Schematic representation (not to scale) of the structure of striated muscle depicting the overlapping actin and myosin filaments: the latter filaments show the cross bridges. Reproduced with permission from Huxley, (*Science, N.Y.* (1969) **164**, 1356). Copyright, 1969, by the American Association for the Advancement of Science.

According to the sliding filament hypothesis of muscle contraction first advanced in 1953 (12–14) and now almost universally accepted (9), shortening of striated muscle depends upon the relative sliding movements of the two filaments; the thicker filaments (diameter ~100 Å) are composed of parallel myosin molecules and the thinner actin filaments are composed of a linear polymeric array of globular actin molecules: cross-bridges, through which actin-myosin interactions occur, originate from the myosin filaments. The detailed X-ray studies by Huxley and Brown (15) of frog sartorius muscle reveal the helical arrangement of

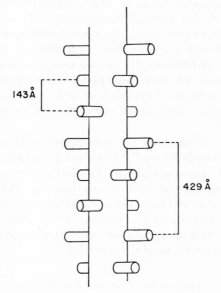

FIG. VII-2. Cross-bridge arrangement of myosin filaments on frog sartorius muscle. Reproduced with permission from Huxley, (*Science, N.Y.* (1969) **164**, 1356). Copyright, 1969, by the American Association for the Advancement of Science.

the cross-bridges with a pitch of 429 Å and a repeat of 143 Å (Fig. VII-2).

The interaction of the myosin cross-bridges with the corresponding binding sites on actin represents the basis of muscle contraction and tension development and the linked hydrolysis of ATP which provides the free energy and driving force of muscle contraction. Myosin itself has ATPase activity which is activated by low Ca^{++} and inhibited by Mg^{++}, but the combination with actin to yield actomyosin results in modification of the ATPase activity to a Mg^{++}-activated state. Neither

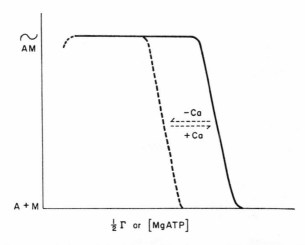

FIG. VII-3. Representation of the effect of ionic strength and MgATP concentration on the response of the contractile system: $\widetilde{AM}$ and A + M represent the contracted and relaxed states respectively. In the presence of the Ca^{++}-regulating factors (troponin and tropomyosin are present) the removal of Ca^{++} from the system causes a shift of the response to the left. Reproduced with permission from Ebashi, Endo and Ohtsuki (8).

myosin nor actin alone possess contractile activity but the addition of ATP to actomyosin results in a contractile state known as super-precipitation (16). Since ATP will cause contraction or relaxation of actomyosin depending upon the conditions of temperature, pH, ionic strength etc. (Fig. VII-3), actin, myosin and ATP constitute the minimum molecular requirements of a contractile-relaxant system. The principal properties of the actomyosin-Mg^{++}-ATP system may be summarized as follows (8):

(a) The interaction of actin and myosin in the presence of Mg^{++} and ATP corresponds to the contracting state in which ATP is converted to ADP.

(b) The absence of this interaction in the presence of Mg^{++} and ATP corresponds to the relaxing state.

The studies by Huxley (9, 15, 17) have provided considerable information about the mechanism by which actin and myosin interact in active contraction and in rigor, which develops in the absence of ATP. These studies reveal first that there is actually substantial disorder in the helical arrangement of the myosin cross bridges suggesting that they possess considerable mobility: furthermore, during rigor or active

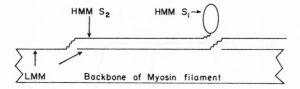

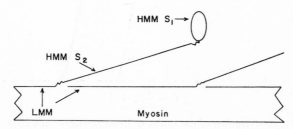

FIG. VII-4. Representation of the attachment of cross-bridges to myosin: the light meromyosin portion (LMM) is bonded into the main filament through a flexible linkage to the heavy meromyosin portion (HMM S_2): flexing at this position enables the globular portion (S_1) to attach to actin. Reproduced with permission from Huxley, (*Science*, N.Y. (1969) **164**, 1356). Copyright, 1969, by the American Association for the Advancement of Science.

contraction the pitch of the cross-bridges of myosin at 429 Å disappears and is replaced by one at 720 Å approximating very closely the helical pitch of the actin chains. However, the cross-bridge repeat of 143 Å remains virtually unchanged. Clearly, the actin-myosin interaction must take place with substantial rearrangement of the cross-bridge and Huxley and Brown (*loc. cit.*) have proposed a model of myosin in which the cross bridges are attached to the main myosin backbone by two flexible areas (known to be sensitive to proteolytic attack) as represented in Fig. VII-4. The flexible character of the cross bridges ensures that the globular heavy meromyosin portion, carrying the ATPase, can move around the circumference of the myosin backbone to interact with specific binding sites on the actin filaments. The most probable origin of the force-developing mechanism is the globular portion of the heavy meromyosin side chain: a mechanism proposed by Huxley to generate the relative sliding movement of action and myosin filaments and based on the above discussion of the mobility of the cross-bridges is shown in Fig. VII-5.

To what extent the geometry and mechanism of muscle contraction outlined above for striated muscle are relevant to other muscle systems

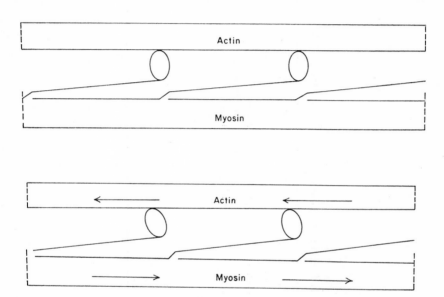

FIG. VII-5. Representation of filament sliding produced by cross-bridge tilting. Reproduced with permission from Huxley (9).

is not wholly established (18). Smooth muscle possesses, of course, well known special properties notably the ability to undergo very extensive shortening and to produce slowly developing and sustained contractions that are absent in striated muscle. There exist also significant structural differences between striated and various smooth muscle (Table VII-1): thus the structural barrier of the Z-column is replaced in smooth muscle by dense bodies, an arrangement which permits more extensive shortening and, furthermore, in many invertebrate smooth muscles the thick filaments are not kept in register and can double-overlap (18).

Double arrays of thick and thin filaments are well documented for invertebrate smooth muscle (for review see ref. 18); there is little doubt

TABLE VII-1. Structural Characteristics of Smooth Muscle (18)

Muscle type	Z-line structure	Thin filaments	Thick filaments	Example
Helical smooth or obliquely striated	Z-column or dense bodies	Actin (12)	Myosin and paramyosin	Earthworm body wall
Invertebrate smooth type I	Dense bodies	Actin (19)	Paramyosin	Anterior byssus retractor muscle of Mytilus
Invertebrate smooth type II	Dense bodies	Actin	Myosin	Pharynx retractor muscle of snail (18)
Vertebrate smooth muscle	Dense bodies	Actin (19, 20)	No thick filaments?	Uterus (21), guinea-pig taenia coli (20, 22–24), chicken gizzard (25)

that the thin filaments are actin but it is not established whether the thick filaments are identical to those from striated muscle or whether they represent some modification. For vertebrate smooth muscle there appears to be no general evidence supporting the existence of a double array of myosin and actin filaments (18, 19, 23, 25–27); an ordered actin array has been observed in the smooth muscle of the guinea-pig taenia coli (20). However, it is possible to obtain myosin filaments from extracted smooth muscle (18, 28, 29) which have properties similar to those from striated muscle, and recently, X-ray data has been provided to support the existence of myosin filaments in guinea-pig taenia coli (30). Furthermore, purified actin and myosin from vertebrate smooth muscle combine to form actomyosin (31, 32) which undergoes superprecipitation in the presence of ATP. Despite the observation that myosin from vertebrate smooth muscle has different composition and solubility properties from skeletal muscle myosin (18) it is probable that the underlying molecular mechanisms of contraction are basically similar in both smooth and skeletal muscle but that in vertebrate smooth muscle the myosin and actin are more highly dispersed (26).

CONTROL OF THE CONTRACTILE PROCESS

Many lines of evidence (for reviews see refs 6 and 8), some of which will be discussed in more detail later, suggest very convincingly that Ca^{++} represents the key controlling factor in the contractile process. However, the purified actin, myosin ATP and Mg^{++} system is not sensitive to Ca^{++} suggesting the absence of some factor or factors. As a result of the work of Ebashi and his colleagues (6, 8, 33–37) it has been

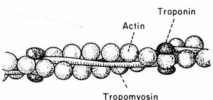

FIG. VII-6. A proposed arrangement of troponin and tropomyosin along the actin filament. Reproduced with permission from Ebashi, Endo and Ohtsuki (9).

established that the Ca^{++}-sensitivity of the actomyosin system is conferred by the presence of two additional proteins, troponin and tropomyosin. These two proteins are distributed along the actin filament with the troponin molecules being bound to tropomyosin which in turn is bound to actin: tropomyosin appears to serve the function of providing a binding environment for the troponin molecule. Several findings (7, 8,

38, 39) suggest an arrangement as shown in Fig. VII-6 in which the fibrous tropomyosin molecule is distributed along the actin chain with two troponin molecules bound at specific loci to tropomyosin.

Of the four proteins involved in the contractile machinery only troponin binds Ca^{++} reversibly at low concentrations (Table VII-2) with a

TABLE VII-2. Exchangeable Ca^{++} Bound to Proteins of Rabbit White Skeletal Muscle† (8)

Proteins	Bound Ca^{++} (moles/10^5 g)	Bound Ca^{++} (mole/mole)	Estimated % of bound Ca^{++} in myofibrils
Myosin	0·006	0·03	6
F-Actin	0·006	0·003	2
Tropomyosin	0·004	0·003	0
Troponin‡	1·78	0·89	87

† Ca^{++} at 3×10^{-6} M.
‡ Binding constants for Ca^{++}: $1\cdot3 \times 10^6$ M^{-1}, 5×10^4 M^{-1}.

binding constant in good accord with that determined from the relationship between Ca^{++} concentration and tension development as shown in Fig. VII-7. Furthermore, the data of Table VII-3 reveal that the sensitivity of contractile systems to Ca^{++} and Sr^{++} are exactly paralleled by the relative affinities of the corresponding isolated troponin systems to Ca^{++} and Sr^{++}.

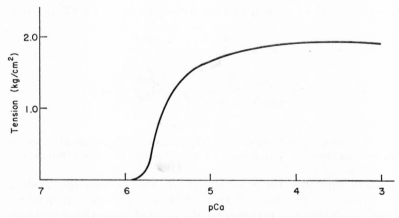

FIG. VII-7. Relationship between isometric tension and Ca^{++} concentration in skinned muscle fibers (Ionic conditions; 1/2 Γ = 015; 4 mM Mg, 4 mM ATP, 20 mM Trismaleate (pH 6·8) and 2 mM EGTA at 4°). Reproduced with permission from Ebashi, Endo and Ohtsuki (9).

TABLE VII-3. Sensitivities of Various Myosin B Preparations and Affinities of Troponins for Ca^{++} and Sr^{++} (8)

Protein	Sensitivity of contractile system to Sr^{++} (relative to Ca^{++})	Affinities of troponin Binding constants $\times 10^5$ M^{-1}		Relative to Ca^{++}
		Ca^{++}	Sr^{++}	
Myosin B (rabbit white skeletal)	1/34	10·2	0·39	1/26
Myosin B (rabbit red skeletal)	1/7	5·0	0·9	1/6
Myosin B (cardiac bovine)	1/5	3·4	1·2	1/3
Myosin B (chicken gizzard)	1/20	—	—	—

Thus troponin appears to be the Ca^{++}-receptive protein of the acto-myosin system and Ebashi and his colleagues have proposed a mechanism for the regulation by Ca^{++} of the actin-myosin interaction through the intermediacy of troponin. According to this model it is proposed that troponin acts through tropomyosin to inhibit the interaction of actin and myosin (Fig. VII-8): the binding of Ca^{++} to troponin serves, through derepression, to permit the actin-myosin interaction and removal of troponin-bound Ca^{++} serves to re-establish the inhibitory

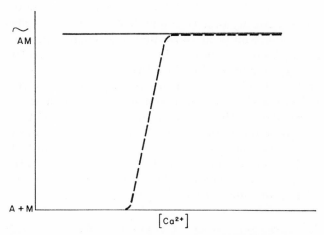

FIG. VII-8. Effect of Ca^{++} ions on the contractile response: solid line—response to actin and myosin: broken line—response to actin, myosin, tropomyosin and troponin. Reproduced with permission from Ebashi, Endo and Ohtsuki (9).

18

interaction and produce relaxation. Thus the troponin and tropo-myosin molecules are to be regarded as the allosteric site and allosteric linkage respectively for the binding of Ca^{++}, the effector ligand.

Some interesting supporting evidence for this proposal that the transmission of information lies in the sequence, $Ca^{++} \rightarrow$ troponin $\rightarrow$ tropomyosin $\rightarrow$ actin is derived from studies using spin-labels (40). Attachment of the maleimide label (VII-1) to tropomyosin, a procedure

VII-1

which did not affect the physiological effectiveness of tropomyosin, gave a mixture of strongly and weakly immobilized signals unaffected by Ca^{++}: addition of troponin and troponin plus actin gave a Ca^{++}-sensitive preparation in which Ca^{++} caused considerable enhancement of the signals from tightly bound labels. Moreover, the Ca^{++} sensitivity of this preparation paralleled that for the superprecipitation of the troponin-tropomyosin-actin-myosin system. The maleimide label attached to actin was insensitive to Ca^{++} save in the presence of relaxing protein (troponin + tropomyosin). Clearly, the attachment of Ca^{++} to troponin produces a conformational change which is transmitted to the fibrous tropomyosin and in turn transmitted to the adjacent actin monomers: the functional state of the actin determines whether or not combination will take place with myosin. Han and Benson (41) have also provided evidence for a Ca^{++}-induced conformational change in troponin from fluorescence emission studies which indicate a cooperative ($n_H = 4$) infolding of tryptophan residues into hydrophobic regions.

This extremely brief and rather superficial discussion of the molecular basis of the contractile process should serve to emphasize the key role of Ca^{++} in regulating this process. In relationship to the actions of neurotransmitters on various muscle types two questions are immediately apparent: how does the neurotransmitter control the access of Ca^{++} to this regulatory system and what is the source of this calcium? The following sections will discuss these questions with respect to skeletal, cardiac and smooth muscle systems.

EXCITATION-CONTRACTION COUPLING IN SKELETAL MUSCLE

Following the presentation of the general role of Ca^{++} in regulating the activity of the actomyosin contractile system attention is now turned to a more detailed discussion of this role in individual muscle systems with particular reference to the regulatory influences of the neurotransmitters, acetylcholine and norepinephrine, upon Ca^{++} mobilization and availability.

Excitation-contraction coupling in skeletal muscle has been reviewed by several authors (2, 4, 6–8, 42): the importance of the role of intracellular Ca^{++} in this process was first directly demonstrated by the experiments of Heilbrunn (43, 44) in which direct injection of Ca^{++} into muscle fibers produced contraction and subsequent work by Portzehl *et al.* (45) showed the extremely low concentrations ($\sim$10^{-6} M) of Ca^{++} that are effective in producing threshold contractions. Podolski and Constantin (46, 47) have been able to demonstrate contraction-relaxation sequences in the Natori "skinned" preparation (48) of skeletal muscle: repeated direct administration of low concentrations of Ca^{++} to the exposed myofibrils produces a cycle of contraction followed by relaxation. Clearly, the cycle of events is produced by the presence of a Ca^{++} concentrating mechanism which serves to continuously reduce the Ca^{++} level to below the threshold concentration necessary for contraction. Considerable evidence now exists that the level of intracellular Ca^{++} is regulated through the sarcoplasmic reticuluum which constitutes part of an internal membranous system (Fig. VII-9) consisting of two distinct divisions; the sarcoplasmic reticuluum which is a longitudinal arrangement of irregularly shaped cisternae enveloping individual myofibrils and the transverse tubules (T-System) which originate at the cell membrane. The transverse tubules end in a pair of lateral sacs, the whole constituting the so called "triads," which are continuous with the sarcoplasmic reticuluum (2, 49). The sarcoplasmic reticuluum in the intact muscle or as microsomal or vesicular preparations possesses a remarkable ability to accumulate Ca^{++} and so reduce the level of free Ca^{++} to 10^{-8} M or less (6, 50, 51).†

Of particular relevance to an understanding of the linkage between membrane excitation and the level of intracellular Ca^{++} are well documented findings that the primary site of Ca^{++} localization is in the lateral sacs (52): the proximity of these latter structures to the transverse tubules through which the membrane depolarization is transmitted (p. 510) suggests that this is the site from which Ca^{++} is released in the contraction-triggering process (2, 52, 53). Further support for this proposal is derived from Winegrad's findings (54, 55) that in resting

---

† The mechanism by which the Ca^{++} is accumulated by the sarcoplasmic reticuluum has not been established completely (6). Ca^{++} is apparently first bound to the membrane and is then transported into the lumen: ATP appears to be absolutely essential to the initial binding and the transport may be associated with the breakdown, by an ATPase, of this ATP.

frog skeletal muscle the Ca^{++} is located principally in the lateral sacs, i.e., at the center of the I bands but that in contracting muscle considerable Ca^{++} is found spread along the A band of the myofibrils.

The elegant studies of A. F. Huxley and his colleagues and H. E. Huxley (56–59) employing highly localized depolarizations of skeletal muscle membranes have revealed that the only loci at which depolarizations are effective in causing localized contractures correspond to the

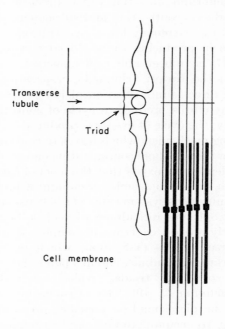

Fig. VII-9. Diagrammatic representation of a portion of frog skeletal muscle fiber. Reproduced with permission from Huxley, (*Science, N.Y.* (1969) **164**, 1356). Copyright, 1969, by the American Association for the Advancement of Science.

location of the triad structure where the transverse tubule extends from the interior to the surface membrane. Thus in frog fast muscle the active patches are distributed around the region of the Z line: the situation is, however, quite different in frog "slow" (tonic fibers) that respond to stimulation with contractures rather than twitches; these fibers possess multiple innervation (Chapter V, p. 402) and do not contain the specialized loci of electrical stimulation found in the twitch fibers.

Many lines of evidence indicate rather clearly that the transverse tubules and the sarcoplasmic reticuluum constitute a functional connection between the membrane and the contractile system (2, 6, 8, 60–62).

The probable sequence of events in this coupling process may be listed as follows (6):

(1) Generation of the endplate potential by acetylcholine.

(2) Initiation of action potential by the endplate potential.

(3) Propagation of the action potential and its spread through the transverse tubules.

(4) Release of Ca^{++} from the sarcoplasmic reticuluum.

(5) Diffusion of Ca^{++} and binding to troponin.

(6) Reaction of the derepressed actin-myosin contractile system.

However much of the underlying molecular basis of these events remains to be determined. Several proposals have been made to account for the spread of depolarizing current down the transverse tubular system (2, 56, 57, 63): at the present time, it does not appear possible to distinguish between electrotonic or regenerative mechanisms for the spread of depolarization. Similarly, the mechanism of release of Ca^{++} from the sarcoplasmic reticuluum remains undefined, although it appears probable that the transverse tubules and the lateral sacs of the sarcoplasmic reticuluum are electrically coupled and that depolarization of the lateral sac membranes results in the release of Ca^{++}. Quite probably this latter process represents the limiting step of the entire sequence of events listed previously. It is well established that the development of maximum tension takes some 40–75 msec whereas the spread of excitation down the transverse tubules can take no more than a few msec. Jöbsis and O'Connor (64) have measured simultaneously changes in intracellular Ca^{++} (by means of the absorption spectrum of the Ca^{++}-murexide complex) and tension development; their data reveal (Fig. VII-10) that the Ca^{++} signal reaches a maximum some 55 msec after the initial stimulus at which time the tension has only reached 20% of the peak value and that at the time of peak tension virtually no free intracellular Ca^{++} remains.†

The source of the calcium involved in skeletal muscle has been the subject of considerable discussion since, during contraction there are increases in both Ca^{++} influx and efflux (66–71). There is little doubt, however, that this Ca^{++} influx cannot be the sole course of Ca^{++} concerned with the contractile mechanism, for the amount entering is far too low to satisfy the Ca^{++} requirements (2, 72). Bianchi and Shanes (67) determined that the Ca^{++} entry during a single twitch of the frog sartorious muscle is $0 \cdot 2 \times 10^{-12}$ moles/cm² which Sandow has calculated (2) to give an intracellular concentration of 8×10^{-8} M, a concentration

---

† A study by Ashley and Ridgway (65) with simultaneous recording of membrane potential, Ca^{++} concentration and tension in single muscle fibers from the barnacle reveals very nicely the sequence of events—depolarization → increased Ca^{++} (free) → increased tension.

some tenfold less than that required for even threshold activation. Presumably this Ca^{++} entry is associated with the depolarizing currents of the action potential. Nevertheless, the contraction of fast skeletal muscle is dependent upon the availability of extracellular Ca^{++}: Frank (73, 74) has shown that removal of extracellular Ca^{++} abolishes the contractile activity of amphibian and mammalian skeletal muscle to potassium depolarization but not to caffeine an agent that induces contraction through mobilization of intracellular Ca^{++} (75, 76). An

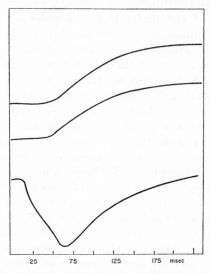

FIG. VII-10. Time relationships in the development of tension (upper trace), light scattering (middle trace) and the formation of the Ca^{++}-murexide complex (bottom trace) in the toad sartorius muscle. Reproduced with permission from Jöbsis and O'Connor (64).

explanation of this role of extracellular Ca^{++} is probably to be found in its function as a membrane stabilizer (Chapter II, p. 164). In the original studies of Hodgkin and Horowicz (77) the relationship between membrane potential and tension in K^+-induced contractures of single muscle fibers was shown to be a steep sigmoid curve and Lüttgau (78) has shown that the shape and position of this curve is dependent upon the Ca^{++} concentration (Fig. VII-11). The mechanical threshold potential is altered from about -60 mV at normal Ca^{++} to -20 mV at 5·0 mM Ca^{++}: in Ca^{++}-free solutions a significant drop in resting potential is observed of some 10–30 mV within a few minutes suggesting that the loss of K^+-induced contractures is related to the reduction in membrane resting potential (79). Edman and Grieve (80) also noted that the decline in membrane potential coincided with the loss of electrically produced contractions. This view is strengthened by several findings that fibers which are unresponsive to high K⁺ in Ca⁺⁺-free media become responsive upon the application of hyperpolarizing stimuli (79, 81). The effect of Ca⁺⁺ lack upon the mechanical responsiveness of fast skeletal muscle is thus the result of a decline in membrane potential and a simultaneous shift of the sigmoid curve relating membrane potential and response towards the hyperpolarized condition and is probably not

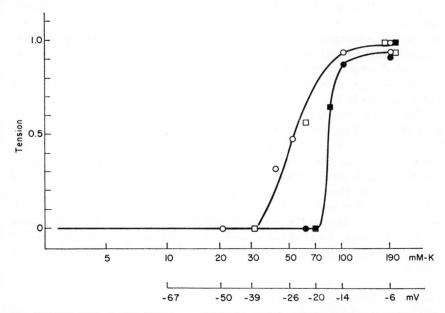

FIG. VII-11. Effect of Ca⁺⁺ upon peak tension and depolarization produced by K⁺. Open symbols, 1·8 and filled symbols, 5·0 mM Ca⁺⁺ respectively. (Circles, 65 μ diameter, squares 70 μ diameter iliofibularis muscle). Reproduced with permission from Lüttgau (78).

indicative of any requirement of the contractile process for extra-cellular Ca⁺⁺. As will be noted, however, in subsequent sections this conclusion may not be generalized to other muscle systems, notably smooth muscle, where a definite requirement for the activation of the contractile machinery by extracellular Ca⁺⁺ appears to exist. Similarly, it will be noted that the role of acetylcholine in excitation-contraction coupling in skeletal muscle, although essential, is but distantly related to any Ca⁺⁺ (intracellular) process: for smooth muscle systems, however, the relationship between the neurotransmitters and Ca⁺⁺ mobilization appears to be rather more intimate.

Excitation-Contraction Coupling in Cardiac Muscle

As with skeletal muscle Ca^{++} represents the link between excitatory events at the cell membrane and the contractile machinery in cardiac muscle. It seems fairly clear (for review see Katz, 82) that regulation of the actin-myosin interaction is through the Ca^{++}-troponin-tropomyosin system extending inward from the Z-line (83), although this system appears less plentiful than in skeletal twitch muscle (84). There exists also in cardiac muscle a well defined sarcoplasmic reticuluum, although most workers agree (82, 83, 85, 86) that is only about 30–50% as extensive as the corresponding system in skeletal muscle: however, cardiac sarcoplasmic reticuluum does appear to have approximately the same Ca^{++}-binding properties and capacity as its skeletal muscle counterpart (82, 86–89). There is also some evidence for the possible involvement of mitochondria in Ca^{++} accumulation and release (89, 90).

The major differences between skeletal and cardiac muscle appear to lie in the coupling mechanisms between membrane excitation and muscle contraction. In skeletal muscle it is well established that the transverse tubules serve as the channels through which electrical excitation is carried inwards to the calcium storage system. It is not fully established to what extent the mechanism is operative in cardiac muscle since these cells are smaller and the rate of contraction much slower than twitch skeletal fibers. Hence the criticism offered by Hill (91) that the time-course of events in skeletal muscle does not permit for diffusion of activating Ca^{++} from an extracellular source is not valid for cardiac muscle.

ORIGIN OF Ca^{++} FOR THE CONTRACTILE PROCESS

It has been established for many years that the contractile activity of cardiac muscle is critically dependent upon the concentration of Ca^{++}_{ext} (76, 92, 93) and several sets of experiments have shown that Ca^{++} influx increases during contraction. In an extensive study of the association between Ca^{++} fluxes and contractile activity in guinea-pig atria Winegrad and Shanes (94) showed that there is a resting Ca^{++} influx unaccompanied by net uptake and that there exists a linear proportionality between the strength of contraction and the uptake of Ca^{++} (Fig. VII-12). From these studies Winegrad and Shanes calculate that the Ca^{++} influx during depolarization increases by a factor of 250 to give a maximum increment of 0.6×10^{-9} moles/g of cardiac muscle. Since it may be calculated (82) that approximately 60×10^{-9} moles of Ca^{++} are needed to achieve full activation of the contractile proteins of cardiac muscle it seems clear that extracellular Ca^{++} cannot represent the sole source of the Ca^{++}

required for contraction and that intracellular Ca^{++}, as in skeletal muscle, is of critical importance.

Considerable effort has been expended in attempts to identify the intracellular Ca^{++} involved. A number of workers have studied Ca^{++} exchange processes in cardiac muscle and have attempted to generate a correlation between contractile activity and the observed parameters of Ca^{++} exchange (95). Langer (96–98) has resolved Ca^{++} exchange in the canine papillary muscle into five, kinetically distinct, components

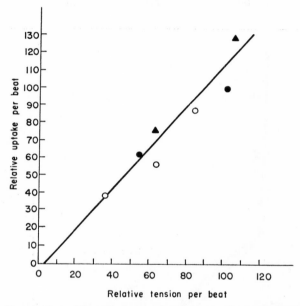

FIG. VII-12. Correlation of Ca^{++} influx and twitch tension per beat in guinea-pig atria ○, 1·25 mM Ca^{++}, 15 and 30 beats/min; ●, 2·5 mM Ca^{++}, 15 and 30 beats/min; ▲, 3·75 mM Ca^{++}, 6 and 15 beats/min. Reproduced with permission from Winegrad and Shanes (94).

(Table VII-4): four of these processes are shown in Fig. VII-13 (component 4 which is not shown here represents very slowly exchangeable and inexchangeable Ca^{++} and appear to have no direct relationship to the activation of the contractile process). Figure VII-13 shows that component 2 (characterized by a time of half exchange $t_{1/2} = 6{\cdot}0$ min) is directly related to tension development since the decline of the latter is directly proportional to the loss of this component and is apparently unaffected by the loss of components 1 and 3. In the isolated cat heart Bailey and Dresel (99) have identified Ca^{++} efflux as characteristic of a three compartment system (Fig. VII-14). Since the kinetics of loss of

18*

TABLE VII-4. Kinetic and Binding Characteristics of Calcium Exchange in Dog Papillary Muscle (96, 97)

Kinetic phase	Rate constant min^{-1}	$t_{1/2}$ exchange min	% Tissue calcium	Probable origin
0	3·5	0·2	4	Vascular
1	0·59	1·2	2·5	Interstitial
2	0·116	6·0	25	Sarcotubular (?)
3	0·021	33	25	Intracellular
4	0·004	170	<20	Connect. tissue, intracellular

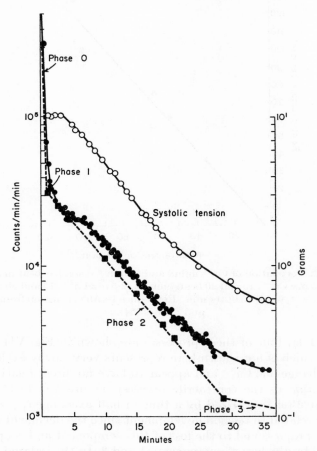

FIG. VII-13. Components of $^{45}Ca^{++}$ efflux from dog papillary muscle and simultaneous loss of systolic tension. Reproduced from Langer (97) with permission of the author and the American Heart Association, Inc.

Ca^{++} from compartment II and the decay of contractile force are identical and since the absolute Ca^{++} concentration of this compartment and the contractile force are closely related it appears that this intracellular store of Ca^{++} is directly involved in the activation of the contractile process. (It should be noted that the rate of loss of Ca^{++} ($k_1 = 0.962$ min^{-1}) from the compartment considered by Bailey and Dresel (*loc. cit.*)

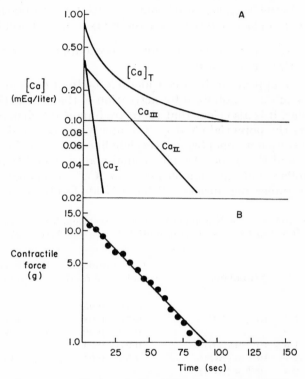

FIG. VII-14. Compartmental analysis of Ca^{++} washout (A) from cat heart ([Ca]$_T$ = total calcium and [Ca]$_I$, [Ca]$_{II}$ and [Ca]$_{III}$ represent calcium concentrations in kinetically defined compartments), and loss of contractile force (B). Reproduced with permission from Bailey and Dresel (99).

to be associated with the contractile process is considerably faster than that obtained by Langer (*loc. cit.*) and Teiger and Farah (100). However, Bailey and Dresel determined Ca^{++} loss into a zero-Ca^{++} medium rather than under steady state conditions. It seems quite probable that all three compartments may well be the same). There is provisional evidence available that the morphological location of this Ca^{++} compartment is the sarcoplasmic reticuluum (98, 101).

The linkage between this store of intracellular Ca^{++} and ionic and potential events at the membrane surface is not defined with any degree of certainty. However, Langer (95, 97, 98) has proposed that the calcium release is related to the temporary increase of Na_{int}^{+} produced by the depolarizing phase of the action potential. The increased level of Na_{int}^{+} is presumed to cause release of Ca^{++} from the sarcoplasmic reticuluum (95, 97, 98, 102, 103) and subsequent activation of the contractile mechanism. As the Na_{int}^{+} is pumped out (95, 104) Ca^{++} will be reaccumulated by the sarcoplasmic reticuluum and relaxation will occur.

THE INFLUENCES OF NOREPINEPHRINE, ACETYLCHOLINE AND THEIR ANALOGS ON Ca^{++} EXCHANGE

Whilst there appears to be a considerable body of evidence that the major source of Ca^{++} mobilized for activation of the contractile process is intracellular, it is also clear that there are important changes in Ca^{++} influx during the potential changes (Chapter V, p. 424) and that these are influenced by norepinephrine, acetylcholine and related agents.

Grossman and Furchgott (105) have analysed the comparative effects of acetylcholine and norepinephrine upon Ca^{++} exchange and contractility in guinea-pig auricles (Table VII-5). Reuter (106, 107) has

TABLE VII-5. Influence of Norepinephrine and Acetylcholine on the Uptake of $^{45}Ca^{++}$ in Electrically Stimulated Guinea-Pig Atria (105)

Rate beats/min	Stimulant	Ca^{++} uptake (μmole/kg/5 min)	Relative contraction amplitude
6	—	0.51 ± 0.05	22 ± 4.0
6	1.6×10^{-6} M (NE)	0.71 ± 0.08	131 ± 14
60	—	0.89 ± 0.02	88 ± 4
60	1.6×10^{-6} M (NE)	0.97 ± 0.04	182 ± 2.8
60	2.4×10^{-6} M (ACh)	0.56 ± 0.04	18 ± 2
60	2.4×10^{-6} M (ACh)+		
60	3×10^{-6} M (atropine)	0.95 ± 0.04	89 ± 4

also compared the effects of sympathomimetic amines on contractility and Ca^{++} uptake in this preparation and has described a generally parallel relationship between the effects of these agents on contractility and their ability to promote Ca^{++} uptake. These effects of acetylcholine and norepinephrine may be related to the inward Ca^{++}-current phase of depolarization (Chapter V, p. 427).

A number of studies have been concerned with the modulating influence of the external ionic concentrations upon the actions of norepinephrine (i.e. 108–112). An increase in the concentration of

Ca$_{ext}^{++}$ brings about an absolute increase but a *relative* decrease in the contractile tension of rat ventricle induced by norepinephrine or Ca$_{ext}^{++}$ (Fig. VII-15). An increase in the concentration of Na$_{ext}^{+}$ markedly reduced the absolute increase in contractile tension although norepinephrine and Ca$_{ext}^{++}$ produce relatively greater tension increases in high Ca$_{ext}^{++}$ media (Fig. VII-16). These data confirm the generally recognized competition between Na^{+} and Ca^{++} at excitable membranes. The implications with regard to the inotropic actions of epinephrine and Ca^{++} are, however, not entirely clear. On the one hand it could be argued

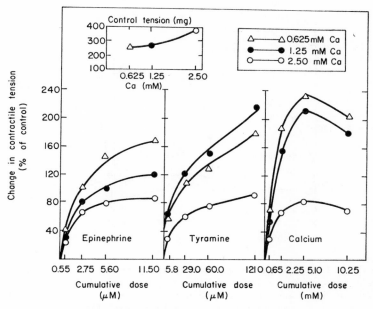

FIG. VII-15. Effects of Ca^{++} concentration on contractile force developed by rat ventricle strips in response to epinephrine, tyramine and calcium. The inset figure shows the effect of Ca^{++} concentration upon base-line tension. In the full figure the increase in contractile force is shown as a percentage of control tension. Reproduced with permission from Dhalla and Braxton (111).

that the interaction of norepinephrine with the receptor is a Ca^{++}-dependent phenomenon being antagonized by high concentrations of Ca$_{ext}^{++}$; on the other hand it could be argued that the relative inotropic effects of norepinephrine become progressively reduced with increased Ca$_{ext}^{++}$ because the latter species alone is able to generate the maximum inotropic response (111–113). Furthermore, despite the findings that epinephrine and Ca^{++} both increase Ca^{++} exchanges and contractile tension it is apparent that they do so by different mechanisms since the effects of epinephrine are antagonized by propranolol while those of Ca^{++} are unaffected (111). A further important difference between Ca^{++} and norepinephrine lies in the findings that the responses to norepinephrine are dependent upon the integrity of metabolic processes and are abolished by iodoacetate, dinitrophenol, fluorodinitrobenzene whilst the responses to Ca^{++} are unaffected. It thus seems plausible that the

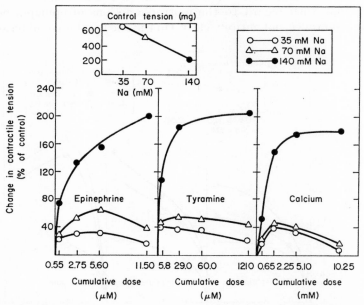

FIG. VII-16. Effects of Na^+ concentration on contractile force developed by rat ventricle strips in response to epinephrine, tyramine and calcium. The inset shows the effect of Na^+ concentration upon base-line tension. Reproduced with permission from Dhalla and Braxton (111).

effects of Ca^{++} and epinephrine, whilst related, are achieved through different mechanisms. In particular the relationships of epinephrine to the activation of adenyl cyclase must be considered (Chapter VI, p. 476).

EXCITATION-CONTRACTION COUPLING IN SMOOTH MUSCLE

Despite the obvious differences between smooth and skeletal muscle, most notably the small size of the smooth muscle cells and the general absence of any well developed sarcoplasmic reticuluum (uterine smooth muscle appears to be exceptional in this regard, 114) and transverse tubule system, it appears highly probable that the molecular events underlying contraction are fundamentally the same in both systems in that the concentration of intracellular Ca^{++} regulates the degree of activation of the contractile process. However, the mechanisms through which events at the cell membrane receptors are coupled to the Ca^{++}-mobilization process appear to be substantially different in the two systems; smooth muscle appears to use a more direct coupling mechanism.

In a number of smooth muscles (Chapter V, p. 430) there appears to be a normal dissociation of contractile and electrical events: furthermore, such dissociation can be readily achieved in other smooth muscles by the use of preparations depolarized in high K^+ media in which stimulant agents continue to produce their normal responses (115–120). However, it must be noted that in K^+-depolarized preparations there can be little doubt that the membrane is at least quantitatively distinct from the polarized cell membrane. It must also be noted, as emphasized in Chapter V, that smooth muscles are not a particularly homogeneous group and that some caution is required in extrapolating data from, for example, intestinal smooth muscle to vascular smooth muscle.

However, regardless of the type of smooth muscle under consideration the identical questions may be posed: what is the source(s) of the Ca^{++} involved in the activation of the contractile process and what is the coupling mechanism between this source(s) and the neurotransmitter-receptor interaction?

ORIGIN OF Ca^{++} FOR THE CONTRACTILE PROCESS

There is ample evidence that Ca^{++} influx and efflux increase during smooth muscle contraction, regardless of whether this is caused by neurotransmitters or K^+-depolarization (116, 121–133). Thus, Briggs and Melvin (122) observed that epinephrine ($1 \cdot 5 \times 10^{-5}$ M) doubled and K^+-depolarization almost tripled Ca^{++} influx into rabbit aortic strips. Many studies have also revealed considerable dependence of smooth muscle contraction, most pronounced for K^+-induced contractions, upon the concentrations of Ca_{ext}^{++} (116, 117–119, 134–142) and it is quite clear that Ca_{ext}^{++} plays an important role in the regulation of smooth muscle contractility.

To what extent intracellular and extracellular Ca^{++} sources are directly involved in the activation of the contractile mechanism cannot be stated definitively at the present time. There appears, however, to be quite convincing evidence that Ca_{int}^{++} and Ca_{ext}^{++} represent two quite distinct sources of Ca^{++}; norepinephrine, acetylcholine and their analogs appear to employ primarily Ca_{int}^{++} and K^+-induced responses to employ primarily Ca_{ext}^{++}.

The evidence that neurotransmitters activate an intracellular Ca^{++} source is derived essentially from findings that the contractile responses

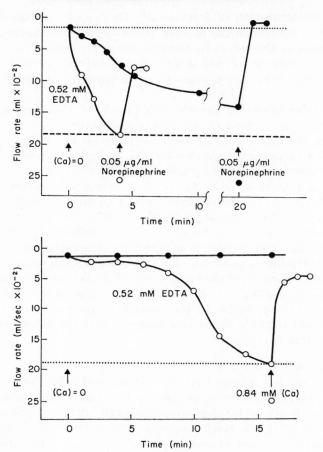

Fig. VII-17. A. Effect of Ca^{++}-free (●) and zero Ca^{++} (○) perfusion of rat tail ventral artery contracted by high K^+ (51 mM) at 37°. Upper dashed line signifies continual response in the presence of 2·1 mM Ca^{++}. Arrows indicate start of experiment and the addition of norepinephrine. B. Effect of Ca^{++} media on the response of artery to norepinephrine (0·05 μg/ml). Reproduced with permission from Hinke (144).

to these agents are maintained, albeit for varying periods of time, in Ca^{++}-free media,† whilst the responses to K^+ are but briefly maintained in Ca^{++}-free media.

Thus, Hurwitz and his co-workers (136) have shown that the response

---

† A careful distinction is to be made between Ca^{++}-free media which are physiological salines without added Ca^{++} and zero-Ca^{++} media in which Ca^{++}-chelating agents are present and where the effective Ca^{++} concentration is much lower than the 10^{-5}–10^{-6} M present in Ca^{++}-free media.

of intestinal smooth muscle to acetylcholine is maintained for some
30–60 min in Ca^{++}-free media: frog stomach muscle remains responsive
to acetylcholine for several hours in similar conditions (140). As other
representative examples, Fig. VII-17 shows the loss of response to
norepinephrine and K$^+$ in the rat tail ventral artery (144) and Fig.
VII-18 the relative loss of response of rat uterus to acetylcholine and
K$^+$: the differential loss of sensitivity of rat uterus to K$^+$ and acetyl-

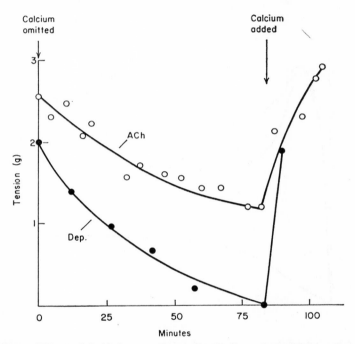

FIG. VII-18. Effect of Ca^{++}-free media on the decline of sensitivity of rat uterus
to acetylcholine (ACh) and K$_2$SO$_4$-depolarization (Dep.). Reproduced with
permission from Edman and Schild (117).

choline has been noted by several workers (117, 145, 146). Rabbit ear
blood vessels remain responsive to norepinephrine for 3–4 h in Ca^{++}-free
media (140) and bovine mesenteric arteries are quite remarkable in
remaining sensitive to norepinephrine for several days (147) whilst K$^+$
sensitivity is lost more rapidly.

Several other lines of evidence also indicate that different sources of
Ca^{++} are employed by neurotransmitters and K$^+$. Schild has demonstrated that K$^+$-depolarized smooth muscle will respond in zero Ca^{++}
media both to Ca$_{ext}^{++}$ and to norepinephrine and acetylcholine. Figure
VII-19 compares the response of depolarized rat uterus to Ca^{++} and to

acetylcholine: there are substantial differences in the responses elicited by these two agents, that due to acetylcholine being more rapid and less well sustained. Furthermore, the effects of the two agents when administered simultaneously are clearly independent and additive indicating that the mechanisms through which acetylcholine and Ca_{ext}^{++} activate the contractile mechanism are different. Similar studies with the depolarized rat seminal vesicle (119) reveal also (Fig. VII-20) that

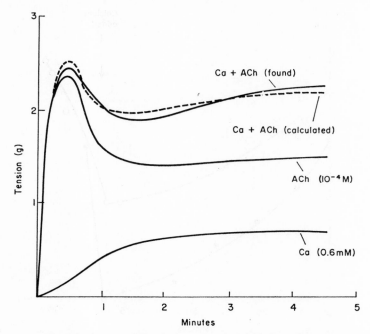

FIG. VII-19. Additivity of effects of calcium and acetylcholine in K_2SO_4-depolarized rat uterus at 24°. Upper dotted line shows calculated additivity. Reproduced with permission from Edman and Schild (117).

the effects of Ca_{ext}^{++}, norepinephrine and acetylcholine are independent and quite distinct in duration and magnitude.

Hinke has also provided (135, 144) evidence for the different Ca^{++} requirements of K^+ and norepinephrine-induced contractions in the ventral artery of the rat tail, in which complete loss of response to norepinephrine and to K^+ results in zero-Ca^{++} media. Restoration of responses can be achieved through perfusion with solutions of increasing Ca^{++} concentration and Fig. VII-21 shows the dependence of response on the Ca^{++} concentration: the magnitude of the K^+-induced contraction is linearly related to $\log[Ca_{ext}^{++}]$ but the magnitude of the response to norepinephrine shows a very steep initial response between 0·5 and 0·75 mM Ca_{ext}^{++}. A further difference in the responses of this system is revealed by the finding that a reduction in the concentration of Na_{ext}^{+} does not alter the ability of Ca^{++} to restore the response to norepinephrine but markedly reduces the magnitude of the K^{+}-induced response.

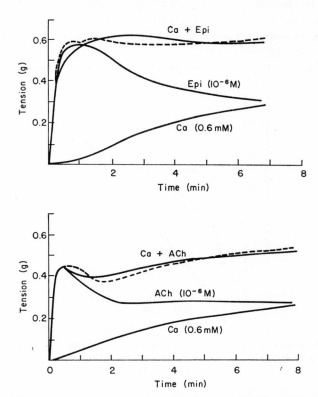

FIG. VII-20. Additivity of effects of calcium and acetylcholine and calcium and epinephrine in the K_2SO_4-depolarized rat uterus. Upper dotted line shows calculated additivity. Reproduced with permission from Edman and Schild (117).

Apparently, neurotransmitters in smooth muscle mobilize a largely intracellular store of Ca^{++} for the activation of the contractile process and several attempts have been made to define more precisely the characteristics of this store. Feinstein and his colleagues (146) have studied $^{45}Ca^{++}$ efflux into zero-Ca^{++} media from preloaded rat uterine muscle: three distinct components of Ca^{++} release were found with $t_{1/2}$'s of 4, 135 and 107 min, these being associated with free and bound Ca_{ext}^{++} and Ca_{int}^{++} respectively. The latter phase accounts for some 35–40%

of the total tissue Ca^{++}. Contractions were induced in this preparation with K^+, acetylcholine and alternating current field stimulation. The response to K^+ was lost quite rapidly ($t_{1/2}$ 29 min) but the responses to acetylcholine were lost more slowly ($t_{1/2} = 72$ min) suggesting that acetylcholine utilizes largely the intracellular Ca^{++} pool. Figure VII-22 compares the loss of response to field stimulation with the loss of Ca^{++}: it is noteworthy that a loss in response to field stimulation only occurs after a lag of some 20–30 min and almost all of the loss of response coincides with the loss of Ca^{++}_{int}.

In studies of $^{45}Ca^{++}$ distribution in rabbit aortic strips Hudgins and

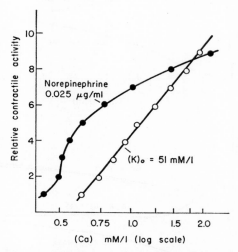

FIG. VII-21. Dependence of norepinephrine and K^+-induced contractions in rat tail ventral artery upon Ca^{++} concentration. Reproduced with permission from Hinke (144).

Weiss (148) have shown that efflux from preloaded strips is a biphasic process with $t_{1/2}$'s of 8 and 105 min for the fast and slow components. The fast process presumably represents loosely and interstitially bound Ca^{++} and the slow process, intracellular Ca^{++}: this latter fraction appears quite readily exchangeable with extracellular Ca^{++}. In a comparison of the effects of norepinephrine, histamine and K^+ upon the contractility and Ca^{++} efflux in this system it is found (20), in common with other tissues, that the responses to histamine, and more particularly norepinephrine, decline relatively slowly in Ca^{++}-free media: in contrast K^+ (25 mM) was unable to induce contractions under these conditions. Whilst there is not complete agreement between the half-times for loss of response and loss of Ca^{++} from the slow component the results do suggest that the latter component is that mobilized by norepinephrine: histamine may use both intra- and extra-cellular sources of Ca^{++}.

Hurwitz and his colleagues (136, 141, 149), working with the longitudinal muscle of the guinea-pig ileum, have shown that preloading of the tissue by exposure to a Ca^{++}-rich medium and subsequent immersion in a zero-Ca^{++} media induces a contraction. The time course of the loss

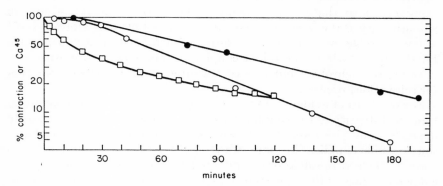

FIG. VII-22. Relationship between ^{45}Ca^{++}-washout and AC field-induced contractions of rat uterus at 21°: □—□, loss of Ca^{++}; ○—○, loss of response of muscles stimulated for 1 sec every 2 min; ●—●, stimulated only at times indicated. Reproduced with permission from Feinstein, Paimre and Lee (146).

of this contraction yields, with the assumption that the loss of response is a hyperbolic function of the concentration of Ca^{++} in an intracellular store,

$$K \frac{R}{R_T - R} = [\text{Ca}_{int}^{++}] \qquad \text{I}$$

where R_T is the maximum response attainable when the intracellular store is fully loaded and K is a proportionality constant. The loss of Ca^{++} from the muscle may be described by,

$$\ln [\text{Ca}^{++}]^t = -kt + \ln [\text{Ca}_{int}^{++}]^0 \qquad \text{II}$$

where $[\text{Ca}_{int}^{++}]^0$ is the initial concentration of stored calcium. Hence

$$\ln K \frac{R}{R_T - R} = -kt + \ln K \frac{R_0}{R_T - R_0} \qquad \text{III}$$

and a plot of $\ln R / R_T - R$ against time yields a straight line of slope $-kt$ ($k = 0.14$ min^{-1}). Comparison of the rates of efflux of ^{45}Ca^{++} from this preparation show two components: the rate constant for the fast component of Ca^{++} efflux ($k = 0.13$ min^{-1}) is in good accord with the rate of loss of the contractile response and Hurwitz and Joiner (149) propose that this component is critical for the development of tension.

NATURE OF THE COUPLING MECHANISM

It appears highly probable that norepinephrine and acetylcholine mobilize an essentially intracellular store of Ca^{++} to activate the contractile process. The location of this store remains undetermined; however, since there is, in general, little sarcoplasmic reticuluum in smooth muscle the very real possibility exists that this store of Ca^{++} is bound to the inner membrane surface. Such location would provide for the apparently rather direct coupling in many smooth muscle cells between the neurotransmitter-receptor interaction and the contraction (or relaxation) process.

Several lines of evidence point, at least tentatively, to the conclusion that the integrity of the coupling mechanism in smooth muscle actually depends upon the integrity of two sources of Ca^{++}: an intracellular source which supplies the major fraction of the Ca^{++} actually needed to activate the contractile process and a much smaller source bound to the external surface of the membrane and which stands in a special relationship to the neurotransmitter recognition site (receptor). These two fractions may be linked so that removal of Ca^{++} from the membrane site promotes mobilization of intracellular Ca^{++}. Daniel has provided (150–153) several discussions which explicitly emphasize the roles of two Ca^{++} binding sites.

Daniel and Irwin (154) have shown in rat uterine muscle that Na_4EDTA produces contractions with a threshold concentration of approximately 3 mM and with maximum contractions being observed at concentrations of 5–10 mM. In marked contrast EGTA, which has a significantly higher affinity for Ca^{++} than Mg^{++}, fails to produce contractions unless Mg^{++} is removed from the incubation medium. Since the concentrations of Na_4EDTA necessary to induce maximum contraction are greater than the total $Ca^{++} + Mg^{++}$ concentration it appears that both Ca^{++} and Mg^{++} need to be removed from the extracellular environment: however, removal of Mg_{ext}^{++} alone does not induce contractions. Since the contractions produced by these chelating species cannot be produced by influx of Ca_{ext}^{++} Daniel and Irwin propose that their mode of action is the removal of Ca^{++} from the external membrane surface which, in turn, is presumed to mobilize Ca_{int}^{++}. Of particular interest is the finding that threshold concentrations of Na_4EDTA very significantly reduce the contractile effects of acetylcholine: the binding and/or activity of acetylcholine apparently require the presence of membrane-bound Ca^{++}. This latter fraction of Ca^{++} may be rather tightly bound for, as noted previously, incubation of uterine tissue in

Ca^{++}-free media neither induces contraction nor affects the initial response to acetylcholine.†

The studies by Hurwitz and his co-workers (155) of the longitudinal muscle of the guinea-pig ileum may also be considered to support the concept outlined above. These workers have observed that the contractions induced by acetylcholine are very dependent upon the con-

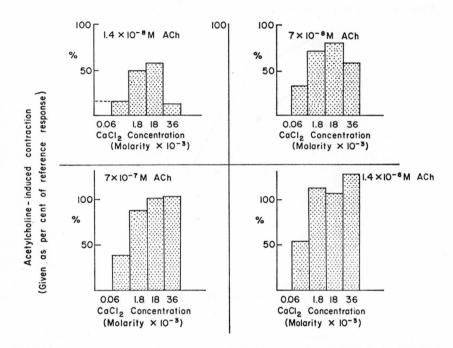

FIG. VII-23. Dependence of contraction of guinea-pig longitudinal muscle as a function of acetylcholine and Ca^{++} concentrations. Reproduced with permission from Hurwitz, von Hagen and Joiner (155).

centration of Ca$_{ext}^{++}$; at low concentrations of acetylcholine high Ca$_{ext}^{++}$ depresses response but this effect is overcome with increased concentrations of acetylcholine (Fig. VII-23). This finding is probably due in part to the general membrane stabilizing effects of high Ca$_{ext}^{++}$ but also suggests an interaction between Ca^{++} and acetylcholine at some binding site or

† There are a number of observations (i.e., 137) that responses to norepinephrine and acetylcholine which are quite persistent in Ca^{++}-free media are rapidly lost when chelating species are added. Of course, this will also deplete Ca$_{int}^{++}$, so the findings are ambiguous from the standpoint of documenting any key role of Ca^{++} bound on the external membrane surface.

sites). Further evidence that removal of membrane-bound Ca^{++} may result in the mobilization of Ca_{int}^{++} has also been provided by Hurwitz (128, 141, 149; p. 523): longitudinal muscle previously incubated in high Ca^{++} (36 mM) undergoes a spontaneous contraction when placed in Ca^{++}-free media (containing 5×10^{-6} M EDTA). Furthermore, acetylcholine will produce a further increase in contraction above that produced by the Ca^{++}-free medium (Fig. VII-24) although the rate of loss of response remains unchanged.

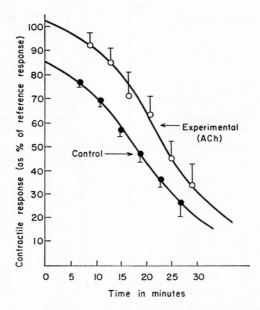

FIG. VII-24. Loss of amplitude of contraction of longitudinal muscle preloaded with Ca^{++} and immersed in Ca^{++}-free media. The experimental curve was obtained in the presence of $1 \cdot 4 \times 10^{-6}$ M ACh. Reproduced with permission from Hurwitz and Joiner (149).

These lines of evidence are at least suggestive that the function of acetylcholine, norepinephrine and their analogs in smooth muscle involves interaction at the neurotransmitter recognition site and removal of specifically bound Ca_{ext}^{++} from the membrane to promote mobilization of Ca_{int}^{++}. As a model for this type of process the observations of Ohki and Papahadjopoulos (Chapter II, p. 170) that bimolecular lipid membranes become very unstable when Ca^{++} is present on one surface only of the membrane are pertinent. We may envisage that neurotransmitters produce highly localized membrane breakdown by this process thus producing Ca^{++}-mobilization and changes in membrane potential and conductances to other ions. In the terminology of Wyman (Chapter I, p. 82) we may regard this process as a linked function.

In principle it appears that two possible mechanisms may be considered for such a process: these may be a direct displacement by the neurotransmitter of Ca^{++} normally bound to the receptor site (Fig. VII-25A). Alternatively, the effect of the neurotransmitter on the membrane bound Ca^{++} may be regarded as an allosteric linkage with the neurotransmitter serving as an effector (when bound to its specific recognition site) to reduce the affinity of the Ca^{++} binding site (Fig.

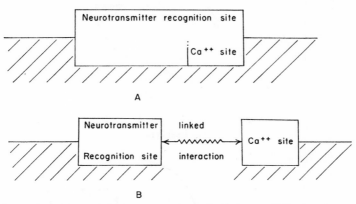

FIG. VII-25. Hypothetical neurotransmitter-Ca^{++} interactions at the excitable membrane level. A: a direct involvement of Ca^{++} at the neurotransmitter recognition site. B: an allosteric arrangement of neurotransmitter and Ca^{++} sites whereby the neurotransmitter-receptor interaction reduces the affinity of the linked site for Ca^{++}.

VII-25B). Which, if either, of these two mechanisms is correct is not easy to say but a certain amount of evidence indicates the latter mechanism to be more plausible.

AN ALLOSTERIC NEUROTRANSMITTER-Ca^{++} INTERACTION

A certain amount of evidence appears to indicate the distinct nature of the proposed neurotransmitter and Ca^{++} binding sites as represented in Fig. VII-25B. Much of this evidence is derived from studies with antagonists whose activities can be argued, with some justification, to produce antagonism to the neurotransmitter-induced responses through interaction at a Ca^{++}-binding site rather than at the neurotransmitter recognition site.

A number of observations have been made that local anesthetics antagonize the responses produced by norepinephrine, acetylcholine, histamine and K^+ (146, 156–163). Of particular significance is that the antagonism of the local anesthetics to the neurotransmitters and their analogs can be described as non-competitive since a reduction in response is observed (Chapter IV, p. 283); this stands in marked contrast to the effects of the classically described competitive antagonists. This is

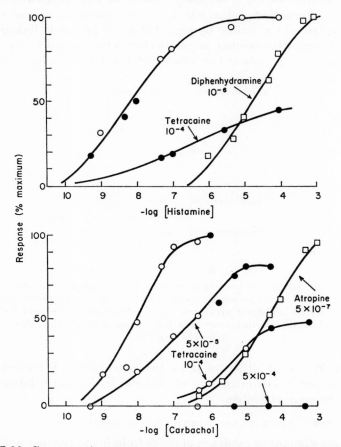

Fig. VII-26. Concentration-response curves for histamine and carbamylcholine in guinea-pig ileum, showing competitive behavior of atropine and diphenhydramine and the noncompetitive behaviour of tetracaine. Reproduced with permission from Feinstein and Paimre (163).

clearly seen in Fig. VII-26 describing the antagonism exhibited by tetracaine, atropine and diphenhydramine towards the responses of the guinea-pig ileum to carbachol and histamine. Similar effects of tetracaine have been described towards the responses of rabbit taenia coli and frog rectus to carbachol, rat uterus to 5-hydroxytryptamine and rabbit aorta to norepinephrine. Since local anesthetics have been well documented as involved in Ca^{++}-binding processes (Chapter II, p. 175) it is probable that these noncompetitive effects of local anesthetics may be attributed to interference at a Ca^{++} site distinct from the neurotransmitter recognition site (146, 159, 163).† Support for this proposal derives from observations that local anesthetics act as competitive antagonists

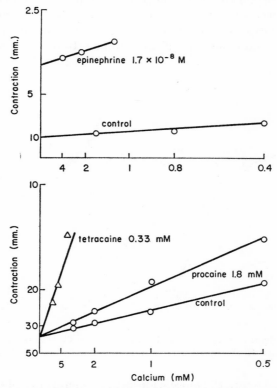

FIG. VII-27. Reciprocal plots showing competitive antagonism by tetracaine and procaine and noncompetitive antagonism by epinephrine of Ca^{++}-induced contractions in depolarized rat uterus. Reproduced with permission from Feinstein (158).

to Ca^{++}-induced contractions in K^{+}-depolarized preparations (Fig. VII-27) and that epinephrine acts as a noncompetitive antagonist of Ca^{++}-induced contractions in the depolarized rat uterus (Fig. VII-27). The differences in action of local anesthetics and epinephrine in this preparation are also revealed by the data in Fig. VII-28 showing that

† Since local anesthetics act as membrane stabilizing species (Chapter II, p. 175) the possibility cannot be ignored that they act by this mechanism and not through involvement with a specific Ca^{++} site linked to the neurotransmitter recognition site (161–163).

only tetracaine inhibits Ca^{++} exchange and presumably local anesthetics prevent the influx of Ca^{++}_{ext} necessary for contraction in the K^{+}-depolarized rat uterus. It is to be recognized, of course, that the antagonism by local anesthetics of neurotransmitter and Ca^{++}-induced contractions cannot be interpreted in terms of a common pathway for elevation of Ca^{++} for there is considerable evidence that, in many smooth muscles, neurotransmitters mobilize intracellular Ca^{++}_{in} for the activation of the contractile process. Rather the data suggest that local anesthetics have a general capacity to compete at sites of Ca^{++} binding and mobilization whether these are specifically linked to the neurotransmitter

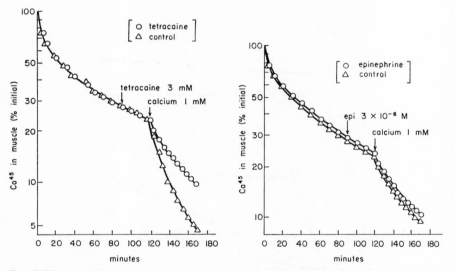

FIG. VII-28. Effects of tetracaine and epinephrine on Ca^{++} efflux from cat uterine horns. Reproduced with permission from Feinstein (158).

recognition site or are the more widespread general sites of Ca^{++} binding on the cell membrane. The difference in behavior of local anesthetics towards Ca^{++} and neurotransmitter-contractions also suggests that, at least in smooth muscle,† they act at a membranal site.

The local anesthetics are, in view of the fairly high concentrations employed, not very specific antagonists of neurotransmitters. However, a number of other agents are known which behave similarly to local anesthetics in distinguishing between neurotransmitter and Ca^{++}-induced processes but appear to be somewhat more specific. Diazoxide

† The action of local anesthetics in skeletal muscle is demonstrably more complex for they can act both at the cell membrane and to inhibit the release of bound Ca^{++} from the sarcoplasmic reticuluum (163–168).

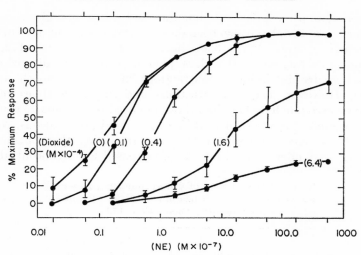

FIG. VII-29. Diazoxide-norepinephrine competition in aortic (rabbit) smooth muscle. Reproduced with permission from Wohl, Hausler and Roth (168a).

(7-chloro-3-methyl-2H-1,2,4-benzothiadiazine-1,1 dioxide), exhibits non-competitive antagonism towards the responses of rat aorta to norepinephrine (Fig. VII-29) but acts competitively towards the responses produced by Ca^{++} (168a–170) in the same preparations (Fig. VII-30). The 2-halogenoethylamines, well established as irreversible antagonists

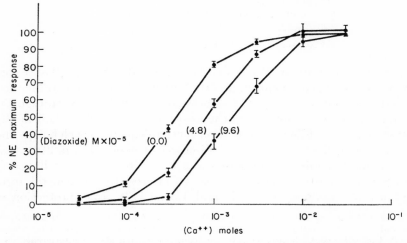

FIG. VII-30. Diazoxide-Ca^{++} interaction in aortic (rabbit) smooth muscle in the presence of constant concentration of norepinephrine. Reproduced with permission from Wohl, Hausler and Roth (169).

at adrenergic α-receptors, cholinergic and histaminergic receptors (Chapter IV, p. 288) have also been demonstrated to act at sites of Ca^{++} involvement (Chapter IV, p. 336). Bevan (171) and Shibata (172, 173) have shown that agents of this class (phenoxybenzamine, dibenzamine, etc.) antagonize K^+-induced contractions in several smooth muscle systems. However, the concentrations and exposure times of the antagonists are much higher than those required to antagonize contractions exhibited by neurotransmitters in polarized preparations. Nevertheless, these agents do reduce Ca^{++} influx during the contractions (Table VII-6),† effects antagonized by increased Ca^{++} concentrations.

TABLE VII-6. Effect of Chlorpromazine, Dibenamine and Phenoxybenzamine on $^{45}Ca^{++}$ Uptake in Guinea-Pig Taenia Coli (173)

Conditions	$^{45}Ca^{++}$ uptake cpm/g $\times 10^4$
Control	$3\cdot4 \pm 0\cdot22$
KCl (40 mM) +	$4\cdot0 \pm 0\cdot2$
Chloropromazine (10^{-5} M)	$2\cdot1 \pm 0\cdot4$
Dibenamine (10^{-4} M)	$2\cdot4 \pm 0\cdot2$
Phenoxybenzamine (10^{-4} M)	$2\cdot2 \pm 0\cdot2$
Phenoxybenzamine (10^{-6} M)	$3\cdot3 \pm 0\cdot4$†
Acetylcholine (10^{-5} M) +	$3\cdot9 \pm 0\cdot1$
Chlorpromazine (10^{-5} M)	$2\cdot5 \pm 0\cdot2$
Dibenamine (10^{-4} M)	$2\cdot5 \pm 0\cdot3$
Phenoxybenzamine (10^{-6} M)	$2\cdot6 \pm 0\cdot2$

† Not significantly different from control.

Of particular interest in Table VII-6 are the data showing that a concentration of phenoxybenzamine (10^{-6} M) which does not antagonize K^+-induced contractures or the associated Ca^{++}-influx does antagonize the actions of acetylcholine and the associated Ca^{++} influx. This neatly distinguishes the different activation mechanisms of acetylcholine and K^+ and emphasizes, as previously discussed (Chapter IV, p. 336), that 2-halogenoethylamines can interact at a Ca^{++} site specifically linked to the neurotransmitter recognition site. Of interest to this general argument are the findings of Tuttle and Moran (178) that protection of

† Table VII-6 indicates that chlorpromazine (Chapter IV, p. 288) also reduces contractions and Ca^{++}-influx and it seems possible that the rather nonselective blocking actions exhibited by this agent towards neurotransmitters are related also to interference with Ca^{++}. Indeed it appears probable that a great number of antagonists to neurotransmitters act, in part, through interference with Ca^{++} (153, 162, 174–177, also see Chapter IV, p. 329).

α-adrenergic and histaminergic receptors by norepinephrine and histamine against inactivation by phenoxybenzamine is prevented by prior severe Ca^{++} depletion (Fig. VII-31 shows the data for norepinephrine: that for histamine is fundamentally similar). Apparently, the interactions of the agonists are Ca^{++}-dependent processes: this finding is certainly consistent with the general representation of Fig. VII-25B in which the agonist-Ca^{++} interaction is represented as a linked function

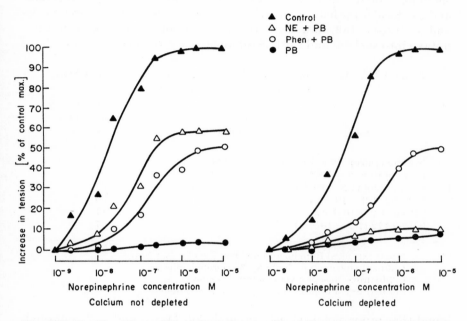

FIG. VII-31. The effect of Ca^{++}-depletion on the ability of norepinephrine and phentolamine (Phen) to protect against phenoxybenzamine (PB) inactivation of α-adrenergic receptors in rabbit aorta. Reproduced with permission from Tuttle and Moran (178).

(179): binding of neurotransmitter will serve to modify the affinity of the Ca^{++}-binding site and, conversely, binding of Ca^{++} will serve to modify the affinity of the neurotransmitter binding site.

Thus far our attention has been devoted exclusively to considerations of the role of Ca^{++} in the smooth muscle contractile process. It is important also to consider neurotransmitter-Ca^{++} interactions in relaxation processes in smooth muscle (β-receptor processes). Relaxation presumably reflects a reduction in the level of free intracellular Ca^{++} although there is little direct evidence relating to mechanisms by which this might be achieved.

However, it is apparent that β-adrenergic agents do interfere with Ca^{++} binding/mobilization processes (180, 181). Some evidence bearing on this point has already been presented (Chapter IV, p. 326) in a previous discussion of the antiarrhythmic activities of β-antagonists, properties which appear correlatable with the local anesthetic properties of these agents. Despite the involvement of local anesthetics with the inhibition of Ca^{++} binding by phospholipids (Chapter II, p. 175) it should be noted that there is a clear dissociation between β-antagonism and the local anesthetic properties of these agents. Nevertheless, Scales and McIntosh (182) in a study of the effects of β-antagonists on Ca^{++} uptake into skeletal and cardiac sarcoplasmic reticuluum fractions have

TABLE VII-7. Effects of Adrenergic Ligands on Lipid-facilitated Transport of Ca^{++} Ions† (180, 183)

Ligand	% Increase in Ca^{++} in $CHCl_3$	% Inhibition of Ca^{++} uptake in $CHCl_3$
Norepinephrine (6×10^{-5} M)	33	—
Epinephrine (5×10^{-5} M)	50	—
Propranolol ($1 \cdot 2 \times 10^{-5}$ M)	—	30
KO-592 ($1 \cdot 2 \times 10^{-5}$ M)‡	—	20
LB-46 ($1 \cdot 2 \times 10^{-5}$ M)§	—	11
ICI 50,172 ($1 \cdot 2 \times 10^{-5}$ M)‖	—	7

† Lipids extracted from microsomal fraction of rabbit hearts.
‡ 1-(3-methylphenoxy)-2-hydroxy-3-isopropylaminopropanol.
§ 4-(2-hydroxy-3-isopropylaminopropoxy) indole.
‖ 4-(2-hydroxy-3-isopropylaminopropoxy) acetanilide.

found that propranolol (IV-64), pronethalol (IV-63) and 4-(2-isopropyl-amino-1-hydroxyethyl) methanesulfonanilide (MJ-1999, IV-65) and 4-(2-isopropylamino-1-hydroxyethyl) nitrobenzene (IV-67), the latter two agents being devoid of local anesthetic activity, all inhibit Ca^{++} uptake at concentrations of 10^{-4} and 10^{-3} M.

Nayler *et al.* (180, 183) have also reported on the effects of catecholamines and β-antagonists on heart lipid-facilitated transport of Ca^{++} in a $H_2O:CHCl_3$ system. Norepinephrine and epinephrine facilitate Ca^{++} transport (Table VII-7): it is of particular interest that the order of effectiveness of the β-antagonists in inhibiting lipid-facilitated Ca^{++} transport is identical with their order of activity as negative inotropic agents.

It might be argued from these few studies that in β-receptor relaxation processes a mutually antagonistic relationship may exist between the agonists and antagonists towards Ca^{++} binding at the cell membrane:

the agonists facilitate Ca^{++} binding and hence stabilize the cell membrane while the antagonists prevent this process perhaps by direct competition for this site. This scheme has obvious analogies to that set up to describe neurotransmitter-Ca^{++} interrelationships in the contractile process save that in the latter (Fig. VII-25B) the excitatory ligands serve to displace the receptor associated Ca^{++} and hence destabilize the membrane.

This suggestion finds some support from considerations of the effects of isopropylnorepinephrine on the depolarized rat uterus (184). This system contracts in response to Ca^{++} (5×10^{-6} M), a response which is antagonized by catecholamines with an activity order, isopropylnorepinephrine > epinephrine > norepinephrine: dichloroisopropylnorepinephrine competitively antagonizes the inhibitory effects of the catecholamines and has identical pA$_2$ values in the polarized and depolarized preparations. Of further interest are findings that EDTA and EGTA (10^{-4}–10^{-3} M) effectively antagonize the relaxant effects of isopropylnorepinephrine: these latter findings are consistent with, but do not prove, the hypothesis that the relaxant effects of isopropylnorepinephrine are achieved through a stabilization of Ca^{++} at a binding site probably located on the membrane.

The Role of Cyclic 3′,5′-AMP in Excitation-Contraction Coupling

In a previous chapter the possible role of cyclic AMP as a second messenger regulating the mechanical events in the sequence initiated by the neurotransmitters was discussed. Whether this is the true role of cyclic AMP remains to be established beyond doubt: in any event there has been, until recently, no mechanism advanced to indicate how cyclic AMP and mechanical events might be linked, although it seems clear that the events are not directly related to any role of cyclic AMP in activating metabolic pathways. There have been recently, however, several independent lines of evidence linking cyclic AMP and Ca^{++}.

Rasmussen has proposed (185, 186) a very general association of cyclic AMP and Ca^{++} such that Ca^{++} may be the more important second messenger in a variety of systems in which cyclic AMP is known to be involved. In the latest expression of this hypothesis (186) it is proposed, in view of the fact that the physiological expression of a number of hormones, including vasopressin (185, 187), MSH (188), ACTH (189), parathyroid hormone (185, 186) known to be mediated through cyclic AMP are reduced or abolished in the absence of Ca^{++} even though cyclic nucleotide levels may be unaffected, that the hormone-induced cyclic AMP causes either an increase in Ca^{++} permeability of the cell membrane

19

TABLE VII-8. Adenyl Cyclase and Ca++-Accumulating Activity in Canine Myocardium Fractions (193, 194)

Conditions	Ca++ accumulation mμmoles/mg protein	Ca++ accumulation % increase min					Adenyl cyclase activity p moles/AMP/10 min
		0	1	2	3	4	
Control	11·6 ± 1·1	—	—	—	—	—	270
Epinephrine, 10^{-6} M	20·2 ± 2·4	1	2	11	23	28	—
Propranolol, 10^{-5} M	12·2 ± 2·4	—	—	—	—	—	—
Epinephrine + propranolol	12·4 ± 0·8	—	—	—	—	—	—
Cyclic 3',5'-AMP, 5×10^{-6} M	22·3 ± 1·6	16	31	32	31	33	—
Cyclic 3',5'-AMP + propranolol	20·8 ± 1·3	—	—	—	—	—	—
Glucagon, 3×10^{-8} M	19·0 ± 3·0	2	3	17	33	36	—
Glucagon + propranolol	19·3 ± 2·1	—	—	—	—	—	—
Epinephrine, 10^{-6} M							305
Epinephrine, 10^{-5} M							405
Epinephrine, 10^{-4} M							450

or a redistribution of intracellular Ca^{++}.† Direct evidence for the involvement of cyclic AMP in mechanical events is provided by the data of Mitznegg, Heim and Meythaler (192) who find that cyclic AMP inhibits the Ca^{++}-dependent oxytocin-induced contractures of rat uterus and will also inhibit the uterine contractions induced by Ca^{++}. It remains to be established, however, to what extent these effects are unique to cyclic AMP (Chapter VI, p. 475).

Certainly the association between Ca^{++} and the contractile process cannot be denied: however, the hypothesis of Rasmussen that cyclic AMP raises the membrane permeability to Ca^{++} produces a number of difficulties: neurotransmitters are believed to mobilize Ca^{++} that is essentially intracellular in origin and furthermore, relaxation processes in smooth muscle are β-receptor mediated events and must involve a reduction in free Ca_{int}^{++}.

Another type of association between Ca^{++} and cyclic AMP has been proposed by Entman, Levey and Epstein (193, 194) who have provided some evidence for the existence of adenyl cyclase in a microsomal fraction of canine myocardium believed to represent sarcoplasmic reticuluum. This fraction possesses the ability to actively accumulate Ca^{++} and both the adenyl cyclase and Ca^{++} accumulating abilities are activated by glucagon or epinephrine but the actions of the latter agent only are abolished by the β-antagonist propranolol (Table VII-8). Cyclic 3',5'-AMP also activates the Ca^{++}-accumulating ability and it will be observed from Table VII-8 that its action is more rapid than epinephrine or glucagon, which is consistent with a mechanism in which the latter agents mediating their effects through cyclic AMP. It is worthy of note that significantly higher concentrations of epinephrine are required to maximally stimulate adenyl cyclase than to maximally stimulate Ca^{++} accumulation. This may mean that very small increases in cyclic 3',5'-AMP levels are quite adequate to trigger subsequent events and could provide one explanation of the findings of Shanfeld et al. (Chapter VI, p. 480) of a dissociation between cyclic AMP levels and increased cardiac contractility. It is clear, however, that much further work is necessary before any relationship of cyclic AMP and Ca^{++} in the excitation-contraction coupling process can be said to be established beyond doubt.

REFERENCES

1. "Muscle—Proceedings of a Symposium" (eds W. M. Paul, E. E. Daniel, C. M. Kay and G. Monckton) (1965). Pergamon, Oxford.
2. A. Sandow, *Pharmacol. Rev.* (1965) **17**, 265.

† The importance of Ca_{ext}^{++} for a variety of hormone induced secretory process has long been realized (190, 191).

3. Symposium on Excitation—Contraction Coupling in Striated Muscle, *Fed. Proc. Fed. Amer. Soc.* (1966) **24**, 1112.
4. "The Contractile Process," Proceedings of a Symposium Sponsored by the New York Heart Association (1967). Little Brown, Boston.
5. "Aspects of Cell Motility", *Symp. Soc. Exp. Biol.*, No. 22. (ed. P. L. Miller) (1968). Academic Press, London and New York.
6. S. Ebashi and M. Endo, *Progr. Biophys. Mol. Biol.* (1968) **18**, 123.
7. J. Hanson, *Quart. Rev. Biophys.* (1968) **1**, 177.
8. S. Ebashi, M. Endo and I. Ohtsuki, *Quart. Rev. Biophys.* (1969) **2**, 351.
9. H. E. Huxley, *Science, N.Y.* (1969) **104**, 1356.
10. M. Young, *Ann. Rev. Biochem.* (1969) **38**, 913.
11. P. Dreizen and L. C. Gershman, *Trans. N.Y. Acad. Sci.* (1970) **32**, 170.
12. J. Hanson and H. E. Huxley, *Nature (London)* (1953) **172**, 530.
13. A. F. Huxley and R. Niedergerke, *Nature (London)* (1954) **173**, 971.
14. H. E. Huxley and J. Hanson, *Nature (London)* (1954) **173**, 973.
15. H. E. Huxley and W. Brown, *J. Mol. Biol.* (1967) **30**, 383.
16. A. Szent-Györgyi, "Chemistry of Muscular Contraction", 2nd Ed. (1951). Academic Press, New York and London.
17. H. E. Huxley, *J. Mol. Biol.* (1968) **37**, 507.
18. J. C. Rüegg, in ref. 5.
19. J. Hanson and J. Lowy, *Proc. Roy. Soc. Ser. B.* (1964) **160**, 449.
20. G. F. Elliot and J. Lowy, *Nature (London)* (1968) **219**, 156.
21. C. F. Schoenberg, *J. Biophys. Biochem. Cytol.* (1958) **4**, 609.
22. D. M. Needham and C. F. Schoenberg, *Proc. Roy. Soc. Ser. B.* (1964) **148**, 517.
23. G. F. Elliot, *J. Gen. Physiol.* (1967) **50**, 171.
24. B. P. Lane, *J. Cell Biol.* (1965) **27**, 199.
25. P. J. Hanner and C. R. Honig, *J. Cell Biol.* (1967) **35**, 303.
26. C. F. Schoenberg, J. C. Rüegg, D. M. Needham, R. H. Schirmer and H. Nemetchek-Gansler, *Biochem. Z.* (1966) **345**, 255.
27. G. F. Elliot, in ref. 4.
28. H. E. Huxley, *J. Mol. Biol.* (1963) **7**, 281.
29. J. Hanson and J. Lowy, *Proc. Roy. Soc. Ser. B.* (1964) **160**, 523.
30. J. Lowy, F. R. Poulsen and P. J. Vibert, *Nature (London)* (1970) **225**, 1053.
31. D. M. Needham and J. M. Williams, *Biochem. J.* (1963) **89**, 552.
32. R. H. Schirmer, *Biochem. Z.* (1965) **343**, 269.
33. S. Ebashi and F. Ebashi, *J. Biochem. (Tokyo)* (1964) **55**, 604.
34. S. Ebashi and A. Kodama, *J. Biochem. (Tokyo)* (1965) **58**, 107.
35. S. Ebashi and A. Kodama, *J. Biochem. (Tokyo)* (1966) **59**, 425.
36. S. Ebashi, H. I. Wakura, H. Nakajima, R. Nakamura and Y. Ooi, *Biochem. Z.* (1966) **345**, 201.
37. S. Ebashi, A. Kodama and F. Ebashi, *J. Biochem. (Tokyo)* (1968) **64**, 465.
38. I. Ohtsuki, T. Masaki, Y. Nonomura and S. Ebashi, *J. Biochem. (Tokyo)* (1967) **61**, 817.
39. S. Higashi and T. Ooi, *J. Mol. Biol.* (1968) **34**, 699.
40. Y. Tonomura, S. Watanabe and M. Morales, *Biochemistry* (1969) **8**, 2171.
41. M. H. Han and E. S. Benson, *Biochem. Biophys. Res. Commun.* (1970) **38**, 378.
42. A. Weber, *in* "Current Topics in Bioenergetics," (ed. D. R. Sanadi) (1966). Academic Press, New York and London.
43. L. V. Heilbrunn, *Physiol. Zoöl.* (1940) **13**, 88.
44. L. V. Heilbrunn and F. J. Wiercinski, *J. Cell. Comp. Physiol.* (1947) **29**, 15.

45. H. Portzehl, P. C. Caldwell and J. C. Rüegg, *Biochem. Biophys. Acta* (1964) **79**, 581.
46. R. J. Podolsky and L. L. Constantin, *Fed. Proc. Fed. Amer. Soc.* (1964) **23**, 933.
47. R. J. Podolsky, *Fed. Proc. Fed. Amer. Soc.* (1965) **24**, 1112.
48. L. L. Constantin and R. J. Podolsky, *Fed. Proc. Fed. Amer. Soc.* (1965) **24**, 1141.
49. K. R. Porter, *J. Biophys. Biochem. Cytol.* (1961) **10**, 219.
50. W. Hasselbach and M. Makinose, *Biochem. Z.* (1961) **333**, 518.
51. A. Weber, R. Herz and I. Reiss, *J. Gen. Physiol.* (1963) **46**, 679.
52. L. L. Constantin, C. Franzini-Armstrong and R. J. Podolsky, *Science, N.Y.* (1965) **147**, 158.
53. E. Anderson-Cedergren, *J. Ultrastruct. Res. Suppl.* (1959) **1**, 5.
54. S. Winegrad, *Fed. Proc. Fed. Amer. Soc.* (1965) **24**, 1146.
55. S. Winegrad, *J. Gen. Physiol.* (1970) **55**, 77.
56. A. F. Huxley and R. E. Taylor, *J. Physiol.* (1958) **144**, 426.
57. A. F. Huxley, *Ann. N.Y. Acad. Sci.* (1959) **81**, 446.
58. A. F. Huxley and R. W. Straub, *J. Physiol. (London)* (1958) **143**, 40P.
59. H. E. Huxley, *Nature (London)* (1964) **202**, 1067.
60. P. W. Gage and R. S. Eisenberg, *Science, N.Y.* (1968) **158**, 1702.
61. J. N. Howell, *J. Physiol. (London)* (1969) **201**, 515.
62. W. H. Barry and L. D. Carnay, *Amer. J. Physiol.* (1969) **217**, 1425.
63. G. Falk and P. Fatt, *Proc. Roy. Soc. Ser. B.* (1964) **160**, 69.
64. F. F. Jöbsis and M. J. O'Connor, *Biochem. Biophys. Res. Commun.* (1966) **25**, 246.
65. C. C. Ashley and E. B. Ridgway, *Nature (London)* (1968) **219**, 1168.
66. C. P. Bianchi and A. M. Shanes, *J. Gen. Physiol.* (1959) **42**, 803.
67. C. P. Bianchi and A. M. Shanes, *J. Cell. Comp. Physiol.* (1960) **56**, 67.
68. C. P. Bianchi, *Fed. Proc. Fed. Amer. Soc.* (1964) **23**, 420.
69. G. B. Weiss and C. P. Bianchi, *J. Cell Comp. Physiol.* (1965) **65**, 385.
70. A. F. Huxley, *Annu. Rev. Physiol.* (1964) **26**, 131.
71. C. P. Bianchi, "Cell Calcium", Chap. 5 (1968). Butterworth, London.
72. S. Winegrad, *Circulation* (1961) **24**, 523.
73. G. B. Frank, *J. Physiol. (London)* (1960) **151**, 518.
74. W. C. Buss and G. B. Frank, *Arch. Int. Pharmacodyn. Ther.* (1969) **181**, 15.
75. A. Weber and R. Herz, *J. Gen. Physiol.* (1968) **52**, 750.
76. C. P. Bianchi, "Cell Calcium", Chap. 6 (1968). Butterworth, London.
77. A. L. Hodgkin and P. Horowicz, *J. Physiol. (London)* (1960) **153**, 404.
78. H. C. Lüttgau, *J. Physiol. (London)* (1963) **168**, 679.
79. D. J. Jenden and J. F. Reger, *J. Physiol. (London)* (1963) **169**, 889.
80. K. A. P. Edman and D. W. Grieve, *Experentia* (1961) **17**, 557.
81. B. A. Curtis, *J. Physiol. (London)* (1963) **166**, 75.
82. A. M. Katz, *Physiol. Rev.* (1970) **50**, 63.
83. D. A. Nelson and E. S. Benson, *J. Cell Biol.* (1963) **16**, 297.
84. L. N. Tice, *in* "Factors Influencing Myocardial Contractility" (eds R. D. Tanz, F. Kavaler and J. Roberts) (1967). Academic Press, New York and London.
85. D. N. Fawcett, *Circulation* (1961) **24**, 336.
86. K. S. Lee in ref. 3.
87. W. G. Nayler, *Amer. Heart J.* (1967) **73**, 379.
88. B. Scales and D. A. D. McIntosh, *J. Pharmacol. Exp. Ther.* (1968) **160**, 249.
89. S. Harigaya and A. Schwartz, *Circ. Res.* (1969) **25**, 781.

90. N. Haugaard, *Pharmacologist* (1968) **10**, 147.
91. A. V. Hill, *Proc. Roy. Soc. Ser. B.* (1949) **136**, 399.
92. S. Ringer, *J. Physiol. (London)* (1883) **4**, 29.
93. G. R. Mines, *J. Physiol. (London)* (1913) **46**, 188.
94. S. Winegrad and A. M. Shanes, *J. Gen. Physiol.* (1962) **45**, 371.
95. G. A. Langer, *Physiol. Rev.* (1968) **48**, 708.
96. G. A. Langer, *Circ. Res.* (1964) **15**, 393.
97. G. A. Langer, *Circ. Res.* (1965) **17**, 78.
98. G. A. Langer, in ref. 2.
99. L. E. Bailey and P. E. Dresel, *J. Gen. Physiol.* (1968) **52**, 969.
100. D. G. Teiger and A. Farah, *J. Pharmacol. Exp. Ther.* (1967) **157**, 8.
101. M. J. Legato, D. Spiro and G. A. Langer, *J. Cell Biol.* (1968) **37**, 1.
102. R. F. Palmer and V. R. Kavalich, *Fed. Proc. Fed. Amer. Soc.* (1966) **25**, 349.
103. R. F. Palmer and V. A. Posey, *J. Gen. Physiol.* (1967) **50**, 2085.
104. J. W. Woodbury, *Fed. Proc. Fed. Amer. Soc.* (1963) **22**, 31.
105. A. Grossman, and R. F. Furchgott, *J. Pharmacol. Exp. Ther.* (1964) **145**, 162.
106. H. Reuter, *Arch. Exp. Pathol. Pharmakol.* (1965) **251**, 401.
107. H. Reuter and U. Wollert, *Arch. Exp. Pathol. Pharmakol.* (1967) **258**, 288.
108. R. Niedergerke and H. C. Lüttgau, *Nature (London)* (1957) **179**, 1066.
109. W. G. Nayler and J. E. Wright, *Arch. Int. Pharmacodyn. Ther.* (1965) **154**, 313.
110. M. Reiter, *Arch. Exp. Pathol. Pharmakol.* (1966) **254**, 261.
111. N. S. Dhalla and A. Braxton, *J. Pharmacol. Exp. Ther.* (1968) **161**, 238.
112. N. Toda, *Brit. J. Pharmacol.* (1969) **36**, 350.
113. F. Kavaler and M. Moradh, *Circ. Res.* (1966) **18**, 492.
114. M. E. Carsten, *J. Gen. Physiol.* (1969) **53**, 414.
115. D. H. L. Evans, H. O. Schild, and S. Thesleff, *J. Physiol. (London)* (1958) **143**, 474.
116. R. P. Durbin and D. H. Jenkinson, *J. Physiol. (London)* (1961) **157**, 74.
117. K. A. P. Edman and H. O. Schild, *J. Physiol. (London)* (1962) **161**, 424.
118. W. H. Waugh, *Circ. Res.* (1962) **11**, 927.
119. K. A. P. Edman and H. O. Schild, *J. Physiol. (London)* (1963) **169**, 404.
120. H. O. Schild, *Brit. J. Pharmacol.* (1967) **31**, 578.
121. P. A. Robertson, *Nature (London)* (1960) **186**, 316.
122. A. H. Briggs and S. Melvin, *Amer. J. Physiol.* (1961) **201**, 365.
123. A. H. Briggs, *Amer. J. Physiol.* (1962) **203**, 849.
124. N. Chujyo and W. C. Holland, *Amer. J. Physiol.* (1962) **202**, 912.
125. N. Sperelakis, *Amer. J. Physiol.* (1962) **203**, 860.
126. N. Urakawa and W. C. Holland, *Amer. J. Physiol.* (1964) **207**, 873.
127. C. van Breemen and E. E. Daniel, *J. Gen. Physiol.* (1966) **49**, 1299.
128. L. Hurwitz, P. D. Joiner and S. Von Hagen, *Proc. Soc. Exp. Biol. Med.* (1967) **39**, 395.
129. N. Urakawa, H. Karaki and M. Ikeda, *Jap. J. Pharmacol.* (1968) **18**, 294.
130. H. Karaki, M. Ikeda and N. Urakawa, *Jap. J. Pharmacol.* (1969) **19**, 291.
131. H. Lüllmann and P. Mohns, *Pflügers Arch. Gesemte Physiol. Menschen* (1969) **308**, 214.
132. H. Karaki, S. S. Ganeshanandan, M. Ikeda and N. Urakawa, *Jap. J. Pharmacol.* (1969) **19**, 569.
133. P. M. Hudgins, *J. Pharmacol. Exp. Ther.* (1969) **170**, 303.
134. N. Sperelakis, *Amer. J. Physiol.* (1962) **202**, 731.
135. J. A. M. Hinke, M. L. Wilson and S. C. Burnham, *Amer. J. Physiol.* (1964) **206**, 211.

136. L. Hurwitz, P. D. Joiner and S. Von Hagen, *Amer. J. Physiol.* (1967) **213**, 1299.
137. B. Johansson, O. Jonsson, J. Axelsson, and B. Wahlström, *Circ. Res.* (1967) **21**, 619.
138. R. S. Alexander, *Amer. J. Physiol.* (1967) **213**, 287.
139. T. F. Burks, T. S. Whitacre and J. P. Long, *Arch. Int. Pharmacodyn. Ther.* (1967) **168**, 304.
140. M. Hiraoka, S. Yamagishi and T. Sano, *Amer. J. Physiol.* (1968) **214**, 1084.
141. L. Hurwitz, P. D. Joiner, S. Von Hagen, and G. R. Davenport, *Amer. J. Physiol.* (1969) **216**, 215.
142. E. Bozler, *Amer. J. Physiol.* (1969) **216**, 671.
143. C. Isojima and E. Bozler, *Amer. J. Physiol.* (1963) **205**, 681.
144. J. A. M. Hinke, *in* "Muscle" (eds W. M. Paul, E. E. Daniel, C. M. Kay and G. M. Monckton) (1965). Pergamon, New York.
145. E. E. Daniel, H. Sehdev and K. Robinson, *Physiol. Rev.* (1962) **42**, Suppl. 5, 228.
146. M. B. Feinstein, M. Paimre and M. Lee, *Trans. N.Y. Acad. Sci.* (1968) **30**, 1073.
147. E. Mohme-Lundholm and N. Vamos, *Acta Pharmacol. Toxicol.* (1967) **25**, 87.
148. P. M. Hudgins and G. B. Weiss, *Amer. J. Physiol.* (1969) **217**, 1310.
149. L. Hurwitz and P. D. Joiner, *Amer. J. Physiol.* (1970) **218**, 12.
150. E. E. Daniel, *Can. J. Physiol. Pharmacol.* (1964) **42**, 453.
151. E. E. Daniel, *Can. J. Physiol. Pharmacol.* (1964) **42**, 497.
152. E. E. Daniel, *in* "Muscle" (eds W. M. Paul, E. E. Daniel, C. M. Kay and G. M. Monckton) (1965). Pergamon, New York.
153. E. E. Daniel, *Annu. Rev. Pharmacol.* (1964) **4**, 189.
154. E. E. Daniel and J. Irwin, *Can. J. Physiol. Pharmacol.* (1965) **43**, 111.
155. L. Hurwitz, S. Von Hagen and P. D. Joiner, *J. Gen. Physiol.* (1967) **50**, 1157.
156. A. Fleckenstein, *Brit. J. Pharmacol.* (1953) **7**, 553.
157. A. Aström, *Acta Physiol. Scand.* (1964) **60**, 30.
158. M. B. Feinstein, *J. Pharmacol. Exp. Ther.* (1966) **152**, 516.
159. M. B. Feinstein and M. Paimre, *Nature (London)* **214**, 151.
160. P. M. Hudgins and G. B. Weiss, *J. Pharmacol. Exp. Ther.* (1968) **159**, 91.
161. Y. Washizu, *Comp. Biochem. Physiol.* (1968) **27**, 121.
162. B. J. Northover, *Brit. J. Pharmacol.* (1968) **34**, 417.
163. M. B. Feinstein and M. Paimre, *Fed. Proc. Fed. Amer. Soc.* (1969) **28**, 1643.
164. M. B. Feinstein, *J. Gen. Physiol.* (1963) **47**, 151.
165. R. Herz and A. Weber, *Fed. Proc. Fed. Amer. Soc.* (1965) **24**, 208.
166. H. C. Lüttgau and H. Oetliker, *J. Physiol. (London)* (1968) **194**, 51'
167. C. P. Bianchi, "Cell Calcium," (1968). Butterworth, London.
168. W. D. Wilcox and F. Richs, *Biochim. Biophys. Acta* (1969) **180**, 210.
168a. A. J. Wohl, L. M. Hausler and F. E. Roth, *J. Pharmacol. Exp. Ther.* (1967) **158**, 531.
169. A. J. Wohl, L. M. Hausler and F. E. Roth, *Life Sci.* (1968) **7**, 381.
170. A. J. Wohl, L. M. Hausler and F. E. Roth, *J. Pharmacol. Exp. Ther.* (1968) **162**, 109.
171. J. A. Bevan, J. V. Osher and C. Su, *J. Pharmacol. Exp. Ther.* (1963) **139**, 216.
172. S. Shibata and O. Carrier, Jr., *Can. J. Physiol. Pharmacol.* (1967) **45**, 587.
173. S. Shibata, O. Carrier, Jr. and J. Frankenheim, *J. Pharmacol. Exp. Ther.* (1968) **160**, 106.

174. S. Imai and K. Takeda, *J. Pharmacol. Exp. Ther.* (1967) **156**, 557.
175. M. Ferrari, *J. Pharm. Pharmacol.* (1964) **16**, 62.
176. M. Ferrari, and F. Carpenedo, *Arch. Int. Pharmacodyn. Ther.* (1968) **174**, 223.
177. M. Ferrari, *J. Pharm. Pharmacol.* (1970) **22**, 71.
178. R. R. Tuttle and N. C. Moran, *J. Pharmacol. Exp. Ther.* (1969) **169**, 255.
179. J. Wyman, *Quart. Rev. Biophys.* (1968) **1**, 35.
180. W. G. Nayler, *J. Pharmacol. Exp. Ther.* (1966) **153**, 479.
181. W. G. Nayler, *Amer. Heart J.* (1967) **73**, 373.
182. B. Scales and D. A. D. McIntosh, *J. Pharmacol. Exp. Ther.* (1968) **160**, 261.
183. W. G. Nayler, J. Stone, V. Carson, I. McInnes, V. Mack and T. E. Lowe, *J. Pharmacol. Exp. Ther.* (1969) **165**, 225.
184. H. O. Schild, *Brit. J. Pharmacol.* (1967) **31**, 578.
185. H. Rasmussen and A. Tenenhouse, *Proc. Nat. Acad. Sci. U.S.A.* (1968) **59**, 1364.
186. N. Nagata and H. Rasmussen, *Proc. Nat. Acad. Sci. U.S.A.* (1970) **65**, 368.
187. H. Rasmussen and I. L. Schwartz, *in "Proc. 1st Int. Pharmacol. Meet."* Vol. 4 (1964). Pergamon, New York.
188. R. R. Novales and W. J. Davis, *Endocrinology* (1967) **81**, 283.
189. F. G. Peron and S. B. Koritz, *J. Biol. Chem.* (1958) **233**, 256.
190. M. Schramm, *Annu. Rev. Biochem.* (1967) **36**, 307.
191. W. W. Douglas, *Brit. J. Pharmacol.* (1968) **34**, 451.
192. P. Mitznegg, F. Heim and B. Meythaler, *Life Sci.* (1970) **9** (I), 121.
193. M. L. Entman, G. S. Levey and S. E. Epstein, *Biochem. Biophys. Res. Commun.* (1969) **35**, 728.
194. M. L. Entman, G. S. Levey and S. E. Epstein, *Circ. Res.* (1969) **25**, 429.

Chapter VIII

THE CHARACTERIZATION OF NEUROTRANSMITTER RECEPTORS

INTRODUCTION

A pleasant task of the final chapter in a monograph such as this would be the summarizing and rationalization of the previous chapters into one coherent picture of the molecular basis of neurotransmitter action. At the present time, however, this task is not possible because there is, quite simply, inadequate information about what neurotransmitter receptors are, how they are integrated into cell membranes and how the events initiated at these receptors may be coupled to ionic, potential, biochemical and mechanical changes. However, it is distinctly possible that this picture will change dramatically over the next few years for there is a rapidly developing awareness of the regulatory significance of cell membrane processes. Whilst progress must be made in all of the areas cited above it is of particular importance to have available some hard information on receptor characterization and composition and this final chapter will, therefore, be concerned with a discussion of current progress in the area of receptor isolation.

In essence there have been two basic techniques with which attempts have been made to isolate receptors: measurements of the ability of various fractions of receptor-containing tissues to bind reversibly neurotropic ligands with affinities appropriate to the receptor system under consideration and the use of agents capable of becoming co-valently attached to the receptor and subsequent tissue fractionation to obtain labeled material. There are certain obvious analogies between the problem of isolation of receptor material and that of isolating and identifying the components of the active sites of enzymes. However, the problem of enzyme isolation and active site determination may be anticipated to be a simpler task since the activity of enzymes can be monitored *in vitro* during isolation and purification procedures. These aims cannot be achieved with receptor systems where the physiological activity, an essential criterion of their existence, is dependent upon the integrity of the cellular system or, at least, of its membrane components.

19* 547

At the present time neither of these approaches has led to the isolation of a pure material or materials that can be unambiguously stated to be the receptor, or portion thereof, for a neurotransmitter.† Each approach has its own disadvantages quite apart from the general disadvantages cited above. The use of the reversible binding technique seems disadvantageous in the sense that conformational and denaturative changes or disaggregation of a receptor mosaic that may take place during the extraction procedure may sufficiently alter the binding characteristics and capacities to an extent that they become totally misleading. On the other hand, the use of irreversible labels, while theoretically extremely attractive, suffers from the known nonspecificity of all of the labeling species thus far employed and, whilst it should be possible to overcome this nonspecificity by appropriate protection techniques this has, as yet, not proved very easy to demonstrate. Furthermore, even if achieved a problem unique to the irreversible labeling technique remains of how to demonstrate and quantitate ligand binding to a presumed receptor fraction in which the recognition site is already occupied by the labeling species. Of the two techniques, that of cellular fractionation and monitoring of receptor "activity" through comparative ligand binding studies has certainly been the more successful.

THE ISOLATION OF RECEPTORS THROUGH COVALENT LABELING

The methodology and techniques of covalent labeling have been established primarily for the area of enzyme active centers. Because this area has been the subject of several recent reviews (4–8a) only a brief outline of these features having the greatest applicability to receptor labeling will be discussed. A general discussion of irreversible adrenergic and cholinergic antagonists has been presented in Chapter IV and some special applications with respect to membrane potentials in Chapter V.

The key problem in the application of this technique to the identification of the functional groups involved in the interaction of substrates, antibodies, activator ligands etc., with their respective macromolecular binding surfaces is that of specificity of interaction. That is, the extent to which any one residue in the catalytic site (cited in the collective sense to define the functional groups of the macromolecule directly involved in the interaction with the ligand) is labeled as compared to residues elsewhere in the macromolecular system.

Great specificity of interaction is possible with those enzyme systems

† Considerable progress has been made, however, with the isolation of, for example, the estrogen-receptor (1–3).

in which a covalently bound intermediate is formed between the ligand and the active site and which is either sufficiently stable to permit isolation (i.e., the phosphorylated intermediates of phosphogluco-mutase (9) and phosphoglyceromutase (10), or to permit trapping by conversion to a stable compound by a mild chemical procedure, i.e., where intermediate Schiff's bases are formed (11, 12). Related to this is the use of substrate-like reagents that generate stable intermediates (13); examples include DFP and other phosphorylating agents (7, 14), the sulfonyl fluorides (15) and carbamylating agents (16) all of which react with seryl residues in the active center. The success of such reagents is dependent upon the presence, in the active center, of uniquely reactive amino acid residues that are, by virtue of their microenviron-ment, far more reactive toward the labeling reagent than the same group in a non-active center environment. Less specific labeling can be achieved with group specific reagents such as iodoacetate, fluoro-dinitrobenzene, carbodiimides etc., which, under carefully controlled conditions, can be used to achieve specific labeling of a single amino acid residue (4, 6, 7). While there are several examples of the application of such reagents to neurotransmitter-receptor systems (17–19) it cannot be said that they have contributed to the isolation or characterization of the receptor systems studied.

Of greater general applicability is a method in which the desired specificity of labeling is introduced, not merely by the the reactivity of the reagent for a given residue or residues, but by the general affinity of the labeling agent for the ligand binding site. The application of this general idea to enzyme chemistry was introduced almost simultaneously by a number of workers including Baker (5, 8, 20), Schoellman and Shaw (21), Wofsy et al. (22), Lawson and Schramm (23) and others (4, 6, 7) and is now generally referred to as affinity, or active-site directed irreversible, labeling. The basic feature of this very general approach is that a potential covalent-bond forming group is attached to a com-petitive inhibitor $(A—B)$ of an active site (X) so that the agent first forms a reversible complex and then, while in the complexed form, undergoes an accelerated covalent-bond forming reaction with one or more appropriately located residues,

$$A—B + \underset{k_2}{\overset{k_1}{\rightleftarrows}} A—B\text{-}\text{-}\text{-}X$$

$$A—B\text{-}\text{-}\text{-}X \xrightarrow{k_3} A—B—X$$

I

It is important to distinguish this process from the corresponding bimolecular event,

$$A—B + X \xrightarrow{k_4} A—B—X$$

which will proceed at a slower rate and with significantly less specificity. A complete rationale of this approach, as it applies to enzyme inhibitors, may be obtained from the many publications of Baker and his colleagues (5, 8, 20) and includes the comprehensive mapping of all potential binding and non-binding areas within and without the active center to ensure optimal placing of the reactive function within the inhibitor molecule.

The choice of labeling agent can have a dramatic influence on the relative extents of specific and nonspecific labeling: if P is the specific product and P' the nonspecific product then it follows from the above equations,

$$P/P' = \frac{k_3 \, K_A (X_e)}{k_4 (X')}$$

where (X_e) is the equilibrium concentration of free X and K_A is the equilibrium constant for the formation of A—B---X. Clearly, the specificity increases with increasing K_A indicating the necessity for high reversible affinity of the labeling ligand.

From the previous discussions (Chapter IV) of irreversible antagonists of adrenergic and cholinergic receptor mediated events, most of which belong to the highly reactive 2-halogenoethylamine class, it is apparent that high specificity of interaction is not a generally prominent feature of their actions. Hence their use as specific labels for neurotransmitter receptors might be expected to pose special problems.

Takagi (24, 25) employed ^{3}H-Dibenamine to attempt to label the cholinergic (muscarinic) receptors of the dog intestine using the procedure of initial treatment with unlabeled Dibenamine in the presence of atropine, presumed to protect only the muscarinic receptors, followed by treatment with the ^{3}H-Dibenamine. Fractionation of the tissues revealed, however, that protection was afforded in all fractions: either all the fractions contain receptor material or, and more probably, nonspecific alkylation and protection is afforded in all fractions. Yong et al. (26, 27) have employed ^{14}C-Dibenamine in attempts to label the α-receptor of rabbit aorta: in experiments in which epinephrine was used as a protecting agent significantly less radioactivity was found in the protected as opposed to the control tissues: similarly in tissues treated with unlabeled Dibenamine in the presence of epinephrine prior to the labeling procedures significant protection was also found. Fractionation of the tissue revealed, in agreement with the data of Takagi (loc. cit.), that labeling had occurred in all fractions: however, in contrast to a previous claim (28), none was found in the lipid fraction. This finding agrees with that of Lewis and Miller (29) who found no protection by phentolamine or norepinephrine of ^{3}H-phenoxybenzamine uptake into the lipid content of the rat seminal vesicle. One of the acute difficulties with this type of approach is revealed by the finding of Yong and Marks (27) that although phentolamine could afford complete pharmacological protection against Dibenamine there was no significant difference in the radioactivity of protected and unprotected tissue. In agreement with this Moran and Triggle concluded, on the basis of a fairly extensive analysis of the action of 2-halogenoethylamines in an adrenergic α-receptor system (30, 31) that "while it is possible to obtain receptor protection and specificity of action with irreversibly acting antagonists at a pharmacologic level, it is not possible to obtain specificity of action at the chemical level with the agents currently available". Nevertheless, the use of such compounds has permitted estimates to be made of the upper number of receptors in tissues. Lewis and Miller (29) assumed that the difference in radioactivity (representing ^{3}H-phenoxybenzamine labeling) of seminal vesicle protected and unprotected by phentolamine corresponded to this upper estimate: their value of $1 \cdot 7 \times 10^{13}$ molecules of phenoxybenzamine per gram of seminal vesicle corresponds to approximately 55,000 "receptors" per smooth muscle cell. For the rabbit aortic strip a rather higher estimate of approximately 200,000 "receptors" per cell was obtained (31) using, however, a different technique in which the amount of radioactivity lost from the tissue following blockade by ^{3}H—N, N-dimethyl-2-bromo-2-phenylethyl-amine, an irreversible antagonist of short duration (Chapter IV, p. 305). Whilst the precise significance of such numbers must remain in doubt because of the known diversity of action of the irreversible α-antagonists studied, it is of some interest that these figures are comparable to earlier estimates provided by Clark (32) of 10^{14} mol/g of tissue for acetylcholine, atropine and norepinephrine, with Waser's estimate (33) of the number of receptors in electric tissue and with the data of Paton and Rang (34) for the uptake of atropine into intestinal smooth muscle.

The Isolation of Receptors Through Reversible Binding Techniques

A second approach, and which in fact was employed first in attempts to achieve receptor isolation, is the fractionation of receptor containing tissues and the isolation of a macromolecule, or macromolecular complex, in an amount that is consistent with present, and rather crude, estimates of receptor concentration and that can bind neurotransmitters, their analogs and antagonists in a manner appropriate both to the physiological responsiveness of the receptor system and to the pharmacological characteristics of the ligands. Because of the high concentration of synaptic material in electric organs much attention has focused on the attempted isolation of receptor material from this source.

The earliest work in this field was associated with Chagas, Ehrenpreis and their respective co-workers (35–40). However, it now appears generally accepted (41–44) that the material isolated by the above and other workers (45) does not represent the cholinergic receptor; because of several reviews of this early work it will not be discussed further here. Nevertheless, this general approach has continued to interest workers and, although the later work has not led to the isolation of any macromolecule or macromolecular system unambiguously determined to be of receptor origin, there is reasonable hope that it will be successful.

O'Brien and his colleagues (46–48) have isolated a particulate fraction from the electric organ of *Torpedo Marmorota* and which appears to accord with several of the characteristics that are anticipated for material involved in the physiological cholinergic receptor. Equilibrium dialysis with the lyophilized particulate fraction reveals reversible binding of muscarone with a binding constant of 7×10^{-7} M and in an amount of 10^{-9} moles/gram of original electroplax tissue. This value of the binding constant appears consistent with values of the affinity of muscarone available from pharmacological experiments (Chapter IV, p. 254) on various neuromuscular systems. It is more difficult to establish whether the quantity of receptor binding material is consistent with its proposed receptor function; however, taking into account the richness of innervation of electric organs this amount approximates to the range suggested for other receptor systems (p. 548). In addition the effectiveness of a number of agents, including acetylcholine, in inhibiting muscarone binding (Table VIII-1) reveals a pattern of activity in which cholinergic ligands are significantly more effective than noncholinergic ligands: clearly from the specificity of action of these ligands the material has, as would be anticipated, the characteristics of the cholinergic receptor of the skeletal neuromuscular junction.

The assignment of "correct" binding constants to appropriate cholinergic ligands is obviously of key importance in the identification of presumed receptor components in tissue preparations (48). It is, therefore, of particular interest that refined studies by O'Brien and his co-workers (48) reveal the existence of multiple binding sites for cholinergic ligands in subcellular preparations from *Torpedo* and *Electrophorus* electric organs (Table VIII-2). The relationship of these various binding sites to the cholinergic receptor is not yet established although it is worth noting that, from different lines of reasoning, the existence of multiple modes and sites of agonist and antagonist ligand binding at the cholinergic receptor has been proposed (Chapter IV). It may be that all

TABLE VIII-1. Ligand Binding to *Torpedo* Plax Extract (47)

Ligand	% blockade of binding of 10^{-6} muscarone	Ligand	% blockade of binding of 10^{-6} muscarone
Curare, 10^{-5} M	79	Flaxedil, 10^{-5} M	58
Win 7758, 10^{-5} M	78	Nicotine, 10^{-5} M	59
Win 7846, 10^{-5} M	70	Decamethonium, 10^{-5} M	77
Win 7789, 10^{-5} M	79	Succinylcholine, 10^{-5} M	86
Win 3317, 10^{-5} M	69	Acetylcholine, 4×10^{-5} M	82
Win 13357, 10^{-5} M	31	(after paraoxon, 10^{-4} M)	
Tetraethylammonium, 10^{-4} M	32	N-Ethylmaleimide, 10^{-4} M	0
Hexamethonium, 10^{-4} M	51	Dithiothreitol, 10^{-3} M	0
Atropine, 10^{-4} M	21	p-Hydroxymercuribenzoate, 5×10^{-4} M	38

TABLE VII-2. Multiple Binding Sites for Cholinergic Ligands in *Torpedo* and *Electrophorus* Preparations (48)

Ligand	*Torpedo*		*Electrophorus*	
	Affinity	Conc. moles $\times 10^{-9}$/g	Affinity	Conc. moles $\times 10^{-9}$/g
Decamethonium	$K_1 = 6.7 \times 10^{-8}$ M	0.5	$K_1 \times 3.2 \times 10^{-9}$ M	0.036
	$K_2 = 5.9 \times 10^{-7}$ M	2.6	$K_2 = 1.9 \times 10^{-8}$ M	0.021
	$K_3 = 2.0 \times 10^{-5}$ M	7.9	$K_3 = 8.3 \times 10^{-7}$ M	0.293
			$K_4 = 5.2 \times 10^{-5}$ M	3.00
Dimethyltubocurarine	$K_1 = 6.5 \times 10^{-8}$ M	0.23	$K_1 = 3.3 \times 10^{-8}$	0.014
	$K_2 = 2 \times 10^{-6}$ M	1.10	$K_2 = 1.1 \times 10^{-7}$	0.10
			$K_3 = 2.9 \times 10^{-5}$	7.1
Muscarone	K_1 2.2×10^{-8} M	0.06	$K_1 = 3.6 \times 10^{-8}$	0.015
	K_2 2.7×10^{-7} M	0.39		

of the sites listed in Table VIII-2 have some receptor or receptor-modulating function, although this remains to be established. It appears unlikely that these sites have any relationship to acetylcholinesterase since O'Brien has demonstrated a number of differences between the two systems including, (a) phospholipase C destroys the binding capacity but does not affect AChE, (b) toluene similarly destroys the binding capacity but leaves AChE activity essentially unchanged, (c) the binding constant of muscarone to AChE is some 1000-fold higher than for the other binding sites and (d) there are profound differences in sensitivity of the two systems to such agents as the organophosphate inhibitors.

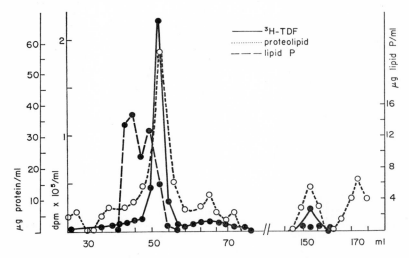

Fig. VIII-1. Sephadex chromatogram (LH 20) of chloroform: methanol (2:1) extract of *Torpedo* material labeled with ^{3}H-TDF (3×10^{-6} M). The peak of radioactivity coincides with the first lipoprotein peak. Reproduced with permission from LaTorre, Lunt and De Robertis (53).

In their search for receptor macromolecules from a variety of chemically excitable tissues De Robertis and his colleagues have described (49, 50) the isolation of two distinct classes of synaptic membrane fragments from brain cortex: one fraction contains high concentrations of acetylcholinesterase and Na$^+$/K$^+$-ATPase whilst the other is devoid of these enzyme activities. The former fragments have been shown to possess significant binding capacity for dimethyl-d-tubocurarine and hexamethonium: this binding appears to be associated with a lipoprotein (extractable with 2:1 CHCl$_3$:MeOH) which may have some function associated with synaptic transmission processes since the abundant proteolipids from myelin have but a very small binding capacity for dimethyl-d-tubocurarine (51). Nevertheless, it appears somewhat paradoxical that the fraction isolated from rat brain cortex should bind both dimethyl-d-tubocurarine and atropine (52).

A similar lipoprotein has been isolated by extraction of the electric tissue of *Torpedo marmorata* and *Electrophorus electricus* (53). Sephadex chromatography of this extract revealed the occurrence of at least four distinct subfractions: studies of the reversible binding of hexamethonium and acetylcholine and the irreversible binding of p-(trimethyl-ammonium)benzenediazonium fluoborate (TDF) revealed maximum

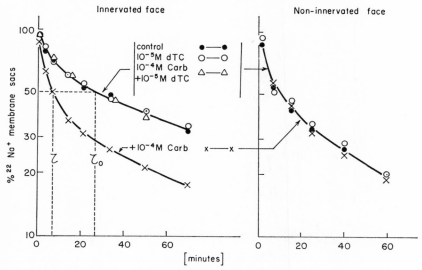

FIG. VIII-2. Effect of carbamylcholine and d-tubocurarine on ^{22}Na$^+$ efflux from membrane sacs prepared from innervated *Electrophorus electricus* membranes. Reproduced with permission from Changeux, Kasai, Huchet, and Meunier (58).

binding to occur only with the first of these lipoprotein fractions (Fig. VIII-1). It is of some interest that O'Brien's data for binding of muscarone and De Robertis's data for binding of hexamethonium both yield figures of approximately 10^{15} binding sites/g of electric tissue.

Changeux, working with electric tissue from *Electrophorus electricus*, has succeeded in fractionating and obtaining a purified fraction of the chemically excited, innervated, membrane of the electroplax and isolating a solubilized protein, which contains significant AChE activity, from these membrane fragments (54–58). Because the membrane fragments can be made to form closed sacs whose permeability characteristics can be studied under the influence of various cholinergic ligands this system affords the possibility of comparing and relating the affinity

TABLE VIII-3. Comparison of Binding Data for Cholinergic Ligands in Receptor Preparations and Acetylcholinesterase (58)

| | Preparation | | | | | |
Ligand	K_D Isolated electroplax (potential) M 22°	Membrane sacs ($^{22}N_a^+$ efflux) M 22°	Membrane sacs ($^{22}N_a^+$ efflux) M 4°	Soluble protein (Deca. dialysis) M 4°	ACh E (Hydrolysis ACTCh) M 4°	ACh E (Hydrolysis ACTCh) M 22°
Decamethonium	$1·2 \times 10^{-6}$	$1·2 \times 10^{-6}$	$1·2 \times 10^{-6}$	$0·8 \times 10^{-6}$	$2·7 \times 10^{-6}$	$2·3 \times 10^{-6}$
Carbamylcholine	$3·0 \times 10^{-5}$	$4·0 \times 10^{-5}$	—	$1·83 \times 10^{-5}$	$4·2 \times 10^{-5}$	$1·7 \times 10^{-5}$
Phenyltrimethylammonium	$1·3 \times 10^{-5}$	$2·0 \times 10^{-5}$	—	$1·3 \times 10^{-5}$	$7·3 \times 10^{-5}$	$5·7 \times 10^{-5}$
d-Tubocurarine	$1·0 \times 10^{-7}$	$1·5 \times 10^{-7}$	$1·5 \times 10^{-7}$	$2·6 \times 10^{-6}$†	$6·1 \times 10^{-5}$	$5·0 \times 10^{-5}$
Gallamine	$2·7 \times 10^{-7}$	$3·0 \times 10^{-7}$	$3·0 \times 10^{-7}$	$2·2 \times 10^{-6}$†	$1·4 \times 10^{-4}$	$1·3 \times 10^{-4}$
Hexamethonium	$5·1 \times 10^{-5}$	$6·2 \times 10^{-5}$	—	$3·5 \times 10^{-4}$	$4·2 \times 10^{-4}$	$4·0 \times 10^{-4}$

† Partial antagonism only.

constants of cholinergic ligands on three separate receptor-containing systems—the intact monocellular electroplax, the membrane sacs and the derived solubilized protein. Thus, preloaded sacs lose $^{22}Na^+$ at a steady rate (Fig. VIII-2) which is accelerated by cholinergic agonists: the effects of agonists are antagonized by d-tubocurarine. That these latter effects may indeed relate to events initiated at the physiological receptor is suggested very strongly by the data of Table VIII-3 which lists the dissociation constants for a series of ligands obtained for the three receptor systems and for acetylcholinesterase, it can be seen that for decamethonium, carbamylcholine and phenyltrimethylammonium the dissociation constants for all four systems are rather similar: however, gallamine and d-tubocurarine have significantly lower affinity for acetylcholinesterase. Additional evidence suggesting that the majority of the decamethonium binding sites in the soluble protein do not represent acetylcholinesterase (to which many cholinergic ligands are known to bind, Chapter VI, p. 460) comes from studies with α-bungarotoxin which blocks irreversibly and specifically the cholinergic receptors of various muscle preparations (59) but has no effect on acetylcholinesterase. Since this toxin irreversibly displaces about 75% of the bound decamethenium it may be inferred that this fraction of the decamethonium binding sites does not represent acetylcholinesterase.

From Table VIII-3 it will also be observed that for the three activator ligands there is good agreement for the dissociation constants obtained in the electroplax, membrane and protein preparations. However, there are significant discrepancies for the antagonist ligands: Changeux has suggested that the protein may contain or represent receptor in a conformational state corresponding to an "excited" level.

CONCLUSIONS

While the successful isolation and characterization of a neurotransmitter remains a goal rather than an achievement it is nonetheless quite clear that substantial progress towards this goal is being made and success may not be too far distant. Certainly, the successful isolation of other cellular and membranal macromolecules including repressors (60) and permeases (61–63) will act as a constant stimulus towards similar achievements in the field of regulatory macromolecules for neurotransmitters. We should not delude ourselves, however, that this success will necessarily solve the problems of receptor activities and mechanisms. Rather we should perhaps view such success in the light and experiences of the now numerous elucidations of enzyme structures: these latter successes, while contributing greatly to our knowledge of enzyme function, have left many questions of major importance to be solved but have also pointed the way to new and sophisticated experiments and hypotheses. We may look for similar progress in the area of neurotransmitter-receptor interactions.

REFERENCES

1. E. V. Jensen, T. Suzuki, T. Kawashima, W. E. Stumpf, P. W. Jungblut and E. R. Sombre, *Proc. Nat. Acad. Sci. U.S.A.* (1968) **59**, 632.
2. G. Shyamala and J. Gorski, *J. Biol. Chem.* (1969) **244**, 1097.
3. J. Gorski, G. Shyamala and D. Toft, *in* "Fundamental Concepts in Drug-Receptor Interactions (eds J. F. Danielli, J. F. Moran and D. J. Triggle) (1970). Academic Press, New York and London.
4. S. J. Singer, *Advan. Protein Chem.* (1967) **22**, 1.
5. B. R. Baker, "Design of Active-Site-Directed Irreversible Enzyme Inhibitors; The Organic Chemistry of the Active Site" (1967). Wiley, New York.
6. L. A. Cohen, *Annu. Rev. Biochem.* (1968) **37**, 695.
7. B. L. Vallee and J. F. Riordan, *Annu. Rev. Biochem.* (1969) **38**, 733.
8. B. R. Baker, *Annu. Rev. Pharmacol.* (1970) **10**, 35.
8a. E. Shaw, *Physiol. Rev.* (1970) **50**, 244.
9. S. Harshman and V. A. Najjar, *Biochemistry* (1963) **4**, 2526.
10. L. I. Pizer, *J. Amer. Chem. Soc.* (1958) **80**, 4431.
11. S. Warren, B. Zeener and F. H. Westheimer, *Biochemistry* (1966) **5**, 817.
12. E. H. Fischer, *in* "Structure and Activity of Enzymes," (eds T. W. Goodwin, J. I. Harris and B. S. Hartley) (1965). Academic Press, New York and London.
13. D. E. Koshland, *Adv. Enzymol.* (1960) **22**, 45.
14. A. K. Balls and E. F. Jansen, *Adv. Enzymol.* (1952) **13**, 321.
15. A. H. Gold, *Biochemistry* (1965) **4**, 897.
16. I. B. Wilson, M. A. Harrison and S. Ginsburg, *J. Biol. Chem.* (1961) **236**, 1498.
17. C. Arezzini, L. Rossini and G. Sergre, *Pharmacol. Res. Commun.* (1969) **1**, 295.
18. C. Edwards, W. Bunch, P. Marfey, R. Marois and D. van Meter, *J. Membrane Biol.* (1970) **2**, 119.
19. K. Chang, J. F. Moran and D. J. Triggle, *Pharmacol. Res. Commun.* (1970) **2**, 63.
20. B. R. Baker, *Cancer Chemother. Rep.* (1959) **4**, 1.
21. G. Schoellman and E. Shaw, *Biochem. Biophys. Res. Commun.* (1962) **7**, 36.
22. L. Wofsy, H. Metzger and S. J. Singer, *Biochemistry* (1962) **1**, 1031.
23. W. B. Lawson and H. J. Schramm, *J. Amer. Chem. Soc.* (1962) **84**, 2017.
24. K. Takagi, M. Akao and A. Takahashi, *Life Sci.* (1965) **4**, 2165.
25. K. Takagi and A. Takahashi, *Biochem. Pharmacol.* (1968) **17**, 1609.
26. M. S. Yong, M. R. Parulekar, J. Wright and G. S. Marks, *Biochem. Pharmacol.* (1966) **15**, 1185.
27. M. S. Yong and G. S. Marks, *Biochem. Pharmacol.* (1968) **18**, 1609, 1619.
28. S. Dikstein and F. G. Sulman, *Biochem. Pharmacol.* (1965) **14**, 881.
29. J. E. Lewis and J. W. Miller, *J. Pharmacol. Exp. Ther.* (1966) **154**, 46.
30. J. F. Moran, M. May, H. Kimelberg and D. J. Triggle, *Mol. Pharmacol.* (1967) **3**, 15.
31. M. May, J. F. Moran, H. Kimelberg and D. J. Triggle, *Mol. Pharmacol.* (1967) **3**, 28.
32. A. J. Clark, "The Mode of Action of Drugs on Cells" (1933). Arnold, London.

33. P. G. Waser, *in* "Bioelectrogenesis" (eds C. Chagas and A. P. De Carvalho) (1961). Elsevier, Amsterdam.
34. W. D. M. Paton and H. P. Rang, *Proc. Roy. Soc. Ser. B.* (1965) **163**, 1.
35. C. Chagas, E. Penna-Franca, K. Nishie, C. Crocker and M. Miranda, *Compt. Rend. H.* (1956) **242D**, 2671.
36. C. Chagas, *Ann. N.Y. Acad. Sci.* (1959) **81**, 345.
37. C. Chagas, *in* "Bioelectrogenesis" (eds C. Chagas and A. P. de Carvhalo) (1961). Elsevier, Amsterdam.
38. S. Ehrenpreis, *Biochim. Biophys. Acta* (1960) **44**, 561.
39. S. Ehrenpreis and M. G. Kellock, *Biochim. Biophys. Acta* (1960) **45**, 525.
40. S. Ehrenpreis, *Proc. 1st Int. Pharmacol. Meet., Stockholm* (1963) **7**, 119.
41. S. Ehrenpreis, *in* "Drugs Affecting the Peripheral Nervous System", Vol. I (ed. A. Burger) (1967). Dekker, New York.
42. S. Ehrenpreis, *Ann. N.Y. Acad. Sci.* (1967) **144**, 720.
43. A. Hasson-Voloch, *Nature (London)* (1968) **218**, 330.
44. S. Ehrenpreis, J. H. Fleisch and T. W. Mittag, *Pharmacol. Rev.* (1969) **21**, 131.
45. T. Namba and D. Grob, *Ann. N.Y. Acad. Sci.* (1967) **144**, 772.
46. R. D. O'Brien and L. P. Gilmour, *Proc. Nat. Acad. Sci. U.S.A.* (1969) **63**, 496.
47. R. D. O'Brien, L. P. Gilmour and M. E. Eldefrawi, *Proc. Nat. Acad. Sci. U.S.A.* (1970) **65**, 438.
48. R. D. O'Brien, M. E. Eldefrawi, A. T. Eldefrawi and J. T. Farrow, *in* "Cholinergic Ligand Interactions," (eds D. J. Triggle, J. F. Moran and E. A. Barnard) (1971). Academic Press, New York and London.
49. G. R. de L. Arnaiz, M. Alberici and E. De Robertis, *J. Neurochem.* (1967) **14**, 215.
50. J. M. Azcurra and E. De Robertis, *Int. J. Neuropharmacol.* (1967) **6**, 15.
51. E. De Robertis, S. Fiszer and E. F. Soto, *Science, N.Y.* (1967) **158**, 928.
52. E. De Robertis, J. Gonzalez-Rodriguez and D. N. Teller, *FEBS Lett.* (1969) **4**, 4.
53. J. L. La Torre, G. S. Lunt and E. De Robertis, *Proc. Nat. Acad. Sci. U.S.A.* (1970) **65**, 716.
54. J.-P. Changeux, J. Gautron, M. Israel and T. R. Podleski, *Compt. Rend. H.* (1969) **269D**, 1788.
55. J.-P. Changeux, M. Kasai, M. Huchet and J.-C. Meunier, *Compt. Rend. H.* (1970) **270D**, 2804.
56. J.-P. Changeux, R. Blumenthal, M. Kasai and T. R. Podleski, *in* "Molecular Properties of Drug Receptors", Ciba Found. Symp. (1970). Churchill, London.
57. M. Kasai and J.-P. Changeux, *Compt. Rend. H.* (1970) **270D**, 1400.
58. J.-P. Changeux, M. Kasai, M. Huchet and J.-C. Meunier, *in* "Cholinergic Ligand Interactions," (eds D. J. Triggle, J. F. Moran and E. A. Barnard) (1971). Academic Press, New York and London.
59. C. Y. Lee and C. C. Chang, *Mem. Inst. Butantan Simp. Int.* (1966) **33**, 555.
60. W. Gilbert and B. Müller-Hill, *Proc. Nat. Acad. Sci. U.S.A.* (1966) **56**, 1891.
61. A. B. Pardee, *J. Biol. Chem.* (1966) **241**, 5886.
62. C. F. Fox and E. P. Kennedy, *Proc. Nat. Acad. Sci. U.S.A.* (1965) **54**, 891.
63. C. A. Homewood, L. R. Smith and W. D. Stein, *in* "Fundamental Concepts in Drug-Receptor Interactions." (eds J. F. Danielli, J. F. Moran and D. J. Triggle) (1970). Academic Press, New York and London.

SUPPLEMENTARY REFERENCES

Chapter I

"A Discussion on The Structures and Functions of Proteolytic Enzymes", *Proc. Roy. Soc. London B* (1970) **257**, 63–266.

B. Belleau and V. DiTullio, "Kinetic Effects of Alkyl Quaternary Ammonium Salts on the Methanesulfonylation of the Acetylcholinesterase Catalytic Center. Significance of Substituent Volumes and Binding Enthalpies", *J. Amer. Chem. Soc.* (1970) **92**, 6320.

D. E. Koshland, "The Molecular Basis for Enzyme Regulation" *in* The Enzymes, Vol. I, (ed. P. D. Boyer) (1970). Academic Press, New York and London.

R. Lumry and S. Rajender, "Enthalpy-Entropy Compensation Phenomena in Water Solutions of Proteins and Small Molecules: A Ubiquitous Property of Water", *Biopolymers* (1970) **9**, 1125.

M. Mares-Guia and A. F. S. Figueiredo, "Thermodynamics of the Hydrophobic Interaction of The Active Center of Trypsin", *Biochemistry* (1970) **9**, 3223.

H. Muirhead and J. Greer, "Three-dimensional Fourier Synthesis of Human Deoxyhemoglobin at 3.5° A Resolution", *Nature (London)* (1970) **228**, 516.

V. A. Parsegian and B. W. Ninham, "Temperature-Dependent Van der Waals Forces", *Biophys. J.* (1970) **10**, 664.

M. F. Perutz, "Stereochemistry of Cooperative Effects in Hemoglobin", *Nature (London)* (1970) **228**, 726.

V. Pirrotta, P. Chadwick and M. Ptashne, "Active Form of Two Coliphage Repressors", *Nature (London)* (1970) **227**, 41.

R. T. Simpson and B. L. Vallee, "Negative Homotropic Interactions in Binding of Substrate to Alkaline Phosphatase of *Escherichia coli*", *Biochemistry* (1970) **9**, 953.

Chapter II

G. Adam and M. Delbrück, "Reduction of Dimensionality in Biological Diffusion Processes", *in* "Structural Chemistry and Molecular Biology" (eds A. Rich and N. Davidson) (1968). Freeman, San Francisco.

L. Bolis, A. Katchalsky, R. D. Keynes, W. R. Loewenstein and B. Pethica (eds) "Permeability and Function of Biological Membranes" (1970). North-Holland Pub. Co., Amsterdam.

R. Blumenthal, J-P. Changeux and R. Lefever, "Membrane Excitability and Dissipative Instabilities", *J. Mem. Biol.* (1970) **2**, 351.

D. A. Cadenhead, M. C. Phillips and H. F. King, "Dipole Interactions in Monomolecular Layers", *J. Colloid Interface Sci.* (in press, 1971).

B. Chance, "Fluorescent Probe Environment and the Structural and Charge Changes in Energy Coupling of Mitochondrial Membranes", *Proc. Nat. Acad. Sci. U.S.A.* (1970) **67**, 560.

M. Glaser, H. Simpkins, S. J. Singer, M. Sheetz and S. I. Chan, "On The Interactions of Lipids and Proteins in the Red Blood Cell Membrane", *Proc. Nat. Acad. Sci. U.S.A.* (1970) **65**, 721.

T. L. Hill and Y-der Chen, "Cooperative Effects in Models of Steady State Transport Across Membranes III. Stimulation of Potassium Ion Transport in Nerve" (and preceding papers). *Proc. Nat. Acad. Sci. U.S.A.* (1970) **66**, 607.

M. T. Laico, E. I. Ruoslahti, D. S. Panermaster and W. J. Dreyer, "Isolation of the Fundamental Polypeptide Subunits of Biological Membranes", *Proc. Nat. Acad. Sci. U.S.A.* (1970) **67**, 120.

A. S. Schneider, M. J. T. Schneider and K. Rosenheck, "Optical Activity of Biological Membranes: Scattering Effects and Protein Conformation", *Proc. Nat. Acad. Sci. U.S.A.* (1970) **66**, 793.

G. Szabo, G. Eisenman and S. Ciani, "The Effects of the Macrotetralide Actin Antibiotics on the Electrical Properties of Phospholipid Bilayer Membranes", *J. Mem. Biol.* (1969) **1**, 346.

G. Vanderkooi and D. E. Green, "Biological Membrane Structure I. The Protein Crystal Model for Membranes", *Proc. Nat. Acad. Sci. U.S.A.* (1970) **66**, 615.

A. S. Waggoner and L. Stryer, "Fluorescent Probes of Biological Membranes", *Proc. Nat. Acad. Sci. U.S.A.* (1970) **67**, 579.

J. H. Wang, "A Possible Role of Phospholipid in Nerve Excitation", *Proc. Nat. Acad. Sci. U.S.A.* (1970) **67**, 916.

CHAPTER IV

W. H. Beers and E. Reich, "Structure and Activity of Acetylcholine", *Nature (London)* (1970) **228**, 917.

B. Belleau, Receptor Mechanisms and Biochemical Rationales. Presented at *Amer. Chem. Soc. Symp.* "The Science of Drug Discovery" (1970) Chicago, U.S.A.

B. Belleau and V. DiTullio, "Kinetic Effects of Alkyl Quaternary Ammonium Salts on The Methanesulfonylation of The Acetylcholinesterase Active Center. Significance of Substituent Volumes and Binding Enthalpies", *J. Amer. Chem. Soc.* (1970) **92**, 6320.

K. Bowden and R. C. Young, "Structure-Activity Relations I. A Series of Antagonists of Acetylcholine and Histamine at the Postganglionic Receptors", *J. Med. Chem.* (1970) **13**, 225.

R. T. Brittain, D. Jack and A. C. Ritchie, "Recent β-adrenoceptor Stimulants", *Advan. Drug. Res.* (1970) **5**, 1970.

A. S. V. Burgen and L. Spero, "The Effects of Calcium and Magnesium on The Response of Intestinal Smooth Muscle to Drugs", *Brit. J. Pharmacol.* (1970) **40**, 492.

"Cholinergic Ligand Interactions" (eds D. J. Triggle, J. F. Moran and E. A. Barnard) (1971) Academic Press, New York and London.

G. G. Hammes and D. E. Tallman, "A Nuclear Magnetic Resonance Study of The Interaction of L-Epinephrine with Phospholipid Vesides", *Biochim. Biophys. Acta* (in press, 1971).

M. I. Kabachnik, A. P. Brestkin, N. N. Godovikov, M. J. Michelson, E. V. Rozengart and V. I. Rozengart, "Hydrophobic Areas on the Active Surface of Acetylcholinesterase", *Pharmacol. Rev.* (1970) **22**, 355.

S. Kalsner, "Enhancement of the α-Receptor Blocking Action of N-Ethoxycarbonyl-2-ethoxy-1,2-dihydroquinoline (EEDQ) by Amines", *Life. Sci.* (1970) **9**(I), 961.

G. Kato, J. Yung and M. Ihnat, "Nuclear Magnetic Resonance Studies on Acetylcholinesterase. The use of Atropine and Eserine to Probe Binding Sites", *Mol. Pharmacol.* (1970) **6**, 588.

C. D. Thron, "Graphical and Weighted Regression Analysis for The Determination of Agonist Dissociation Constants", *J. Pharmacol. Exp. Ther.* (1970) **175**, 541.

CHAPTER V

E. Bartels, W. Deal, A. Karlin and H. G. Mautner, "Affinity Oxidation of the Reduced Acetylcholine Receptor", *Biochim. Biophys. Acta* (1970) **203**, 568.

G. W. Beeler and H. Reuter, "Membrane Calcium Current in Ventricular Myocardial Fibres", *J. Physiol. (London)* (1970) **207**, 191.

E. Bülbring and T. Tomita, "Calcium and the Action Potential in Smooth Muscle", *in* "Calcium and Cellular Function" (ed. A. W. Cuthbert) (1970). St. Martins Press, New York.

E. Bülbring and T. Tomita, "Effects of Ca Removal on the Smooth Muscle of the Guinea-pig *Taenia Coli*", *J. Physiol. (London)* (1970) **210**, 217.

E. Bülbring, A. F. Brading, A. W. Jones and T. Tomita, (eds) "Smooth Muscle", (1970), Williams and Wilkins, Co., Baltimore.

W. G. Davis, "The Effects of Beta Adrenoceptor Blocking Agents on the Membrane Potential and Spike Generation in the Smooth Muscle of Guinea-pig *Taenia Coli*", *Brit. J. Pharmacol.* (1970) **38**, 12.

K. Krnjević, "Glutamate and α-Aminobutyrate in Brain", *Nature (London)* (1970) **228**, 119.

A. Portela, R. J. Perez, J. Vaccari, J. C. Perez and P. Stewart, "Muscle Membrane Depolarization by Acetylcholine, Choline and Carbamylcholine, Near and Remote from Motor End Plates", *J. Pharmacol. Exp. Ther.* (1970) **175**, 476.

A. Portela, J. Vaccari, P. A. Stewart, R. J. Perez and J. C. Perez, "Cesium Effects on Muscle Membrane Responses to Quaternary Ammonium Ions", *J. Pharmacol. Exp. Ther.* (1970) **175**, 483.

H. Reuter *in* "Calcium and Cellular Function" (ed. A. W. Cuthbert) (1970). St. Martins Press, New York.

G. R. Siggins, A. P. Oliver, B. J. Hoffer and F. E. Bloom, "Cyclic Adenosine Monophosphate and Norepinephrine: Effects on Transmembrane Properties of Cerebellar Purkinje Cells", *Science, N.Y.* (1971) **171**, 192.

D. B. Taylor, J. Steinborn and T-C. Lu, "Ion Exchange Processes at the Neuromuscular Junction of Voluntary Muscle", *J. Pharmacol. Exp. Ther.* (1970) **175**, 213.

CHAPTER VI

G. Burnstock, G. Campbell, D. Satchell and A. Smythe, "Evidence that Adenosine Triphosphate or a Related Nucleotide is the Transmitter Substance Released by Non-adrenergic Inhibitory Nerves in the Gut", *Brit. J. Pharmacol.*, (1970) **40**, 668.

G. Cehovic, I. Marcus, A. Gabbai and T. Posternak, "Etude de l'action de certains nouveaux analogues de l'AMP cyclique sur la liberation de l'hormone de croissance et de la prolactine *in vitro*", *Compt. Rend. H* (1970) **271D**, 1399.

D. B. P. Goodman, H. Rasmussen, F. DiBella and C. E. Guthrow, Jr., "Cyclic Adenosine 3', 5'-Monophosphate Stimulated Phosphorylation of Isolated Neurotubule Subunits", *Proc. Nat. Acad. Sci. U.S.A.* (1970) **67**, 652.

H. Hilz and W. Tarnowski, "Opposite Effects of Cyclic AMP and its Dibutyryl Derivative on Glycogen Levels in Hela Cells", *Biochem. Biophys. Res. Commun.* (1970) **40**, 973.

F. A. Kuehl, J. L. Humes, J. Tarnoff, V. J. Cirillo and E. A. Ham, "Prostaglandin Receptor Site: Evidence for an Essential Role in the Action of Luteinizing Hormone", *Science, N.Y.* (1970) **169**, 883.

J. F. Kuo and P. Greengard, "Cyclic Nucleotide Dependent Protein Kinases IV. Widespread Occurrence of Adenosine 3', 5'-Monophosphate-Dependent Protein Kinase", *Proc. Nat. Acad. Sci. U.S.A.* (1969) **64**, 1349.

A. Langslet and I. Øye, "The Role of Cyclic 3', 5'-AMP In the Cardiac Response to Adrenaline", *Eur. J. Pharmacol.* (1970) **12**, 137.

I. Pastan and R. Perlman, "Cyclic Adenosine Monophosphate in Bacteria", *Science, N.Y.* (1970) **169**, 339.

H. Rasmussen, "Cell Communication, Calcium Ion and Cyclic Adenosine Monophosphate", *Science, N.Y.* (1970) **170**, 404.

H. Rasmussen and N. Nagata, "Hormones, Cell Calcium and Cyclic AMP", *in* "Calcium and Cellular Function" (ed. A. W. Cuthbert) (1970). St. Martins Press, New York.

H. Rasmussen and A. Tenenhouse, "Parathyroid Hormone and Calcitonin", *in* "Biochemical Actions of Hormones" (ed. G. Litwack) (1970). Academic Press, New York and London.

"Role of Cyclic AMP in Cell Function" (ed. P. Greengard and E. Costa) (1970). Raven Press, New York.

S. S. Solomon, J. S. Brush and A. E. Kitabchi, "Divergent Biological Effects of Adenosine and Dibutyryl Adenosine 3', 5'-Monophosphate On the Isolated Fat Cell", *Science, N.Y.* (1970) **169**, 387.

CHAPTER VII

A. S. V. Burgen and L. Spero, "The Effects of Calcium and Magnesium on The Response of Intestinal Smooth Muscle to Drugs", *Brit. J. Pharmacol.* (1970) **40**, 492.

M. Endo, M. Tanaka and Y. Ogawa, "Calcium Induced Release of Calcium from the Sarcoplasmic Reticuluum of Skinned Skeletal Muscle Fibers", *Nature (London)* (1970) **228**, 34.

M. Lièvremont, M. Czajka and F. Tazieff-Depierre. "Cycle du Calcium à La Jonction Neuromusculaire", *Compt. Rend. H* (1969) **268**D, 379.

M. Lièvremont and M. Pascaud, "Intervention du Calcium, des Phospholipides et des Cholinestérases dans la sensibilité cholinergique à la Jonction Neuromusculaire", *Compt. Rend. H* (1970) **271**D, 1779.

A. Manthey, "Further Studies of the Effect of Calcium on the Time Course of Action of Carbamylcholine at the Neuromuscular Junction", *J. Gen. Physiol.* (1970) **56**, 407.

W. D. M. Paton and A. M. Rothschild, "The Effect of Varying Calcium Concentration on the Kinetic Constants of Hyoscine and Mepyramine Antagonism", *Brit. J. Pharmacol.* (1965) **24**, 432.

R. J. Podolsky and L. E. Teichholz, "The Relation Between Calcium and Contraction Kinetics in Skinned Muscle Fibers", *J. Physiol. (London)* (1970) **211**, 19.

H. Rasmussen, "Cell Communication, Calcium Ion and Cyclic Adenosine Monophosphate", *Science, N.Y.* (1970) **170**, 404.

J. M. Stewart and H. M. Levy, "The Role of The Calcium-Troponin-Tropomyosin Complex in the Activation of Contraction", *J. Biol. Chem.* (1970) **245**, 5764.

K. Takagi, I. Takayanagi, K. Kubota and F. Taga, "Effect of Calcium Ions and Phospholipids on Antiacetylcholine Action of Acetone and Phospholipids", *Jap. J. Pharmacol.* (1970) **20**, 398.

F. Tazieff-Depierre, M. Lièvremont and M. Czajka, "Nouvelle Méthode d'étude des substances actives sur la Transmission Neuromusculaire", *Compt. Rend. H* (1968) **267**D, 2383.

R. J. P. Williams, "The Biochemistry of Sodium, Potassium, Magnesium and Calcium", *Quart. Rev. Chem. Soc.* (1970) **24**, 331.

CHAPTER VIII

J.-P. Changeux, M. Kasai and C-Y. Lee, "Use of a Snake Venom Toxin to Characterize the Cholinergic Receptor Protein", *Proc. Nat. Acad. Sci. U.S.A.* (1970) **67**, 1241.

H. Kiefer, J. Lindstrom, E. S. Lennox and S. J. Singer, "Photo-affinity Labeling of Specific Acetylcholine-Binding Sites on Membranes", *Proc. Nat. Acad. Sci. U.S.A.* (1970) **67**, 1688.

R. J. Lefkowitz, J. Roth, W. Pricer and I. Pastan, "ACTH Receptors in the Adrenal: Specific Binding of ACTH-^{125}I and its Relation to Adenyl Cyclase", *Proc. Nat. Acad. Sci. U.S.A.* (1970) **65**, 745.

J. C. Meunier, M. Huchet, P. Boquet and J.-P. Changeux, "Se'paration de la protéine réceptrice de l'acétylcholine et de l'acétylcholinestérase", *Compt. Rend. H* (1971) **274**D, 117.

R. Miledi, P. Molinoff and T. L. Potter, "Isolation of the Cholinergic Receptor Protein of Torpedo Electric Tissue", *Nature (London)* (1971) **229**, 554.

AUTHOR INDEX

Numbers in Parentheses are reference numbers and are included to assist in locating references in which authors' names are not mentioned in the text. Numbers in italics indicate the page on which the reference is listed.

A

Abe, K., 471(111), *495*
Aberg, G., 327(422), *397*
Abildskow, J. A., 326(412), *396*
Ablad, B., 324(403), *396*
Abram, D., 120(47), 121(47), *193*
Abramson, F. B., 368(529), 369(529), *400*
Abramson, M. B., 167(340, 342), 168(342), *201*
Aceves, J., 164(295), 176(295), *200*
Adam, N. K., 145(190), 187(414), *197, 203*
Adelman, R. C., 63(213), *111*
Agin, D. P., 170(346), *201*
Ahluwalia, J. C., 246(135), *389*
Ahn, C. S., 471(137), *495*
Akao, M., 550(24), *559*
Alberici, M., 555(49), *560*
Albuquerque, E. X., 466(28), 467(28), *493*
Alden, R. A., 54(180), *110*
Alexander, A. E., 187(415), *203*
Alexander, J., 67(229), *112*
Alexander, R. S., 521(138), *545*
Alfassi, Z. B., 34(102), *108*
Al Katib, H., 298(317, 338), *394*
Allen, G., 478(211), *497*
Allen, J. F., 291(287, 288), 292(287, 288), 308(288), 311(288), *393*
Allen, L. C., 9(29), *107*
Alles, G. A., 252(169), 262(169), *390*
Allinger, N., 273(225), *391*
Allmann, D. W., 138(152), 141(152), *196*
Almirante, L., 320(376), *395*
Alonso, D., 471(114), *495*
Alonso de la Sierra, B. G., 228(87), *388*

Amatnieck, E., 175(364), 176(364), *201*
Ammar, I. A., 2(7), *106*
Anderson, H. L., 246(144), *389*
Anderson, N. C., Jr., 449(154), *457*
Anderson, S. M., 28(84), *108*
Anderson-Cedergren, E., 509(53), *543*
Andon, R. J. L., 39(125), *109*
Andreoli, T. E., 153(215), 180(377, 378), 181(383), *198, 202*
Angelini-Kothny, H., 353(483, 484), *398*
Angyal, S. J., 273(225), *391*
Ansell, G. B., 467(35), 469(35), *493*
Antonini, E., 80(268, 269), 104(307), *113, 114*
April, S. A., 319(393), *396*
Archer, S., 274(234), *392*
Archibald, F. M., 123(68), *194*
Arel, M., 246(140), *389*
Arezzini, C., 549(17), *559*
Ariëns, E. J., 211(6), 213(11, 12), 214(11), 215(15, 16), 216(12), 213(6, 16), 220(61, 62), 223(62), 224(61), 225(61, 62), 236(12), 238(12), 239(12), 240(12), 241(12), 249(159), 252(167, 168), 258(189), 259(189), 260(159, 193, 194), 284(12), 286(12), 288(270), 289(12), 312(386), 331(15), 335(12), 347(464), 350(12, 472), 351(12, 472, 475), 352(12), 367(526), 376(12), 383(550, 551), 384(550), *385, 386, 387, 389, 390, 393, 398, 399, 400,* 410(35), *454*
Armitage, A. K., 255(176), 256(176), 260(176), *390*
Armstrong, M. D., 233(95), *388*
Armstrong, P. D., 274(236, 237), *392*
Arnaiz, G. R., de, 555(49), *560*

C

E

21

M

SUBJECT INDEX

A

Acetylcholine, alkylammonium analogs 239, 252

akyltrimethylammonium analogs, 277

bisquaternary analogs, 240, 347, 349, 354, 360, 361, 362, 363, 364

calcium exchange in cardiac muscle, 518

calcium exchange in smooth muscle, 521

carbonyl analogs, 251

cyclic AMP, 471

1, 3-dioxolane analogs, 238, 256, 275

effect on phospholipid turnover, 467–470

epp, 407

equilibrium potential, 404

ester analogs, 237, 248, 249, 258, 366, 367, 384

ether analogs, 250, 364

furan analogs, 252

induced ionic changes, 404

induced potential changes, 404

minimum effective quantity, 407

muscarine analogs, 253

muscarone analogs, 254

piperidine analogs, 360

quaternary ammonium analogs, 359

structure–activity, 236–282

tropanol analogs, 366

Acetylcholine analogs, 209, 236–282

action at electroplax, 414

1, 3-dioxolanes, 275

effect on Rb^+ permeability, 445

MO calculations, 273

PMR analysis, 273

rigid structures, 271–276

stereoselectivity of, 257–276, 384

superdelocalizability, 249

X-ray structures, 272

Acetylcholine receptor, 236–282

Acetylcholine receptor—*continued*

and adenyl cyclase, 489

alkylation, 339–344

allosteric antagonism, 339–344, 377–385

allosteric antagonists, 418

analogies to AchE, 460–467

antagonists, structure–activity relationship, 344–385

as lattice array, 248–352, 364

"5-atom" rule, 262

atropine uptake, 377–383

bifunctional antagonists, 346–365

binding of R in R^+NMe_3, 247–251

biophase model, 382

bisonium antagonists, 346–365

calcium, 408, 411, 413, 469

cardiac muscle, 426

cation binding to, 241–247

chirality of, 257–276

classification, 236–276

comparison with AChE, 276–282

comparative stereoselectivity, 259, 264

competitive ganglion antagonists, 358–365

conformation of bound ligand, 271–276

conformational change, 276–282

cooperative binding, 350–352

cooperative effects, 415–420

cyclic AMP, 489

depolarizing antagonists, 346–352

depolarizing ganglion antagonists, 356–358

distinction from AChE, 555

effect of α-bungarotoxin, 558

effects of tubocurarine, 409

electric organs and ionic events, 413–424

free energy of cation binding, 241

ganglionic antagonists, 356–365

ganglionic antagonists, formulae, 357